Nutrition & Diet Therapy
Principles and Practice
SECOND EDITION

Nutrition & Diet Therapy
Principles and Practice
SECOND EDITION

Corinne Balog Cataldo

Jacquelyn R. Nyenhuis

Eleanor Noss Whitney

West Publishing Company

St. Paul   New York   Los Angeles   San Francisco

Copyediting/Index   Deborah Cady
Interior/Cover design   Lois Stanfield
New illustrations   Barbara Barnett
Page layout   David J. Farr, Imagesmythe, Inc.
Composition   Carlisle Communications, Ltd.
Cover image   Detail of *Still Life Painting, 30* by Henry Church, late 1870s. Collection of Miriam
               Church Stem. Reprinted with permission.

PHOTO CREDITS

6 Table 1–2 a) Courtesy of the U.S.D.A., b) Ray Stanyard, c) d) The International Diabetes Center, Minneapolis, MN; **25** Ray Stanyard; **31** ©Tony Freeman, PhotoEdit; **66** ©SB Productions, The Image Bank; **80** ©Robert George Gaylord; **100** FourByFive/Tom Rosenthal; **104** Ray Stanyard; **106** (bottom) ©Alan Oddie, PhotoEdit; **113** (center) Lester V. Bergman & Associates; **118** (top) ©Tony Freeman, PhotoEdit; (bottom) Ray Stanyard; **119** ©Tony Freeman, PhotoEdit; **120** Ray Stanyard; **121** Tony Freeman, PhotoEdit; **128** Mike Mazzaschi, Stock Boston; **138** Courtesy of Gjon Mill; **140** Courtesy of the U.S.D.A.; **142** Ray Stanyard; **146** ©Tony Freeman, PhotoEdit; **148** Reproduced with permission of *Nutrition Today* magazine, P.O. Box 1829, Annapolis MD, 21404, March 1968; **150** Ray Stanyard; **151** (top) Courtesy of FAO; **152** Courtesy of H. Kaplan and V.P. Rabbach; **163** Jacquelyn Nyenhuis; **164** Jacquelyn Nyenhuis; **188** Photos courtesy of Ann Pytkowicz Streissguth, University of Washington. Reprinted with permission from CIBA

(continued after index)

Printed in the United States of America

96 95 94 93 92 91 90 89   8 7 6 5 4 3 2 1

Library of Congress Cataloging-in-Publication Data

Cataldo, Corinne Balog.
  Nutrition and diet therapy.

  Includes index.
  1. Diet therapy.   2. Nutrition.   I. Whitney, Eleanor Noss.   II. Nyenhuis, Jacquelyn.   III. Title.
RM216.C36   1989   615.8′54   88-27778
ISBN 0-314-47825-6

Corinne Balog Cataldo, MMSc, RD, LD, CNSD, received her BS in Community Health Nutrition from Georgia State University in 1976 and her MMSc in Clinical Dietetics from Emory University in 1979. She has worked in private practice in Atlanta, as a clinical dietitian and metabolic support nutritionist at Georgia Baptist Medical Center in Atlanta, as a faculty member and dietetic internship coordinator at Emory University, and as a nutritionist with the Infant Formula Council. She has made numerous presentations, and in addition to this book, she has published a tube feeding manual and the book *Understanding Normal and Clinical Nutrition.* She has recently become a certified nutrition support dietitian and continues to do consulting work.

Jacquelyn R. Nyenhuis, MS, RD, received her BS in food science from Iowa State University in 1981 and her MS in nutrition from Louisiana State University in 1985. She was a nutrition instructor at Louisiana State University and has taught community classes and workshops in foods, health, and weight control. She has published articles in *Biochemical Archives,* newsletters, and popular magazines and has written a correspondence study guide *Advanced Nutrition: Nutrition and Disease.* Previously she had her own cable television show and currently is a nationally syndicated newspaper columnist.

Eleanor Noss Whitney, PhD, RD, received her BA in biology from Radcliffe College in 1960 and her PhD in biology with an emphasis on genetics from Washington University, St. Louis, in 1970. Formerly an associate professor at Florida State University, she now devotes full time to research, writing, and consulting in nutrition and health. Her publications include articles in *Science,* the *Journal of Nutrition, Genetics,* and other journals and the textbooks *Understanding Nutrition, Understanding Normal and Clinical Nutrition, Nutrition: Concepts and Controversies,* and *Life Choices.* She is president of Nutrition and Health Associates, an information resource center in Tallahassee, Florida.

Dedication

*To Tony who has given me the love, laughter, and
confidence to help me through good times and bad.*
Corkie Cataldo

*To the one who gives me the discipline of tenacity
and to Dave who helps keep my priorities right.*
Jacque Nyenhuis

*To Fran, Linda, Sharon, and Lori, who share my
joy and dedication to learning and communicating
about nutrition and health.*
Ellie Whitney

CONTENTS IN BRIEF

CONTENTS

In contents listings for chapters 16–22, conditions discussed appear in blue.
A table showing a summary of modified diets by organ system follows the contents.

Summary of Modified Diets by Organd System

Disorders	Possible Diet Modifications	Page Reference
Conditions affecting or involving the GI tract, liver, and exocrine pancreas[a]		
Blind loop syndrome	Low-fat	458
Broken jaw	Mechanical soft	353
Celiac disease	Gluten-restricted	505
Cirrhosis	Protein-restricted, sodium-restricted, fluid-restricted	494
Constipation	High-fiber, increased fluids	360
Dental caries	Mechanical soft	353
Difficulty swallowing (dysphagia)	Mechanical soft, tube feeding, total parenteral nutrition (TPN)	345
Diverticulitis	Low-fiber	361
Diverticulosis	High-fiber	361
Dry mouth	Mechanical soft	353
Dumping syndrome	Carbohydrate-restricted; no concentrated sugars; small, frequent feedings; fluid and electrolyte replacement	436
Gallbladder disease	kCalorie-restricted, regular	460
Gastritis	Low-fiber, bland	355
Hepatic coma	Protein-restricted, sodium-restricted, fluid-restricted	496
Hepatitis	Regular, high-kcalorie, high-protein	493
Hiatal hernia	Small, frequent feedings; low-fat; bland; weight loss	362
Ill-fitting dentures	Mechanical soft	353
Indigestion (dyspepsia)	Low-fiber; bland; small, frequent feedings	350
Inflammatory bowel diseases	Low-fiber, low-fat, high-kcalorie, high-protein, fluid and electrolyte replacement, lactose-restricted, tube feeding, TPN	456
Irritable bowel syndrome	High-fiber	361
Lactose intolerance	Lactose-restricted	441
Malabsorption	Low-fat, high-kcalorie, high-protein, fluid and electrolyte replacement	452
Missing teeth	Mechanical soft	353
Nausea	Low-fiber; bland; small, frequent feedings	350
Oral surgery	Mechanical soft	353
Pancreatitis	Low-fat; regular; small, frequent feedings; tube feeding; TPN	454
Peptic ulcer	Bland	356
Periodontal disease	Mechanical soft	353
Plastic surgery of head of neck	Mechanical soft, tube feeding, TPN	353
Reflux esophagitis	Small, frequent feedings; low-fat; bland; weight loss	362
Short bowel syndrome	Low-fat, high-kcalorie, high-protein, fluid and electrolyte replacement	458
Ulcers of mouth or gums	Mechanical soft, bland	354
Vomiting	Fluid and electrolyte replacement	351

(continued)

Disorders	Possible Diet Modifications	Page Reference
Conditions of the endocrine pancreas[a]		
Diabetes mellitus	Carbohydrate-controlled, kcalorie-restricted, fat-controlled, high-fiber	423
Hypoglycemia	No concentrated sweets; small, frequent feedings	435
Conditions affecting the heart, blood vessels, and lungs		
Atherosclerosis	Fat-controlled, kcalorie-restricted, sodium-restricted, high-fiber	467
Chronic obstructive pulmonary disease	High-kcalorie, high-protein	384
Congestive heart failure	Sodium-restricted; kcalorie-restricted; low-fiber; bland; small, frequent feedings; fluid-restricted	479
Coronary heart disease	(see *Atherosclerosis*)	467
Hyperlipidemias	Fat-controlled, kcalorie-restricted, carbohydrate-controlled	469
Hypertension	Low-sodium, kcalorie-restricted, high-potassium; fat-controlled	475
Myocardial infarction	Low-sodium; kcalorie-restricted; low-fiber; bland; small, frequent feedings; moderate-temperature foods; fat-controlled	478
Conditions affecting the kidneys		
Acute renal disease	Protein-restricted, high-kcalorie, fluid-controlled, sodium-controlled, potassium-controlled, fat-controlled, carbohydrate-controlled	504
Chronic renal disease	Protein-restricted, low-sodium, fluid-restricted, potassium-restricted, phosphorus-restricted, fat-controlled, carbohydrate-controlled	499
Kidney stones	Increased fluid intake, calcium-controlled, low-oxalate	509
Nephrotic syndrome	Sodium-restricted, high-kcalorie, high-protein, potassium-restricted	480
Conditions affecting many organ systems		
Acquired immune deficiency syndrome	High-kcalorie, high-protein, increased fluid intake, mechanical soft, tube feeding, TPN	386
Burns	High-kcalorie, high-protein, increased fluid intake	376
Cancer	High-kcalorie, high-protein (see also specific related conditions: dry mouth, indigestion, malabsorption, nausea, plastic surgery of head or neck, ulcers of mouth or gums, vomiting, and so on)	379
Cystic fibrosis	Low-fat, high-kcalorie, high-protein	455
Food sensitivities	Elimination of offending substance	222
Galactosemia	Galactose-restricted	441
Obesity, overweight	kCalorie-restricted, high-fiber	407
Phenylketonuria (PKU)	Phenylalanine-restricted	505
Stroke	Mechanical soft, regular, tube feeding	354
Surgery	Regular, high-kcalorie, high-protein, increased fluids	346
Underweight	High-kcalorie, high-protein	375

[a]The pancreas produces both external (exocrine) and internal (endocrine) secretions. The external secretions (enzymes) play an important role in the digestion of food; the internal secretions (insulin and other hormones) play a primary role in the regulation of glucose metabolism.

PREFACE

In revising this textbook, we have been amazed at the amount of information about nutrition that has surfaced in the three years since this book was first published. This second edition incorporates many new discoveries and highlights areas of research that may change the practice of nutrition. No doubt in the three years after this book is published, additional information will continue to become available. To help you sort through new information, this book provides not only simple facts and figures but also focuses on developing the skills you need in order to judge and interpret nutrition information. With these skills, you can apply what you learn about nutrition in the future.

Each chapter deals with subjects of importance to health care professionals. At the end of each chapter, a *Nutrition in Practice* section deals with practical questions you may have about nutrition, and questions you may be asked by people you work with. Within the chapters are *digressions* on topics of current or personal interest, to make the subject more relevant to personal lives and more enjoyable in the classroom. Technical terms are defined in *page margins*, and notes pertinent to the discussion can also be found there. This arrangement permits you to go on reading if you already know the term; to stop and learn it if it is new to you; and to return easily for a review of all the terminology at any later time.

The first nine chapters introduce you to nutrition as it relates to all healthy people. A new chapter dealing with nutrition and wellness has been added. This chapter describes the importance of nutrition, exercise, and other health habits in helping individuals achieve optimal health. New information that appears in the first nine chapters includes omega 3-fatty acids, fat substitutes, and world hunger. Chapter 5 contains a new figure that completely and succinctly summarizes the process of digestion.

Chapters 10, 11, and 12 apply the principles of nutrition to people at different stages in life from before birth through old age. Expanded information on pediatric nutrition, complications of pregnancy, teenage pregnancy, osteoporosis, and the impact of fast foods on nutritional health can be found in these life cycle chapters and Nutrition in Practice sections.

Chapter 13 replaces the Chapter 9 of the first edition of this book. It contains new information about anthropometric measures, laboratory indices, hydrostatic weighing, bioelectrical impedance techniques, nutrition care plans, and medical records.

Chapters 14 through 22 address the nutrition concerns of people who are ill or who have medical conditions that require modification of the diet. This edition of the text continues to approach diet therapy based on diet rather than on organ systems. Each diet is described once. Disorders for which the diets are used are then discussed so you can understand the rationale for using the diet.

A good deal of new information can be found in the diet therapy chapters of the book. Some of the areas that have been revised include protein-kcalorie malnutrition and illness, nutrition screening, nutrition for nursing home residents, enteral and parenertal nutrition, ethical issues in clinical nutrition, computers in clinical nutrition, cost containment, chronic obstructive pulmonary disease, acquired immune deficiency syndrome (AIDS), and cancer cachexia. The revised exchange lists have been incorporated into the discussion of diabetes, and the dietary recommendations for the management of hyperlipidemias are completely revised. The discussion of the dietary management of hypertension has also been updated.

The appendices have all undergone changes. A new appendix of enteral formulas has been included. A revised and more extensive food composition table is included. A glossary of all the words found in the margins has been added so that you can quickly look up words of interest.

As you can see from this preface, our writing style is informal and conversational. We know that textbooks often present material in a more formal fashion than this one does, but we have found that most readers of our books appreciate the relaxed-sounding pace, and still respect and trust the book's contents for their accuracy.

We hope you find this book pleasant to read, interesting, and easy to use. We believe nutrition is an important subject for study, not only for the sake of your clients, but also for the enhancement of your own life and health. We hope that, by the time you have finished reading, you will wholeheartedly agree that this is true.

Acknowledgements

The completion of this book would not have been possible without the assistance and support of many individuals who contributed in many ways to its publication. Our sincerest appreciation goes to the many reviewers who have consistently provided us with excellent suggestions for improving the text. Our reviewers include:

Isabelle Anderson—Cuyahoga Community College
Mary Butler—Huntsville Memorial Hospital
Jacque Coulson—Iowa Methodist School of Nursing
Kathryn Daughton—Asheville-Buncombe Technical Community College
Jan Dowell—Olivet Nazarene University
Vicki Erdmann—Normandale Community College
Mary Beth Gilboy—Community College of Philadelphia
Mary Hubbard—Grossmont College
Suzanne Little—San Jacinto College
Frieda Muwakkil—Gateway Community College
Beatrice Phillips—Tuskogee University

Linda Picklesimer—Greenville Technical College
Helen Reid—Southwest Missouri State University
Janet Rodeghiero—Eastern Montana College
Marilyn Rowe—South Suburban College
Maureen Sanderson—Pan American University
Netta Schwartz—Broward Community College
Margaret Seymour—Medicine Hat College School of Nursing
Jo Taylor—Southeast Community College
Samantha Vacendak—Meredith College
Simin Vaghefi—University of North Florida

Special thanks to Deborah Cady for her meticulous work on the index, to Jana Kicklighter for the excellent *Instructor's Manual* and *Student Study Guide*, and to Betty and Bob Geltz for the extensive and thorough food composition table and computerized diet analysis program that goes with this book. We also wish to express our gratitude to our editors Peter Marshall, Jane Bacon, and Jean Cook for their tireless efforts in guiding us through this project. To students who give us the motivation to write and to our families and friends who support us in ways too numerous to mention we offer our heartfelt appreciation.

Nutrition & Diet Therapy
Principles and Practice

SECOND EDITION

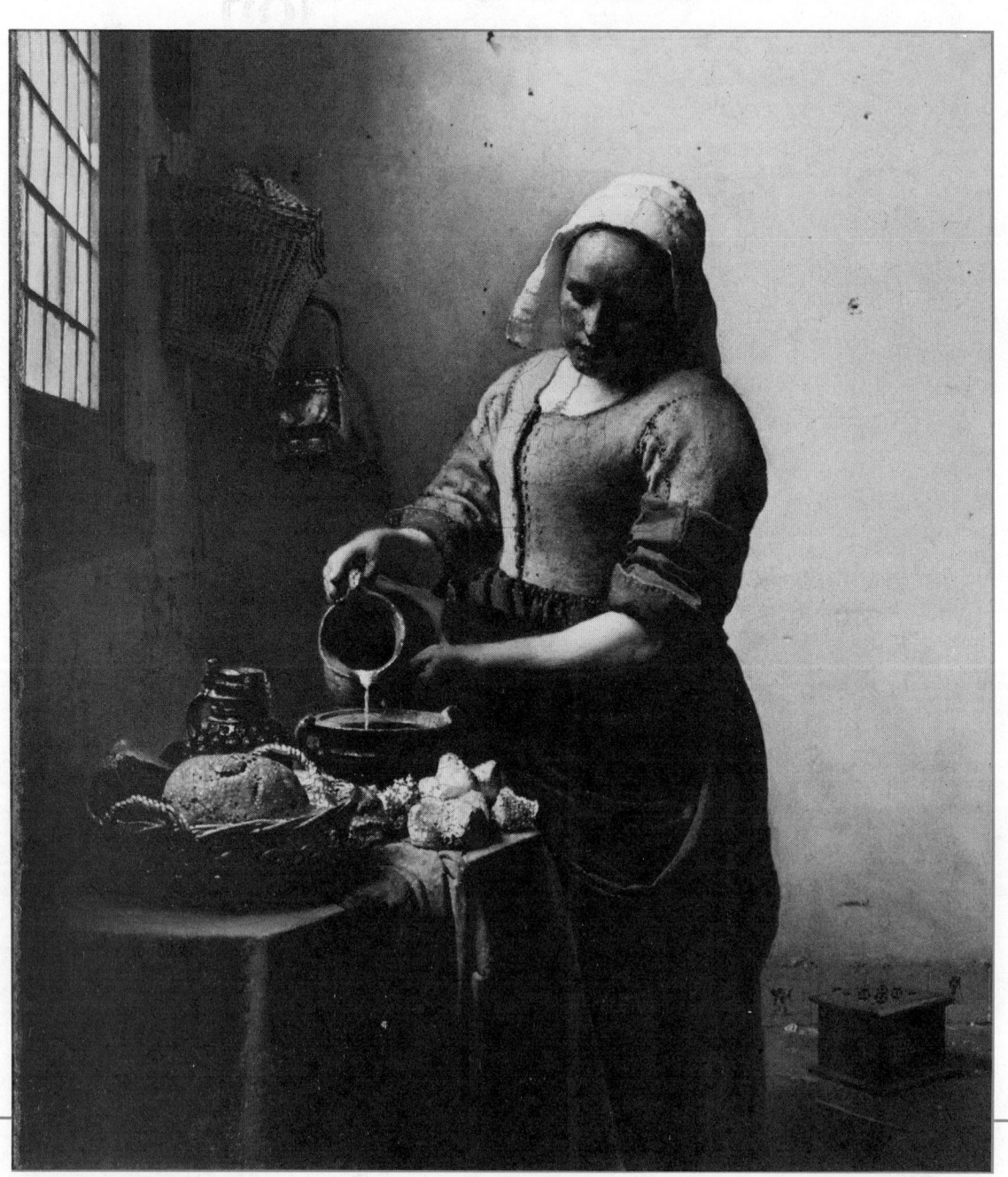

Perspective On Nutrition

CONTENTS

The Milkmaid by Johannes Vermeer. The Rijksmuseum,
Amsterdam.

You are a collection of molecules that move. All these moving parts are arranged into patterns of extraordinary complexity and order—cells, tissues, and organs. The arrangement is constant, but the parts are continually being replaced by a carefully regulated process using nutrients and energy derived from nutrients. To maintain your body systems therefore, you must regularly replenish the *energy* you burn and replace the *pieces* you lose.

Your energy and all the pieces you are made of come from the food you ingest. For optimum health, you need not only adequate amounts of the essential nutrients, but also an assortment of nutrients in good proportion to each other. The science of nutrition is the study of the nutrients in food and the body's handling of these nutrients.

Despite the fact that we need the nutrients in food to maintain health, we do not choose our foods just for their nutrient contributions. Food choices are influenced by media and peer pressure to a great extent and they resist change. Before undertaking diet planning, the planner must understand the dynamics of food choices, because people will alter their eating habits only if their preferences are honored.

Food Choices

Whether a person chooses a traditional, ethnic or vegetarian meal is influenced by many factors. For example, consider the foods you ate today. The reasons you chose the foods you did may be any of the following:

- Personal preference (you like them).
- Habit or tradition (they are familiar; you always eat them).
- Social pressure (they were offered; you couldn't refuse).
- Availability (there were no others to choose from).
- Convenience (you were too rushed to prepare anything else).
- Economy (they were within your means).
- Nutritional value (you thought they were good for you).

Of these seven possible reasons, only one has to do with nutrition directly. Even people who pride themselves on obtaining the proper nutritional value in their meals will admit that the other six factors listed also influence their food choices. No matter how nutritious a meal is, it cannot benefit a person's health until it is eaten.

Why do we like certain foods? One reason, of course, is our preferences for certain tastes. Two of these preferences are widely shared: the taste for sugar and salt. We also like foods with which we have happy associations—those we eat in the midst of a warm family gathering on traditional holidays, those given to us as children by someone who loved us, or those eaten by people whom we admire. By the same token, we can attach an intense and unalterable dislike to foods that we ate when we were sick, foods that were forced on us when we weren't hungry, or foods that are eaten by people we don't respect. Your parents may have taught you to like and dislike certain foods for reasons of their own without even being aware of it.

science of nutrition:
the study of nutrients and of their ingestion, digestion, absorption, transport, metabolism, interaction, storage, and excretion. A broader definition includes the study of the environment and of human behavior as it relates to these processes.

The practical application of nutrition is called **dietetics**: the assessment of nutrition status, recommendation of appropriate diets, nutrition education, and the planning and servicing of meals.

registered dietitian (R.D.):
a trained professional in dietetics with a bachelor's degree in nutrition or food science, a year's internship or the equivalent, and a passing score on the four-hour qualifying exam administered by the American or Canadian Dietetic Association.

dietetic technician, registered (G.T.R.):
a trained professional who has earned an associate degree or higher, has completed an ADA-approved Dietetic Technician program, has passed a national registration exam, and who assists in planning, implementing, and evaluating nutritional care.

The influence of availability, convenience, and economy on our food selections is clear. You cannot eat foods if they are not available, if you cannot prepare them, or if you cannot afford them.

A growing trend in food selection is to include a variety of foods other than those found in the typical North American diet. Each country—and even regions of countries—have their own food preferences and favorite combinations of foods for meals. Many of these foods have become ethnic specialties in our menus such as tacos, egg rolls, lasagna, and gyros, to name just a few. Other foods with ethnic origins such as pizza, spaghetti, and croissants, have become integrated into our food habits and are accepted as a part of traditional North American meals. North American regional cuisines like Cajun and TexMex foods may seem more foreign to many than some actual ethnic foods.

The vegetarian diet is an alternative diet that may be adopted for a variety of religious, ethical, social, or economic reasons. A well planned vegetarian diet can provide all the essential nutrients needed, although there are a few nutrients that the vegetarian must be careful to obtain. Nutrition in Practice 4 provides additional information about vegetarian diets.

Because excluding or including specific foods in your diet or subscribing to the diet of a particular ethnic group does not guarantee adequacy, the nutritional value of food is an important consideration in addition to the factors mentioned. Consumers today are interested in selecting foods that will provide the nutrients they need to achieve optimal health.

The Nutrients

Almost any food you eat is composed of dozens or even hundreds of different kinds of materials—atoms and molecules tinier than anything that can be seen with the most powerful microscope. The complete chemical analysis of food such as spinach shows that it is composed mostly of water (95 percent) and that most of the solid materials are organic compounds—carbohydrate, fat, and protein. If you could remove these materials, you would find a tiny residue of minerals, vitamins, and other items. Water, carbohydrate, fat, protein, vitamins, and some of the minerals are nutrients. Some of the other materials are not.

Four of the six classes of nutrients (carbohydrate, fat, protein, and vitamins) are organic. On being oxidized during metabolism, three of these four (carbohydrate, fat, and protein) provide energy the body can use. The energy-yielding nutrients are vital, for without continual replenishment of the energy you spend daily, you would soon die. When metabolized in the body, these nutrients break down to smaller compounds and release energy.

In contrast, minerals and water are inorganic nutrients and do not yield energy in the human body. Vitamins are organic, but do not provide energy. They catalyze the release of energy from the other three organic nutrients.

The amount of energy that energy-yielding nutrients release can be measured in calories (or more properly, kilocalories), which are familiar to everyone as those things that make foods "fattening." The kcalorie content of a food therefore depends on how much carbohydrate, fat, and protein the food contains. If you know the number of grams of these nutrients in a food, you can derive

---

ethnic diets:
diets associated with particular national origins, races, cultural heritages, or geographic locations.

vegetarian diets:
diets that omit meat or all animal flesh or all animal products.
The **lacto-ovo vegetarian** uses milk and eggs (animal products) but excludes meat, fish, and poultry (animal flesh) from the diet. The **vegan** excludes all these foods and uses only plant foods.

nutrient:
a substance obtained from food and used in the body to promote growth, maintenance, or repair.
The **essential nutrients** are those the body cannot make for itself in sufficient quantity to meet physiological needs, and so have to be obtained from food.

The six classes of nutrients are carbohydrate, fat, protein, vitamins, minerals, and water.

oxidation:
a type of chemical reaction. Oxidation reactions usually result in the release of energy. In chemical oxidation of nutrients, the energy released is largely chemical and mechanical; in oxidative combustion (burning), the energy released is mostly heat and light energy.

Metabolism, the set of processes by which nutrients are rearranged into body structures or broken down to yield energy, is described in Chapter 6.

The major energy-yielding nutrients are carbohydrate and fat. Protein is used only when other fuels are unavailable.

calorie:
a unit in which energy is measured. Most people, even nutritionists, speak of these units simply as calories, but on paper they should be prefaced by a k for kilocalorie. We use *kcalories* and *kcal* throughout this book. Food energy can also be measured in kilojoules (KJ). One kcalorie equals 4.2.KJ. The kilojoule is not in popular use yet.

To calculate the kcal in a slice of bread with 1 teaspoon of butter (15 g carbohydrate, 2 g protein, 5 g fat):

15 g carbohydrate	× 4 kcal/g	=	60 kcal
2 g protein	× 4 kcal/g	=	8 kcal
5 g fat	× 9 kcal/g	=	45 kcal
	Total		113 kcal

the number of kcalories. Simply multiply the carbohydrate grams times 4, the fat grams times 9, and the protein grams times 4 and add them together. Any alcohol consumed is multiplied by 7 kcalories for each gram.

If you don't need the energy-yielding nutrients immediately after you eat them, your body rearranges them (and the energy they contain) into storage compounds, such as body fat, and puts them away for later use. Thus an excess intake of any energy-yielding nutrient can lead to overweight. Too much meat (a protein-rich food) is just as fattening as too many potatoes (a carbohydrate-rich food).

Although alcohol is not called a nutrient since it does not promote growth, maintenance or repair in the body, it shares several characteristics with the energy-yielding nutrients. The body metabolizes alcohol into energy just as it metabolizes the other energy-yielding nutrients. When taken in excess of energy need, alcohol is converted to body fat and stored. When alcohol contributes a substantial portion of the energy in a person's diet, its effects are damaging. Nutrition in Practice 6 discusses more about alcohol and nutrition.

Practically all foods contain mixtures of the energy-yielding nutrients, although they are sometimes classified by the predominant nutrient. To speak of meat as "a protein" or of bread as "a carbohydrate," therefore, is incorrect. Each is a *food* rich in a particular nutrient, but a protein-rich food such as beef contains a lot of fat along with protein; a carbohydrate-rich food such as corn also contains fat (corn oil) and protein. Only a few foods are exceptions to this rule, the common ones being sugar (which is pure carbohydrate) and oil (which is almost pure fat).

The typical North American diet is very high in energy-rich foods, especially fatty processed meats, fried foods, and simple sugars. Energy-rich foods are not bad in themselves, but can be detrimental when consumed to the point that they displace other valuable vitamins and minerals or when the kcalories exceed the number needed to maintain ideal body weight.

How We Rate Nutritionally

One of the first nutrition surveys, taken before World War II, suggested that up to a third of the U.S. population might be eating poorly. Programs to correct nutrition problems have been evolving ever since.

During the 1970s, public awareness of the nutrition status of U.S. citizens reached a new high. The Senate's Poverty Subcommittee and the Select Committee on Nutrition and Human Needs held hearings, widely broadcast on national television, that projected pictures of poor families unable to feed their children. Hunger and malnutrition in the United States became a controversial, political issue, disclaimed by some who said the findings were exaggerated and singled out by others who considered them a scandal and a national disgrace. The findings that generated the controversy arose from the Ten-State Survey conducted in the late 1960s (1968–1970). Other important nutrition surveys include the Health and Nutrition Examination Survey (HANES) and the Nationwide Food Consumption Survey.

The Nationwide Food Consumption Survey was conducted in 1977 and 1978 and is the most current survey available. This survey confirmed the suspicion that food consumption appears to be quite modest in spite of wide-

TABLE 1–1. Nationwide Food Consumption Survey Findings

| Nutrient | Percentage of Persons with Nutrient Intakes at or below 70% of RDA[a] | | | |
	Income to $6,000	Income $6,000– $9,999	Income $10,000– $15,999	Income $16,000 and Over
Vitamin A	36%	33%	32%	29%
Vitamin B₆[b]	59	51	49	48
Vitamin C	30	29	27	23
Calcium	49	43	39	39
Iron	29	31	33	33
Magnesium	48	40	36	35

[a]Data represent percentage of persons in each income group with intakes at or below 70% of RDA. Example: 36% of all those surveyed whose incomes were at or below $6,000 per year had vitamin A intakes below 70% of the RDA.
[b]Vitamin B₆ intakes may not be as deficient as they appear. People who get along on minimum protein intakes need less than the RDA of vitamin B₆ to handle the amount of protein they consume.
Source: USDA Food Consumption Survey, 1977–1978.

spread obesity. This must mean that people are extraordinarily inactive. The average woman who consumes the foods available to her and who stays within the kcalorie allowance that will maintain her weight will fail to obtain her needs of several nutrients.

The Nationwide Food Consumption Survey showed dietary adequacy related to income. Table 1–1 shows the results for six nutrients. Because 19 million people in the United States are now living at or below the poverty line, nutrition problems are quite widespread.

The Nationwide Food Consumption Survey did not assess folacin and zinc, because sufficient information was not available on the food contents of these nutrients and on the factors in food that affect their absorption and use by the body. This is unfortunate, because deficiencies of both nutrients are suspected in our population.

Food Group Plans

How can food choices be juggled to create a diet that supplies all the needed nutrients in appropriate amounts for good health? The principle is simple enough: select a variety of foods that present the nutrients your body needs. The essential minerals calcium and iron illustrate the importance of dietary balance. Foods that are rich in iron (meats and meat substitutes) are often poor sources of calcium and most foods that are rich in calcium (milk and milk substitutes) are poor in iron. In fact, milk (except breast milk) and milk products are so poor in iron that the overuse of these foods can actually cause iron-deficiency anemia if they displace iron-rich foods from the diet. The anemia even has a special name: milk anemia.

The Four Food Group Plan, one of the most familiar systems of classifying foods to provide a balanced diet, is shown in Table 1–2. Each of the four

Diet-planning principles are ABCMV—adequacy, balance, kcalorie control, moderation, and variety.

adequacy:
the characteristic of a diet that provides all the essential nutrients and kcalories necessary to maintain health and body weight. Ideally, a diet will be more than just adequate; it will be optimal, providing an assortment and balance of nutrients and kcalories that maintain a favorable body weight and the best possible state of health.

TABLE 1–2. The Four Food Group Plan

Food Group	Servings/Day (Adult)	Sample Foods	Main Nutrient Contributions
Milk and milk products	2[a]	(A) Nonfat milk, buttermilk, lowfat milk, plain yogurt; (B) whole milk, cheese, fruit-flavored yogurt, cottage cheese; (C) custard, milkshake, pudding, ice cream	Protein, riboflavin, vitamin B_{12},[b] calcium, magnesium
Fruits and vegetables	4[c]	(A) Apricot, bean sprouts, broccoli, Brussels sprouts, cabbage, cantaloupe, carrots, cauliflower, cucumber, grapefruit, green beans, green peas, leafy greens (spinach, mustard, and collard greens), lettuce, mushrooms, orange, orange juice, peach, strawberries, tomato, winter squash; (B) apple, banana, canned fruit, corn, pear, potato; (C) avocado, dried fruit, sweet potato	Vitamins A and C[d] folacin, fiber
Grains (whole-grain and enriched bread and cereal products)	4[e]	(A) Whole grain and enriched breads, rolls, tortillas; (B) rice, cereals, pastas (macaroni, spaghetti), bagel; (C) pancake, muffin, cornbread, biscuit, presweetened cereals	Thiamin[f] niacin, iron, zinc, fiber
Meat and meat alternates	2	(A) Poultry, fish, lean meat (beef, lamb, pork), dried peas and beans, eggs; (B) beef, lamb, pork, luncheon meats, refried beans; (C) hot dogs, peanut butter, nuts	Protein, thiamin, riboflavin, niacin, vitamins B_6 and B_{12},[c] folacin, magnesium, zinc.

[a]For children up to 9, 2–3 c; for children 9–12; 3–4 c; for teenagers and pregnant women, 3–4 c; for nursing mothers, 4c or more; for women past 50, 3–5 c.
[b]Vitamin B_{12} is contributed only by foods that come from animals.
[c]One should be rich in vitamin C; at least one every other day should be rich in vitamin A.
[d]Dark green and deep orange vegetables are especially reliable vitamin A sources; other fruits and vegetables are not. For vitamin C, citrus fruits, green leafy vegetables, and selected other fruits and vegetables are superior sources. See Chapter 7 for more details.
[e]Enriched or, preferably, whole-grain products only. Whole grains include wheat, oats, rice, barley, millet, rye, and bulgur.
[f]One serving is not a significant source of any of these nutrients, but if the recommended four or more servings are eaten, they contribute significant quantities to the diet. This group also contributes most of the complex carbohydrate of the diet. Whole-grain products are highly recommended in place of refined enriched products. For more details, see Chapter 2.

Note: Foods labeled (A) are lowest in kcalories. (C) highest, (B) in between. A miscellaneous category includes foods that tend to be high in fat, salt, sugar, alcohol, and in most cases, calories. Foods high in fat include margarine, salad dressing, oils, mayonnaise, cream, cream cheese, butter, gravy, and sauces. Foods high in salt include potato chips, corn chips, pretzels, pickles, olives, bouillon, prepared mustard, soy sauce, steak sauce, salt, and seasoned salt. Foods high in sugar include cake, pie, cookies, doughnuts, sweet rolls, candy, soft drinks, fruit drinks, jelly, syrup, gelatin desserts, sugar, and honey. Alcoholic beverages include wine, beer, and liquor. Other miscellaneous foods, not high in kcalories, include spices, herbs, coffee, tea, and diet soft drinks.

Sources: Adapted from *Building a Better Diet,* Food and Nutrition Service, USDA Program Aid No. 1241, 1979, and Food Group Chart 4, Dairy Council of California (0020N, 1983, distributed by National Dairy Council).

groups contains foods that are similar in origin and nutrient content. The nutrients named in the table are representative of all nutrients. Once you have adequate amounts of these representative nutrients, it is assumed that you will have enough of the two dozen or so essential nutrients as well, because they occur in the same groups of foods. This is not an entirely safe assumption, however, when fortified foods are involved. Some eight or ten nutrients may be listed on a fortified food label, making the food appear nutritious, but the other essential nutrients (ten or more) may be missing. When most of the foods chosen are whole foods, the Four Food Group Plan provides a suitable foundation for diet planning.

The Four Food Group Plan specifies that a certain quantity of food must be consumed from each group. The recommended amount for the adult is two servings of meat and meat alternates, two servings of milk and milk products, four servings of fruits and vegetables, and four servings of bread and cereal products.

Many foods don't fit into any of the four food groups. Consider butter, margarine, cream, sour cream, salad dressing, mayonnaise, jam, jelly, broth, coffee, tea, alcoholic beverages, synthetic products, and others. Although some of these items do contribute nutrients to the day's intake, they don't qualify as foods to be used frequently, either because they do not convey significant amounts of enough different nutrients or because their nutrient content has been greatly diluted by fat, sugar, or water.

The original Four Food Group Plan was devised several decades ago. Despite much study and effort on its behalf, it has never worked perfectly. Few people follow it exactly and those who do, often overconsume kcalories, especially from fat. More importantly, a person can follow all its rules and still fail to meet the daily needs for some nutrients—especially for vitamin B_6, magnesium, zinc, and vitamin E. Obtaining enough iron has always been a problem.

In use of the food group plan, variety is important. The safest way to ensure that nutrient needs are met is to eat a variety of foods within each food group. Some good choices would be milk, fish, green beans, applesauce, and bread for one meal and yogurt, nuts, spinach, cantaloupe, and a bagel for the next.

The Four Food Group Plan appears quite rigid but becomes flexible once its intent is understood. For example, cheese can be substituted for milk because it supplies protein, calcium, and riboflavin in about the same amounts. Legumes and nuts are alternative choices for meats. The lacto-ovo vegetarian can adapt the Four Food Group Plan by making a change in the meat group (see Table 1–3).

TABLE 1–3. Four Food Group Plan for the Vegetarian

2 servings milk or milk products (or soy milk fortified with vitamin B_{12})

2 servings protein-rich foods (include 2 cups legumes daily to help meet iron requirements for women; count 4 tbsp peanut butter as 1 serving)

4 servings whole-grain foods

4 servings fruits and vegetables (include 1 cup dark greens to help meet iron requirements for women)

Source: Adapted from *Vegetarian Food Choices* (Gainesville: Shands Teaching Hospital and Clinics, Food and Nutrition Service, University of Florida, 1976).

Nutrient Density

How can a person get all the essential nutrients without overeating? The answer lies in selecting the foods within each group that deliver the most nutrients at the lowest kcalorie cost: foods with high nutrient density. Consider foods containing iron: a 3-ounce portion of either sirloin steak or sardines provides 2.5 milligrams of iron; but the beef contains 330 kcalories, and the sardines contain only 175 kcalories (see items 170 and 154 in Appendix C). The sardines, then, are more iron dense; that is, they have the same amount of iron

nutrient density:
a characteristic of a food. A nutrient-dense food provides a high quantity (relative to need) of one or (preferably) several essential nutrients, with a small quantity (relative to need) of kcalories.

Example of nutrient density: Whole milk and nonfat milk contain the same nutrients, but nonfat milk has them in half the kcalories. Nonfat milk is a more nutrient-dense food and thus a better choice for the dieter.

for a smaller number of kcalories. If asked whether beef or sardines are more nutritious, you would have to say both are nutritious in the sense that both provide valuable, needed nutrients. But based on the amount of iron they offer for a given kcalorie amount, sardines are more nutrient dense than beef. The idea of nutrient density can help the weight-conscious consumer make informed choices.

Another case in point is honey, a well advertised "health-food" product widely believed to be more nutritious than white sugar. Honey does provide small amounts of a few B vitamins and trace minerals compared to white sugar, which does not supply them at all. But to say that honey is nutritious is misleading. On the other hand, wheat germ, another favorite "health-food" item, provides abundant B vitamins, iron, and other nutrients relative to its kcalories. If the two should enter a contest for being the most nutrient dense, the wheat germ would win hands down.

Recommended Nutrient Intakes

Nutrient intake recommendations all have the same objective—to offer a rough guideline for diet adequacy. Here, we will discuss the RDA of the United States as an example of recommended intakes. (The U.S. RDA used on food labels are different and are described in Nutrition in Practice 3.)

RDA:
Recommended Dietary Allowances. The RDA are daily recommended intakes of nutrients intended to provide for individual variations among most normal, healthy people in the United States under usual environmental stresses.

Different nations and international groups have published different sets of standards similar to the RDA. The Canadian equivalent is called the **RNI: Recommended Nutrient Intakes for Canadians.** Among the most widely used recommendations are a set developed by two international groups, the Food and Agricultural Organization and the World Health Organization (the FAO/WHO recommendations). For more information see Appendix A.

The main RDA table includes recommendations for protein, ten vitamins, and six minerals, while another table specifies energy needs for people of different ages and still another presents tentative recommendations for twelve more vitamins and minerals. The main table is used and referred to so often that it is presented on the inside front cover of this book. Other standards are given in Appendix A.

The RDA have been much misunderstood. One person, on first learning of their existence, was outraged: "You mean Uncle Sam tells me that I must eat exactly 45 grams of protein every day?" This is not the government's intention, and the RDA are not laws, just suggestions. The following facts will help put the RDA in perspective:

- They are published by the government, but the study group that determines them is composed of highly qualified scientists selected by the National Academy of Sciences.

- RDA are based on available scientific evidence to the greatest extent possible, and the committee reviews them about every five years, taking into account new findings and revising them if necessary.[1]

- RDA are not absolute requirements. *R* stands for *recommended*, not for *required*. They are allowances, and except for energy (see Figures 1–1 and 1–2), they are generous. Even so, they do not necessarily cover every individual for every nutrient.

- RDA take into account the differences among individuals and define a range within which most healthy persons' intakes of nutrients probably should fall. Individuals whose needs are higher than the average are included within this range, too.

- RDA are for healthy persons only. Medical problems alter nutrient needs.

requirement:
the minimum amount of a nutrient that will just prevent the development of specific deficiency signs; distinguished from the RDA, which are recommended allowances that include a safety factor to provide for individual variability.

Separate recommendations are made for different sets of people. Children aged 4 to 6 are distinguished from men aged 19 to 22, for example. Each individual can look up the recommendations for his or her own age and sex group.

With the understanding that they are approximate, flexible, and generous, we can use the RDA as a yardstick, not to assess the adequacy of individual diets but to measure the adequacy of diets in entire populations, such as those of the United States. Diets of individuals are often assessed by comparing them to the RDA, but this is only an estimation because individuals' needs differ unpredictably. The RDA are in the process of being revised. Controversies about how to interpret available research have delayed the revision process considerably.

Dietary Guidelines

Since the mid-1960s, there has been increasing concern that overnutrition may be contributing to the illnesses many people suffer from, including heart disease, cancer, diabetes, and liver disease. These diseases may arise in part from excesses in fat, salt, sugar, and even protein intakes. Government authorities are now as much concerned about people who consume too much of these substances as they once were about people who had deficient intakes. In the past decade, the governments of several developed countries have published recommendations that people reduce their intakes of fat, salt, and sugar and turn toward diets based more on whole foods.

Among the new sets of recommendations have been the *Dietary Goals for the United States (1977), the Dietary Guidelines for Americans (1980), Toward Healthful Diets (1980)* and others directed at preventing diseases, such as the National Academy of Sciences' *Diet, Nutrition, and Cancer* report (1982). These sets of guidelines differ somewhat from each other, but they agree in most areas. All emphasize prevention of overnutrition and disease.

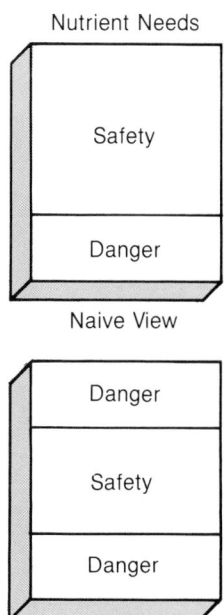

FIGURE 1–1
Nutrient needs. The RDA are not minimum amounts but represent the approximate midpoint ranges within which nutrient intakes probably should fall. Nutrient intakes above or below these ranges might be equally harmful.

overnutrition:
overconsumption of energy or nutrients.

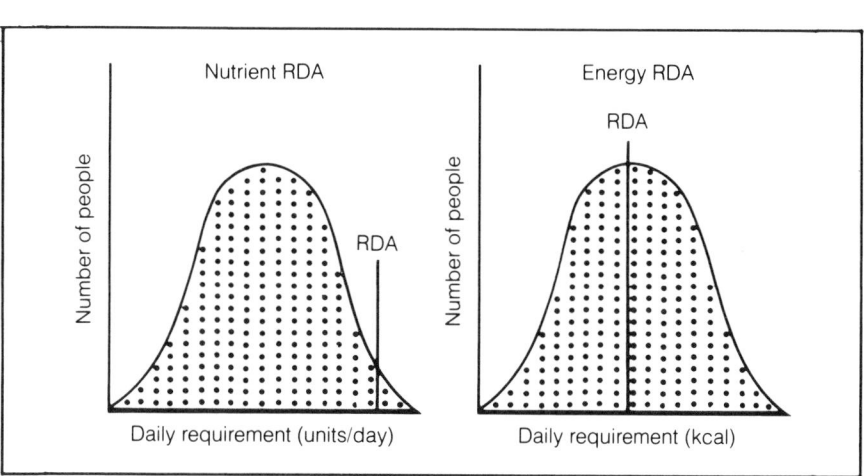

FIGURE 1–2
The RDA. The nutrient RDA are set so that only a few people's requirements will exceed them. The energy RDA are set so that half the population's requirements will fall below and half above them.

The progress of science is marked by the development of a continually changing *picture* of nutrition and health. Observations that don't quite fit in the old picture keep coming to light. We cannot, therefore, be dogmatic in stating nutrition facts because they aren't facts. Observations are only findings from which we try to generalize.

Some people are fully aware that science is an evolving process, but many are uncomfortable on the shifting ground and resent having to adjust constantly in order to integrate new information. We need to become comfortable with the tasks of adjusting and integrating, even enjoy the process, if we are to adopt a realistic attitude toward nutrition information.

Nutrition scientists have divergent opinions about advising the public on diet. Some feel that no advice can reasonably be given; others feel justified in

---

Dietary Guidelines for Americans and Suggestions for Food Choices

1. *Eat a variety of foods daily.* Include these foods every day: fruits and vegetables; whole-grain and enriched breads and cereals; milk and milk products; meats, fish, poultry, and eggs; dried peas and beans.

2. *Maintain ideal weight.* Increase physical activity; reduce kcalories by eating fewer fatty foods and sweets and less sugar and by avoiding too much alcohol; lose weight gradually. Eat more foods that are low in kcalories and high in nutrients.

3. *Avoid too much fat, saturated fat, and cholesterol.* Choose low-fat protein sources, such as lean meats, fish, poultry, dry peas, and beans; use eggs and organ meats in moderation; limit intake of fats on and in foods; trim fats from meats; broil, bake, or boil—don't fry; read food labels for fat content.

4. *Eat foods with adequate starch and fiber.* Substitute starches for fats and sugars; select whole-grain breads and cereal, fruits and vegetables, dried beans and peas, and nuts to increase fiber and starch intake.

5. *Avoid too much sugar.* Use less sugar, syrup, and honey; reduce concentrated sweets, such as candy, soft drinks, cookies, and the like; select fresh fruits or fruits canned in light syrup or in their own juices; read food labels—sucrose, glucose, dextrose, maltose, lactose, fructose, syrups, and honey are all sugars; eat sugar less often to reduce dental caries.

6. *Avoid too much sodium.* Reduce salt in cooking; add little or no salt at the table; limit salty foods like potato chips, pretzels, salted nuts, popcorn, condiments, cheese, pickled foods, and cured meats; read food labels for sodium or salt contents especially in processed and snack foods.

7. *If you drink alcohol, do so in moderation.* Individuals who drink should limit all alcoholic beverages (including wine, beer, liquors, and so on) to one or two drinks per day. Note that the use of alcoholic beverages during pregnancy can result in the development of birth defects and mental retardation called fetal alcohol syndrome.

offering very concrete advice. The *Dietary Guidelines* are presented here because they represent a compromise between the two extremes.[2]

Unlike the food group plans described earlier, the Dietary Guidelines focus not on "getting enough" but rather on "not getting too much." Some diets are close to the Guidelines, but the typical North American diet, high in meat, would need to be altered. The recommendations state not only what we should eat but also what we should avoid. In addition, they make reference to weight maintenance and exercise.

We have seen that surveys undertaken to assess the nutrition status of families in the United States have revealed that getting the proper nutrients and adequate exercise and not overconsuming food energy are still real concerns. There is, then, a need for all of us to choose our foods intelligently in the interest of our nutritional health.

SELF-STUDY:

How Balanced Is Your Diet?

Make a record of your typical food intake and analyze it for the nutrients it contains. You will use the results over and over again in succeeding Self-Studies, so invest time and effort now to achieve maximum accuracy. You can undertake this analysis before you have learned about the nutrients; having the results in front of you as you work will help make the reading significant.

1. Use three copies of Form 1 and record on them all the foods you eat for a three-day period. If, like most people, you eat differently on weekdays than on weekends, then you should probably record for two weekdays and one weekend day to get a true average, or record your food intake for a week. You will learn the most from these Self-Studies if you select days that are truly typical of your food intake and physical activity.

    As you record each food, make careful note of the measure. Estimate the amount to the nearest ounce, quarter cup, tablespoon, or other common measure. In guessing at the sizes of meat portions, it helps to know that a piece of meat the size of the palm of your hand weighs about 3 or 4 ounces. If you are unable to estimate serving sizes in cups, tablespoons, or teaspoons, try measuring out servings in those proportions to see how they look. It also helps to know that a slice of cheese (like sliced "American" cheese) or a 1½-inch cube of cheese weighs about one ounce.

    You may have to break down mixed dishes to their ingredients. Many mixed dishes, however, including soups, are listed in the miscellaneous section at the end of Appendix C. Other mixtures are simple to analyze. A ham and cheese sandwich, for example, can be listed as two slices of bread, one tablespoon of mayonnaise, two ounces of ham, one ounce of cheese, and so on. If you can't identify all the ingredients, just estimate the amounts of the major ones, like the beef, tomatoes, and potatoes in a beef-vegetable soup.

    You will, of course, make errors in estimating amounts. In calculations of this kind, errors of up to 20 percent are expected and tolerated. Still, your rough approximation will enable you to compare your nutrient intakes with the recommended ones.

Do not record any nutrient supplements you take. It is important for you to discover whether your food choices alone deliver the nutrients you need. If they don't, you'll have the first clues to a solution, perhaps one that involves better food choices rather than supplements. An exercise in the last Self-Study provides an opportunity for you to reevaluate your need for supplements.

2. Using Appendix C, calculate for each day your total intakes of kcalories, protein, fat, carbohydrate, calcium, iron, zinc, vitamin A, thiamin, ribo-flavin, niacin, folacin, and vitamin C.

   If a food you have eaten does not appear in Appendix C, read the label on the package. If you eat a packaged food in which the nutrient amounts are listed on the label as "percent of U.S. RDA," use the table on the inside back cover of the text to convert to grams, milligrams, micrograms, or retinol equivalents. Suppose a food label states that a serving contains 25 percent of the U.S. RDA of iron, for example. The table shows that the U.S. RDA for iron is 18 milligrams. The food portion therefore contributes 25 percent of 18 milligrams, or 4.5 milligrams of iron.

   If a food you eat offers no information on the label, use your ingenuity to guess the composition. Use the most similar food you can find as a guide. For example, if you ate halibut (which is not listed in Appendix C), you would not be far off in using the values for haddock or perch. If you ate cream of celery soup, you might substitute the values for cream of mushroom soup.

   Be careful in recording the nutrient amounts in odd-size portions. For example, if you used ¼ cup of milk, you will have to divide the amount of every nutrient listed for a cup of milk by four. Also note the units in which the nutrients are measured:

   • Energy is measured in kcalories.

   • Protein, fat, and carbohydrate are measured in grams (g).

   • Calcium, iron, zinc, thiamin, riboflavin, niacin, and vitamin C are measured in milligrams (mg)—thousandths of a gram (0.001 g). Folacin is measured in micrograms (mcg or μg)—thousandths of a milligram or millionths of a gram (0.001 mg or 0.000001 g). Thus 800 mg calcium is the same as 0.8 g calcium, and 400 μg folacin is the same as 0.4 mg folacin. Be sure to convert all calcium amounts to milligrams and all folacin amounts to micrograms before calculating.

   • Vitamin A can be measured in international units (IU) or retinol equivalents (RE). Appendix C lists vitamin A in RE to ease comparison with the recommended intake, which is also in RE. If you eat a packaged food in which vitamin A is listed in IU on the label, be sure to convert to RE before calculating. (For more details, see Chapter 7.)

3. Now total the amount of each nutrient you've consumed for each day, and transfer your totals to Form 2. Form 2 provides a convenient means of deriving an average intake for each nutrient.

4. As a final step, transfer your average intakes to Form 3 for future reference. For comparison, enter the intakes recommended for a person of your age and sex, using either the RDA (on the inside front cover of the text) or the *Recommended Nutrient Intakes for Canadians* (in Appendix A), whichever you prefer. Note that no recommendations are made for intakes of fat or carbohydrate. Guidelines for these nutrients and for others, like cholesterol

and fiber, are presented and discussed later. Succeeding Self-Studies will guide you in focusing on each of the nutrients provided by your diet.

Suspend judgment about the adequacy of your intakes for the moment. You have much to learn about your individuality, the nutrients, and the recommendations before you can reach any reasonable conclusions.

5. Now, check your overall food intake for balance. You can get an indication of whether you are choosing a balanced selection of foods by using the Food Group Plan Scorecard (Form 4—one copy for each day). How does your diet score by these criteria?

_____

_____

_____

6. Another way to check for balance is to evaluate your diet using the guideline that about 58 percent of your kcalories should come from carbohydrate, about 12 percent from protein, and not more than 30 percent from fat. Use Form 5 to calculate these percentages. What percentage of the kcalories you consume comes from protein? _____ percent. Fat? _____ percent. Carbohydrate? _____ percent. Is your diet balanced by these criteria?

Notes

1. Food and Nutrition Board, Committee on Recommended Allowances, *Recommended Dietary Allowances*, 9th ed. (Washington, D.C.: National Academy of Sciences, 1980).

2. A. E. Harper and E. V. McCollum, Recommended Dietary Allowances in perspective, *Food and Nutrition News,* March/April 1986.

FORM 1
Nutrient Intakes (Use One Form for Each Day)

Food	Approximate Measure or Weight	Energy[a] (kcal)	Pro- tein[b] (g)	Fat[b] (g)	Carbo- hydrate[b] (g)	Cal- cium[a] (mg)	Iron[c] (mg)	Zinc[b] (mg)	Vitamin A[a] (RE)	Thia- min[c] (mg)	Ribo- flavin[c] (mg)	Niacin[b] (mg)	Fola- cin[a] (µg)	Vitamin C[b] (mg)
Total														

[a]Compute these values to the nearest whole number.
[b]Compute these values to one decimal place.
[c]Compute these values to two decimal places.

FORM 2
Average Daily Energy and Nutrient Intakes

Day	Energy (kcal)	Protein (g)	Fat (g)	Carbo-hydrate (g)	Calcium (mg)	Iron (mg)	Zinc (mg)	Vitamin A (RE)	Thiamin (mg)	Riboflavin (mg)	Niacin (mg)	Folacin (μg)	Vitamin C (mg)
1													
2													
3													
Total													
Average daily intake (divide total by 3)													

FORM 3
Comparisons with a Standard Intake

Day	Energy (kcal)	Protein (g)	Fat (g)	Carbo-hydrate (g)	Calcium (mg)	Iron (mg)	Zinc (mg)	Vitamin A (RE)	Thiamin (mg)	Riboflavin (mg)	Niacin (mg)	Folacin (μg)	Vitamin C (mg)
Average daily intake (from Form 2)													
Standard[a]	[b]		✕	✕									
Intake as percentage of standard[c]													

[a]Taken from RDA tables (inside front cover) or *Recommended Nutrient Intakes for Canadians* (Appendix A).
[b]Use YOUR calculation for energy from Self-Study 6, the RDA tables, or *Recommended Nutrient Intakes for Canadians* (Appendix A).
[c]For example, if your intake was 50 g and the standard for a person your age and sex was 46 g, you consumed (50 ÷ 46) × 100, or 109 percent of the standard.

FORM 4
Food Selection Scorecard

Food Group and Recommended Intake	Your Intake from Group (Specify Food and Amount)	Your Score
FRUITS & VEGETABLES—4 or more portions (½ cup cooked edible portion or 3–4 oz[100 g] raw.) Have at least 1 raw daily.		
1 serving DARK GREEN or DEEP ORANGE—Vitamin A source (any food with more than RDA). 1 serving = 10 points (no more than 10 points allowed).		
1 serving VITAMIN C-RICH fruit or vegetable (any food with more than your RDA). 1 serving = 10 points (no more than 10 points allowed).		
Other fruits and vegetables including potatoes = 2.5 each.		
SUBTOTAL (no more than 25 points allowed.)		
GRAINS (BREADS & CEREALS)—4 or more servings of whole-grain or "enriched" (serving = 1 oz dry-weight cereal or 1-oz slice bread or equivalent grain product).		
1 serving cereal or 2 bread equivalents = 10 points (No more than 10 points allowed).		
Other bread equivalents = 5 points each		
SUBTOTAL (no more than 25 points allowed.)		
MILK & MILK PRODUCTS—2 or more servings (serving = 8 oz fluid milk. Calcium equivalents would be 1⅓ oz hard cheese, 1⅓ cup cottage cheese, 1 pint ice milk, or 1 pint ice cream).		
1 serving = 12.5 points		
SUBTOTAL (no more than 25 points allowed).		
MEAT & MEAT ALTERNATES—2 or more servings (serving = 2–3 oz. cooked *lean* meat, fish, poultry. Protein equivalents would be 2 eggs; 2 oz hard cheese; ½ cup hard cheese; ½ cup cottage cheese; 1 cup cooked legumes; 4 tbsp peanut butter; 1 oz nuts or sunflower seeds). Count cheese *either* in milk group or in meat group, not both.		
1 serving = 12.5 points		
SUBTOTAL (no more than 25 points allowed).		
GRAND TOTAL (no more than 100 points).		

The above are FOUNDATION FOODS. ADDITIONAL FOODS are those that do not fit into the above groupings but add flavor, interest, variety, and (often) kcalories. List those eaten.

_____   _____   _____   _____

_____   _____   _____   _____

_____   _____   _____   _____

Percentage of kCalories from Protein, Fat, and Carbohydrates

Average Daily intakes from Form 2:

Protein: g/day × 4 kcal/g = (P)_____ kcal/day

Fat: g/day × 4 kcal/g = (F)_____ kcal/day

Carbohydrate: g/day × 4 kcal/g = (C)_____ kcal/day

Total kcal/day = (T)_____ kcal/day

Percentage of kcalories from protein: $\dfrac{(P)}{(T)} \times 100 =$ _____ % of total kcalories

Percentage of kcalories from fat: $\dfrac{(F)}{(T)} \times 100 =$ _____ % of total kcalories

Percentage of kcalories from carbohydrates: $\dfrac{(C)}{(T)} \times 100 =$ _____ % of total kcalories

Note: The three percentages can total 99, 100, or 101, depending on the way in which figures were rounded off earlier.

Note: If you used an alcoholic beverage, you have to add a line for kcalories from alcohol. To find out how many kcalories in the beverage were from alcohol, look the beverage up in Appendix C. Figure out how many kcalories were from carbohydrate (multiply carbohydrate grams times 4), fat (fat grams times 9), and protein (protein grams times 4). The remaining kcalories were from alcohol.

Nutrition and the Health Care Professional

With nutrition receiving so much attention in the popular press, it is easy to be overwhelmed with conflicting information. Everyone seems to be giving advice on the subject and it can be difficult to know whom to listen to. In fact, determining what nutrition information is accurate may be one of the most challenging tasks you will face. It should also be one of the most important, since nutrition is important to you in both your professional and your personal life. We hope that this discussion will help make your study of nutrition meaningful.

Why are people so interested in nutrition?
One reason is that the idea of health has evolved from merely being free from disease to the idea of optimal health. Instead of simply treating diseases, people are encouraged to achieve a higher level of wellness so they can feel their best and avoid illness. Chapter 9 provides more information about this subject.

A natural consequence of the desire to achieve optimal health is an increased interest in nutrition. Since an appropriate diet is a cornerstone of good health, people are becoming aware of the need for learning more about nutrition.

Many nutrition products are on the market that I do not know much about. Are people who sell nutrition products (health food store owners, for example)

qualified to provide nutrition information to their customers?
Nutrition products abound on the market because the sellers make big money from them. More time may go into designing the package than researching the claims that the package makes.

A health food store owner may be in the nutrition business simply because it is a lucrative market. Such a person may have a background in business or sales and no education in nutrition at all. Such a person is not qualified to provide nutrition information to customers.

To effectively communicate nutrition information requires a trained professional with a working knowledge of nutrition.

Tell me more about professionals with proper training in nutrition.
Registered dietitians or nutrition professionals with advanced degrees are experts in nutrition and are probably in the best position to answer your nutrition questions.

A "nutritionist" is any individual who claims a career connection with the nutrition field, and is *not* necessarily a nutrition expert. Anyone can call himself a "nutritionist"

What about other health care professionals?
The health care team shares responsibility for helping each client to achieve optimal health. Nutrition education and direct nutrition services

are often part of the care the client needs. Health care professionals, especially nurses and dietetic technicians, often assist dietitians in providing nutrition information as well as in administering direct nutrition care. Nurses play central roles in client care management and client relationships. Other primary care assistants such as dietetic technicians assist the dietitian in nutritional care. A physical therapist can provide an individualized exercise program to control obesity. A social worker may provide practical and emotional support.

Can you give me more examples of specific roles these health professionals might be responsible for in nutrition care?
Yes. Some of the responsibilities of the health care professional might be

- Helping people understand why nutrition is important to them.

- Answering questions about food and diet.

- Explaining to a client how a modified diet works.

- Spotting a client at risk for poor nutrition status (see Chapter 13) and taking appropriate action.

- Recognizing when a client needs more help with a nutrition problem (in such a case, the problem should be referred to someone who can help, a dietitian or physician).

The following are some specific nutrition-related tasks that a health care professional might routinely perform:

- Obtaining diet histories.
- Feeding clients who cannot feed themselves.
- Recording what a client eats or drinks.
- Helping a client mark menus.
- Monitoring weight changes.
- Encouraging clients to eat.

As you can see, although the dietitian assumes the primary role as the nutrition expert on a health care team, other health care professionals play important roles in administering nutrition care.

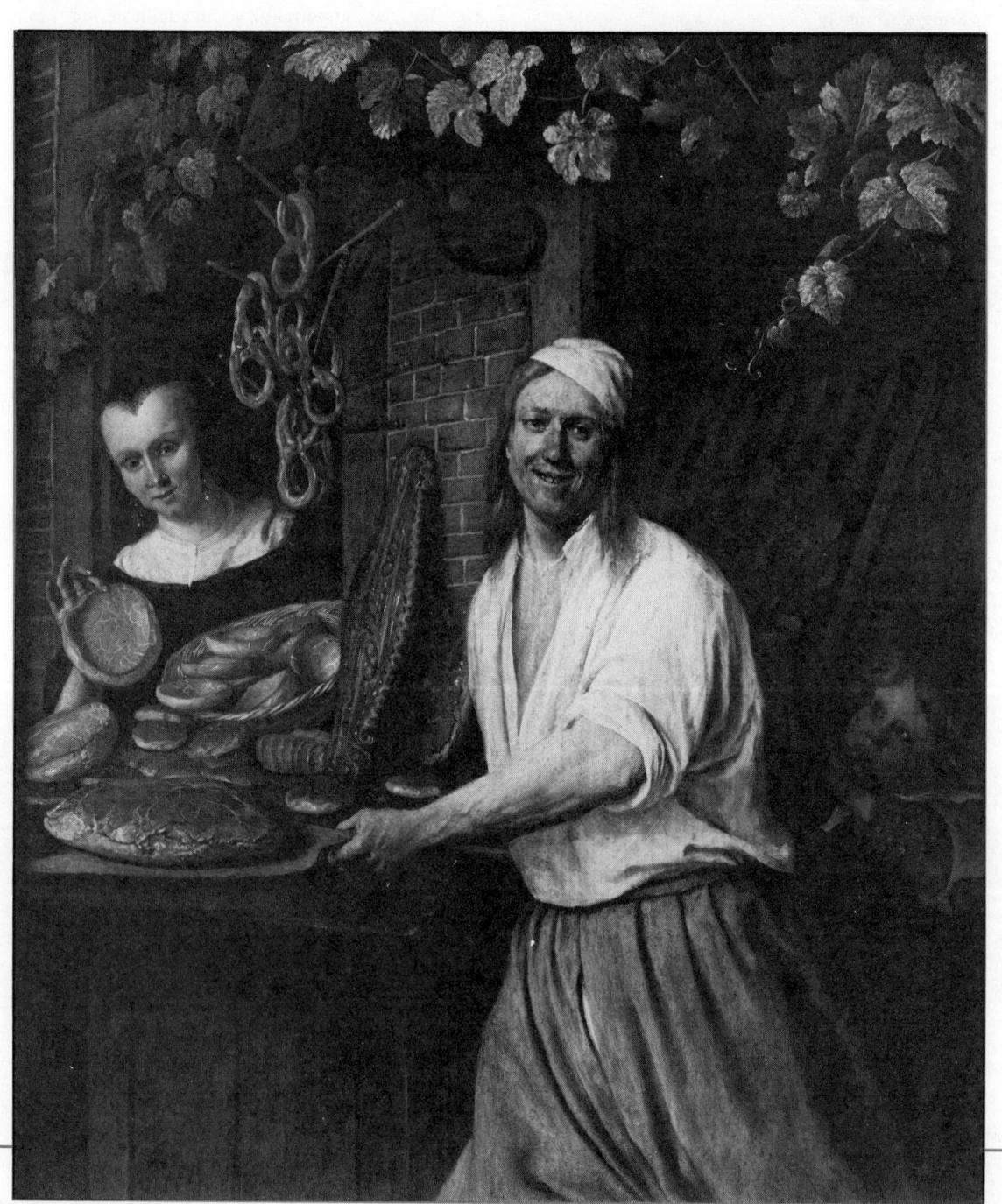

2

Carbohydrates

CONTENTS

Baker Oostwaard by Jan Steen. The Rijksmuseum, Amsterdam.

Glucose

Glucose: the body's principal energy fuel.

carbohydrate:
an energy nutrient composed of
monosaccharides.
carbo = carbon
hydrate = water

simple carbohydrates:
the monosaccharides (glucose, fructose, and
galactose) and the disaccharides (sucrose,
lactose, and maltose); also called the sugars.

complex carbohydrates:
the polysaccharides (starch, glycogen, and
cellulose).

monosaccharide:
a single sugar unit.

disaccharide:
a pair of sugar units bonded together.

polysaccharide:
many sugar units bonded together.

TABLE 2–1. The Major Simple
Carbohydrates

Monosaccharides	Disaccharides
Glucose ●	Maltose ●—●
Fructose ▲	Sucrose ●—▲
Galactose ■	Lactose ●—■
(found only in lactose)	

Most of us would like to feel good all the time. The enjoyment available in a day, no matter what the day may bring, can be tremendous if our bodies and minds are tuned for it. The feeling of well-being that comes with energy, alertness, clear thinking, and confidence is so rewarding that if you know how to produce it, you will probably make the necessary effort.

Of the three energy nutrients, carbohydrates provide the most readily available source of energy. You will see that carbohydrates have diverse roles and power tremendous tasks in our bodies. For example, whenever carbohydrate is available to the body, the human brain depends exclusively on it as an energy source. Athletes eat a "high carb" diet to store as much muscle fuel as possible, and dieters are told that eating foods high in complex carbohydrate can help them lose weight.

The Chemist's View of Carbohydrates

Chemists divide the carbohydrates into two categories: simple and complex. The simple carbohydrates are monosaccharides and disaccharides, also known as sugars (see Table 2–1). White table sugar is one of the disaccharides. Starch, glycogen, and some fibers are complex carbohydrates, also known as polysaccharides. All of these carbohydrates are composed of the simple sugar glucose and other compounds that are much like glucose in composition and structure.

Monosaccharides

Glucose is the monosaccharide that serves as the chief energy source for all the body's cells. Most of the other carbohydrates (except fructose) are split or converted to glucose before the cells use them. Nearly all plant foods contain glucose.

Fructose, the sweetest of the sugars, is the sugar of fruit. Fructose can be converted to glucose in the body, or broken down, like glucose, to fragments from which fat can be made. Most plants, especially fruits and saps, contain fructose.

Glucose and fructose are the most common single sugars or monosaccharides. A third, galactose, is seldom found free in nature but occurs as part of milk sugar (lactose).

Disaccharides

Sucrose (table sugar) is the most familiar of the three disaccharides. This sugar is usually obtained by refining the juice from sugar beets or sugar cane to provide the brown, white, and powdered sugars available in the supermarket, but it is found naturally in many fruits and vegetables.

When you eat a food containing sucrose, enzymes in your digestive tract split the sucrose to yield glucose and fructose. One molecule of sucrose can ultimately yield two molecules of glucose.

It ultimately makes no difference whether you eat monosaccharides bonded together as in table sugar or broken apart as in honey. This doesn't mean that there are no differences between sugar sources. Fruit sugars contain the same monosaccharides and about the same kcalories as table sugar and honey, but what you get along with that sugar does make a difference. For example, in an orange or other fruit, the sugars are diluted in large volumes of water, packaged in fiber and mixed with valuable vitamins and minerals. Table 2–2 shows the vitamin and mineral contents of some sugar sources.

Sucrose is often the principal energy-nutrient ingredient of carbonated beverages, candy, cakes, frostings, cookies, and other concentrated sweets. Nutrition in Practice 2 addresses questions often asked about sucrose in the diet.

Lactose is the principal carbohydrate of milk. A human baby is born with the digestive enzymes necessary to split lactose into its two monosaccharide parts, glucose and galactose, so that it can be absorbed. Breast milk or formula provides a simple, easily digested carbohydrate to meet a baby's energy needs.

Some people lose the ability to digest lactose and become lactose intolerant. Lactose intolerance arises at about the age of four and is found in 70 percent of Native American, Asian, African, Mediterranean, and Middle Eastern people. Lactose intolerance is not the same as the commonly observed milk allergy, which is caused by an immune reaction to the protein in milk. Lactose intolerance is discussed further in Chapter 19, and milk allergy in Chapter 11.

The third disaccharide, maltose, consists of two glucose units. Maltose is found at only one stage in the life of a plant—when the plant is digesting its stored starch for energy and sprouting. The malt found in beer contains maltose.

Polysaccharides

While the sugars contain three monosaccharides in different combinations, the polysacchrides are composed almost entirely of only one—glucose. The differences between them have to do with the bonds that link glucose into the large molecules of glycogen, starch, and cellulose. Glycogen is not important as a nutrient but is the body's storage form of glucose. Starch is a branch chain

glucose:
a monosaccharide, the sugar common to all disacchrides and polysaccharides; sometimes known as blood sugar, sometimes as grape sugar; also called *dextrose*.

fructose:
a monosaccharide; sometimes known as fruit sugar. Slightly sweeter than glucose and requires less energy to metabolize than glucose.
fruct = fruit

galactose:
a monosaccharide; part of the disaccharide lactose.

lactose:
a disaccharide composed of glucose and galactose; commonly known as milk sugar.
lact = milk

An enzyme is not a hormone. Enzymes are large protein molecules; hormones are small or medium-sized molecules, usually made of protein or lipid. Enzymes facilitate specific chemical reactions; hormones act as master controllers, often regulating enzymes.

sucrose:
a disaccharide composed of glucose and fructose; commonly known as table sugar, beet sugar, or cane sugar.
sucro = sugar

maltose:
a disaccharide composed of two glucose units; sometimes known as malt sugar.

TABLE 2–2. Vitamins and Minerals Supplied by Some Sugar Sources

	Calcium (mg)	Iron (mg)	Vitamin A (IU)	Thiamin (mg)	Riboflavin (mg)	Vitamin C (mg)
1 tbsp sugar (white granulated)	0	trace[a]	0	0	0	0
1 tbsp honey (strained or extracted)	1	0.1	0	trace[a]	0.01	trace[a]
Possible daily nutrient need[b]	1,000	18	5,000	1.5	1.7	60

[a]A trace is an amount large enough to be detectable in chemical analysis but too small to be significant in comparison to the amounts recorded in these tables.

[b]These are amounts that an adult might typically need in a day. Not all the vitamins and minerals are listed.

starch:
a plant polysaccharide composed of glucose and digestible by humans.

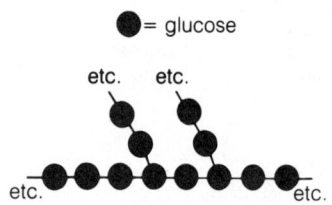

= glucose

etc.   etc.

etc.   etc.

Portion of a starch molecule.

Starch can be broken down to shorter chains of glucose units known as **dextrins**. The word sometimes appears on food labels, because dextrins can be used as thickening agents in foods.

fiber:
a loose term denoting the substances in plant foods that are not attacked by human digestive enzymes. The terms *crude fiber* and *dietary fiber* are more precise.

cellulose (CELL-you-loce):
a plant polysaccharide composed of glucose, indigestible by humans; one of the fibers.

pectin and **hemicellulose:**
carbohydrate fibers found in plant foods. Like cellulose, they are not attacked by human enzymes.

of 300 to 1,000 glucose units are linked together. These giant molecules are packed side by side in the rice grain or potato root—as many as a million per cubic inch of food. When we consume the plants, we receive that energy in the form of complex carbohydrates such as wheat, potatoes, or rice. Glucose can also be bonded in another way to form chains of glycogen and cellulose. Glycogen is the body's storage form of energy just as starch stores energy for plants.

All starchy foods are plant foods. Seeds are the most concentrated source. Most societies have a staple grain, which is the seed of the plant, that provides a majority of their food energy. Rice is the staple grain of Asia. In Canada, the United States, and Europe, the staple grain is wheat. Consider all the products that we eat that are made with wheat: flour, bread, pasta, and cereals. The staple grains of other peoples include corn, millet, rye, barley, and oats.

A second important source of starch is the legume family, including such beans and peas as butter beans, kidney beans, "baked" beans, black-eyed peas (cowpeas), chickpeas (garbanzo beans), and soybeans. These vegetables are about 40 percent starch by weight and also contain abundant protein. A third major source of starch is root vegetables such as potatoes and yams, which serve as the primary starch sources in many non-Western societies. When any of these foods are eaten, the starch molecules are digested to yield glucose units.

The Fibers

Plant foods contain many fibers, predominantly as constituents of their cell walls. Cellulose is one such fiber. Other fibers include gums, pectin, hemicelluloses, and mucilages. Until recently, lignins have been classified as a fiber, but since they are non-carbohydrate components of plants they are no longer considered a fiber.[1]

Although cellulose and other fibers are not attacked by human enzymes, some fiber, notably hemicellulose, can be digested by bacteria in the human digestive tract, and can yield some absorbable products. Food fibers are therefore not totally kcalorie free, although their energy contribution can be considered negligible.

Some fibers in the GI tract function like a sponge, holding water, binding minerals, and binding acidic materials such as the bile salts used by the body to prepare fat for digestion. Dietary fibers exercise the intestinal muscles so that they retain their health and tone. The major impact of dietary fiber is on the colon, the last part of the GI tract, where colon cancer and diverticular disease can arise. The addition of fibrous foods to the diet increases the bulk of food all along the intestine.

Fiber may play a beneficial role in the management of medical problems such as overweight, constipation and diarrhea, hemorrhoids, appendicitis, diverticulosis, colon cancer, raised blood lipids and cardiovascular disease, and diabetes control. Fiber is discussed further in Nutrition in Practice 16A. Even with all these advantages, carbohydrate in the form of raw fiber is not a wonder cure. In some cases it can be detrimental. When too much fiber is consumed, essential vitamins and minerals are bound and excreted without ever being available for the body to use. Also, consuming purified fiber such as cellulose may not confer the same health benefits as consuming cellulose from a food source such as whole grains.[2]

Not all fibers have similar effects. For example, wheat bran, which is composed mostly of cellulose, has no cholesterol-lowering effect, whereas oat bran and the fiber of apples (pectin) do lower blood cholesterol. On the other hand, wheat bran seems to be one of the most effective stool-softening fibers, especially if larger particle sizes are used. Fibers that form gels in water (pectin and guar) prolong the time of transit of materials through the intestine, whereas the insoluble fibers (cellulose) tend to reduce the time.

The Carbohydrates in Foods

Starches are often one of the first things that dieters mistakenly eliminate from their menu plans when trying to lose weight. Dieters have heard and often believe the myth that carbohydrates are fattening. Other misguided individuals have heard so much about the benefits of fiber that they force themselves to eat oat groats and alfalfa pellets while excluding meals that contain even small amounts of meat.

So what is the truth about carbohydrates? Are they "bad" for us because they are fattening or are they the wonder cure of the decade? The truth lies somewhere between these two extremes. Since carbohydrates contain the same number of kcalories per gram as protein and fewer kcalories than fat, it is erroneous to say that they are more fattening. This point was emphasized by the Senate committee that produced the Dietary Goals for the United States when it made the observation that a young man could include as many as 12 slices of bread in a day's meal plan and still lose over one pound a week.[3]

Foods that contain carbohydrate, such as grains, vegetables, fruits, and milk, are useful in our diets for many reasons. They are easy to digest, absorb, and use, not to mention economical and readily available. Most importantly, you need some carbohydrate daily as a source of glucose.

The dietary goals and guidelines offered to the public by various agencies in the United States and Canada all agree that it would do no harm, and that it might do some good, for people to reduce their intake of some sugars and increase their intake of foods containing complex carbohydrates. This advice is based on two distinctions. First, not all sugars need to be restricted; those in ordinary foods such as fruits, vegetables, and milk are excepted. *Concentrated* sweets, relatively empty of nutrients and high in kcalories, are the ones singled out for avoidance. Second, the concentrated sweets are to be replaced, not just with complex carbohydrates, but with foods containing carbohydrates. The major additions to the diet would be foods containing starch and fiber—vegetables, grains, legumes, and fruits.

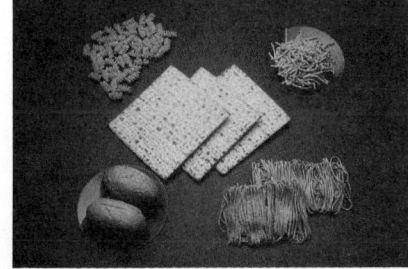

Grains are a source of fiber.

The health benefits to be expected from such a change would be many. Before enumerating them, though, let us hasten to say that it is difficult to sort out just what dietary factors might contribute to each health benefit. A diet lower in pure sugars and higher in foods containing complex carbohydrates would almost certainly be lower in fat, lower in kcalories, and higher in fiber as well. The combination of all these factors working together might be expected to bring about, or contribute to, lower rates of obesity, cardiovascular disease, diabetes, cancer, malnutrition, and tooth decay.

There is no RDA for carbohydrate, nor is there one for fiber. It is left to you to make sure that you plan to get enough. Most authorities agree that 55 to 60 percent of total kcalories should come from carbohydrate. A minimum of 100 grams of carbohydrate a day is essential.[4] To be safe, at least 125 grams is needed; and 300 grams might be an ideal intake for many people. At four kcalories per gram, that would be 1,200 kcalories from carbohydrate, or 60 percent of the kcalories in a 2,000 kcalorie diet. The carbohydrate content of a diet can be determined by using a nutrient composition table as found in Appendix C or by using the exchange list system described in Chapter 18.

Sugar Intake

Food group plans do not make allowances for sugary foods such as candy, jam, and soft drinks because they are not considered desirable in diet plans. But people do consume them, and such foods certainly contain carbohydrate. To estimate how much carbohydrate is consumed as sugar, the following concentrated sweets can be treated as equivalent to 1 teaspoon of white sugar:

- 1 teaspoon brown sugar, candy, jam, jelly, corn sweeteners, syrups, honey, molasses, or maple sugar
- 1 tablespoon catsup (ketchup)
- 1 ½ ounces carbonated soft drink

These portions of sugar all provide about the same number of kcalories. Some are closer to 10 kcalories (for example, 13 kcalories for sucrose), while some are over 20 (22 kcalories for honey); an average figure of 20 kcalories is an acceptable approximation. The accompanying miniglossary presents the multitude of names that denote sugar on food labels.

One of the reasons people are told to restrict their intakes of concentrated sweets is that sugars have a greater glycemic effect on the body than complex carbohydrates do. The glycemic effect of a food is the effect that food has on a person's blood glucose and insulin response—how fast and how high the blood glucose rises, and how quickly the body responds by bringing it back to normal. Most simple sugars produce a major surge in blood glucose while complex carbohydrates produce a flatter response curve—but the difference is not altogether clear-cut. The effects of different foods on blood glucose apparently depend on many factors.

The glycemic effect of a food is important to people with abnormalities of blood glucose regulation, notably diabetes and hypoglycemia. More about the glycemic effect of food is covered in chapter 19.

Fiber Intake

The amounts of dietary fiber in food are hard to estimate. Chemists can analyze food for crude fiber content in the laboratory by digesting it with acids and bases, but if you eat the same food, subjecting it to the action of your own enzymes, the undigested residue will be greater, because the body's enzymes are less harsh than the laboratory treatment. What we really need to know is the dietary fiber content of foods, but it is difficult to measure.

crude fiber:
the residue of plant food remaining after extraction with dilute acid followed by dilute alkali in a laboratory procedure; that is, the fiber that remains in food after a harsh chemical digestive procedure.

Miniglossary of kCaloric Sweeteners

brown sugar sugar crystals contained in molasses syrup with natural flavor and color; 91% to 96% pure sucrose. (Some refiners add syrup to refined white sugar to make brown sugar.)

confectioners' sugar finely powdered sucrose; 99.9% pure.

corn sweeteners corn syrup and sugars derived from corn.

corn syrup a syrup produced by the action of enzymes on cornstarch, containing mostly glucose. See also *high-fructose corn syrup*.

dextrose glucose (an older name).

fructose, galactose, glucose already defined (pp. 23).

granulated sugar crystalline sucrose; 99.9% pure.

high-fructose corn syrup (HFCS) the predominant sweetener used in processed foods today. HFCS is mostly fructose; glucose makes up the balance.

honey sugar formed from nectar (mostly sucrose) gathered by bees. An enzyme splits the sucrose into glucose and fructose. Composition and flavor vary, but honey always contains a mixture of sucrose, fructose, and glucose.

invert sugar a mixture of glucose and fructose formed by the splitting of sucrose in a chemical process. Sold only in liquid form, sweeter than sucrose, invert sugar is used as an additive to help preserve food freshness and prevent shrinkage.

lactose already defined. (p. 23).

levulose fructose (an older name).

maltitol, mannitol, sorbitol, xylitol sugar alcohols, which can be derived from fruits or commercially produced from dextrose; absorbed more slowly, and metabolized differently than other sugars in the human body, and not readily utilized by ordinary mouth bacteria.

maltose already defined. (p. 23).

maple sugar a sugar (mostly sucrose) purified from concentrated sap of the sugar maple tree. Maple sugar is expensive compared with other sweeteners.

molasses a thick brown syrup, left over from sugar cane juice during sugar refining. It retains residual sugar and other by-products and a few minerals; blackstrap molasses contains significant amounts of calcium and iron—the iron from the machinery used to process it.

raw sugar the first crop of crystals harvested during sugar processing. Raw sugar cannot be sold in the United States because it contains too much filth (dirt, insect fragments, and the like). Sugar sold domestically as raw sugar has actually gone through about half of the refining steps.

sucrose already defined. (p. 23).

turbinado (ter-bih-NOD-oh) **sugar** raw (brown) sugar from which the filth has been washed; legal to sell in the United States.

white sugar pure sucrose, produced by dissolving, concentrating, and recrystallizing raw sugar.

dietary fiber:
the residue of plant food resistant to human digestive enzymes; that is, the fiber that remains from food after digestion in the body.

1 g crude fiber ≈ 2–3 g dietary fiber

With all the uncertainties, it is probably true to say that about 20 to 30 grams of dietary fiber daily is a desirable intake. The diet can supply that amount, given ample choices of whole foods. However, it involves eating such quantities of fruits, vegetables, legumes, and grains that little room is left for meats and dairy products—a way of eating to which some people find it hard to adjust.

Energy Nutrients in Perspective

An uninterrupted flow of energy is so vital to life that other functions are sometimes sacrificed to maintain it. For example, when a child is fed too little food, the food he or she does consume will be used for energy to keep the heart and lungs going, but growth will come to a standstill. To go totally without an energy supply, even for a few minutes, is to die. Over the course of evolution, the urgency of the need for energy has ensured that all creatures have built-in reserves to protect themselves from being deprived of energy. Our provision against this sort of emergency is glycogen, the storage form of glucose.

When you do not eat carbohydrate, your body rapidly devours first its glycogen stores and then its own protein to generate glucose. The body needs its protein, however, for other vital purposes. This protein-sparing effect of carbohydrate is important. It is protection against an emergency when the body runs short of glucose, because glycogen can return glucose to the blood whenever the supply runs short. The liver cells, however, can store only a limited amount of energy as glycogen. Once this supply is depleted, the body must turn to the other energy nutrients—fat and protein—to meet its energy needs.

Unlike the liver, the body's fat mass has a virtually unlimited storage capacity, and fat supplies two thirds of the body's energy needs. During a prolonged period of food deprivation, fat can provide energy for most tissues. However, fat cannot provide energy in the form of glucose, the substance needed as fuel by the brain and nerves. After a long period of glucose deprivation, brain and nerve cells develop the ability to derive about half of their energy from a special form of fat known as ketones, but they still require glucose as well. With the available glycogen long gone, brain and nerve cells demand this glucose from the only alternative source—protein. Because no protein is coming in from food, the only supply is in the muscles and other lean tissues. These tissues give up their protein and atrophy, bringing on weakness, loss of function, and ultimately death after using half of the body protein. Death from loss of lean body tissues will occur even in an obese person who fasts too long. It should be clear, then, that although carbohydrate is an ideal energy source, fat and sometimes protein are extremely important in meeting energy demands.

ketones (KEY-tones):
a condensation product of fat metabolism produced when carbohydrate is not available (see Chapter 3).

atrophy (ATT-ro-fee):
to waste away.
a = without
trophy = growth

SELF-STUDY:

How's Your Carbohydrate Intake?

From the forms you filled out for Self-Study 1, answer the following questions and complete Form 6.

1. How many grams of carbohydrate do you consume in an average day?
   _____ grams

2. How many kcalories does this represent? _____ kcalories (Remember, 1 gram of carbohydrate contributes 4 kcalories.)

3. It is estimated that you should have 125 grams or more of carbohydrate in a day. How does your intake compare with this minimum? _____

4. What percentage of your total kcalories is contributed by carbohydrate (carbohydrate kcalories divided by total kcalories times 100-or use the answer you obtained on Form 5)? _____ percent

5. How does this figure compare with the dietary goal stating that about 55 to 60 percent of the kcalories in your diet should come from carbohydrate? _____ (Note: If you are on a diet to lose weight, this goal does not apply to you. See the exercises in Self-Study 6: Diet Planning.)

6. Another dietary goal is that no more than 10 percent of total kcalories should come from refined and other processed sugars and foods high in such sugars. To assess your intake against this standard, sort the carbohydrate-containing food items you ate into three groups:

   • Group A: Foods containing complex carbohydrate (foods found among the grains, starchy foods, and vegetables in the exchange lists, Chapter 18) contributed _____ kcalories.

   • Group B: Nutritious foods containing simple carbohydrate (foods on the milk and fruit lists) contributed _____ kcalories.

   • Group C: Foods containing mostly concentrated simple carbohydrate (sugar, honey, molasses, syrup, jam, jelly, candy, cakes, doughnuts, sweet rolls, cola beverages, and so on) contributed _____ kcalories.

   Does your concentrated sugar intake (Group C) fall within the recommended maximum of 10 percent of total daily kcalories? _____ If not, what food choices account for the excess sugar? _____
   _____

7. Estimate the number of pounds of sugar (concentrated simple carbohydrate) you eat in a year (1 pound = 454 grams):

   _____ kcalories from Group C divided by 4 = _____ grams/day
   _____ grams/day × 365 days/year = _____ grams/year
   _____ grams/year divided by 454 grams/pound = _____ pounds/year

   How does your yearly sugar intake compare with the estimated U.S. and Canadian average of about 75 pounds per person per year? _____ Comment on this. _____
   _____

Notes

1. D.A.T. Southgate, The relation between composition and properties of dietary fiber and physiological effects, in *Dietary Fiber: Basic and Clinical Aspects,* eds. G.V. Vahouny and D. Kritchevsky (New York: Plenum Press, 1986), pp. 35–48.

2. J.L. Slavin, Dietary fiber: Classification, chemical analyses, and food sources. *Journal of the American Dietetic Association* 87 (1987): 1164–1171.

3. U.S. Senate, Select Committee on Nutrition and Human Needs, *Dietary Goals for the United States.* 2d.ed. (Washington, D.C.: Government Printing Office, 1977).

4. *Recommended Dietary Allowances*, 9th ed. (Washington, D.C.: National Academy of Sciences, 1980), 33.

FORM 6
Carbohydrate and Sugar kCalories

Average daily carbohydrate intake: _____ grams

Total kcalories from carbohydrate: _____ kcalories (grams × 4)

Total kcalories from all sources: _____ kcalories

Total kcalories from carbohydrates should equal 60 percent of total kcalories from all sources.

Percentage of kcalories from carbohydrate: _____ %

Breakdown of carbohydrate kcalories:

A. _____ complex   B. _____ nutritious simple

C. _____ concentrated simple

kCalories from concentrated simple sugars should equal 10 percent or less of total kcalories from all sources. Percentage of kcalories from concentrated simple sugars: _____ %

Is Sugar the Adversary?

Most children are generally oblivious to diet fads, but that doesn't mean they are immune to prevailing nutrition ideas. A generation ago, thin children were given milkshakes and candy so they would look healthier. Today the style is ultra thin, and many a mother starts worrying immediately after childbirth that her child is going to have a weight problem. Having absorbed the message to change her own diet, she is wondering about her child's diet.

A mother asks you about her one-year-old daughter. The child is healthy with bright, inquisitive eyes. You comment on what a great job the mother has done. The mother wants to continue giving her child the best nutrition possible and is facing new concerns about sugar now that her child is eating table foods. Answers to some of the questions she may ask are found in this section.

It seems that every time I read the newspaper, I see something negative about sugar. Is the same low-sugar diet for adults recommended for children? Children need a well-rounded, balanced diet but not necessarily the same diet as their parents. Children have high energy demands and must eat enough to meet their demands.

Failure to thrive (FTT), which is a failure for a child to grow at an appropriate rate, has many causes, but it has been seen in children whose parents are conscientious about their own diet. Researchers found that

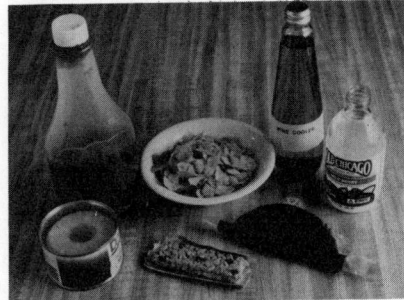

Sugar is concealed in many common products.

because some parents feared that their children would become obese, they sought to give their children what they believed was ideal—a low-kcalorie diet. The children's failure to thrive reversed itself when the children were given a more liberalized diet, including moderate amounts of sugar.[1]

This is just one example of how accusations made against sugar can be misleading. Another case in which accusations are unproved is in the argument that a high sugar intake leads to diabetes.[2] Similarly, the accusation that sugar causes atherosclerosis is not yet proven.[3] All this does not mean that sugar is off the hook as a causative factor in these disorders. More research may give a clearer picture of the relationship of sugar, if any, to these disorders.

In other instances, sugar can be bad for you. If eating a lot of sugar means that you eat fewer foods containing essential nutrients, malnutrition can result. Conversely, if you eat a lot of sugar without eating less of something else, you will get too many kcalories. Obesity can result which does contribute to many diseases. Furthermore, sugar does promote tooth decay, or dental caries in susceptible people—and that means most of us.

How does sugar promote tooth decay? Dental caries are caused by the acid by-product of bacterial growth in the mouth. Because bacteria thrive on food particles, especially those that contain carbohydrate, we can logically implicate sugar as the cause of cavities. Any carbohydrate, however, including starch, can support bacterial growth. Equally important is the length of time the food stays in the mouth, and this depends on how soon you brush your teeth after eating and how sticky the food is. The damage sugar does relates to both the amount and the stickiness of the sugar. A sticky, sugary food, such as raisins or granola, causes more caries than an easily rinsed off sugary food, such as a sweetened beverage.

Sugar can be eaten and then removed from tooth surfaces soon enough to prevent decay. A rule of thumb is that bacterial action is maximal within the first 20 minutes after the first contact. If immediate brushing is not possible, milk or other beverages swished in the mouth after a meal can effectively rinse the teeth. Once-a-day flossing may also effectively control formation of caries, regardless of carbohydrate content of the diet. Some people may *never* get cavities because they have inherited resistance to them.

From what you've said, I gather that sugar in reasonable amounts is acceptable for normal-weight children, but should an overweight child be put on a sugar-free weight-loss diet?

In direct contrast to children who suffer from inadequate food energy intakes, obesity among children is becoming a serious problem. The first thing that comes to mind when a person mentions weight loss is to reduce sugar in the diet, but recall that sugar is only one of the energy nutrients. Protein and fat also contribute kcalories to the diet. Secondly, weight gain is caused by greater energy consumption than energy expenditure. Some researchers have found that obesity stems from inactivity as much as from overeating.[4] Sugar may not be the problem. Often, obese children do not consume more kcalories than nonobese children. The obese children are just less active. Reducing sugar, then, would not be as beneficial as increasing the children's activity levels.

Even if a child is mildly obese, the psychological risks of putting the child on a diet might be too severe. You might substitute low-kcalorie foods for snacks and desserts but only to help the child maintain his or her weight until height catches up with weight.

How much sugar would be acceptable in an otherwise balanced diet?

There is no reason to believe that a moderate consumption of sugar (5 to 10 percent of kcalories) is in any way dangerous to a normal, healthy human being. The guideline to restrict sugar to less than 10 percent of total kcalories does not apply to *all* sugars in the diet. Don't confuse the diluted sugars found in milk and fruits with concentrated refined sugars, such as table sugar and its relatives. Avoid these concentrated sweets. There's no room for sugar in the diet if it displaces needed nutrients.

What are some ways in which I can cut down on sugar?

A lot of good ideas come to mind. The American Friends Service Committee suggests that alternatives to sweet desserts might be cheese and whole-grain crackers and yogurt, and that snacks for children need not be sugar-water drinks. Instead, children can have fruits, raw vegetables, popcorn, unsalted nuts, homemade fruit-juice popsicles, and other wholesome foods.[5] Here are some other suggestions:

- Substitute fruit *juices* or plain water for fruit *drinks*, regular soft drinks, punches, and ales that contain considerable amounts of sugar. Children love fruit juices that come in small boxes with straws.
- Go easy on candy, pies, cakes, pastries, and cookies.
- Fruits are often canned in heavy syrup, a high-sugar product. Buy fruit canned in its own juice, other fruit juice, or light syrup.

- Many cereals are presweetened. Check labels. Some list sugar first—or second and third—among their ingredients. Buy *unsweetened* kinds so you can control the amount of sugar added.
- Experiment with reducing the sugar in your favorite recipes. Some recipes taste the same even after a 25 percent reduction in sugar content. Others taste different but just as delicious if not more so.

The sweet spices—allspice, anise, cardamom, cinnamon, cloves, fennel, and ginger—can replace substantial sugar in recipes. Use half as much sugar and half again as much spice as the recipe calls for.

Note also that sugar is hidden in many supposedly healthful products. Chocolate milk, gelatin, catsup, breakfast bars, and flavored yogurt are high in sugar.

Notes

1. M. Pugliese and coauthors, Parental diet beliefs causing failure to thrive, *Pediatrics* 80 (1987): 175–178.
2. D.B. Peterson and coauthors, Sucrose in the diet of diabetic patients—Just another carbohydrate? *Diabetologia* 29 (1986): 216–220, as cited by *Modern Medicine,* October 1986, pp. 117, 120.
3. D.J.A. Jenkins and coauthors, Low glycemic index carbohydrate foods in the management of hyperlipidemia, *American Journal of Clinical Nutrition* 42 (1985): 604–617.
4. W. H. Dietz Jr., Obesity among children: It's growing bigger, *Tufts University Diet and Nutrition Letter,* November 1987, p. 7.
5. L. Warschoff, *What Betty Crocker doesn't tell you about sugar!* (Baltimore: American Friends Service Committee, 1976), p. 1.

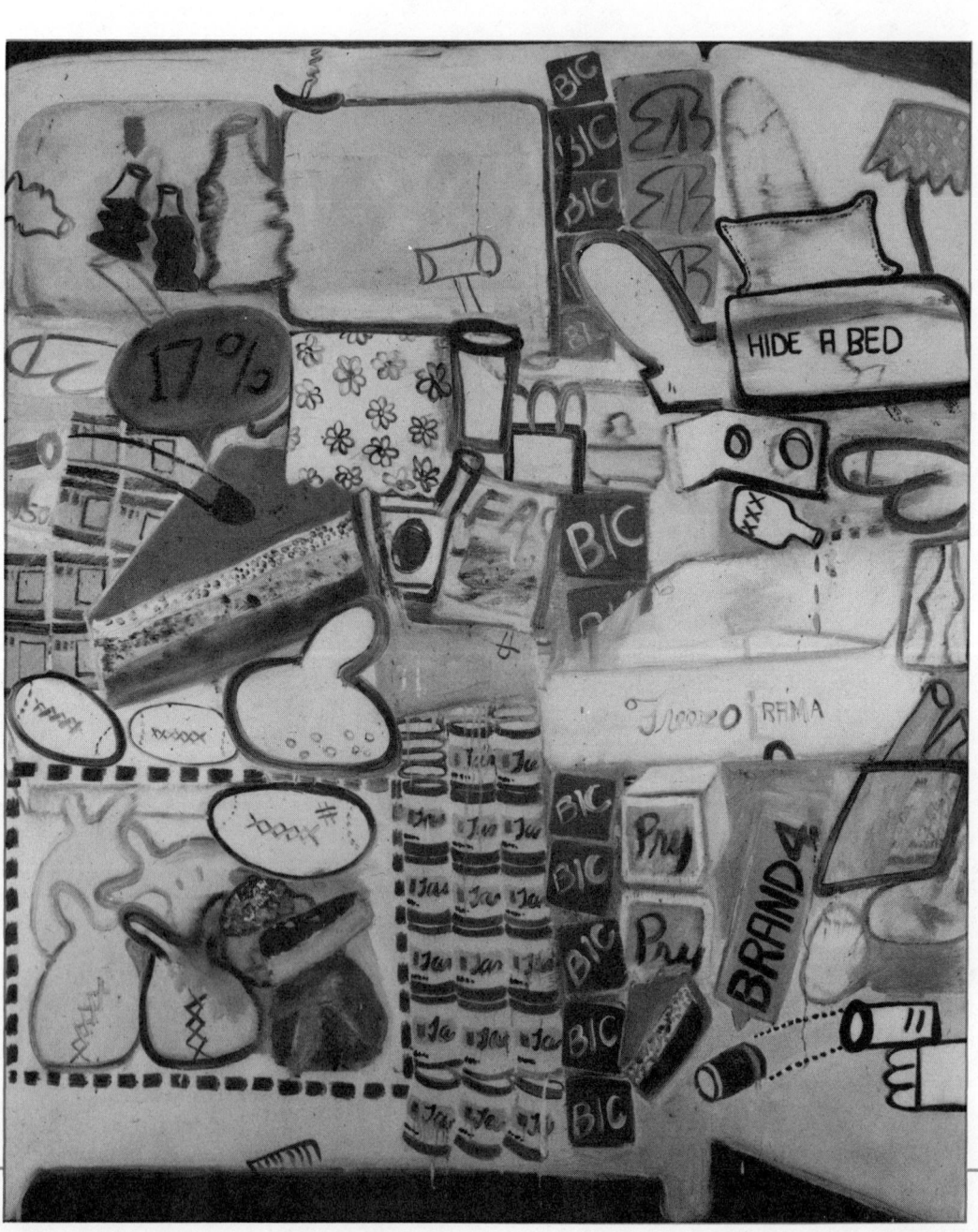

3

Fats

CONTENTS

"Icebox" by Peter Saul, 1960. Oil on canvas 69" × 58¼". Courtesy of Frumkin/Adams Gallery, New York.

Remember, fat is a more concentrated energy source than the other energy nutrients: 1 g carbohydrate or protein = 4 kcal, but 1 gram fat = 9 kcal

We often hear of the potential harm of excess fats in the diet, but those same fats are indispensable to life. The fats are more properly called lipids, which is a classification that includes fats, sterols and oils. Lipids serve many functions in addition to their role in energy metabolism and occur in your body to help keep it healthy. Natural oils in the skin provide a radiant complexion; in the scalp, they help nourish the hair and make it glossy. The layer of fat beneath the skin insulates the body from extremes of temperature. A pad of hard fat beneath each kidney protects it from being jarred and damaged, even during a motorcycle ride on a bumpy road. The soft fat in the breasts of a woman protects the mammary glands from heat and cold and cushions them against shock. The fat that lies embedded in muscle tissue shares with muscle glycogen the task of providing energy when the muscles are active.

Not only is fat important in the body, it is also important in foods. Many of the compounds that give foods their flavor and aroma are found in fats and oils. The delicious aromas associated with bacon, ham, and other meats, as well as with onions being fried, come from fats. Four vitamins—A, D, E, and K—are soluble in fat. When the fat is removed, so are these vitamins.

When fat is removed, kcalories also are lost. A medium pork chop with the fat trimmed to within a half-inch of the lean contains 260 kcalories; with the fat trimmed off completely, it contains 130 kcalories. A baked potato with butter and sour cream (one tablespoon each) has 215 kcalories; a plain baked potato has 90 kcalories. The single most effective step you can take to reduce the number of kcalories in a food is to trim the fat. To keep the kcalorie count low, refrain from adding fat, too.

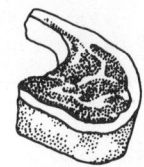

Pork chop with 1/2 inch fat (260 kcal).

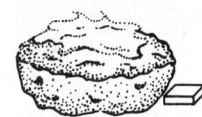

Potato with 1 tbsp butter and 1 tbsp sour cream (215 kcal).

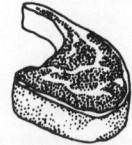

Pork chop with fat trimmed off (130 kcal).

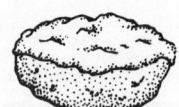

Plain potato (90 kcal).

fatty acid glycerol

HO HO HO

fatty acid:
a chain of carbon atoms with hydrogen attached.

glycerol (GLISS-er-ol):
a small compound related to carbohydrates that can form the backbone of triglycerides and phospholipids.

fat:
a mixture of triglycerides.

Fatty acids and triglycerides make up 95 percent of all the fats we eat. The other 5 percent consists of phospholipids and sterols.

The Fatty Acids and Triglycerides

When energy from any energy-yielding nutrient is stored as fat, fragments derived from that nutrient are linked together into chains known as fatty acids.

Fatty acids are then packaged in threes with glycerol to make triglycerides, the material of fat.

Fatty acids may differ from each other in two ways—in chain length and in degree of saturation. Chain length affects the way the fatty acid is absorbed (see Chapter 5). Saturation refers to the chemical structure—specifically to the number of hydrogens the fatty acid chain is holding. If every available bond from the carbons is holding a hydrogen, the chain is called a saturated fatty acid, meaning that the chain is filled to capacity with hydrogen.

Sometimes, especially in plants, hydrogen atoms are missing in the fatty acid chains. These missing hydrogen atoms are points of unsaturation, and such a chain is called an unsaturated fatty acid. An example is oleic acid. If there is one point of unsaturation, the chain is monosaturated. If there are two or more points of unsaturation, then the fatty acid is polyunsaturated. You sometimes see polyunsaturated fatty acids abbreviated on food labels as PUFA. Plants make most of the unsaturated fatty acids, which help form the protective coating of leaves and the skin of seeds. For example, olive oil contains abundant monounsaturated fatty acids, while many nuts, seeds, and leaves contain polyunsaturated fatty acids.

The human body can synthesize all the fatty acids it needs from carbohydrate, fat, or protein except for linoleic and linolenic acid. These fatty acids cannot be made from the breakdown of other substances and so must be provided in the diet. They are therefore considered essential fatty acids. Linoleic acid is an omega-6, polyunsaturated fatty acid found in leafy vegetables and soybean oil. Infants especially need linoleic acid, and it is no coincidence that human breast milk has a much higher percentage of it than cow's milk.

Another class of polyunsaturated fatty acids is the omega-3 fatty acids which are found in fish oils or are derived from dietary linolenic acid. The importance of omega-3 fatty acids is just now being realized as fatty acids are studied in more depth as protectors against hypertension.[1] Eicosanoids—compounds that have regulatory functions in the body—are made from both the omega-6 and omega-3 fatty acids, but their effects are subtly different.

Research has shown that when the omega-3 fatty acids are present in the diet many desirable health effects occur. Some that are being investigated include reduced blood triglycerides and cholesterol, slowed clotting time, slowed progression of atherosclerotic heart disease, enhanced defenses against cancer, and reduced inflammation in arthritis and asthma sufferers.

Whenever research suggests that a compound is a protective factor against heart disease, manufacturers start producing it as a supplement without regard for the best interest of the consumer. Omega-3 fatty acids are available in supplement form, although supplements may not be the best vehicle for delivering these fatty acids.

The omega-3 and omega-6 fatty acids compete for the same enzymes in the body. The possible consequences of taking supplements of one is that a deficiency of the other could easily be induced. Another problem is that it is possible that the supplement form does not function the same way as the form available directly from fish oils. There are still questions about how much is the right amount, and the problem is compounded

A saturated fatty acid.

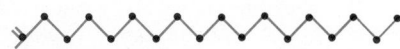

saturated fatty acid:
a fatty acid carrying the maximum possible number of hydrogen atoms, for example, stearic acid. A saturated *fat* is composed of triglycerides in which all, or virtually all, of the fatty acids are saturated.

Oleic acid, an unsaturated fatty acid.

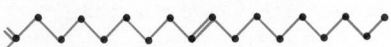

monounsaturated fatty acid:
a fatty acid that has one point of unsaturation where hydrogens are missing, for example, oleic acid.

Linoleic acid, a polyunsaturated fatty acid.

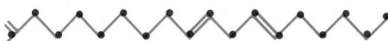

polyunsaturated fatty acid (PUFA):
a fatty acid with two or more points of unsaturation. For example, linoleic acid has two such points and linolenic acid has three. Thus, a polyunsaturated *fat* is composed of triglycerides containing a high percentage of PUFA.

linoleic acid, linolenic acid:
polyunsaturated fatty acids, essential for human beings

essential fatty acids:
fatty acids that cannot be synthesized in the body in amounts sufficient to meet physiological need.

omega:
the last letter of the Greek alphabet (ω), used by chemists to refer to the position of the last double bond in a fatty acid. The *omega-6* fatty acids have their last double bond six carbons back along the chain; the *omega-3* acids, three carbons back.

eicosanoids (eye-COSS-a-noids):
derivatives of a 20-carbon fatty acid; hormonelike compounds that regulate blood pressure, clotting, and other body functions.

by the fact that the quantities of omega-3 fatty acids in supplements vary widely from what the labels say they contain.

The best way to increase your intake of omega-3 fatty acids is to increase consumption of fatty fish. The darker flesh of fish has the highest fat content and this is where most omega-3 fatty acids are found.

triglyceride (try-GLISS-uh-ride): a compound composed of glycerol with three fatty acids attached to it.
tri = three
glyceride = a compound of glycerol

Very few free fatty acids are found in the body or in foods. Usually, the fatty acids have been incorporated into the larger, more complex compounds, triglycerides. Usually when we refer to fat, such as when we say, "I am fat" or "That meat is fatty," it is triglycerides that we are discussing. The name has been explained: three fatty acids (*tri*) are attached to a molecule of glycerol.

Any combination of fatty acids can be incorporated into a triglyceride—long chain or short chain, saturated or polyunsaturated. Each animal species (including human beings) has its own characteristic kinds of triglycerides, but animals raised for food can be fed certain diets to give them softer or harder fat, whichever the consumer demands. The degree of saturation determines the softness or hardness of fats (discussed later in the chapter).

The Phospholipids and Sterols

Phospholipids and sterols don't contribute many kcalories to our diet because they form such a small percentage (five percent) of total dietary fat. Two are of particular interest nutritionally—lecithin among the phospholipids and cholesterol among the sterols.

The Phospholipids: Lecithin

phospholipid: a compound similar to a triglyceride but having choline or another phosphorus-containing acid in place of one of the fatty acids.

lecithin: one of the phospholipids.

Like the triglycerides, the lecithins and the other phospholipids have a backbone of glycerol; they are different because they have only two fatty acids attached to them. In place of the third fatty acid is a molecule of choline or a similar compound. Lecithin is the best known phospholipid.

Lecithin and other phospholipids are important constituents of cell membranes. They also act as emulsifying agents, helping to keep other fats in solution in the blood and body fluids.

Lecithin periodically receives noisy attention in the popular press and is credited with great deeds. You may have heard that it is a major constituent of cell membranes (true), that the functioning of all cells depends on the integrity of the cells' membranes (true), and that you must therefore purchase bottles of lecithin and give yourself daily doses (false). The body digests lecithin before it absorbs it, so the lecithin you eat does not reach the body tissues intact. The liver then makes from scratch the lecithin you need for building cell membranes. In other words, the lecithins are not essential nutrients. Furthermore, large doses of lecithin have been seen to cause digestive upsets, sweating, salivation, and loss of appetite.[2]

Before buying bottles of lecithin or any other wonder substance, ask yourself, "Do I really need this? What is the evidence that my body is likely to be deficient?"

The Sterols: Cholesterol

Like the lecithins, cholesterol is needed metabolically but is not an essential nutrient. Your liver is manufacturing it now, as you read, at the rate of perhaps 50,000,000,000,000,000 molecules per second. The raw materials that the liver uses to make cholesterol can all be taken from glucose or saturated fatty acids. Another way of saying the same thing is that cholesterol can be made from either carbohydrate or fat. More than nine-tenths of all the body's cholesterol ends up in the cells, where it performs vital structural and metabolic functions.

After being made, cholesterol either leaves the liver or is transformed into related compounds such as the sex hormones (for example, testosterone) or the adrenal hormones (for example, cortisone). The cholesterol that leaves the liver has three possible destinations:

1. It may be made into bile and move into the intestine where some may then be excreted in the feces.

2. It may be deposited in the body's cells.

3. It may accumulate in arteries, contributing to arterial disease(atherosclerosis).

Bile, made from cholesterol by the liver, is released into the intestine to aid in the digestion and absorption of fat (see Chapter 5). After doing its job, some of the bile reenters the body with absorbed products of fat digestion. Cholesterol is thus recycled—back to the liver, once again into bile, back to the intestine, again into the body, and once more back to the liver.

Once out in the intestine, however, some of the bile can be trapped by certain kinds of dietary fibers or by some medications, which carry it out of the body in feces. The excretion of bile reduces the total amount of cholesterol remaining in the body.

Some cholesterol leaves the liver packaged with other lipids and protein for transport to the body tissues. The packages are the lipoproteins. The blood carries lipoproteins through all the body's arteries, and any tissue can extract lipids from them. Some cells take lipoproteins up whole. To pass into the cells, lipids must first cross the artery walls, and some are deposited there. Lipids have been implicated ·in artery disease because of this association with the artery wall.

sterol:
a class of lipids. Cholesterol, vitamin D, and steroid hormones are examples.

cholesterol:
one of the sterols.

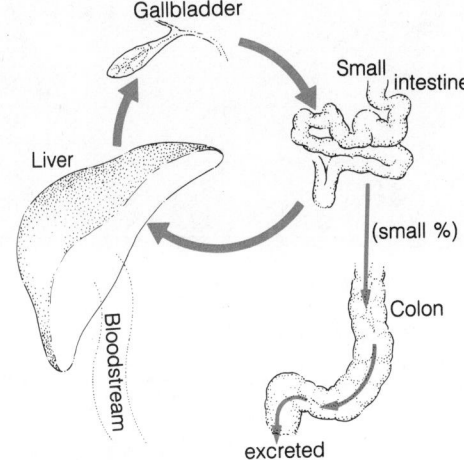

The circulation of bile from the liver to the gallbladder to the intestine and back to the liver is known as the **enterohepatic circulation** of bile.
enteron = *intestine*
hepat = *liver*

Lipoproteins are made by both the intestine and the liver. Chapter 5 tells the story of lipid transport.

Artery disease—atherosclerosis—is discussed in Chapter 21.

The Fats in Foods

The basic dietary principle of reducing blood lipids and blood cholesterol, which are contributing factors in heart and artery disease, is to restrict saturated fat intake.[3] The cholesterol that accumulates in arteries is manufactured largely from fragments derived from saturated fat. Thus, limiting your consumption of saturated fat may help. On the assumption that some of the body's cholesterol may come from the diet, it may make sense to limit your cholesterol intake as well, but dietary saturated fat is much more important in this connection than dietary cholesterol. In any case, many health care professionals recommend that you limit your intakes of both saturated fat and cholesterol. In effect, you will achieve this if you limit your intake of total fat.

Total Fat

In the 1970s, there was a slight downward shift in the saturated fat and cholesterol consumption of people in this country.[4] This may have been the result of an intensive campaign to show the public the relationship between dietary fat and the development of cardiovascular disease. However, there has not been a reduction in total fat intake. Fat consumption today is one-sixth higher than it was at the turn of the century. Even though people eat less red meat and trim more fat from the meat that they eat, there has been an overall increase in fat intake from fats that are not as visible as the ones just mentioned.

Most people recognize that butter, margarine, shortening, and oils contain only fat, and many consumers are aware of the high fat content of red meats. Those same consumers, however, have increased their consumption of fat from such products as convenience foods, fried foods, and luncheon and other prepared meats. The fats in these foods are sometimes referred to as invisible fat, because they do not have the obvious appearance of fat. An ounce of lean meat supplies 28 kcalories from its protein and 27 kcalories from its fat. An ounce of a high-fat meat (such as bologna) supplies 28 kcalories from protein and 72 kcalories from fat. Two tablespoons of peanut butter, also with 28 kcalories from protein, supply 140 kcalories from fat! Foods that are usually thought of as protein-rich foods may actually contain more fat energy than protein energy. Note that the values for meat given here are for one-ounce portions. An average serving of hamburger is usually 3 or 4 ounces. An average dinner steak may be 6 to 8 ounces or larger.

Other foods contain a considerable amount of fat. An eighth of an avocado, one strip of bacon, or five small olives contain as much fat as a pat of butter (45 kcalories from fat).

Saturated Fat and Cholesterol in Foods

The fat in milk is about 62 percent saturated fat; the cholesterol content is 25 milligrams per cup of whole milk or 7 milligrams per cup of nonfat milk. Thus, choosing nonfat in place of whole milk reduces your intake of saturated fat as well as your intake of cholesterol.

The fats in meats and eggs are about half saturated; those in poultry and fish have a healthier balance between saturated and unsaturated fats. The foods that contain the highest amounts of cholesterol are eggs, organ meats such as liver and kidneys, and high-fat dairy products. Shellfish have been thought to contain high concentrations of cholesterol, but the findings on which this idea

1 g protein = 4 kcal
1 g fat = 9 kcal
1 oz = about 30 g

Remember that an ounce of meat is not an ounce of protein. An ounce (30 g) of lean meat contains 7 g protein and 3 g fat. The other 20 g are largely water with associated vitamins and minerals.

was based have been called into question. Shellfish contain sterols, but possibly not the kind that have metabolically negative effects, and they contain much less cholesterol than has been thought in the past.

As a general rule, a meat eater wishing to reduce both saturated fat and cholesterol intake could accomplish these objectives by eating less high-fat meat and dairy foods, fewer eggs, and more poultry and fish. A vegetarian who uses animal products could shift to nonfat milk and low-fat cheeses and could limit butter and egg intake. Vegetarians who do not consume any animal products eat a diet low in fat and consume no cholesterol because plant foods do not contain cholesterol.

To the extent that a person does eat fats, the fats to choose are the unsaturated ones. The hardness of fats at room temperature is an indicator: the harder it is, the more saturated it is. Chicken fat is softer than pork fat, which is softer than beef tallow. Of the three, chicken fat is the most unsaturated, and beef tallow is the most saturated. Unsaturated fats melt more readily. Generally speaking, vegetable and fish oils are rich in polyunsaturates, olive oil is rich in monounsaturates, and the harder fats—animal fats—are more saturated.

Saturated fats are solid at room or body temperature. Polyunsaturated fats are liquid at room or body temperature.

If you wish to make choices consistent with current recommendations, you should learn how to read food labels, avoid fat in general, and seek out the poly- and monounsaturated fats in preference to the saturated ones. But beware: *vegetable fat* or *vegetable oil* doesn't always mean *unsaturated fat*. Coconut oil and palm oil, for example, are often used in nondairy creamers, and both are saturated fats. Vegetable oils that are hydrogenated may have lost their polyunsaturated character.

hydrogenation:
the process of adding hydrogen to unsaturated fat to make it more solid and resistant to chemical change.

Each culture has its own favorite food sources of fats and oils. In Canada, rapeseed oil is widely used. In the Mediterranean area, Greeks, Italians, and Spaniards rely heavily on olive oil. Asians use the polyunsaturated oil of soybeans. Jewish people traditionally employ chicken fat, whereas U.S. southerners rely heavily on pork fat—lard and bacon. Everywhere in North America, butter and margarine are widely used, and with the recent popularity of fast foods, the use of vegetable oil has also been increasing.

In the past, the fat that foods were fried in was not a health concern. As research discovers more unhealthy links between saturated fats and heart disease and cancer, people have a reason to be concerned about the types of fats used to fry the foods ordered at restaurants. With fast foods becoming a major portion of many people's diets, it is important to know whether the origin of the fats is animal or vegetable. All fats have the same number of kcalories per spoon, but the animal fats are saturated and have increased health risks associated with them. Some fast-food restaurants are beginning to take consumers' concerns into account and are frying foods in polyunsaturated vegetable oils. However, some of the most popular fast-food establishments continue to use beef tallow, because it is more economical. If consumers are concerned enough to avoid foods fried in animal fats, establishments may change the types of fats they use.

Artificial Fats

Artificial fats are attracting public attention. One fat substitute is sucrose poly-ester (SPE), invented in the late 1960s. It is a synthetic combination of sucrose and fatty acids that looks, feels, and tastes like food fat. Unlike either sucrose or fatty acids, SPE is indigestible; the body has no way to take it apart. Sucrose polyester can therefore be substituted for fats without adding kcalories or promoting a rise in a person's blood lipid level.

Another fat substitute made from protein is marketed under the name of Simplesse.[6] The protein, either egg white or milk, is disintegrated into mistlike particles similar in consistency to fat. This fat substitute mimics the rich taste and texture of fat but cuts the kcalorie content up to 80 percent. Since proteins coagulate at high temperatures, this fat substitute cannot be used for frying or cooking. It can be used in ice creams, yogurts, salad dressings, mayonnaise, and butter.

Unlike sucrose polyesters, Simplesse does not require regulatory approval, since it is made up of proteins already in use. The FDA is appraising these substitutes to see if they present any safety issues. SPE is a synthesis of sugar and edible oils that must pass regulatory approval before it is marketed. So far, tests with animals and human beings indicate that SPE is a safe and acceptable substitute for fat and oil.

Undesirable side effects of these fat substitutes might yet be discovered. For example, fat-soluble vitamins might be carried out of the body with SPE, causing deficiencies. Further tests will give us this information, but given that high blood cholesterol and obesity are two of our major health problems, artificial fats are being viewed with hope as a possible help in the treatment of both.

Chapters 2 and 3 looked briefly at the two major energy fuels in the body—carbohydrate and fat. When used for energy, each has desirable characteristics. The glucose we derive from carbohydrate is needed by the brain and nerve tissues and is easily used for energy in other cells. Fat is a particularly useful fuel because it is stored in generous amounts and can be used by some parts of body for energy if carbohydrate is not available. Chapter 4 looks at protein, a nutrient that can be used as fuel, but whose primary role is to provide machinery for gettings things done.

SELF-STUDY:

How's Your Fat Intake?

From the forms you filled out for Self-Study 1, answer the following questions:

1. How many grams of fat do you consume in a day (from Form 1)? _____ grams

2. How many kcalories does this represent? _____ kcalories (Remember, 1 gram of fat contributes 9 kcalories.)

3. What percentage of your total kcalories is contributed by fat? _____ percent (To figure this, divide fat kcalories by total kcalories, then multiply by 100, or use the answer you obtained in Self-Study 1, Form 5.)

4. A dietary guideline says that fat should contribute not more than 30 percent of total kcalories. How does your fat intake compare with this recommendation? _____ If it is higher, look over your food records. What specific foods could you cut down on or eliminate, and what foods could you add to your diet to bring your total fat intake into line?

_____

_____

5. You may not be aware of how much fat you are eating when you eat meat. Weigh your meat portions for a day or so, then calculate how much fat you derive from meat in a day (use Appendix C). To visualize this amount of fat, weigh out an equal amount from a bottle of oil, a can of cooking fat, or a tub of butter or margarine. Try the same demonstration with a fast-food meal that includes fried foods. How much fat do you eat in a day?

Notes

1. E.M. Berry and J. Hirsch, Does dietary linolenic acid influence blood pressure? *American Journal of Clinical Nutrition* 44 (1986): 336–340.
2. J. L. Wood and R. G. Allison, Effects of consumption of choline and lecithin on neurological and cardiovascular systems, *Federation Proceedings* 41 (1982): 3015–3021.
3. G. Rivellese and coauthors, The use of diet to lower plasma cholesterol levels, *European Heart Journal* Supplement E (1987):79–85.
4. R. Goor and coauthors, Nutrient intakes among selected North American populations in the Lipid Research Clinics Prevalence Study: Composition of fat intake, *American Journal of Clinical Nutrition* 41 (1985): 299–311.
5. Simplesse fat supplement, *Nutrition and the M.D.*, March, 1988.

NUTRITION IN PRACTICE

3

Nutrition Labeling

The nutrition scene in the United States is changing. Many new kinds of foods have come into the picture since the 1940s: fast foods, convenience foods, fabricated foods, engineered foods. All of them are prepared by people other than ourselves, and we are relying on them more and more. They are easy to store and carry along and quick to prepare. It is important for people who use these foods daily to understand what sorts of nutrient contributions they make. Learning how to read nutrition labels can be a big help.

What will the label tell me?
First of all, according to law, all labels must state the following information:

- The common name of the product.
- The name and address of the manufacturer, packer, or distributor.
- The net contents in terms of weight, measure, or count.
- The ingredients listed in descending order of predominance by weight.

If you know how to read the front and side of a package, you're already a step ahead of the naive buyer. This is particularly true in regard to the ingredient list. The ingredient listed first is the one that the package contains the largest amount of. Consider the following ingredient lists:

- An orange powder that contains "sugar, citric acid, orange flavor . . ." versus a juice can that contains "water, tomato concentrate,

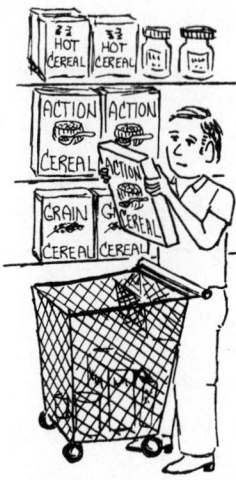

Consumers who can read labels are a step ahead.

concentrated juices of carrots, celery. . . ."

- A cereal that contains "puffed milled corn, sugar, corn syrup, molasses, salt . . ." versus one that contains "100 percent rolled oats."

Wherever additives are listed on labels, their functions must be stated. If you read the label, you know what you're getting and what the main ingredient is. Figure NP3–1 demonstrates the reading of a label, and the Miniglossary of Food Types defines terms that relate to food labels.

Sometimes labels include more than that. Why?
The nutrition labeling section of the law states that if any nutrition claim is

made on the label of a food package, the label must conform to the following format under the heading "Nutrition Information":

- Serving or portion size.
- Servings or portions per container.
- kCalorie content per serving.
- Carbohydrate grams per serving.
- Fat grams per serving.
- Protein, vitamins, and minerals as percentages of the U.S. RDA. Protein is also given in grams per serving. (No claim may be made that a food is a significant source of a nutrient unless it provides at least 10 percent of the U.S. RDA of that nutrient in a serving.)

If a nutrient is added to a food (for example, if vitamin D is added to a breakfast drink), or if an advertising claim is made (for example, that orange juice is a good source of vitamin C), the package must provide an information panel that complies *fully* with the nutrition labeling requirement. Without a complete information panel, nutrition claims could deceive the consumer about the true nutritional value of a food.

What is the U.S. RDA?
The U.S. RDA table is shown on the inside *back* cover of this book. The U.S. RDA were designed to provide one recommended amount for each nutrient. (You may recall that the RDA table lists different recommendations for each sex and age group.) The set of U.S. RDA most

often used on labels is the one designed for adults. Another set of U.S. RDA is used for infants and children under four, and still another set of U.S. RDA is used for labeling prenatal vitamin and mineral supplements.

The U.S. RDA for adults used on food package labels are usually the highest of the regular RDA. For most nutrients, the U.S. RDA are the same as the RDA for an adult man. Because a woman's need for iron is greater than a man's, though, the women's RDA is used as the recommended amount for iron. The RDA for pregnant and lactating women are not used, because they are too high for a general standard.

The U.S. RDA table includes two values for protein: 45 grams if the protein is of high quality, and 65 grams if it is of lower quality. This rule enables the consumer to "buy protein" in appropriate amounts, without having to understand the concept of protein quality.

How can I use the label to see how well the food meets my nutrient needs?
If you just want to know generally what amounts of nutrients are in the package, the percentage of the U.S. RDA will tell you that without your having to do any calculating. If you read, for example, that a serving of breakfast cereal provides "25 percent of calcium," you can be sure it provides at least a quarter of *your* calcium allowance for a day (unless you are pregnant or lactating). If you want to know exactly how many grams of calcium are in a serving, you can look at the U.S. RDA table, find out that the U.S. RDA is 1 gram of calcium, and figure that 25 percent of that is .25 gram. For the nutrients included in the RDA tables then, all the information that most consumers might want is listed there.

I have to watch my weight, so I look for foods labeled "low in calories." Are these foods really low in kcalories?
Foods labeled *low in calories* must state the absolute number of kcalories on the label and must contain no more than 40 kcalories per serving. Any food calling itself a *reduced calorie food* must be at least a third lower in kcalories than the food it most closely resembles and must carry a nutrition label. The terms *lite* or *light* on a food label have no legal meanings. These terms often imply that foods are low in kcalories, light in color, low in alcohol content, or low in sodium content. The Miniglossary of Terms on Food Labels defines the meaning of other terms on food labels.

From what you've said, I think I can deal with nutrition labels on foods like breakfast cereals. But what about foods that simply say "TV dinner" or "macaroni and cheese"?
The Food and Drug Administration (FDA) has devised nutritional quality guidelines for the nutrient contents of many kinds of convenience foods:

Miniglossary of Food Types

convenience food   a food prepared or packaged in such a way that it is easy to cook and serve at home.

empty-calorie food   a popular term used to denote foods that contain no nutrients, only kcalories. Actually, since almost all foods contain some nutrients, most nutritionists prefer to say "food of low nutrient density."

engineered food   a food subjected to a complex technical process, such as extraction of certain components.

fabricated food   a food put together from highly processed ingredients, such as meat-substitute burgers made from textured vegetable protein.

fast food   food prepared quickly in a fast-food restaurant, such as a hamburger stand or fried-chicken place.

imitation food   a food nutritionally inferior to the food it imitates. By law, this term must appear on the label of a food if it contains less than 10 percent of the U.S. RDA of an essential nutrient found in the food it imitates.

junk food   a popular term used to denote foods that are "bad" for you, for example, foods high in salt, sugar, or fat.

natural food   an unprocessed food; a term often mistakenly used synonymously with "good for you."

nutritious food   a food with high nutrient density.

processed food   any food subjected to a process, such as enrichment, refinement, fortification, alteration of texture, mixing, or cooking.

FIGURE NP3–1
How to read a food label.

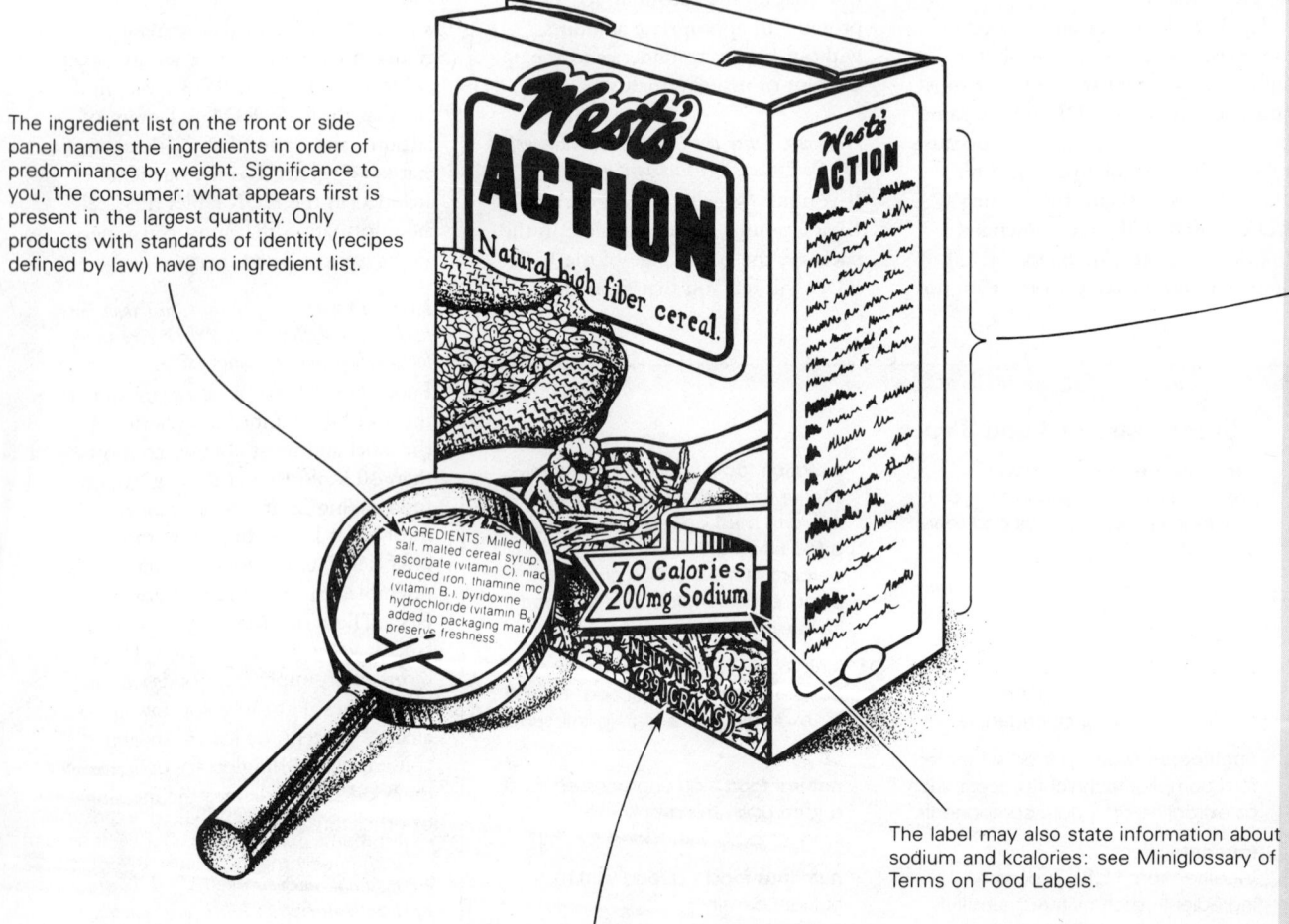

The ingredient list on the front or side panel names the ingredients in order of predominance by weight. Significance to you, the consumer: what appears first is present in the largest quantity. Only products with standards of identity (recipes defined by law) have no ingredient list.

The label may also state information about sodium and kcalories: see Miniglossary of Terms on Food Labels.

The front of the package must always tell you the product name, the name and address of the company, and the weight or measure; and it may list the ingredients.

The nutrition information panel tells you the nutrients in a serving.

The serving size may or may not be the same as the amount you eat. Check the servings per container to get an idea if it is.

FIGURE NP3–1 **(continued)**

Nutrition Information (per serving)
Serving Size = 1 C
Servings Per Container = 24

The nutrient contents are listed in the food as served (after cooking, in this example).

	Cereal	Cereal + Butter, Milk, Water, Salt
Calories	140	280
Protein (g)	4	6
Total carbohydrates (g)	30	32
Simple sugars (g)	25	27
Complex carbohydrates	5	5
Fat (g)	0	14
Sodium	460 mg	975 mg

The kcalorie-bearing ingredients are given in grams (units of weight). This is especially meaningful with respect to protein, because you need 40 to 80 g a day, depending on your size and other factors. Protein is also given in percentage of U.S. RDA in the list below.

The carbohydrate breakdown tells you how much simple sugar and how much starch is in the product. A fat breakdown may also be listed, including saturated fat, polyunsaturated fat, and cholesterol.

Sodium is listed in milligrams. About 1,000 to 3,000 mg/day is considered a safe intake, but the average U.S. citizen consumes 5,000 to 7,000 mg/day. A teaspoon of salt contains nearly 2,000 mg sodium.

Percentage of U.S. Recommended Daily Allowances (U.S. RDA)

Protein	4	8
Vitamin A	2	10
Vitamin C	80	80
Thiamin	10	15
Riboflavin	2	8
Niacin	10	10
Calcium	2	4
Iron	4	4

Protein, vitamins, and minerals are given in percentages of U.S. RDA (see inside back cover). Significance to you, the consumer: if it meets 10% of the U.S. RDA, it almost undoubtedly meets at least 10% of your daily needs.

*Prepared according to recipe on back of package.

Miniglossary of Terms on Food Labels

Sodium terms

sodium free   less than 5 mg per serving.

very low sodium   35 mg or less per serving.

low sodium   140 mg or less per serving.

reduced sodium   processed to reduce the usual level of sodium by 75%.

unsalted   processed without the normally used salt.

low salt   made with less salt than the regular variety of the same food.

Energy terms

diet, dietetic   terms used to indicate that a food is either *low in kcalories* or a *reduced kcalorie* food.

low in calories   no more than 40 kcal per serving or 0.9 kcal/g.

reduced calorie   containing at least a third fewer kcalories than the food is most closely resembles.

Fat terms

low fat   made with less fat than the regular variety of the same food.

lean   90% fat-free.[a]

extra lean   95% fat-free.

[a]The word *lean* as part of the brand name (as in "Lean Supreme") indicates that the product is 25 percent lower in fat than the regular variety.

frozen dinners, breakfast cereals, meal replacements, certain beverages, and prepared main dishes such as pizza. If a product complies with the guidelines, it may carry on its label a statement that says so without spelling out the details.

For some items, the law provides standards of identity and excuses manufacturers from the requirement of listing ingredients. Standards of identity exist for such foods as bread and mayonnaise—common foods that at one time were often prepared at home, so the basic recipe was understood by almost everyone. Certain ingredients must be present in a specific percentage before the food may use the standard name.

Another class of foods that concerns consumers is made up of inferior foods developed in imitation of and as substitutes for familiar foods. Regulations require that the word *imitation* must be used on the label if the product is a substitute for and resembles another food but is nutritionally inferior to the food imitated. Nutritional inferiority is defined as a reduction in the content of an essential vitamin or mineral or of protein that amounts to 10 percent or more of the U.S. RDA. Thus if you read *imitation* on a label, you may conclude that the food is a poor imitation nutritionally.

Many of the convenience foods I use are either enriched or fortified. Does this mean that they are more nutritious than ordinary foods?

Not necessarily. A fortified breakfast cereal may have such large quantities of nutrients added that one serving provides 100 percent of the U.S. RDA for all of them. Yet, the shrewd consumer will realize that the word *fortified* sometimes conveys an emptiness of other nutrients. The nutrients named on the label are added, yes, but others may be missing altogether (see Chapter 7). Fruit *juice* is more nutritious than fortified fruit *drink,* even though the drink may be higher in vitamin C content. The fruit juice is likely to contain important trace minerals, fiber and vitamins, other than vitamin C, that are not found in the fortified fruit drink.

To distinguish between nourishing foods (those that provide some nutrients besides kcalories) and *nutritious foods,* you have to apply the concept of nutrient density. Consider these two questions:

1. How much of the nutrients does a serving of this food supply in relation to my need?

2. How many kcalories does a serving supply in relation to my need?

If the food is of high nutrient density—for example, if it supplies half your daily allowance for a vitamin and at the same time only one tenth of your daily allowance for kcalories—it is a good source of that vitamin. You could obtain a substantial quantity of the vitamin from it at a low kcalorie cost, and it is a nutritious food.

Is there anything else I should know about labels?

Yes, you need to know how to see through misleading claims. As they presently appear, food labels provide useful information, but the law still allows some loopholes. You might be interested in trying your skill at detecting misleading claims by taking the nutrition label quiz.

When a package with an artificially constituted food or dietary supplement claims that the food contains all the vitamins and minerals

---

Nutrition Label Quiz

All three of the label claims below are true. Which two claims are misleading?

1. A label says one serving of a food provides 35 times as much iron as an 8-ounce glass of whole milk.
2. A label says a fortified product contains "more vitamin C than fresh orange juice."
3. A label says a brand of instant nonfat dry milk has "all the calcium, protein, and B vitamins of whole milk."

The answers are:

1. True but misleading because milk is a poor source of iron.
2. True but misleading because orange juice contains so many *other* nutrients not provided by the fortified drink.
3. True and responsible.

Source: L. Schwartzberg, C. George, and M. C. Phillips, Issues in food advertising: The nutrition educator's viewpoint, *Journal of Nutritional Education* 9 (1977): 60–63.

---

known to be essential in human nutrition, it is also misleading because the claim implies a completeness that may be overestimated. We really do not know everything that should be included in such foods.

Finally, consumers may be misled by a label that claims that a breakfast bar or drink has the same amounts of protein, fat, carbohydrate, vitamins, and minerals as those found in a breakfast of milk, egg, toast, and orange juice. The label fails to mention that the carbohydrate is sugar (versus the complex carbohydrate in toast), that the fat is saturated fat (versus the polyunsaturated oil in which the egg might have been fried), or that the salt content is considerable. Furthermore, there are other nutrients in milk, egg, toast, and orange juice that the breakfast bar does not contain. Consumers are putting pressure on legislators to provide labeling laws that will make such misleading claims illegal.

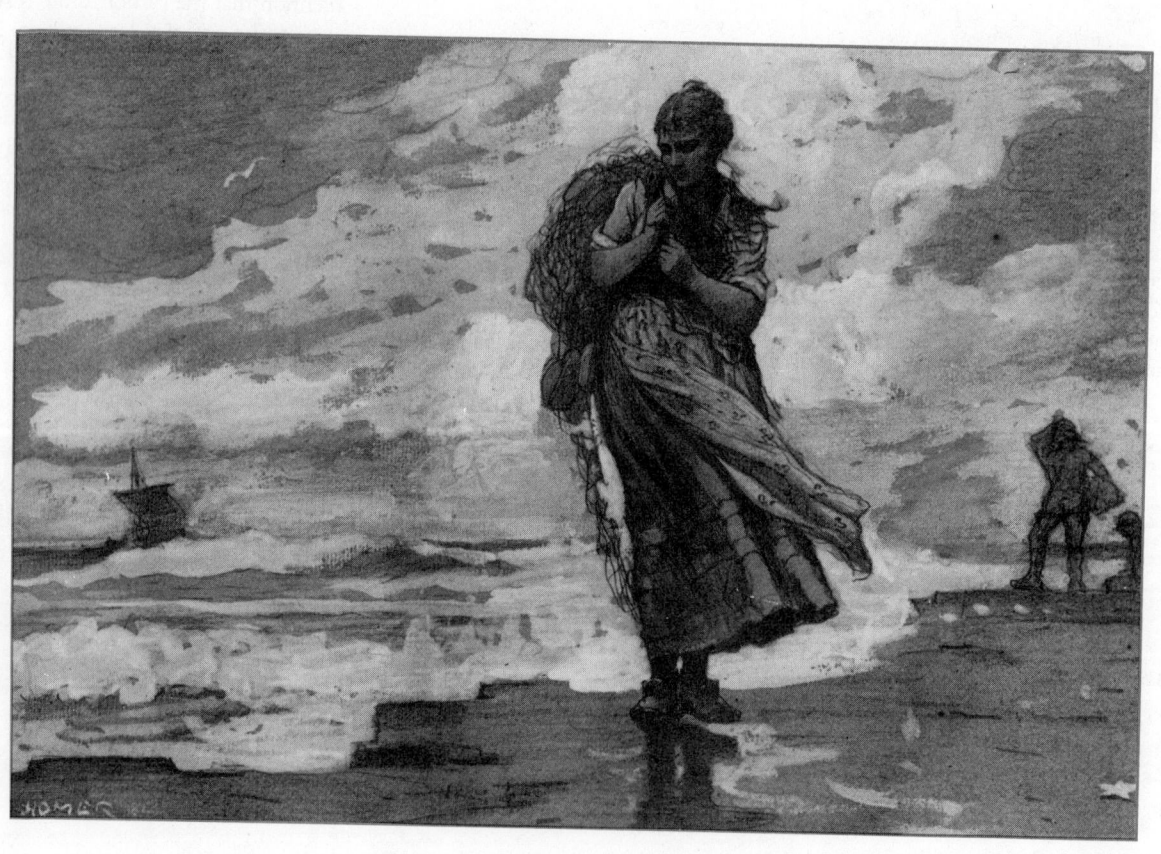

Proteins and Amino Acids

"Fisher Girl with Net," by Winslow Homer, 11⅜" × 16⅛." From the collection of European and American drawings, 16th–19th centuries. Courtesy the Sterling and Francine Clark Art Institute, Williamstown, Massachusetts.

Although protein can serve as an energy-yielding nutrient, the roles it plays in the body are far more varied than those of carbohydrate or lipid. In fact, its other functions are so important that using protein for energy is undesirable, as mentioned earlier (see p. 28).

The Chemist's View of Protein

A protein is a compound that contains the same atoms as carbohydrate and lipid—carbon, hydrogen, and oxygen—but also contains nitrogen atoms. These atoms are arranged into amino acids, which are linked into chains to form proteins.

All amino acids share a common chemical "backbone" through which they can be linked together. Twenty-two different amino acids may appear in proteins.* With their attached structures, amino acids make proteins varied in comparison with either carbohydrates or lipids (see Figure 4–1).

The 22 common amino acids can be linked together in a great variety of ways to form proteins. Most proteins are polypeptides, 100 to 300 amino acids long. Because of the different properties of the amino acids in them, polypeptide chains fold and intertwine into intricate coils (see Figure 4–2). The sequence of amino acids in a protein determines which specific way the chain will fold.

The variety of sequences in which the 22 amino acids can be linked together is even greater than that possible for letters in a sentence, because proteins do not have to be pronounced as do words. This gives amino acids a tremendous range of possible surface structures, which in turn enables them to perform distinct, individual, and specialized functions. The human body contains an estimated 10,000 to 50,000 different kinds of proteins. Of these thousands, only about 1,000 have been identified.

*It is often said that there are 20 amino acids, but if cystine and ornithine are counted, there are 22. Related forms of amino acids occur in nature, and chemists can make others.

protein:
a compound composed of amino acids linked in a chain.

amino (a-MEEN-oh) **acid:**
a building block of protein; a compound containing an amino group and an acid group attached to a central carbon, which also carries a distinctive side chain.
amino = containing nitrogen

dipeptide:
two amino acids bonded together.
di = two
peptide = amino acid

tripeptide:
three amino acids bonded together.
tri = three

polypeptide:
many amino acids bonded together. *Many* refers to ten or more. An intermediate string of between four and ten amino acids is an *oligopeptide.*
poly = many
oligo = few

FIGURE 4–1

Examples of amino acids.

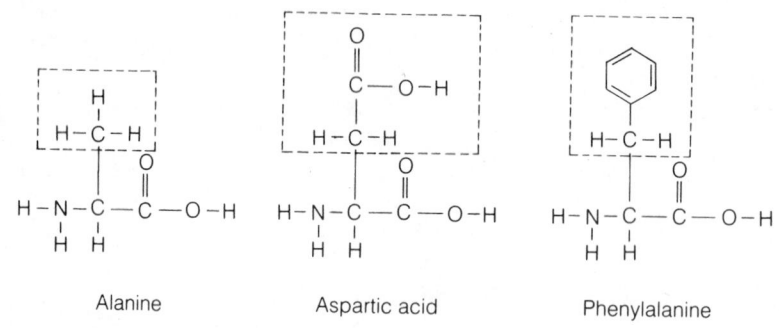

Alanine   Aspartic acid   Phenylalanine

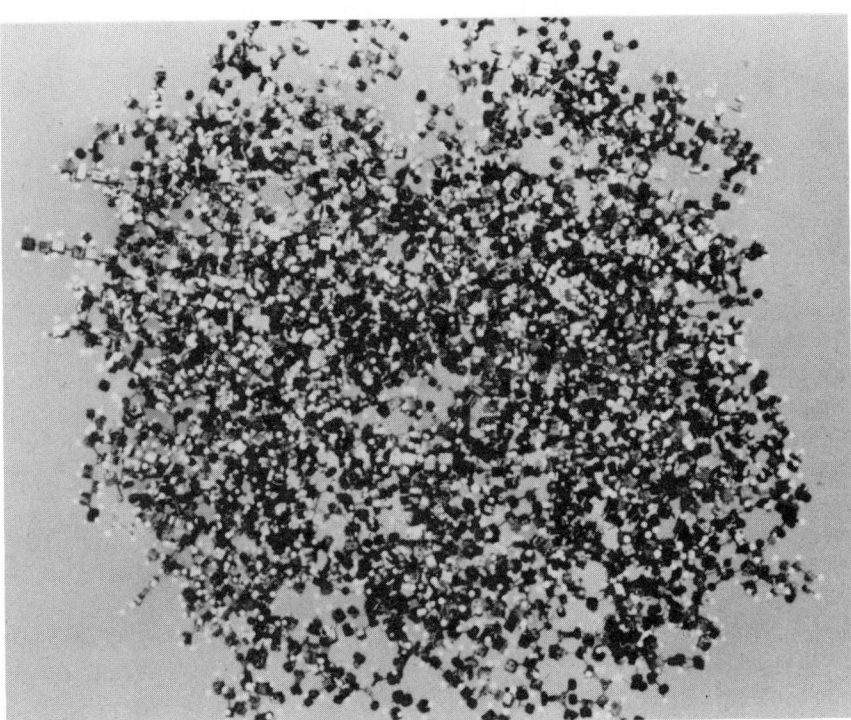

FIGURE 4–2
**The intricate structure of a protein
molecule.** This molecule represents one
molecule of hemoglobin, magnified 27
million times.

Source: Human hemoglobin model constructed
by Dr. Makio Murayama, National Institutes of
Health (NIH), Bethesda, Maryland (scaled to ½
inch to an angstrom). Atomic coordinates were
supplied for the model by Dr. Max F. Perutz,
Cambridge, England.

The Functions of Proteins

What distinguishes you chemically from any other human being is minute
differences in your body proteins (enzymes, antibodies, and others). These
differences are determined by the amino acid sequences of your proteins, and
these sequences are written into the genes you inherited from your parents
and ancestors. The genes direct the making of all the body's proteins. Let's
now focus on one type of these proteins, the enzymes.

Enzymes

All enzymes are proteins. They are catalysts that facilitate the rate at which
compounds in the body are put together or taken apart. Enzymes are essential
to all life processes.

The protein story moves in a circle. To follow the circle in nutrition, start
with a person eating protein. The proteins are broken down by proteins (enzymes) into amino acids. The amino acids enter the cells of the body, where
proteins (enzymes) put the amino acids together in long chains with sequences
specified by the genes. Some of the chains fold and become enzymes themselves.
These enzymes may then be used to break apart other compounds or to put
other compounds together. Day by day in billions of reactions, these processes

catalyst (CAT-uh-list):
a compound that facilitates chemical
reactions without itself being destroyed in the
process.

enzyme:
a protein catalyst.

repeat themselves, and life goes on. Only living systems work with such self-renewal. A broken toaster cannot be fixed by another toaster; a car cannot make another car. Only living creatures and the parts they are composed of—the cells—can duplicate themselves.

Fluid and Acid-Base Balance

Proteins help maintain the body's fluid balance. Fluid is present in several body compartments, chief among them the spaces inside the blood vessels, within the cells, and between the cells outside the blood vessels. Fluids flow back and forth between these compartments, and proteins in the fluids, together with minerals, help to maintain the needed distribution of these fluids.

The reason that proteins in fluids can help determine their distribution in living systems is that they are large and attractive to water (hydrophilic). Being large, proteins cannot pass freely across the membranes that separate body compartments. Being hydrophilic, they attract the water molecules near them, which in effect makes them even larger. A cell that "wants" to keep a certain amount of water in its interior space can't move the water around directly, but it can manufacture proteins and these proteins will hold water. Thus the cell uses protein to regulate the distribution of water indirectly. Similarly, the body makes proteins to keep in the bloodstream and in the intercellular spaces. These proteins help maintain the fluid volume in those spaces.

Proteins also help maintain the balance between acids and bases in body fluids. If the body's fluids become too acidic, the structure of vital proteins can be disrupted. When this happens, the proteins are pulled out of shape and can no longer function, resulting in acidosis or alkalosis. Either of these imbalances can be fatal.

Proteins, such as albumin, in plasma help to prevent these imbalances from arising. In a sense, the proteins protect one another by gathering up extra acid (hydrogen) ions when there are too many in the surrounding medium and by releasing them when there are too few. This ability to regulate the acid-base balance of the medium is known as the buffering action of proteins.

Antibodies and Hormones

Other major proteins found in the blood—the antibodies—act against viruses, bacteria, and other foreign agents. The antibodies work so efficiently that if a million bacterial cells are injected into the skin of a healthy person, fewer than ten are likely to survive for five hours. Without sufficient protein, the body cannot maintain its resistance to disease.

The blood also carries hormones, of which some are made of amino acids. (Recall that other hormones are sterols.) Among the hormones composed of amino acids are the thyroid hormone and insulin. Hormones have many profound effects, which will become evident in subsequent chapters.

Transport Proteins

A specific group of the body's proteins specializes in moving nutrients and other molecules in and out of cells. They act as "pumps," picking up compounds

Minerals are helper nutrients. The attractiveness of protein and mineral particles to water creates a force known as osmotic pressure (see Chapter 8).

The space in the blood vessels is the **intravascular space;** the space between the cells is the **intercellular** or **interstitial** (inter-STISH-ul) **space;** the space inside the cells is the **intracellular space.**
intra = inside
inter = between
interstice = space between

acid-base balance:
the balance maintained in the body between too much and too little acid. Blood pH, for example, is regulated normally between 7.38 and 7.42.

pH:
the concentration of hydrogen ions. The lower the pH, the stronger the acid. Thus pH 2 is a strong acid; pH 6 is a weak acid; pH 7 is neutral; a pH above 7 is alkaline.

The change in a protein's shape brought about by heat, acid, or other conditions is known as **denaturation** (dee-nay-cher-AY-shun). Past a certain point, denaturation is irreversible.

acidosis:
too much acid in the blood and body fluids.

alkalosis:
too much base in the blood and body fluids.

buffer:
a compound that can reversibly combine with hydrogen ions to help maintain a constant pH.

on one side of the membrane and depositing them on the other, thereby "deciding" what substances cells will take up and what they will release. The protein machinery of cell membranes can be switched on or off in response to the body's needs. Often hormones do the switching with marvelous precision.

Other transport proteins move about in the body fluids, carrying nutrients and other molecules from one organ to another. Those that carry lipids in the lipoproteins are an example. Special proteins also can carry fat-soluble vitamins, water-soluble vitamins, and minerals.

All the body's tissues and organs—muscles, bones, blood, skin, nerves—are made of protein. One important protein, collagen, helps make scar tissue, forms the protein matrix of bones and teeth, forms the material of ligaments and tendons, and is a strengthening constituent of artery walls.

The list of protein functions mentioned here is by no means exhaustive, but it does give you some sense of the immense variety and importance of proteins in the body. With this information as background, you are in a position to appreciate the need for protein in the diet.

Protein in Foods

The role of protein in food is not to provide body proteins directly but to supply the amino acids from which the body can make its own proteins. The body can make some amino acids itself, but there are others that the body cannot make at all. The body also cannot make some amino acids fast enough to meet its needs. Those the body cannot make or make fast enough are the essential amino acids. Nine amino acids are essential for adults. The amino acid arginine is not essential, although health food stores sell it in bottles with various claims.

To make body protein, a cell must have all the needed amino acids available simultaneously. Therefore, the first important characteristic of dietary protein is that it should supply at least the nine essential amino acids and enough nitrogen and energy for the synthesis of the other thirteen.

A complete protein is a protein that contains all the essential amino acids in amounts adequate for human use; it may or may not contain all the others. A high-quality protein is not merely complete but contains the essential amino acids in amounts proportional to the body's need for them. Such protein is easily digestible, so that these amino acids reach the body's cells in the needed amounts.

Ideally, dietary protein supplies each amino acid in the amount needed for protein synthesis in the body. If one amino acid is supplied in an amount smaller than is needed, the total amount of protein that can be synthesized from the others will be limited. By analogy, suppose that a sign maker plans to make 100 identical signs, each saying Left Turn Only. She needs 200 Ls, 200 Ns, 200 Ts, and 100 of each of the other letters. If she has only 20 Ls, she can make only 10 signs even if all the other letters are available in unlimited quantities. Furthermore, the sign maker has no place to keep leftover letters (just as the body has no storage place for extra amino acids). If she doesn't get some more Ls right away, she will have to throw away all the other letters.

antibody:
a large protein of the blood and body fluids, produced in response to invasion of the body by unfamiliar molecules (mostly proteins); it inactivates the invaders and so protects the body. The invaders are called *antigens*.
anti = against

hormone:
a chemical messenger. Hormones are secreted by a variety of glands in the body in response to altered conditions. Each affects one or more target tissues or organs and elicits specific responses to restore normal conditions.

essential amino acid:
an amino acid that the body cannot synthesize in amounts sufficient to meet physiological need. Nine amino acids are known to be essential for human adults:
methionine (meh-THIGH-oh-neen)
threonine (THREE-oh-neen)
tryptophan (TRIP-toe-fane)
leucine (LOO-seen)
isoleucine (eye-so-LOO-seen)
lysine (LYE-seen)
valine (VAY-leen)
phenylalanine (fee-nul-AL-uh-neen)
histidine (HISS-tuh-deen)

complete protein:
a protein containing all the amino acids essential in human nutrition in amounts adequate for human use.

high-quality protein:
an easily digestible, complete protein whose amino acids fit the pattern needed by human beings.

limiting amino acid:
the amino acid found in the shortest supply relative to the amounts needed for protein synthesis in the body.

A convenient way to distinguish among proteins is to think of animal proteins as being of higher quality generally than plant proteins. The educated vegetarian, with careful planning, can design a perfectly acceptable diet around plant foods alone by choosing a variety of plant foods. (Vegetarian diets are discussed further in Nutrition in Practice 4.)

Foods that supply protein in abundance are milk and milk products, eggs, meats, fish, poultry, and legumes. Other vegetables and grain products contribute small but significant amounts of protein to the diet.

Dietary protein—no matter how high the quality—will not be used efficiently by the body and will not support growth when energy from carbohydrate and fat is lacking. The body assigns top priority to meeting its energy need and, if necessary, will break down protein to meet this need. After stripping off and excreting the nitrogen from the amino acids, the body will use their carbon skeletons in much the same way it uses those from glucose or from fat. The major reason why we must have ample carbohydrate and fat in the diet is to prevent this wasting of protein.

Carbohydrate and fat allow amino acids to be used to build body proteins. This is known as the **protein-sparing action** of carbohydrate and fat.

Recommended Protein Intakes

Cells are lost daily. To replace cells' protein, we must ingest amino acids from food. If the body is growing, it needs more protein than is necessary just for maintenance. Children end each day with more blood cells, more muscle cells, and more skin cells than they had at the beginning of the day. Body builders, during the time when their muscles are growing, need more protein too, but only a very little more than when they are maintaining a constant muscle mass.

Normally, healthy adults are in nitrogen balance; that is, they have the same amount of protein in their bodies at all times. They use what nitrogen they need and excrete the excess. Growing children and pregnant women are in positive nitrogen balance, because they are adding protein to their bodies as new blood, bone, and muscle cells. People in negative nitrogen balance are losing body protein. People who are fasting or starving, such as anorexics or people with burns (see Chapter 17) are in negative nitrogen balance, because they must use protein for energy.

nitrogen balance:
the amount of nitrogen consumed (N in) as compared with the amount of nitrogen excreted (N out) in a given period of time. The laboratory scientist can estimate the protein in a sample of food, body tissue, or excreta by measuring the nitrogen in it. Chapter 13 provides additional information about N balance.

The Committee on RDA states that a generous daily protein allowance for a healthy adult would be 0.8 gram of high-quality protein per kilogram of appropriate or average body weight for height. Protein RDA for people of average height at all ages are presented in the RDA Table (inside front cover). If your height is not average, you can compute your own individualized RDA for protein (see Self-Study).

In setting the RDA, the committee assumes that the protein eaten will be of high quality, that it will be consumed with adequate kcalories from carbohydrate and fat, and that other nutrients in the diet will be adequate. The committee also assumes that the RDA will be used to apply only to healthy individuals with no unusual metabolic need for protein.

It is possible to consume too much protein. Animals fed high-protein diets experience a protein overload effect, seen in the hypertrophy of their livers and kidneys. Infants are placed at risk in many ways if fed excess protein.[1]

People who wish to lose weight may be handicapped in their efforts if they consume too much protein.[2] The higher a person's intake of such protein-rich foods as meat and milk, the more likely it is that fruits, vegetables, and grains will be crowded out of the diet, making it inadequate in other nutrients. Diets high in protein necessitate higher intakes of calcium as well, because such diets promote calcium excretion.[3] Protein from animal, as opposed to vegetable, food sources may raise serum cholesterol and thus the risk of heart disease; at least as much vegetable as animal protein should be eaten (a 1 to 1 ratio).[4] There are evidently no benefits to be gained by consuming a diet that derives more than 15 percent of its kcalories from protein, and there are possible risks as intakes rise to 20 or more percent of kcalories when kcalories are adequate.[5]

Protein-kCalorie Malnutrition

When people are deprived of food and suffer a kcalorie deficit, they degrade their own body protein for energy and indirectly suffer a protein deficiency as well as an energy deficiency. Because protein and kcalorie deprivation thus go hand in hand, public health officials have adopted an abbreviation for the overlapping pair: protein-kcalorie malnutrition (PCM). Cases of PCM are observed at both ends of the spectrum. The classic protein deficiency disease is kwashiorkor, and the kcalorie deficiency disease is marasmus. The consequences of PCM as a world health problem are considered here. PCM can also occur during illness, affecting adults as well as children. The problems associated with PCM in illness are described in Chapter 14.

Hunger wastes the most precious of all the world's resources—the human being. Despite numerous development programs, malnutrition is not disappearing; the tragic number of malnourished people continues to grow. The United Nations Food and Agriculture Organization (FAO) estimates that there are at least a half-billion undernourished people in the world today. These people lack the nutrients to support healthy, active lives. The marks of undernutrition include blindness, swollen bellies, skin irritations, general listlessness, and stunted physical growth.

Of all population groups, children are most seriously affected by malnutrition. Children who are thin for their height may be suffering from acute PCM or recent severe food restriction, whereas children who are short for their age may have experienced long-term chronic PCM. Stunted growth due to PCM rather than symptoms of vitamin and mineral deficiency diseases may be the most common sign of malnutrition in the developing countries.

Pregnant or lactating women, together with their small children, have a greater need for nutrients for their size than other groups because of the higher demand for nutrients during periods of rapid growth. When family food is limited, these women and their children are the first to show the signs of undernutrition. In developing countries, these women and their children are the least able to demand their share and are least recognized by other family members as deserving a fair share.

While cultural and social beliefs limit food intake, in some instances, so does inappropriate modernization such as replacing breast milk with formula feeding

protein-kcalorie malnutrition: a deficiency of protein or kcalories or both, often referred to as *PCM* and also as *PEM,* for *protein-energy malnutrition.*
mal = bad, poor

kwashiorkor (kwash-ee-OR-core, or kwash-ee-or-CORE): malnutrition caused by protein deficiency in the presence of adequate kcalories.

marasmus: (ma-RAZZ-mus): malnutrition caused by simple starvation.

in environments where it is impossible to formula feed safely. Breast milk, the recommended food for infants, is sterile and contains antibodies that enhance an infant's resistance to disease. On the other hand, mixing contaminated water with milk powder and feeding it to infants often causes infections leading to diarrhea, dehydration, and decreased absorption of nutrients from the foods the children are given.

Kwashiorkor

The word kwashiorkor originally meant "the evil spirit that infects the first child when the second child is born." You can easily see how this superstitious belief arose among the Ghanians who named the disease by considering how kwashiorkor often develops. When a mother who has been nursing her first child bears a second child, she weans the first and puts the second on the breast. If fed an inadequate diet, the first child soon begins to sicken and die. Breast milk provides a child with sufficient protein, but the child is generally weaned to a starchy, protein-poor gruel. The gruel does not supply enough amino acids even to maintain a child's body, much less enough to enable the child to grow.

Kwashiorkor occurs not only in Africa but also in Central America, South America, the Near East, the Far East, and in wealthy and poor countries on every continent. It is probably a mixture of deficiency symptoms from lack of both protein and zinc and possibly other nutrients as well. Wherever mother's milk is the only reliable and readily available source of protein and zinc for infants, kwashiorkor threatens them at weaning time. It typically sets in at about the age of two. The child's growth slows down, so that by the time she is four, she is no taller than she was at two. Her hair loses its color, her skin is patchy and scaly, sometimes with ulcers and sores that fail to heal. The child's limbs and face become swollen with edema; her belly bulges with a fatty liver; she sickens easily and is weak, fretful, and apathetic.

The body follows a priority system when there is not enough protein to meet all its needs. It abandons its less vital systems first. When it cannot obtain enough amino acids from dietary sources, the body switches to a "metabolism of wasting"; it begins to digest its own protein tissues. In this way, it can supply the amino acids needed to continuously maintain the vital, internal organs and thus keep itself alive. Hair and skin pigments (which are made of amino acids) are the first to go. They begin to lose their color, and skin sores fail to heal. Many antibodies are also degraded so that their amino acids can be used as building blocks for heart, lung, and brain tissue. A child with a depleted supply of antibodies cannot resist infection and readily contracts dysentery, a disease of the digestive tract. Dysentery causes diarrhea, leading to rapid loss of many nutrients, including amino acids, that the child may be receiving in food. Thus, dysentery worsens the protein deficiency, and the protein deficiency in turn increases the likelihood of a second or third or tenth attack of dysentery.

Marasmus

Whereas kwashiorkor seems to occur in individuals who receive food but too little protein, marasmus occurs in those who receive little or no food at

edema (e-DEE-muh): an accumulation of fluid. In PCM, protein in the blood is depleted and water cannot be held there. Instead, water seeps into the interstitial space and accumulates. Hormonal imbalances in protein deficiency also contribute to edema.

fatty liver: an accumulation of fat in the liver. In PCM, fat accumulates in the liver because there is no protein available to form the lipoproteins that normally escort fat molecules in the blood.

dysentery (DIS-en-terry): an infection of the gastrointestinal tract caused by an amoeba or bacterium that gives rise to severe diarrhea.

dys = bad
entery = intestine

all; it is simple starvation. A marasmic child looks like a wizened little old person—just skin and bones. He is often sick because his resistance to disease is low. All his muscles are wasted, including the heart muscle, and the heart is weak. Reduced synthesis of key hormones leads to a metabolism so slow that the child's body temperature is subnormal. Unlike the kwashiorkor child, he has no fat accumulation in the liver, and little or no fat under the skin to insulate against cold. Hospital workers see that the primary need of marasmic victims is to be wrapped up and kept warm.

Unlike the kwashiorkor child who has been fed milk until weaning, the marasmic child typically has been neglected from early infancy. The disease occurs most commonly in children from 6 to 18 months of age in all the overpopulated city slums of the world and in rural children who have been fed inadequate formulas for too long. Because the brain normally grows to almost its full adult size within the first two years of life, marasmus impairs brain development and so may have a permanent effect on learning ability.

Protein-kcalorie malnutrition affects not only infants but also pregnant and lactating women, infants, just-weaned children, and children in periods of rapid growth. These groups have a great need for protein, and they need ample kcalories to protect it. In many cultures, however, these groups are the very ones who are denied nourishing food.

Experts assure us that we possess the knowledge, technology, and resources to end hunger. Some success has rewarded local efforts where programs involved the local people in the process of identifying the problem and devising its solution. To fight the war on hunger, it is going to take the will to do so by those who have the food, technology, and resources.

> When two variables interact so that each increases the other, **synergism** (SIN-er-jiz-um) is said to be acting. Malnutrition and infection are a deadly combination because they work in this way.
> *syn* = with, together
> *ergism* = work

SELF-STUDY

How's Your Protein Intake?

These exercises make use of the information you recorded on Forms 1 to 5.

1. How many grams of protein do you consume in a day? _____ grams

2. How many kcalories does this represent? _____ kcalories

3. What percentage of your total kcalories is contributed by protein?
   _____ percent

   A dietary guideline suggests that protein should contribute about 10 to 15 percent of total kcalories. How does your protein intake compare with this recommendation? (Note: if you are on a kcalorie-restricted diet, a higher percentage of your kcalories should come from protein. See Self-Study 8.) If your protein intake is out of line, what foods could you consume more or less of to bring it into line?_____

   _____

   _____

   _____

5. Compare your recommended protein intake (from 1) with the recommendation for an "average" person of your age and sex as shown in the RDA

Tables (inside front cover) or in the Canadian recommendations (Appendix A)? _____ If you are not of average height or weight, figure your protein RDA:

a. Look up the weight for a person your height (inside back cover). Assume this weight is "ideal" for you.

b. Change pounds to kilograms (kg); 2.2 pounds equal 1 kilogram.

c. Multiply kilograms by 0.8 g/kg.

   Example (for a 5'8" medium-frame male):

a. "Ideal" weight: about 150 lb.

b. 150 lb × 1 kg/2.2 lb = 68 kg (rounded off).

c. 68 kg × 0.8 g/kg = 54 g protein (rounded off).

6. Compare your average daily protein intake with the recommendation. About what percentage of that intake are you consuming each day? _____ percent. If you are "average" and healthy, the recommendation is probably generous for you, yet you are probably eating more protein than that. This means that you may be spending protein prices for an energy nutrient. What substitutions could you make in your day's food choices for you to derive the kcalories you need for energy from carbohydrate rather than from protein? _____

_____

7. How many of your protein grams are from animal foods? _____ How many from plant foods? _____ Assuming that the animal protein is of high quality, no more than 20 percent of your total protein has to come from this source. Should you alter the ratio of plant to animal protein in your diet? _____ If you were to do so, what effect would this have on the total *fat* content of your diet? _____

_____

Notes

1. Infections and undernutrition, *Nutrition Reviews* 40 (1982): 119–128.
2. Dietary protein and body fat distribution, *Nutrition Reviews* 40 (1982): 89–90.
3. A. A. Licata, Acute effects of increased meat protein on urinary electrolytes and cyclic adenosine monophosphate and serum parathyroid hormone, *American Journal of Clinical Nutrition* 34 (1981): 1779–1784.
4. K. K. Carroll, Dietary protein and heart disease, *Nutrition and the MD*, June 1985.
5. High protein diets and bone homeostatis, *Nutrition Reviews* 34 (1981): 11–13.

4

The Vegetarian Diet

More and more people are following vegetarian diets. Their reasons for becoming vegetarian vary widely. Some have religious reasons, others ethical. Some believe that vegetarianism is ecologically sound, and others believe that it is less costly than the meat-eating alternative. Whatever the reasons, vegetarians and health professionals who work with them should be aware of the nutrition and health implications of the vegetarian diet. The Miniglossary defines vegetarian diets.

I've been thinking about becoming a vegetarian myself, but I'm still not sure whether vegetarianism is nutritionally sound. Is it?

The answer is *yes* if the vegetarian carefully plans his diet. Specifically, the tasks for a vegetarian diet planner are

* To obtain neither too few nor too many kcalories, that is, to maintain a desirable weight.
* To obtain adequate quantities of complete protein.
* To obtain the needed vitamins and minerals.

Balancing the diet: that sounds familiar. How can vegetarians adjust their diets so that they can obtain needed nutrients?

The idea of balancing the diet to obtain need nutrients is as important for vegetarians as it is for everyone. Vegetarians can use the special food group plan (Table 1–3 in Chapter 1) to help them plan a balanced diet.

Isn't it important, too, to obtain adequate amounts of complete protein?

Yes it is, but the task may be difficult only for the person who is eating only plant foods. You may recall from Chapter 4 that all the essential amino acids must be eaten within the same time period to meet the body's protein needs. The proteins of meat, fish, poultry, cheese, eggs, and milk contain ample amounts of the essential amino acids. The lacto-ovo vegetarian who consumes two cups of milk or the equivalent in milk products and two cups of legumes each day is guaranteed an adequate intake of complete protein. The vegan, who does not use milk, milk products, or eggs, must combine plant proteins to achieve a balance of all the needed amino acids.

Combining two protein foods, each of which supplies amino acids missing from the other is called *mutual supplementation*. The two protein foods that mutually supplement each other are called *complementary proteins*. The accompanying box gives examples of how mixtures of foods can be combined to form complete proteins. The vegetarian should adopt a strategy of eating a wide variety of protein sources in generous servings. In so doing, he can be virtually assured of an adequate protein intake.

Miniglossary of Vegetarian Diet Terms

complementary proteins two or more proteins whose amino acid assortments complement each other in such a way that the essential amino acids missing from each are supplied by the other.

lacto-ovo vegetarians vegetarians who omit meat, fish, and poultry from their diets but use eggs, cheese, milk, and milk products.

meat replacements textured vegetable protein products formulated to look and taste like meat, fish, or poultry. Many of them are designed to match the known nutrient contents of animal-protein foods, but sometimes they fall short.

mutual supplementation the strategy of combining two protein foods in a meal so that each food provides the essential amino acid(s) lacking in the other.

nutritional yeast a food supplement containing B vitamins, iron, and protein that can be used to improve the quality of a vegetarian diet; also called brewer's yeast.

vegans vegetarian who omits all animal products (including eggs, cheese, and milk) from the diet; also called strict vegetarian.

Mixtures That Provide Complete Protein

Legumes, including peanuts and soy products   +   Grains (corn, oats, rice, and wheat)
Legumes, including peanuts and soy products   +   Seeds (sesame or sunflower seeds)
Leafy vegetables   +   Grains (corn, oats, rice, and wheat)

If I go on a vegetarian diet, will I need to take vitamin supplements?

That depends on the kind of vegetarian diet you follow. The lacto-ovo vegetarian diet can be complete in all vitamins, but several vitamins may be a problem for the vegan. One such vitamin is B_{12}, which doesn't occur in plant foods except for special nutritional supplements, such as yeast grown in a vitamin B_{12}-enriched environment. The vegan needs a reliable source, such as vitamin B_{12}-fortified soy milk or meat replacements. Some vegetarians use seaweeds, fermented soy, and other products in the belief that such foods provide vitamin B_{12} in adequate amounts. These products are not currently recommended as reliable sources. A pregnant or lactating woman who is eating a vegan diet should be aware that her infant can develop a vitamin B_{12} deficiency even if the mother remains healthy. The mother can remain healthy because vitamin B_{12} is stored in the body, and it may take years for a deficiency to develop. Since deficiency of vitamin B_{12} severely damages the infant's nervous system, all vegan mothers must be sure to use vitamin B_{12}-fortified products or take the appropriate supplements.

What other vitamins do vegans need?

Another vitamin of concern is vitamin D. The milk drinker is protected, provided the milk is fortified with vitamin D, but there is no practical source of vitamin D in plant foods. Regular exposure to the sun will prevent a deficiency, but the homebound or vegan living in a northern climate or smoggy city probably should take vitamin D supplements. Excesses of vitamin D are toxic and one should not exceed the recommended daily amount of 5 micrograms.

Riboflavin, another vitamin often obtained from milk, is not a problem for the vegan who uses dark greens frequently in ample servings. The vegan who doesn't use a lot of greens, however, may not meet riboflavin needs. Nutritional yeast is a rich source of riboflavin for the vegetarian.

So on a vegan diet, vitamin B_{12}, vitamin D, and riboflavin can be problems if I'm not careful. What about minerals?

Two minerals may be of concern for all vegetarians, not just the vegan. These are iron and zinc. Legumes are an important source of iron in the vegetarian diet. The iron in legumes, however, is not as absorbable as that in meat. In fact, people absorb three times as much iron from a meal that includes meat as from one that does not (see p. 000). Because vitamin C in fruits and vegetables also can triple iron absorption from other foods eaten at the same meal, vegetarian meals should be rich in foods offering vitamin C.

As for zinc, it too may be a problem nutrient for vegetarians. It is widespread in plant foods, but its availability may be hindered by the fibers and other binders found in fruits and vegetables. The zinc needs of vegetarians and the effects of mineral binders are subjects of intensive study at the present time. While research continues, vegetarians are advised to eat varied diets that include whole-grain breads well leavened with yeast, which improves the availability of their minerals.

What about minerals for the vegan? Would calcium be a problem?

Good thinking. Yes, of course calcium is of concern. The milk-drinking vegetarian is protected from deficiency, but the vegan must find other sources of calcium. Some good calcium sources are *regular* and *ample* servings of stone-ground meal; self-rising flour and meal; legumes; calcium-fortified soy milk; some nuts, such as almonds; and certain seeds, such as sesame seeds. The choices should be varied because absorption of calcium from some of these foods is hindered by binders in the foods. The vegetarian is urged to use *calcium-fortified* soy milk *in ample quantities regularly*. This is especially important for children. Infant formula, based on soy, is fortified with calcium and can easily be used in cooking foods even for adults.

It sounds as if I can do well with a vegetarian diet as long as I do a little planning. Are there any nutritional advantages to the vegetarian diet?
Yes. Vegetarian protein foods are often higher in fiber, richer in certain vitamins and minerals, and lower in fat than meats. Vegetarians can enjoy a nutritious diet very low in fat provided that they limit other high-fat foods such as butter, cream cheese, sour cream, and nuts. If vegetarians follow the guidelines presented here and plan carefully, they can support their health as well as, or perhaps better than, nonvegetarians.

Are you saying that vegetarians may actually be healthier than meat eaters?
Yes, abundant evidence supports that idea. Informed vegetarians are more likely to be at the desired weights for their heights and to have lower blood cholesterol levels, lower rates of certain kinds of cancer, better digestive function, and better health in other ways as well. Even among people who are health conscious, vegetarians experience fewer deaths from cardiovascular disease. Since vegetarianism often goes with a clean-living lifestyle (no smoking, abstinence from alcohol, emphasis on supportive family life), it is unlikely that dietary practices *alone* account for all the aspects of improved health. Clearly, however, they contribute significantly to it.

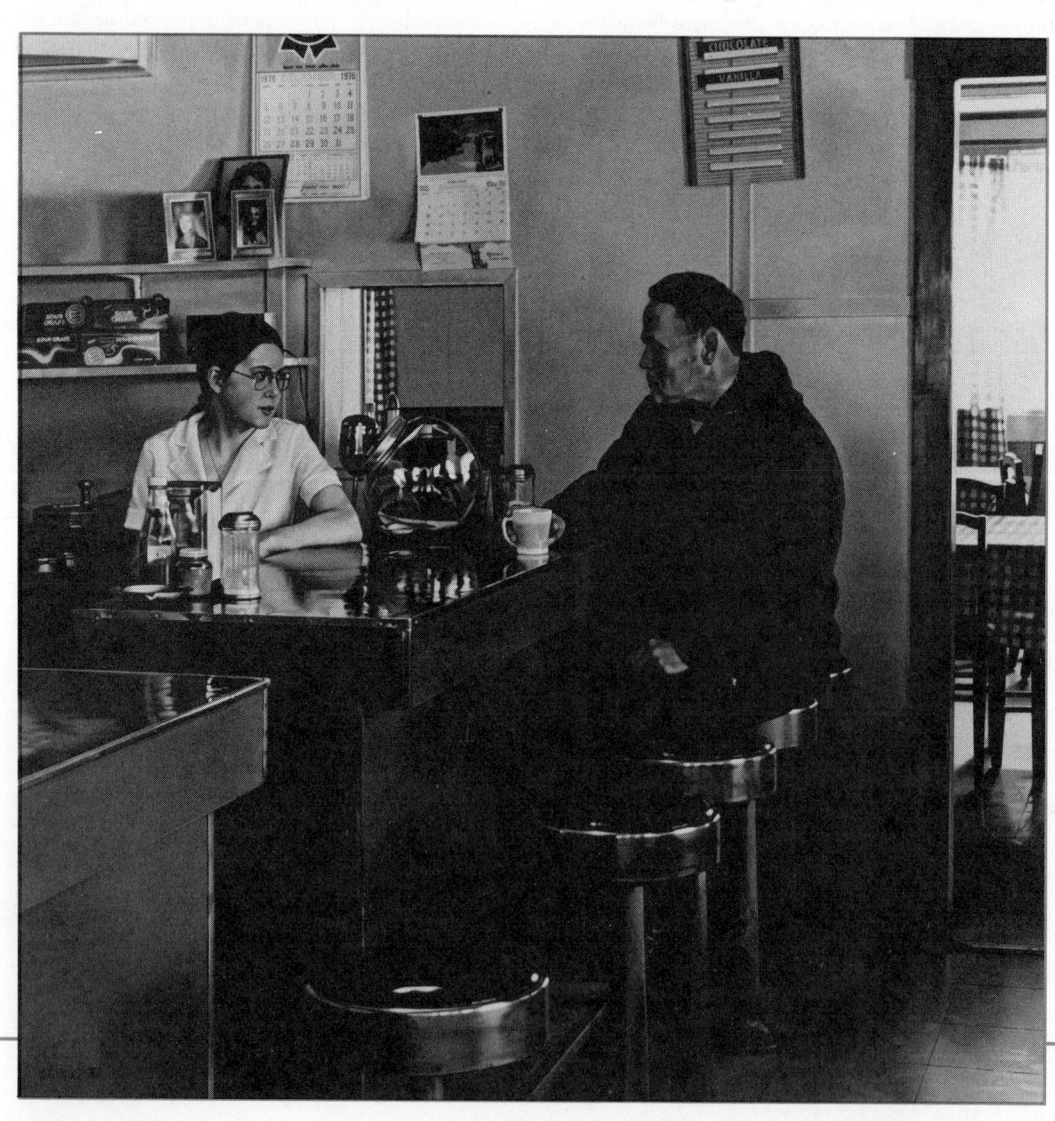

CHAPTER

5

Digestion and Absorption

CONTENTS

"Pee Wee's Diner, Warnerville, New York," by Ralph Goings, 1977.
Oil on canvas, 48" × 48". Courtesy The Pollock Family Collection.

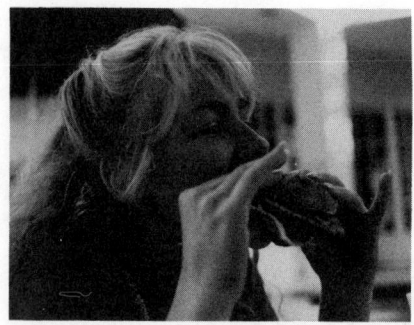

The problems of food contaminants, which may be absorbed defenselessly by the body, are presented in Nutrition in Practice 14.

GI tract:
the gastrointestinal tract or alimentary canal; the principal organs are the stomach and intestines.
gastro = stomach
aliment = food

gland:
a cell or group of cells that secrete materials for special uses in the body. Glands may be *exocrine glands,* secreting their materials "out" (into the digestive tract or onto the surface of the skin) or *endocrine glands,* secreting their materials "in" (into the blood).
exo = outside
endo = inside
krine = to separate

One of the beauties of the digestive tract is that it is selective. Materials that are nutritive for the body are broken down into particles that can be assimilated into the bloodstream. Most of the nonnutritive materials are left undigested and pass out the other end of the digestive tract. In a sense, the human body is doughnut shaped, and the digestive tract is the hole through the doughnut.

Anatomy of the Digestive Tract

The gastrointestinal (GI) tract is a flexible muscular tube measuring about 26 feet in length from the mouth to the anus. Figure 5–1 traces the path followed by food from one end to the other.

The Digestive Organs

When you swallow a mouthful of food, it first slides across your epiglottis, bypassing the entrance to your lungs. Whenever you swallow, the epiglottis closes off your air passages so that you do not choke.

Next the food slides down the esophagus, which conducts it through the diaphragm to the stomach. There it is retained for a while. The cardiac sphincter, a band of muscle at the stomach's entrance, closes behind the food so that it cannot slip back. Then bit by bit, it pops through the pylorus, which opens into the small intestine, and the pylorus, too, closes behind it. At the top of the small intestine the food bypasses an opening (entrance only, no exit) from the common bile duct, which conveys secretions into the small intestine from two organs outside the GI tract—the gallbladder and the pancreas. It travels on down the small intestine through its three segments—the duodenum, the jejunum, and the ileum—a total of 20 feet of tubing coiled within the abdomen.

Having traveled through these segments of the small intestine, the chyme arrives at another sphincter, the ileocecal valve, at the beginning of the large intestine (colon) in the lower right-hand side of the abdomen. Then it travels along the large intestine up the right-hand side of the abdomen, across the front to the left-hand side, down to the lower left-hand side, and finally below the other folds of the intestines to the back side of the body above the rectum.

During chyme's passage through the colon, water is withdrawn, leaving semisolid waste. This waste is held back by the strong muscles of the rectum. When it is time to defecate, these muscles relax, and the last sphincter in the system, the anus, opens to allow the wastes to pass.

In summary, the path followed by food is as shown in the margin. This is not a very complex route, considering all that happens on the way.

The Involuntary Muscles and the Glands

You are usually unaware of all the activity that goes on between the time you swallow and the time you defecate. As is the case with so much else that goes on in the body, the muscles and glands of the digestive tract meet internal needs without your having to exert any conscious effort to get the work done.

Miniglossary of GI Terms

epiglottis (epp-ee-GLOT-tiss)   cartilage in the throat that guards the entrance to the trachea and prevents fluid or food from entering it when a person swallows.
epi = upon (over)
glottis = back of tongue

trachea (TRAKE-ee-uh)   windpipe.

esophagus (e-SOFF-uh-gus)   food pipe.

cardiac sphincter (CARD-ee-ack SFINK-ter)   sphincter muscle at the junction between the esophagus and the stomach.
sphincter = band (binder)

pyloric (pie-LORE-ic) **sphincter**   sphincter muscle separating the stomach from the small intestine.
pylorus = gatekeeper

gllbladder and pancreas   see pp. 000.

duodenum (doo-oh-DEEN-um or doo-ODD-num)   the top portion of the small intestine (about "12 fingers' breadth" long, in ancient terminology).
duodecim = twelve

jejunum (je-JOON-um)   the first two-fifths of the small intestine beyond the duodenum.

ileum (ILL-ee-um)   the last segment of the small intestine.

ileocecal (ill-ee-oh-SEEK-ul) **valve**   sphincter muscle separating the small and large intestines.

colon (COAL-un)   the large intestine. Its segments are the ascending colon, the transverse colon, the descending colon, and the sigmoid colon.
sigmoid = shaped like the letter S (*sigma* in Greek)

appendix   a narrow blind sac extending from the beginning of the colon; a vestigial organ with no known function.

rectum   the muscular terminal part of the intestine from the sigmoid colon to the anus.

anus (AY-nus)   terminal sphincter muscle of the GI tract.

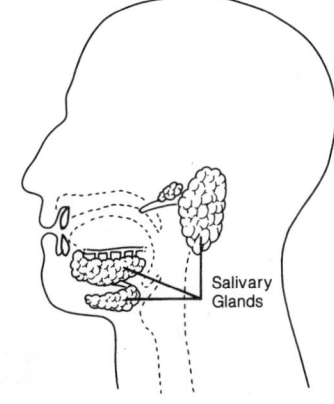

The salivary glands are exocrine glands.

Chewing and swallowing are under conscious control, but even in the mouth there are some automatic processes you can't control. The salivary glands secrete just enough saliva to moisten each mouthful of food so that the food can easily pass down your esophagus. After you have swallowed a mouthful of food, the food mass is called a bolus.

Peristalsis begins when the bolus enters the esophagus. The entire GI tract is ringed with muscles that can squeeze it tightly. Within these rings of muscle lie longitudinal muscles. When the rings tighten and the long muscles relax, the tube is constricted. When the rings relax and the long muscles tighten, the tube bulges. These actions follow each other so that the intestinal contents are continuously pushed along. If you have ever watched a bolus of food pass along the body of a snake, you have a good picture of how these muscles work. The waves of contraction ripple through the GI tract all the time, at the rate of about three a minute, whether or not you have just eaten a meal. Peristalsis,

saliva:
the secretion of the salivary glands; the principal enzyme is salivary amylase.

bolus (BOH-lus):
the portion of food swallowed at one time.

peristalsis (peri-STALL-sis):
successive waves of involuntary muscular contraction passing along the walls of the intestine.
peri = around
stellein = wrap

FIGURE 5-1
The gastrointestinal tract.

Fiber	Carbohydrate

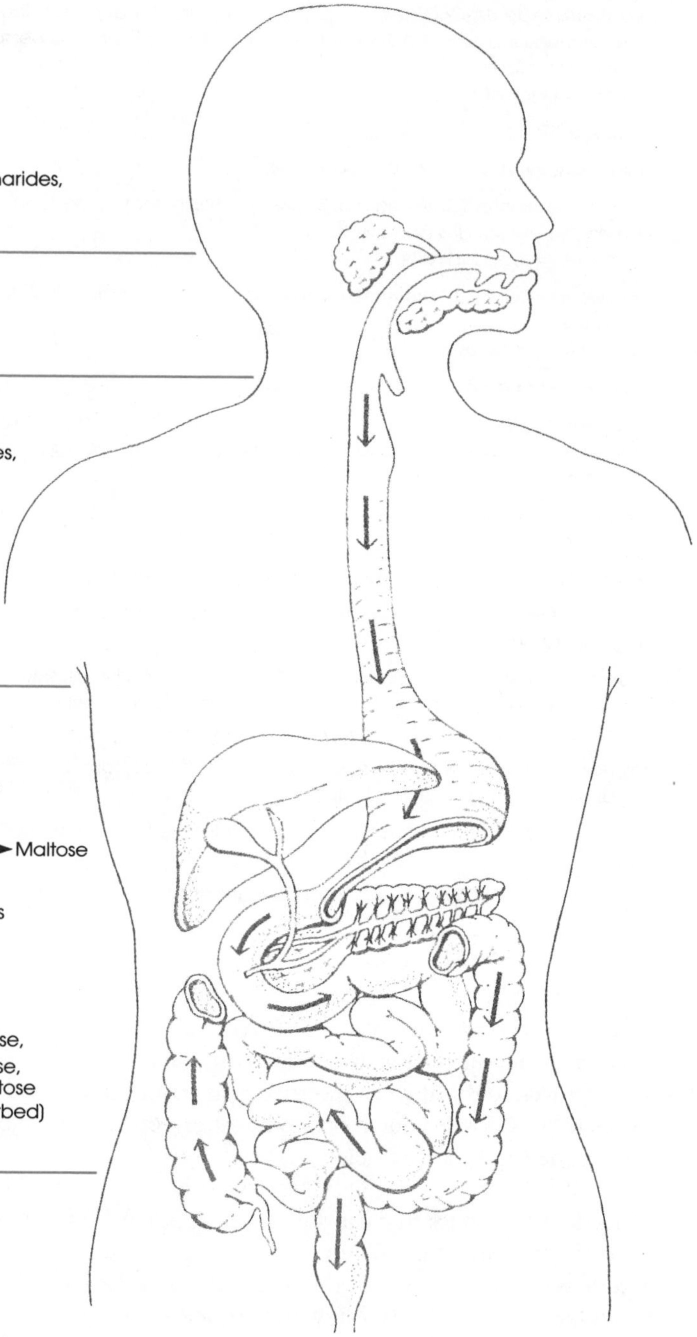

Mouth

The mechanical action of the mouth crushes and tears fiber in food and mixes it with saliva to moisten it for swallowing.

The salivary glands secrete a watery fluid into the mouth to moisten the food. The salivary enzyme amylase begins digestion:

$$\text{Starch} \xrightarrow{\text{amylase}} \text{Small polysaccharides, maltose}$$

Esophagus

Fiber is unchanged.

Digestion of starch continues as swallowed food moves down esophagus.

Stomach

Fiber is unchanged.

Stomach acid and enzymes start to digest salivary enzymes, halting starch digestion. To a small extent, stomach acid hydrolyzes maltose and sucrose:

$$\text{Maltose} \xrightarrow{\text{HCl}} \text{Glucose}$$

$$\text{Sucrose} \xrightarrow{\text{HCl}} \text{Glucose and fructose}$$

Small intestine

Fiber is unchanged.

The pancreas produces carbohydrates and releases them through the pancreatic duct into the small intestine:

$$\text{Polysaccharides} \xrightarrow{\text{pancreatic amylase}} \text{Maltose}$$

Then enzymes on the surfaces of the small intestinal cells break these into monosaccharides and the cells absorb them:

$$\text{Maltose} \xrightarrow{\text{maltase}}$$
$$\text{Sucrose} \xrightarrow{\text{sucrase}} \left.\begin{array}{c}\end{array}\right\} \text{Glucose, fructose, galactose (absorbed)}$$
$$\text{Lactose} \xrightarrow{\text{lactase}}$$

Large intestine

Most fiber passes intact through the digestive tract to the large intestine. Here, bacterial enzymes digest some fiber:

$$\text{Some fiber} \xrightarrow{\text{bacterial enzymes}} \text{Glucose (absorbed)}$$

Fiber holds water, regulates bowel activity, binds cholesterol and some minerals, carrying them out of the body.

Fat	Protein	Vitamins	Minerals and Water
Mouth Glands in the base of the tongue secrete a lipase known as lingual lipase. Some hard fats begin to melt as they reach body temperature.	Chewing and crushing moistens protein-rich foods and mixes them with saliva to be swallowed.	No action on vitamins takes place in the mouth or esophagus.	The salivary glands add water to disperse and carry food.
Esophagus Fat is unchanged.	No action.	No action.	No action.
Stomach The lingual lipase hydrolyzes one bond of triglycerides to produce diglycerides and fatty acids. The degree of hydrolysis of fats by lingual lipase is slight for most fats but may be appreciable for milk fats.	Stomach acid uncoils protein strands and activates stomach enzymes: Protein $\xrightarrow[\text{HCl}]{\text{pepsin}}$ Smaller polypeptides	Intrinsic factor (see Chapter 7) attaches to vitamin B_{12}.	Stomach acid (HCl) acts on iron to reduce it, making it more absorbable (see Chapter 8). The stomach secretes enough watery fluid to turn moist, chewed mass of solid food into liquid chyme.
Small intestine The stomach's churning action mixes fat with water and acid. A gastric lipase accesses and hydrolyzes a very little fat. Bile flows in from the liver (via the common bile duct): Fat $\xrightarrow{\text{bile}}$ Emulsified fat Pancreatic lipase flows in from the pancreas: Emulsified fat $\xrightarrow[\text{lipase}]{\text{pancreatic}}$ Monoglycerides, glycerol, fatty acids (absorbed)	Pancreatic and small intestinal enzymes split polypeptides further: Polypeptides $\xrightarrow[\substack{\text{and intestinal}\\\text{proteases}}]{\text{pancreatic}}$ Dipeptides, tripeptides, and amino acids Then enzymes on the surface of the small intestinal cells hydrolyze these peptides and the cells absorb them: Peptides $\xrightarrow[\substack{\text{di- and tri-}\\\text{peptidases}}]{\text{intestinal}}$ Amino acids (absorbed)	Bile emulsifies fat-soluble vitamins and aids in their absorption with other fats. Water-soluble vitamins are absorbed.	The small intestine, pancreas, and liver add enough fluid so that the total secreted into the intestine in a day approximates 2 gallons. Many minerals are absorbed. Vitamin D aids in the absorption of calcium.
Large intestine Some fat and cholesterol, trapped in fiber, exits in feces.		Bacteria produce vitamin K, which is absorbed.	More minerals and most of the water are absorbed.

Tube with longitudinal (L) and circular (C) muscles.

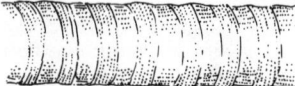

Peristalsis.

bolus

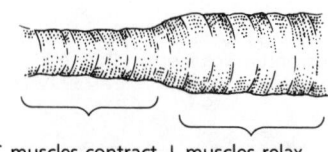

C muscles contract, L muscles relax.
L muscles contract, C muscles relax.

bolus

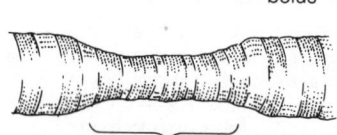

Wave moves along, pushing bolus ahead of it.

segmentation:
a periodic squeezing or partitioning of the intestine by its circular muscles.

chyme (KIME):
the semiliquid mass of partly digested food expelled by the stomach into the duodenum.
chymos = juice

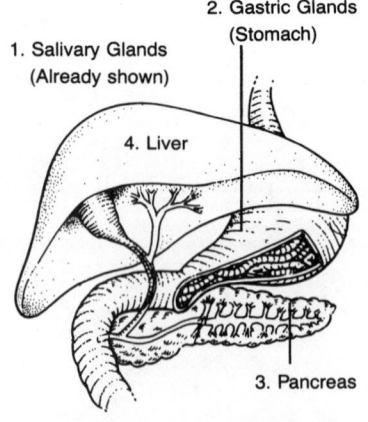

1. Salivary Glands (Already shown)

2. Gastric Glands (Stomach)

4. Liver

3. Pancreas

Organs that secrete digestive juices.

along with the sphincter muscles that surround the tract at key places, prevents anything from backing up.

The intestines not only push but also periodically squeeze their contents at intervals as if you had put a string around them and pulled it tight. This motion, called segmentation, forces their contents backward a few inches, mixing them and allowing the digestive juices and the absorbing cells of the intestinal walls to make better contact with them.

Besides forcing the bolus along, the muscles of the GI tract help to liquefy it so that the digestive enzymes will have access to all the nutrients in it. The first step in this process takes place in the mouth where chewing, the addition of saliva, and the action of the tongue reduce the food to a coarse mash suitable for swallowing. A further mixing and kneading action then takes place in the stomach.

The stomach has a third layer of transverse muscles that also alternately contract and relax. While these three sets of muscles are all at work forcing the bolus downward, the pyloric sphincter usually remains tightly closed, preventing the bolus from passing into the duodenum. Meanwhile, the gastric glands release juices that mix with the bolus. As a result, the bolus is churned and forced down, hits the pyloric sphincter, and bounces back. When the bolus is thoroughly liquefied, the pyloric sphincter opens briefly, about three times a minute, to allow small portions through. From this point on, the intestinal contents are called chyme, which no longer resemble food in the least.

The Process of Digestion

One person eats nothing but vegetables, fruits, and nuts; another, hardly anything other than meat, milk, and potatoes. How is it that both people wind up with essentially the same body composition? It all comes down to the fact that the body renders food—whatever it is to start with—into the carbohydrate, fat, protein, vitamins, and minerals of which it is composed. The body absorbs these units and builds its tissues from them.

For this purpose, five different body organs secrete digestive juices: the salivary glands, the stomach, the small intestine, the liver, and the pancreas. Each of the juices has a turn to mix with the intestinal contents and promote their breakdown to small units that can be absorbed into the body.

Digestion in the Mouth

Digestion of carbohydrate begins in the mouth where enzymes found in the saliva break down the starch chains. Saliva also has the role of protecting the tooth surfaces and linings of the mouth, esophagus, and stomach from attack by molecules that might harm them.[1] The chemicals in the mouth do not affect fats, proteins, vitamins, minerals, and fiber that are present in the foods we eat.

Digestion in the Stomach

Gastric juice is composed of water, enzymes, and hydrochloric acid. The acid is so strong that it burns the throat if it chances to reflux into the mouth. The strong acidity of the stomach prevents bacterial growth and kills most bacteria that enter the body with food. You might expect that the stomach's acid would attack the stomach itself, but the cells of the stomach wall secrete mucus, a thick, slimy, white polysaccharide that coats the stomach's lining.

Other than being crushed and mixed with saliva, nothing happens to protein until it comes in contact with the gastric juices found in the stomach. There, the acid helps to uncoil (denature) the protein's tangled strands so that the stomach enzymes can attack the bonds.

All proteins are responsive to acidity, and stomach enzymes work most efficiently in the stomach's strong acid. However, salivary amylase, which is swallowed with food, does not work in acid this strong, so the digestion of starch gradually ceases as the acid penetrates the bolus. In fact, salivary amylase becomes just another protein to be digested. The amino acids in amylase end up being absorbed and recycled into other body proteins.

amylase (AM-uh-lace): an enzyme that splits amylose (a form of starch). Amylase is a *carbohydrase*. The ending *-ase* indicates an enzyme; the root tells what it digests. Other examples: protease, lipase.

gastric glands: exocrine glands in the stomach wall that secrete gastric juice into the stomach. *gastro* = stomach

gastric juice: the secretion of the gastric glands. The principal enzymes are rennin (curdles milk protein, casein, and prepares it for pepsin action), pepsin (acts on proteins); and lipase (acts on emulsified fats).

mucus (MYOO-cuss): a mucopolysaccharide (relative of carbohydrate) secreted by cells of the stomach wall. The cellular lining of the stomach wall with its coat of mucus is known as the mucous membrane. (The noun is *mucus*; the adjective is *mucous*.)

Note that the strong acidity of the stomach is a desirable condition, TV commercials for antacids notwithstanding. People who overeat or who bolt their food are likely to suffer from indigestion. The muscular reaction of the stomach to unchewed particles or to being overfilled may be so violent as to cause regurgitation (reverse peristalsis). When this happens, the overeater may taste the stomach acid in her mouth and think she is suffering from "acid indigestion." Responding to TV commercials, she may take antacids to neutralize the stomach acid. The consequence of this action is a demand on the stomach to secrete more acid to counteract the neutralizer and enable the digestive enzymes to do their work. The consumer ends up with the same amount of acid in her stomach but has had to work against the antacid to produce it.

Antacids are not designed to relieve the digestive discomfort of the hasty eater. Their proper use is to correct an abnormal condition, such as that of the person with ulcers whose stomach or duodenal lining has been attacked by acid. To avoid falling into the same trap as our misguided consumer, remember that what such a person needs to do is to chew food more thoroughly, eat it more slowly, and possibly eat less at a sitting.

The major digestive event in the stomach is the initial breakdown of proteins. Both the enzyme pepsin and the stomach acid itself act as catalysts in the process. Minor events are the digestion of some fat by a gastric lipase, the digestion of sucrose (to a very small extent) by the stomach acid, and the attachment of a protein carrier to vitamin B$_{12}$.

Digestion in the Small Intestine

By the time the energy-yielding nutrients enter the small intestine, they are already broken into smaller sized pieces. In the small intestine, the pancreas and liver contribute three additional digestive juices through ducts into the duodenum. Glands situated in the intestinal wall secrete a water juice containing all three kinds of digestive enzymes—carbohydroses, lipases, and proteases—and others as well. In addition, both the pancreas and the liver make contributions by way of ducts leading into the duodenum.

The pancreatic juice contains enzymes to break down fats, proteins, and carbohydrates. The pancreatic juice also contains sodium bicarbonate which neutralizes the acidic chyme as it enters the small intestine. From this point on, the contents of the digestive tract are neutral or slightly alkaline. The enzymes of both the intestine and the pancreas work best in this environment.

Food evidently needs to be digested completely. The sharing of this task by several organs underscores the body's determination to get the job done. Such distribution of labor is seen in nature whenever the job to be done is absolutely vital, as it is in this case.

Bile, a secretion from the liver, also flows into the duodenum. The gallbladder concentrates and stores bile and squirts it into the duodenum whenever fat arrives there. Bile is not an enzyme but an emulsifier that brings fats into suspension in water. After the fats are emulsified, enzymes can work on them and they can be absorbed. Thanks to all these secretions, the digestion of the energy nutrients is completed in the small intestine.

Most proteins are broken down into dipeptides, tripeptides, and amino acids before they are absorbed. With this in mind, you will be in a position to refute certain untrue claims made about foods. For instance, "Don't eat food A. It contains enzyme B that will harm you." Any enzyme you eat becomes but one among thousands of different proteins in your digestive tract. Except for digestive enzymes, whose design prevents them from being digested while they work, enzymes you eat are simply proteins that are broken down to amino acids. Don't be fooled by claims implying that enzymes you eat will act as enzymes in your body.

The rate of digestion of the energy nutrients depends upon the contents of the meal. If the meal is high in simple sugars, the process of digestion will be fairly rapid. On the other hand, if the meal contains a considerable amount of fat, the digestive process will be slower. The fact that fat slows digestion is also why fat increases the satiety value of a meal.

The story of how food is broken down into nutrients that can be absorbed is now nearly complete. Carbohydrate, fat, and protein are disassembled to basic building blocks before they are absorbed. Most of the other nutrients—vitamins, minerals, and water—are absorbable as they are. The function of undigested residues, such as some fibers, is to provide a semisolid mass that can stimulate the muscles of the GI tract so that they will remain strong and perform peristalsis efficiently. Fiber also retains water, keeping the stools soft, and carries bile acids, sterols, and fat with it out of the body.

For the moment, let us assume that the digested nutrients simply disappear from the GI tract as they are ready. Virtually all are gone by the time the contents of the GI tract reach the end of the small intestine. Little remains but water, a few undissolved salts and body secretions, and undigested materials such as fiber. These enter the large intestine (colon).

In the colon, intestinal bacteria degrade some of the fiber to simpler compounds. Another function of the colon is to retrieve from its contents the materials that the body is designed to recycle—water and dissolved salts. The waste that is finally excreted has little or nothing of value left in it. The body has extracted all that it can use from the food. The colon also contains bacteria that produce a variety of vitamins, including biotin and vitamin K. The GI bacteria also protect us from infections. Provided that the normal intestinal flora are thriving, infectious bacteria have a hard time getting established and launching an attack on the system. In addition, the small intestine, and in fact the entire GI tract, manufactures and maintains a strong arsenal of defenses against foreign invaders. Several different types of defending cells are present there and confer specific immunity against intestinal diseases.

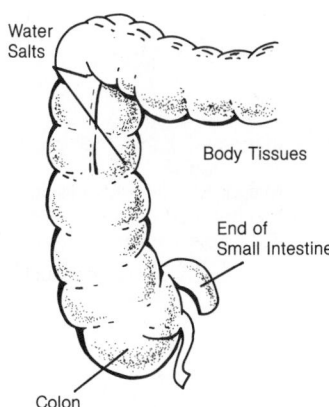

The large intestine reabsorbs water and salts.

intestinal flora:
the bacterial inhabitants of the GI tract.
flora = plant growth

The Absorptive System

Within three or four hours after you have eaten a meal, your body must find a way to absorb some two hundred thousand, million, million, million amino acid molecules one by one, and an equivalent number of monosaccharide, monoglyceride, glycerol, fatty acid, vitamin, and mineral molecules as well. The absorptive system is ingeniously designed to accomplish this task.

The Small Intestine's Lining

The small intestine provides a surface whose extent is comparable to a quarter of a football field in area. Nutrient molecules make contact with this surface and are absorbed. To remove these molecules rapidly and provide room for more to be absorbed, a rush of circulation continuously bathes the underside of the surface, washing away the absorbed nutrients and carrying them to the liver and other parts of the body.

The small intestine is a tube about 20 feet long and an inch or so across. Its inner surface looks smooth and slippery, but viewed through a microscope, it turns out to be wrinkled into hundreds of folds. Each fold is covered with thousands of finger-like projections as numerous as the hairs on velvet fabric. Each of these small intestinal projections is a villus. A single villus, magnified still more, turns out to be composed of hundreds of cells, each covered with microscopic hairs called microvilli (see Figure 5–2).

villi (VILL-ee or VILL-eye):
fingerlike projections from the folds of the small intestine. The singular form is *villus*.
villus = shaggy hair

microvilli (MY-cro-VILL-ee or MY-cro-VILL-eye):
projections from the membranes of the cells of the villi. The singular form is *microvillus*.

FIGURE 5–2
Surface features of the small intestinal wall.

A. Folds in the wall of the small intestine. Each is covered with villi.
B. Villi (detail of A). Each villus is composed of several hundred cells.
C. Cells of a single villus (detail of B). Each cell is coated with microvilli.

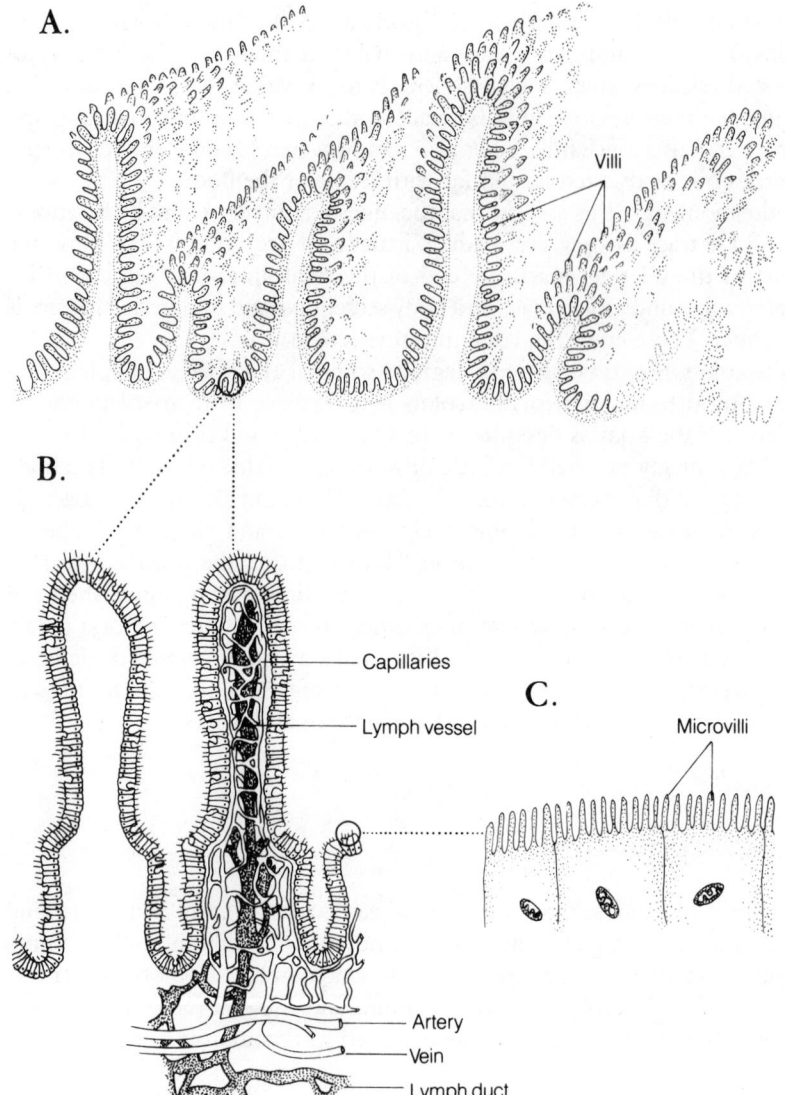

A.

Villi

B.

Capillaries

Lymph vessel

C.

Microvilli

Artery

Vein

Lymph duct

    The villi are in constant motion. Each villus is lined by a thin sheet of muscle so that it can wave, squirm, and wiggle like the tentacles of a sea anemone. Any nutrient molecule small enough to be absorbed is trapped in the microvilli and drawn into the cells beneath them. Some partially digested nutrients are caught in the microvilli, digested further by enzymes there, and then absorbed into the cells.

    Once a molecule has entered a cell in a villus, the next problem is to transport it to its destination elsewhere in the body. Everyone knows that the blood-stream performs this function, but you may be surprised to learn that there is a second transport system—the lymphatic system. Both of these systems supply vessels to each villus, as shown in Figure 5–2. When a nutrient molecule has crossed the cell of a villus, it may enter either the lymph or the blood. In either case, the nutrients end up in the blood, at least for a while.

As you can see, the intestinal tract is beautifully designed to perform its functions. A further refinement of the system is that the cells of successive portions of the tract are specialized to absorb different nutrients. The top portion of the duodenum is specialized for the absorption of calcium and several B vitamins, such as thiamin and riboflavin. The jejunum accomplishes most of the absorption of fats, and vitamin B_{12} is absorbed at the end of the ileum. The rate at which the nutrients travel through the GI tract is finely adjusted to maximize their availability to the appropriate absorptive segment of the tract when they are ready. The lowly "gut" turns out to be one of the most elegantly designed organ systems in the body.

Release of Absorbed Nutrients

Once inside the intestinal cells, the products of digestion must be released for transport to the rest of the body. The water-soluble nutrients, including the smaller products of lipid digestion, are released directly into the bloodstream. The larger lipids and the fat-soluble vitamins, however, find access directly into the capillaries impossible because they are insoluble in water. The cells assemble the monoglycerides and long-chain fatty acids into larger molecules called triglycerides. These triglycerides, fat-soluble vitamins (when present), and other large lipids (cholesterol and the phospholipids) are then made

lymph (LIMF):
the body's interstitial fluid, located between cells and outside the vascular system. Lymph consists of all the constituents of blood that can escape from the vascular system. It circulates in a loosely organized system of vessels and ducts known as the *lymphatic system.*

Delivery of Nutrients into Blood

Water-soluble nutrients	
Carbohydrates	
Monosaccharides	Directly into blood
Lipids	
Glycerol	Directly into blood
Short-chain fatty acids	Directly into blood
Medium-chain fatty acids	Directly into blood
Proteins	
Amino acids	Directly into blood
Vitamins	
Vitamins B and C	Directly into blood
Minerals	Directly into blood
Fat-soluble nutrients	
Lipids	
Long-chain fatty acids	Made into triglycerides
Monoglycerides	Made into triglycerides
Triglycerides	To lymph, then blood
Cholesterol (in chylomicrons)	To lymph, then blood
Phospholipids	To lymph, then blood
Vitamins	
Vitamins A, D, E, K	To lymph, then blood

into bundles with special proteins to form chylomicrons, one kind of lipoprotein (lipoproteins are described beginning on page 75). Finally, the cells release the chylomicrons into the lymphatic system. They can then glide through the lymph spaces until they move to a point of entry into the bloodstream near the heart.

Transport of Nutrients

Once a nutrient has entered the bloodstream or the lymphatic system, it may be transported to any part of the body and thus becomes available to any of the cells, from the tips of the toes to the roots of the hair. The circulatory systems are arranged to deliver nutrients wherever they are needed.

The Vascular System

The vascular or blood circulatory system is a closed system of vessels through which blood flows continuously in a figure eight, with the heart serving as a pump at the crossover point. Blood travels a simple route: heart to arteries to capillaries to veins to heart.

The routing of the blood through the digestive system is different, however. The blood is carried to the digestive system (as it is to all organs) by way of an artery, which (as in all organs) branches into capillaries to reach every cell. Blood leaving the digestive system, however, goes by way of a vein, not back to the heart but to the liver. This vein *again* branches into capillaries so that every cell of the liver also has access to the blood it carries. Blood leaving the liver then returns to the heart by way of a vein. The route is heart to arteries to capillaries (in intestines) to vein to capillaries (in liver) to vein to heart.

An anatomist studying this system knows there must be a reason for this special arrangement. The liver is placed in the circulation at this point so that it will have the first chance at the materials absorbed from the GI tract. In fact, the liver is the body's major metabolic organ. It must prepare the absorbed nutrients for use by the body and has many jobs to perform in this process. Furthermore, the liver stands as gatekeeper to waylay intruders that might otherwise harm the heart or brain. Chapter 22 offers more information about this noble organ.

The Lymphatic System

The lymphatic system is an open system that can be compared to the water-filled spaces in a sponge. The system has no pump, rather lymph is squeezed from one portion of the body to another as muscles contract and create pressure here and there, much like water in a sponge. Ultimately, the lymph collects in a large duct behind the heart. This duct terminates in a vein that conducts the lymph into the heart. Thus, some materials from the GI tract enter the lymphatic system at first, then later enter the bloodstream.

artery:
a vessel that carries blood away from the heart.

capillary (CAP-ill-ary):
a small vessel that branches from an artery. Capillaries connect arteries to veins. Exchange of oxygen, nutrients, and waste materials takes place across capillary walls.

The blood arriving at the intestines flows through the **mesentery** (MEZ-en-terry), a strong, flexible membrane that surrounds and supports the abdominal organs.
mes = middle

The vein that collects blood from the mesentery and conducts it to capillaries in the liver is the **portal vein.**
portal = gateway

The vein that collects blood from the liver capillaries and returns it to the heart is the **hepatic vein.**
hepat = liver

The duct that conveys lymph toward the heart is the **thoracic** (thor-ASS-ic) **duct.** The **subclavian vein** connects this duct with the right upper chamber of the heart, providing a passageway by which lymph can be returned to the vascular system.

Transport of Lipids: Lipoproteins

Within the circulatory system, lipids always travel from place to place bundled with protein, that is, as lipoproteins. Lipoproteins are very much in the news these days. In fact, when the doctor measures a person's blood lipid profile, she is interested not only in the types of fat she finds (triglycerides and cholesterol) but also in the types of protein they travel with. Newly absorbed lipids leaving the intestinal cells are mostly packaged in the lipoproteins known as chylomicrons. As the chylomicrons circulate through the body, cells remove their lipid contents. The liver picks up and dismantles the remnants and assembles new lipoproteins, which are known as very-low-density lipoproteins (VLDL) and low-density lipoproteins (LDL). Lipids returning to the liver from other parts of the body are packaged in lipoproteins known as high-density lipoproteins (HDL). The composition of the lipoproteins is shown in Figures 5–3 through 5–5. We present more about the lipoproteins and heart disease in Chapter 21.

chylomicron (kye-lo-MY-cron):
The lipoprotein formed in the intestinal wall cells following digestion and absorption of fat. Released from these cells, chylomicrons transport ingested fats to all cells of the body which remove the ones they need, leaving chylomicron remnants to be picked up by the liver cells. The liver cells dismantle the chylomicron remnants and construct other lipoproteins for further transport of lipids.

VLDL:
very-low-density lipoprotein. This type of lipoprotein is made by liver cells and to some extent by intestinal cells. An alternative name is *pre-beta* (pre-BAY-tuh) *lipoprotein.*

LDL:
low-density lipoprotein. This type of lipoprotein may be made by liver cells or derived from VLDL as cells remove triglycerides from them. An alternative name is *beta lipoprotein.*

HDL:
high-density lipoprotein. These lipoproteins seem to transport cholesterol back to the liver from peripheral cells. An alternative name is alpha *lipoprotein.*

FIGURE 5–3
A chylomicron.

The density of these particles is very, very low because they contain so little protein and so much triglyceride. If a laboratory report reveals that a person has "high blood triglycerides," this might easily reflect a high concentration of chylomicrons in his blood.

FIGURE 5–4
VLDL and LDL.

Compare these particles with chylomicrons and HDL. Note that high blood cholesterol might easily reflect a high LDL concentration.

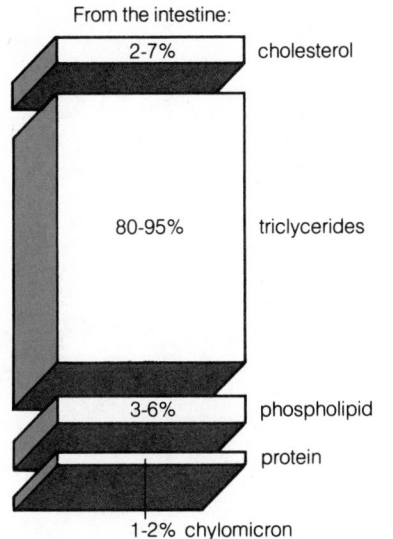

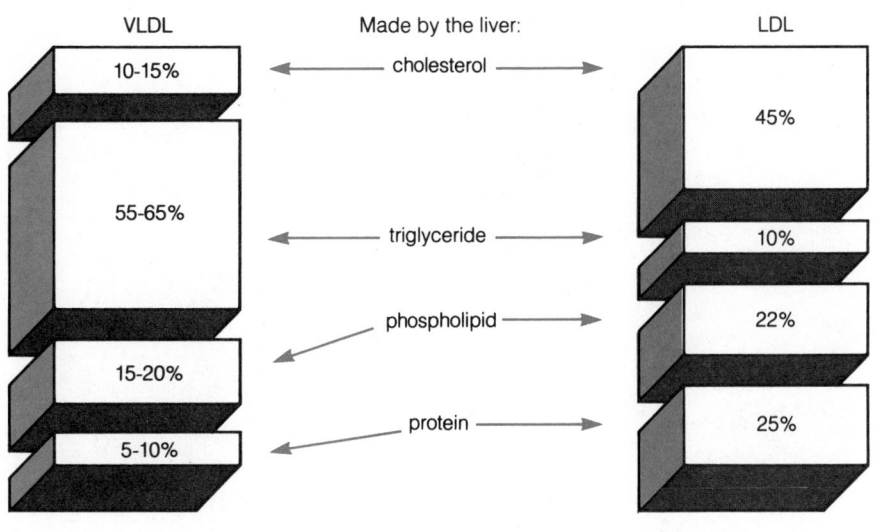

Returned to the liver:

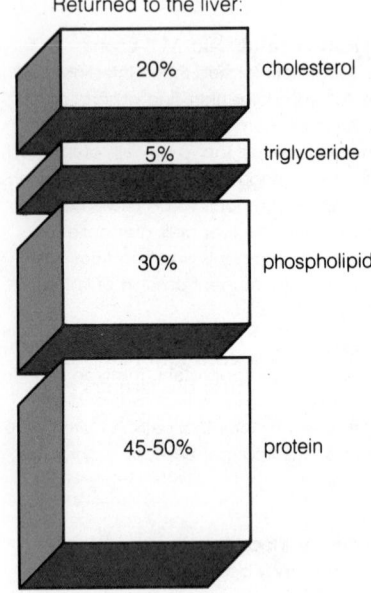

20%	cholesterol
5%	triglyceride
30%	phospholipid
45-50%	protein

FIGURE 5–5
HDL.

These particles are denser than the others because they contain such a high percentage of protein.

The System at Its Best

The intricate architecture of the GI tract makes it sensitive and responsive to conditions in its environment. A condition indispensable to its performance is good health. Such lifestyle factors as sleep, exercise, state of mind, and nutrition affect the health of the GI tract. For example, in a person under stress, digestive secretions are reduced and the blood is routed to the muscles more than to the digestive tract. This impairs efficient absorption of nutrients. To digest and absorb food best, one should be relaxed and tranquil at mealtimes.

Among the characteristics of meals that promote optimal absorption of nutrients are balance, variety, adequacy, and moderation, because every nutrient depends on every other. They all work together and all are present in the cells of a healthy digestive tract.

Notes

1. R. J. Gibbons and I. Dankers, Inhibition of lectin-binding to saliva-treated by hydroxyapatite, to buccal epithelial cells, and to erythrocytes by salivary components, *American Journal of Clinical Nutrition* 36 (1982): 276–283.

Organic, Natural, and Health Foods

In this Nutrition in Practice, we deal with something close to many people's hearts—the foods we choose to buy and eat. No one will be completely in agreement with all that is said here. If we do not present your own view here, please be aware that it will probably receive fair treatment later on.

I'm confused. What exactly is an organic food?

Your confusion is understandable, because the term *organic food* has two meanings. A food fertilized with natural organic matter (such as manure) rather than with chemical fertilizers, grown without application of pesticides, and processed without the use of food additives is one meaning. As defined by chemists, however, the term *organic* merely means containing organic compounds or molecules with carbon atoms in them. By the latter definition, all foods are organic. Your body cannot tell whether the nutrients it receives come from an "organic" food or any other food. When you read the word *organic* on a food label it usually conveys the popular meaning: free of chemical fertilizers, pesticides, and additives.

Are natural and health foods the same as organic foods?

Not exactly. The word *natural* has similar connotations but more generally means foods altered as little as possible from their original farm-grown state. *Health foods* encompass both organic and natural foods. They include ordinary, little-processed foods, such as whole-grain breads, and special foods, such as brewer's yeast, sunflower seeds, and wheat germ. The latter items are popularly, but wrongly, believed to have special power to promote health. None of these words has any legal meaning, so they may express different intents when used on different labels.

Does the consumer obtain any advantage by buying health foods?

When the foods themselves are studied, no evidence shows that they confer any special physical benefit. However, they may confer a psychological benefit to people who believe in them. People who eat health foods are often people who long for purity, who distrust technology, especially "chemicals," and who are concerned about their health. Some health food store operators have been seen to play the role of doctors. They "diagnose" the ailments their customers complain of and "prescribe" foods or pills or powders to relieve the symptoms. For this service, customers may pay prices inflated by 50 percent or more above the prices of comparable grocery-store items.

The terms *organic, natural,* and *health food* are considered so misleading that the Federal Trade Commission has proposed to prohibit their use on labels. *Organic*—meaning pesticide free—may sometimes be an outright lie. Many foods sold as organic contain pesticide residues at the same levels as conventional foods, in some cases because the farmers secretly spray them and in others because pesticide residues remain in the environment from previous uses. Moreover, organic foods in several experiments have been found not to differ chemically from conventional foods. It is not surprising, even if it is disappointing, that some sellers will label their products organic just to be able to sell them at twice the price they would get for the same foods without the label. Even though this is unethical, it is not illegal, nor is it false advertising, because *organic* has not been legally defined.

Can health foods actually be dangerous?

In some cases, yes. When people postpone obtaining sound medical advice because they believe they can be "cured" using a health food, the results can be serious. As an example, consider an herb that is claimed to correct "miscarriage even after hemorrhaging and pain have begun."[1] Imagine a woman with an impending miscarriage, beginning to bleed and delaying her trip to the doctor or hospital in order to take an herbal preparation! Yet, it is easy to see why a young woman fearful of doctors and hospitals and trusting of "nature" would make such a choice, even against all reason and evidence.

Taking herbal products is risky for several other reasons. Such products

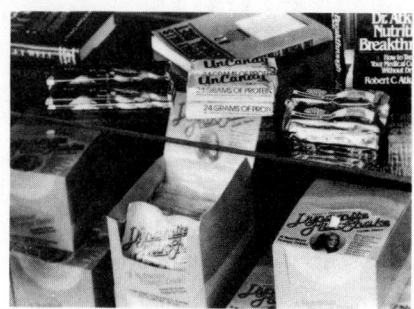

cannot be monitored or held to defined standards by government agencies as can packaged, labeled foods. The *Journal of the American Medical Association* has warned physicians that when they see food poisoning symptoms, they should keep in mind the possibility that herbal teas from natural food stores may be involved.[2] Seven hundred different plants have been reported to cause deaths or serious illnesses in the Western hemisphere.[3]

I have heard that organic farming is better for the ecology than conventional farming. Is that true?
Organic foods are grown in soil fertilized only with natural waste materials, such as manure and compost (rotted vegetable matter and garbage). Like "chemical" fertilizers, these waste materials are composed of chemicals, and they support the growth and health of plants only to the extent that they provide the chemicals the plants need: potassium, nitrogen, phosphate, and others. There is nothing superior about organic fertilizer from that standpoint.

There may, however, be fringe benefits to the use of natural fertilizers such as compost. For example, such fertilizers affect the structure (tilth) of the soil to give a mechanical advantage to the plant. Moreover, organic material returned to the soil is recycled in the natural way. It might otherwise be burned (polluting the air) or dumped to wash into the rivers, lakes, and oceans (polluting the water). Organic farming conserves energy and doesn't pollute. In contrast, conventional agriculture consumes vast amounts of energy and produces fully *half* of the more than four billion tons of solid waste the United States generates each year.

Is there really no health advantage to natural foods?
There is no advantage to foods *labeled* "natural," but there may be an advantage to foods that really are natural. Generally speaking, the more a food resembles the original, farm-grown product, the more nutritious it is likely to be. During processing, nutrients are lost, and often nutrient-empty additions such as sugar, salt, and fat are added. A potato contains 20 milligrams of vitamin C; French fries with the same number of kcalories contain only about 7 milligrams; and potato chips with the same number of kcalories contain only 2 milligrams of vitamin C. By this

Miniglossary

ginseng (JINN-seng) one of a number of plants whose leaves, flowers, or other parts are popularly used for the making of herbal teas. Hazards are associated with this and many other herbs.

health food a misleading term used on labels, usually of organic or natural foods, to imply unusual power to promote health. This term has no legal definition as of 1989.

natural food a food that has been altered as little as possible from the original farm-grown state. As used on labels, this term may misleadingly imply unusual power to promote health and has not been legally defined as of 1989.

organic (chemist's definition) containing carbon atoms or, more precisely, containing carbon-carbon or carbon-hydrogen bonds.

organic (popular definition) referring to foods produced without the use of chemical fertilizers, pesticides, or additives; may also refer to nutrients extracted from natural sources as opposed to those that are chemically synthesized. As used on labels, this term may misleadingly imply unusual power to promote health and has not been legally defined as of 1989.

staple with respect to food, one that is used frequently or daily in the diet; for example, wheat bread in North America, potatoes in Ireland, or rice in the Far East.

standard, it isn't fair to call potato chips "natural" even if the potatoes are organically grown! An apple contains 12 RE of vitamin A; applesauce with the same number of kcalories contains about 5; and apple jelly contains less than 1. Regardless of where these products were purchased—whether at the health food store or at the grocery store—there is something to be said for buying the potato and the apple. Both *are* natural. The more you depend on a food as a staple item, the more important this quality is.

Something else to keep in mind is that some food choices are simply neutral. If you happen to know an organic farmer locally and want to buy his produce, there is certainly no reason not to. His products may be more attractive, more flavorsome, and more desirable to you as a consumer than the same kind of foods available elsewhere. You may want to support his "ecologically sound agriculture" even if it means paying a higher price to do so. If you have taken a fancy to a particular food sold at the local health food store, whatever it may be, there is no reason why you should not buy it and use it. Some foods sold as natural, such as the local baker's whole-grain bread, are truly delicious, nourishing, and worth the extra price if you have the money to spend.

If you don't have the money or don't have a personal preference for specific foods in these special categories, there is no reason that you should make any effort in that direction. It is possible to obtain all the wholesome, nutritious foods you need for a balanced and adequate diet by making educated choices in the regular grocery store.

Notes

1. B. McPherrin, Mail order health fraud, *ACSH News and Views* 1 (September/October 1980): 10.
2. W. H. Lewis, Reporting adverse reactions to herbal ingestants (letter to the editor), *Journal of the American Medical Association* 240 (1978): 109–110.
3. A. Brynjolfsson, Food irradiation and nutrition, *Professional Nutritionist,* Fall 1979, pp. 7–10.

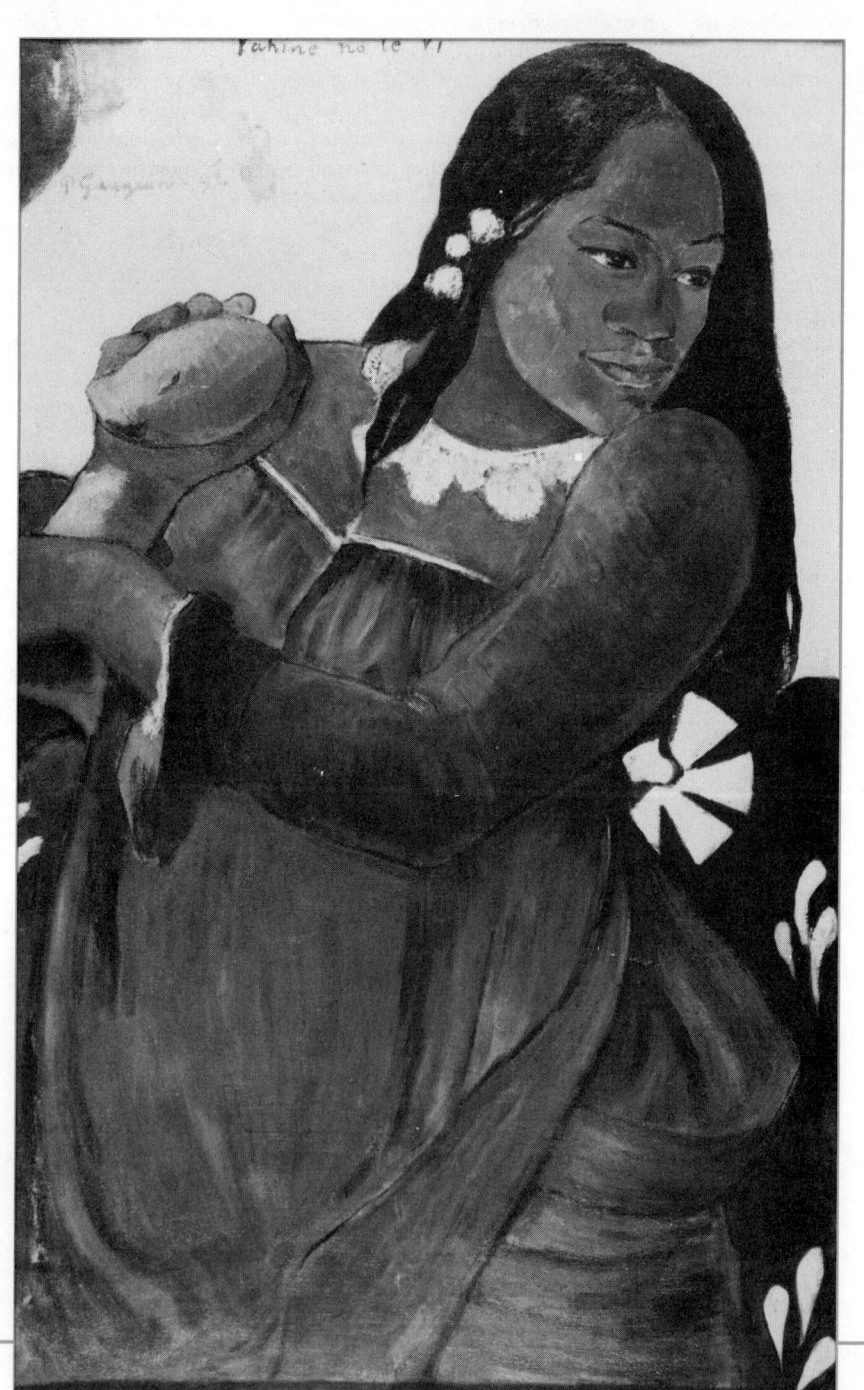

6

Metabolism
and Energy Balance

CONTENTS

"Woman With Mango" by Paul Gauguin, 1892. The Baltimore
Museum of Art: The Cone Collection, formed by Dr. Claribel Cone
and Miss Etta Cone of Baltimore, Maryland.

The way the body manages its energy supply is amazing. Consider, for example, that a 1 percent error in energy intake could cause a person to become more than 200 pounds overweight in her lifetime. Yet most of us maintain our weight, fluctuating only about 10 or 20 pounds, throughout our life. This miraculous energy maintenance system is puzzling in many ways. For instance, when we see two people of the same size who both maintain their ideal weight, it doesn't seem fair that one can eat twice as much as the other. Why does our weight seem to stay the same no matter how hard we try to gain or lose? Are carbohydrate-rich foods more fattening than other foods? What's the best fuel for an athlete? What's the best way to lose weight? Is fasting dangerous? Are low-carbohydrate diets dangerous? The answers to these and many other questions lie in an understanding of metabolism.

In earlier chapters, we introduced the energy-yielding nutrients—carbohydrate, fat, and protein—as they are found in the human body. We then followed the nutrients through digestion to the simpler units they are composed of and showed these units entering the body. Here we will see what becomes of them within the body. The basic units on which metabolism centers are: (1) *glucose* from carbohydrate, (2) *glycerol* from lipids, (3) *fatty acids* from lipids, and (4) *amino acids* from protein.

Metabolism can be defined as the way in which the body handles the energy-yielding nutrients; vitamins and minerals assist in this task. The body can use the energy-yielding nutrients to build new compounds or for energy.

Building Body Compounds

When the basic units are not needed by the cells for energy, they can be used to build body compounds. Glucose units can be strung together to make glycogen chains. Glycerol and fatty acids can be assembled into triglycerides. Amino acids can be used to make protein. These larger compounds have many uses, and they can be used for energy if energy is needed later.

Breaking Down Nutrients for Energy

If the body needs energy, it may break apart any or all of the basic units into smaller fragments. Glucose is broken down first to pyruvate and then to a smaller compound, acetyl CoA. In a series of metabolic reactions called the tricarboxylic acid (TCA) cycle, acetyl CoA splits and donates its energy to storage compounds, or to do the body's work, or to produce heat.

Like glucose, glycerol can be converted to pyruvate and then acetyl CoA, finally releasing energy through the TCA cycle. Fatty acids are not converted to pyruvate; instead they are converted directly into acetyl CoA. The sequence

glucose $\leftrightarrow$ pyruvate $\rightarrow$ acetyl CoA $\rightarrow$ energy

is central to an understanding of metabolism. Notice the two-way arrow between glucose and pyruvate and the one-way arrows after pyruvate. They show that pyruvate can be reconverted to glucose but acetyl CoA cannot. Anything that can be converted to pyruvate can be used to make glucose. Anything broken down to acetyl CoA cannot be used to make glucose.

---

metabolism:
the sum total of all the chemical reactions that go on in living cells. *Energy metabolism* includes all the reactions by which the body obtains and uses energy from food or body stores.
meta = among
bole = change

pyruvate (PIE-roo-vate):
pyruvic acid, a compound derived from glucose and certain amino acids in metabolism. The term *pyruvate* means a salt of pyruvic acid. (Throughout this book the ending *ate* is used interchangeably with *-ic acid*; for our purposes they mean the same thing.)

The metabolic breakdown of glucose to pyruvate is **glycolysis** (gligh-COLL-uh-sis).
glyco = glucose
lysis = breakdown

CoA (coh-AY):
nickname for a small molecule that participates in metabolism. As pyruvate breaks down to the smaller compound *acetic acid,* a molecule of CoA is attached to it, making *acetyl CoA* (ASS-uh-teel or uh-SEET-ul co-AY).

The reactions by which the complete oxidation of acetyl CoA is accomplished are those of the **TCA cycle** or **Krebs cycle** and **oxidative phosphorylation.** The net result is that acetyl CoA splits, and the energy it contained is made available for the body's use.

Fatty acids are converted to acetyl CoA, and for this reason, they *cannot* be used to make glucose. Glycerol can yield glucose, but that represents only about five percent of the weight of a triglyceride molecule. Thus, fat is a poor and inefficient source of glucose. About 95 percent of it cannot be converted to glucose at all; therefore fat, for the most part, cannot normally provide energy for the organs (brain, nervous system) that require glucose for energy metabolism.

Ideally, amino acids will be used to replace needed body proteins and will not be used for energy. If they are needed for energy, they are first stripped of their nitrogen, which can be used to make other compounds, including the nonessential amino acids, or can be excreted. With nitrogen removed, about half of the amino acids can be converted to pyruvate and can therefore provide glucose. The other amino acids are converted to acetyl CoA directly or enter the TCA cycle at another point. Thus protein, unlike fat, is a fairly good source of glucose when carbohydrate is not available. Figure 6–1 depicts these metabolic pathways.

Removal of the amino (NH_2) group from a compound, such as an amino acid, is called **deamination.**

The principal nitrogen-excretion product of metabolism is **urea** (you-REE-uh).

The making of glucose from protein or fat is **gluconeogenesis** (gloo-co-nee-o-JEN-uh-sis). About 5 percent of fat (the glycerol portion of triglycerides) and about 50 percent of protein (the **glycogenic** amino acids) can be converted to glucose.
gluco, glyco = glucose
neo = new
genesis = making

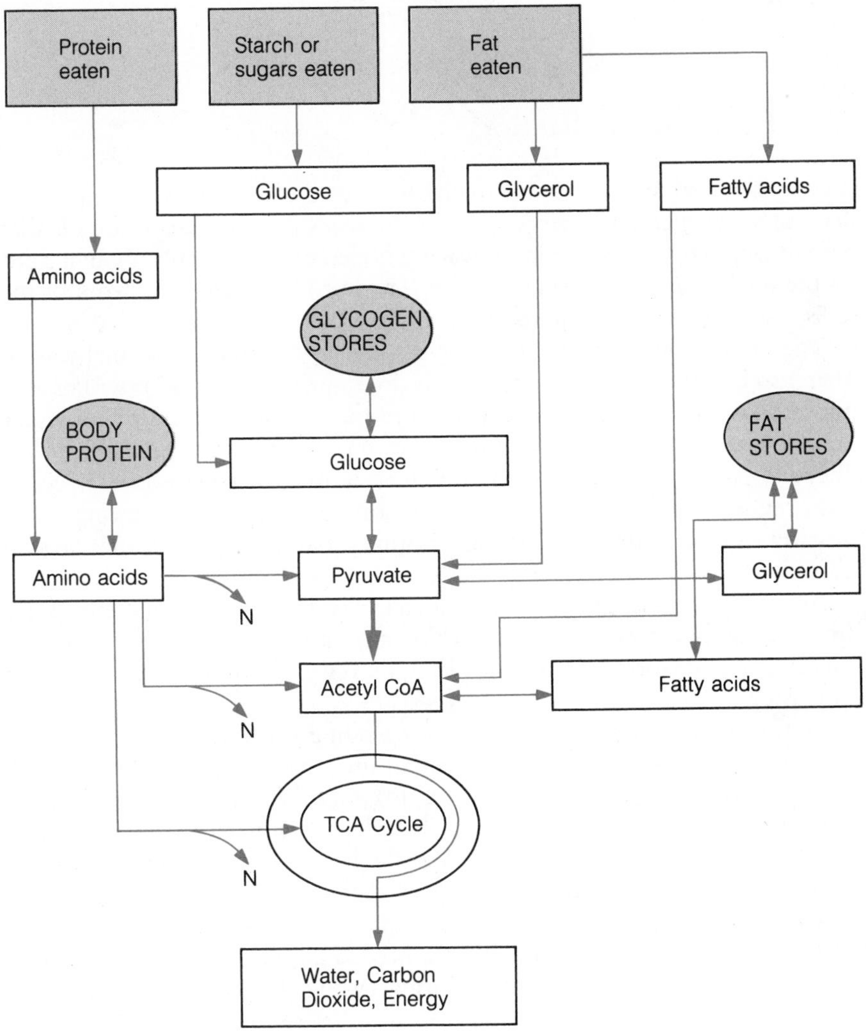

FIGURE 6–1
The central pathways of energy metabolism. Carbohydrate via glucose yields glycogen, fat, or energy. Some amino acids via pyruvate can yield glucose/glycogen. The glycerol from fat (5 percent of total fat) can also yield glucose/glycogen. The remainder of energy stores are found in body fat.

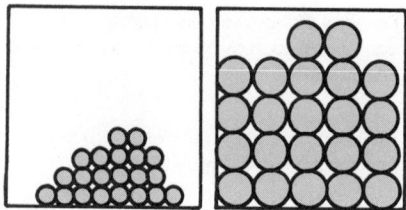

Fat cells enlarge.

The Economy of Feasting

Fat can be made from an excess of any energy-yielding nutrient that you eat. Fat cells enlarge as they fill with fat, and the body's fat-storing capacity seems to be able to expand indefinitely.

Surplus *carbohydrate* (glucose) is first stored as glycogen, but the glycogen-storing cells have limited capacity. Once glycogen stores are filled, the overflow is routed to fat. Thus, excess carbohydrate can contribute to obesity.

In the same way, surplus dietary *fat* can contribute to the fat stores in the body. Fat may break down into fragments, such as acetyl CoA, but if energy flow is already rapid enough to meet the demand, these fragments will not be broken down further. Instead, they will be routed to the assembly of tri-glycerides and stored in the fat cells.

Finally, surplus *protein* may encounter the same fate. If protein is consumed in excess of the need for protein, or is not needed to meet energy needs, amino acids will lose their nitrogens and will be converted through the intermediates, pyruvate and acetyl CoA, to triglycerides. These, too, swell the fat cells and increase body weight.

The Economy of Fasting

Even when you are asleep and totally relaxed, the cells of many organs are hard at work spending energy. In fact, the work that you are aware of, that you do with your muscles during waking hours, represents only about a third of the total energy you spend in a day. The rest is the metabolic work of the cells, which constantly require fuel.

The body's top priority is to meet these energy needs. Its normal way of doing so is by periodic refueling, that is, by eating. When food is withdrawn, the body must find other fuel sources in its own tissues. If people choose not to eat, we say they are fasting; if they have no choice (as in a famine), we say they are starving; but no metabolic difference exists between the two. In either case, the body is forced to switch to a wasting metabolism by drawing on its reserves of carbohydrate and fat and, within a day or so, on its vital protein tissues as well.

As the fast begins, glucose from the liver's stored glycogen and fatty acids from the body's stored fat are both flowing into cells, delivering energy to power the cells' work. Several hours later, however, the liver glycogen is being exhausted.

At this point, most of the cells are depending on fatty acids to continue providing their fuel. The brain cells cannot use fatty acids, however; they still need glucose, which is their energy fuel. Even if other energy fuel is available, glucose has to be present to permit the brain's energy-metabolizing machinery to work. Normally, the nervous system (brain and nerves) consumes about two thirds of the total glucose used each day—about 400 to 600 kcalories' worth.[1]

Because fat stores cannot provide the needed glucose, body protein tissues always break down to some extent during fasting. In the first few days of a

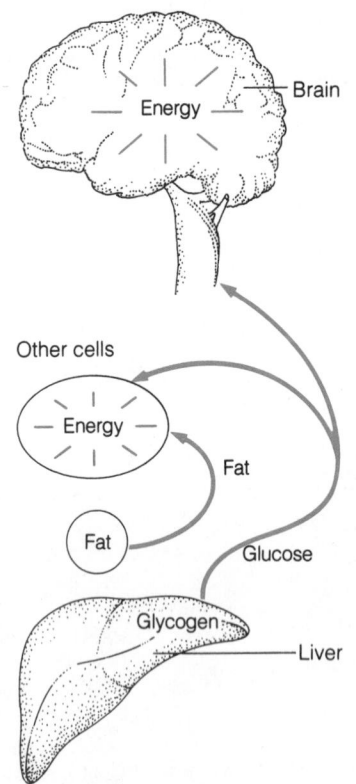

The liver releases glucose, and the fat cells release fat to be used as fuel by the body's cells, but the brain can use only glucose.

fast, body protein provides about 90 percent of the needed glucose, and glycerol provides about 10 percent. If body protein loss were to continue at this rate, death would ensue within three weeks. However, as the fast continues, the body adapts by condensing together acetyl CoA fragments derived from fatty acids to produce ketones, an alternative energy source. Normally produced and used only in small quantities, ketones can serve some brain cells as fuel. Ketone production rises until, at the end of several weeks, it is meeting about half or more of the nervous system's energy needs. Still, many areas of the brain rely exclusively on glucose, and body protein continues to be sacrificed to produce it.[2] Figure 6–2 shows the metabolic events that occur during fasting.

As fasting continues and the body is shifting to the use of ketones, the body simultaneously reduces its energy output and conserves both its fat and lean tissue. Because of the slowed metabolism, the loss of fat falls to a bare minimum. Thus, although weight loss during fasting may be quite dramatic, fat loss may actually be less than when some food is supplied.

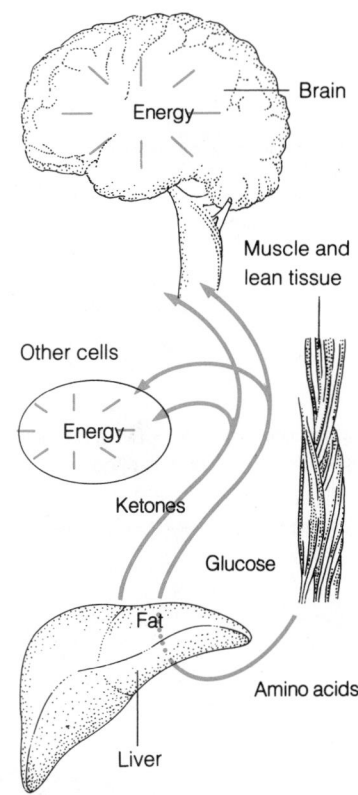

In prolonged fasting, muscle and lean tissue atrophy to supply amino acids for conversion to glucose. This glucose, with ketones produced from fat, fuels the brain's activities.

ketone (KEE-tone):
a compound formed from fatty acids. Small amounts of ketones are a normal part of the blood chemistry, but when their concentration rises, they spill into the urine. The combination of high blood ketones (ketonemia) and ketones in the urine (ketonuria) is termed *ketosis*.

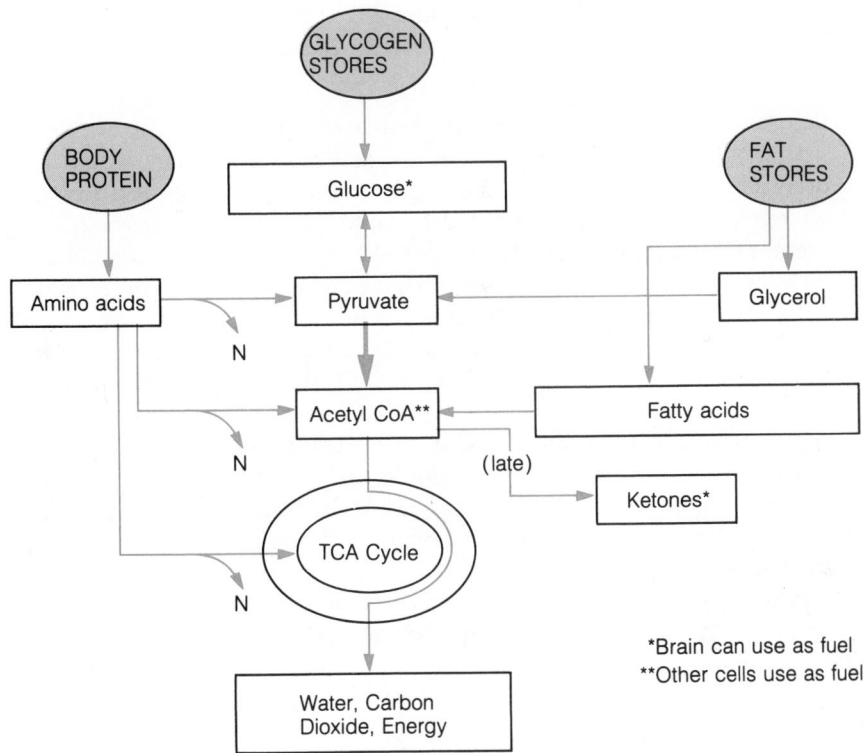

*Brain can use as fuel
**Other cells use as fuel

FIGURE 6–2

Fasting. All body stores break down. Glycogen is soon exhausted. Some amino acids and 5 percent of body fat are used to provide fuel for the brain. The other amino acids and 95 percent of fat provide fuel for other cells by way of acetyl CoA.

In late fasting, acetyl CoA condenses to ketones, which the brain can use as fuel. The brain continues to require glucose from body proteins as well.

The body's adaptations to fasting are sufficient to maintain life for a long period. Mental alertness need not be diminished. Even physical energy may remain unimpaired for a surprisingly long time. Still, fasting is not without its hazards. Wasting, impaired resistance to disease, and lowered body temperature occur. Physician-supervised fasting has revealed many other changes, including disturbances of the body's salt and water balance.

Similar alterations are seen in low-carbohydrate dieting (discussed in the next section). Renewed food intake, especially of carbohydrate, results in dramatic changes in the body's salt and water balance, accounting for most of the wide swings in body weight seen in people on fasts or low-carbohydrate diets.[3]

Fasting = Living on the body's fat and protein.

The Low-Carbohydrate Diet

An economy similar to that of fasting prevails when a low-carbohydrate diet is consumed; ketosis occurs. Advocates of the low-carbohydrate diet would have you believe there is something magical about ketosis, something that promotes faster weight loss than a regular low-kcalorie diet. In fact, however, the low-carbohydrate diet presents the same problem as a fast. Once the body's available glycogen reserves are spent, the only significant remaining source of energy in the form of glucose is protein. The low-carbohydrate diet provides a little protein from food, but some must still be taken from body tissue. The onset of ketosis is the signal that this wasting process has begun.

Low-carbohydrate diet = Living on (dietary and body) fat and protein almost exclusively.

Low-kcalorie diet = Living on limited food and body fat.

People are attracted to the low-carbohydrate diet because of the dramatic weight loss it brings about within the first few days. They would be disillusioned if they realized that much of this weight loss is a loss of glycogen and protein accompanied by large quantities of water and important minerals. A dieter who boasts of losing seven pounds in two days on a low-carbohydrate diet must be unaware that a pound or two, at best, is fat and five or six pounds are lean tissue, water, and minerals. Once "off" the diet, the dieter's body will avidly devour and retain these needed materials, and weight will zoom back to within a few pounds of the starting point.

The person who wishes to lose body *fat* will select a balanced diet of 1,200 kcalories or more, one containing carbohydrate, fat, *and* protein. At this level, body protein will be spared, ketosis will not occur, vital lean tissues (including both muscle and brain) will not starve, and unwanted *fat* will be lost.

A warning is suggested by these facts. Beware of those who promote quick weight-loss schemes. Learn to distinguish between loss of *fat* and loss of *weight*.

The Protein-Sparing Fast

A variant on fasting is the technique of eating only protein. The hope is that the protein will spare lean tissue and that body fat will be broken down at a maximal rate to meet other energy needs. You may suspect that this is not

Protein-sparing fast = Eating only protein.

so different from the low-carbohydrate diet and will guess that this protein, together with the body's lean tissues, will be used to provide glucose. You are probably right. The protein-sparing idea sounded good when it was first advanced, but it has met with mixed results.

Two approaches have been used with protein-sparing fasting: the medical approach and the popular approach. The first has been safe, but the second has been dangerous. The medical approach allows only carefully screened people to participate. They consume 400 to 600 kcalories a day of protein-rich foods, such as lean meat, fish, or a high-quality complete amino acid preparation supplemented with vitamins and minerals, and their progress is accompanied by conscientious monitoring, especially of critical water and mineral balances. This fast has been successful in promoting large weight losses in people who might not otherwise lose weight, although it is not an ideal approach. It seems to become effective only after considerable lean tissue has already been lost, at which time the body may be conserving itself quite efficiently anyway. The protein-sparing fast has not been shown more effective than a diet containing a mixture of protein and carbohydrate. Furthermore, it doesn't seem to "stick" very well; that is, most people regain the lost weight.

The popular use of the protein-sparing fast has been an entirely different matter. *The Last Chance Diet,* a popular paperback published in 1977, led thousands of people to follow a so-called protein-sparing regimen in which several important principles were ignored. The Last Chance Diet required that people purchase and use only a predigested liquid protein product named Prolinn while they were fasting. Fad dieters, usually without any medical supervision, drank liquid protein potions prepared from low-quality sources, or consumed very low kcalorie, high-protein diets and lost dramatic amounts of weight—including, of course, lean tissue, water, and vital minerals. Within the year, 11 deaths had been ascribed to the fad, and since then, many more have died. High-biological-value protein supplements were used by some of the victims—so the quality of the protein was not alone responsible for the deaths.[4] Mineral deficiencies were suspected as contributing factors.

As a result of its investigation, the FDA ruled that liquid protein and other protein products promoted for use in weight reduction or as dietary supplements have to carry warning labels. We have learned a hard lesson at great cost.

The term *protein-sparing* has also been used in another connection. Malnourished people in the hospital also lose body protein. Such loss is likely to occur and is especially dangerous if the person is simultaneously fighting infection. Physicians make every effort to prevent the loss of vital lean tissue by supplying amino acids as well as glucose in some form—through a vein if the person can't eat. The effort to provide protein-sparing *therapy* in such circumstances should not be confused with the profiteering of faddists who promote the protein-sparing *fast*.

Moderate Weight Loss

Someone who wants to lose body fat must reconcile himself to the hard fact that there is a limit to the rate at which this tissue will break down. The maximum rate, except for a very large, very active person, is one to two pounds a week. The most effective means to achieve weight loss that actually reflects body-fat loss, is to adopt a balanced, low-kcalorie diet supplying all three energy nutrients in reasonable amounts while increasing energy expenditure by getting more exercise.[5] In effect, this means adjusting the energy budget so that intake is 500 to 1,000 kcalories per day less than output. Safe and effective weight reduction diets are covered in Chapters 9 and 18.

The Body's Energy Output

How can you count the kcalories you expend in a day? To answer this question, let's first take a look at the ways you use energy.

Human energy is spent in two major ways—on the basal metabolic processes and on voluntary activities. A way of estimating the total energy you spend is to estimate these components individually, then add them together.

The first component, basal metabolic energy, is by far the largest item in most people's energy budgets. It consists of the energy spent to keep the heart beating, the lungs inhaling and exhaling air, the cells conducting their metabolic activities, and the nerves generating their continuous streams of electrical impulses—in short, it consists of the energy spent to support life.

The basal metabolic rate (BMR) is the rate at which kcalories are spent for these maintenance activities, usually expressed as kcalories per hour. The BMR varies from one person to the next as well as for one individual with changed circumstances, physical condition, or age. The BMR is lowest when someone is lying down in a room at a comfortable temperature and not digesting any food. These are the conditions under which it is measured.

Basal metabolic rate is higher in people with greater lean body mass, in people with fever or under stress, and in people with high thyroid gland activity. It is lowered by loss of lean tissue due to inactivity, fasting, or malnutrition. The following box shows how basal metabolic energy can be estimated from a person's weight and sex.

basal metabolism:
the total energy output of a body at rest after a 12-hour fast; also called *basal metabolic rate* or *BMR*.

Shortcut for Estimating Energy Output: Basal Metabolism

Use the factor 1.0 kcalorie per kilogram of body weight per hour for men or 0.9 for women. The following is an example for a 150-pound man.

1. Change pounds to kilograms:
$$\frac{150 \text{ lb}}{2.2 \text{ lb}} \times 1.0 \text{ kg} = 68 \text{ kg.}$$

2. Multiply weight in kilograms by the BMR factor:
68 kg × 1 kcal/kg/hr = 68 kcal/hr

3. Multiply the kcalories used in one hour by the hours in a day:
68 kcal/hr × 24 hr/day = 1632 kcal/day.

Energy for BMR equals 1,632 kcalories per day.

The second component of energy output is physical activity. As disheartening as it may be to discover, intense mental activity requires only slightly more energy than normal nervous system activity, even though it may make you very tired. Vigorous, prolonged muscular activity, on the other hand, uses up a great many kcalories. In addition to the muscles involved in moving the body, the heart must beat faster to send nutrients and oxygen to the muscles, and the lungs must move faster to get rid of the carbon dioxide and bring in additional oxygen.

The amount of energy needed for a physical activity depends on two factors: body weight and duration of the activity. A heavier person needs more kcalories than a lighter person does when performing the same task in the same amount of time, because it takes extra effort to move the additional body weight. Also, the longer a person continues an activity, the more kcalories it will cost. You can estimate the energy needed for activities by using the rules of thumb offered in the following box.

Shortcut for Estimating Energy Output: Voluntary Muscular Activity

The figures we use are crude approximations based on the amount of muscular work a person typically performs in a day. To select the one appropriate for you, remember to think in terms of the amount of *muscular* work performed. Don't confuse being *busy* with being *active*.

- For sedentary (mostly sitting) activity (a typist), add 50 percent of the BMR.
- For light activity (a teacher), add 60 percent.
- For heavy work (a roofer), add 100 percent or more.

If the man we used in the previous example were a typist, we would estimate the energy he needed for physical activities by multiplying his BMR kcalories per day by 50 percent:

1,632 kcal/day × 50% = 816 kcal/day. His energy need for activities equals 816 kcalories per day.

The total energy a person spends in a day is derived by adding the two components together.

Shortcut for Estimating Energy Output: Total

In a day, the man in our example spends 1,632 kcal/day + 816 kcal/day = 2,448 kcal/day. Because the exact figure is based on several estimates, it's probably best to express his needs as falling within about a 100-kcalorie range: total energy equals about 2,400 to 2,500 kcalories per day.

Some energy expenditure not taken into account in this estimate is that required for the body to manage food. When food is taken into the body, many cells that have been dormant begin to be active. The muscles that move the food through the intestinal tract speed up their rhythmic contractions; the cells that manufacture and secrete digestive juices begin their tasks. All these and other cells need extra energy as they come alive to participate in the digestion, absorption, and metabolism of food. This stimulation of cellular activity is called diet-induced thermogenesis, and is generally thought to represent about 6 to 10 percent of the total food energy taken in. For purposes of rough estimates, diet-induced thermogenesis can be ignored; the 10 percent it might contribute to total energy output is smaller than the probable errors involved in estimating energy input from food or output for activities.

Diet-induced thermogenesis is also sometimes called the **specific dynamic effect (SDE)** or **specific dynamic activity (SDA)** of food.

Energy Balance: Weight Loss and Gain

In the average person of average height, a deficit of 500 kcalories a day brings about a loss of body fat at the rate of a pound a week; a deficit of 1,000 kcalories brings about a loss of two pounds a week. Extraordinarily active people, by virtue of their high energy expenditures, or extremely obese persons, by virtue of the high energy cost of maintaining and moving their bodies, can lose weight faster. For those who are only moderately obese, the maximum possible rate of fat loss is one to two pounds a week, which for most people means an intake of about 1,000 to 1,500 kcalories a day. Below 1,000 to 1,200 kcalories a day, the dieter will be losing lean tissue. It is difficult for the diet planner to achieve adequate vitamin and mineral intake at such a restricted kcalorie level.

1 lb = 3,500 kcal. A pound of body fat is actually composed of a mixture of fat, protein, and water and yields 3,500 kcal when metabolized. A pound of pure fat (454 g) would yield 4,086 kcal at 9 kcal/g.

Although these principles are simple, putting them into practice is more difficult than you might imagine. Obesity and underweight are complex problems with social and psychological ramifications as well as the metabolic ones just described. Chapters 17 and 18 deal with the problems of underweight and overweight and provide some practical pointers for the person who wants to lose or gain weight.

SELF-STUDY

How Much Energy Do You Spend in a Day?

Use the boxes in Chapter 6 (Shortcut for Estimating Energy Output) to estimate the energy you spend in a day. Form 7 will help you record your calculations.

Notes:

1. G. F. Cahill, T. T. Aoki, and A. A. Rossini, Metabolism in obesity and anorexia nervosa, in *Nutrition and the Brain,* vol. 3, eds. R. J. Wurtman and J. J. Wurtman (New York: Raven Press, 1979), pp. 1–70.

2. R. A. Hawkins and J. F. Biebuyck, Ketone bodies are selectively used by individual brain regions, *Science* 205 (1979): 325–327.

3. Cahill, Aoki, and Rossini, 1979.

4. T. B. Van Itallie and M. U. Yang, Cardial dysfunction in obese dieters: A potentially lethal complication of rapid, massive weight loss, *American Journal of Clinical Nutrition* 39 (1984): 695–702.

5. C. M. Tipton, Exercise, training and hypertension, *Exercise and Sports Sciences Reviews* 12 (1984): 245–306.

Form 7:
Shortcut for Estimating Energy Output

1. Basal metabolism
   - Step 1: My weight in pounds (_____ lb) divided by 2.2 pounds per kilogram equals my weight in kilograms: _____ kg.
   - Step 2: My weight in kilograms (_____ kg) times 1.0 kcal/kg/hr for men or 0.9 kcal/kg/hr for women equals the number of kcalories I spend on basal metabolism in an hour: _____ kcal/hr.
   - Step 3: My energy expenditure per hour (_____ kcal/hr) times the hours in a day (24) equals the number of kcalories I spend on basal metabolism in a day: _____ kcal/day.

2. Activities (check one)

   _____ I am sedentary, so my activities cost 50 percent of my basal metabolic energy each day. Fifty percent of my basal metabolic energy (step 3) equals _____ kcal/day.

   _____ I am lightly active, so my activities cost 60 percent of my basal metabolic energy each day. Sixty percent of my basal metabolic energy (step 3) equals _____ kcal/day.

   _____ I am very active, so my activities cost 100 percent of my basal metabolic energy each day. One hundred percent of my basal metabolic energy (step 3) equals _____ kcal/day.

3. Total energy spent in a day
   - Energy for basal metabolism: _____ kcal/day.
   - Energy for activities: _____ kcal/day.
   - Total: _____ kcal/day.

Nutrition and the Alcohol Abuser

Alcohol is one of the most widely abused drugs in the world. Alcoholism takes a heavy toll on the health of the 10 million adults and 3.3 million teenagers who are considered problem drinkers in the United States.[1] Alcoholism is a serious and debilitating disease that frequently results in illness, disability, and death. Furthermore, the effects of alcohol on nutrition and metabolism—both as a direct effect and as a consequence of alcohol-related diseases—are significant. Every alcohol abuser should be considered at risk for poor nutrition status.

Before we go any further, I would like you to clarify exactly what alcoholism is. That's an important starting point because many people have misconceptions about alcoholism. Most people feel that they can take alcohol or leave it, but about one in every ten drinkers, for unknown reasons, becomes an addict and develops a risky relationship with alcohol. Although these people may be able to drink moderately on some occasions, on others they drink far more than they intend to, exhibiting loss of control. These occasions occur unpredictably at first, but more and more often the first drink becomes the first of too many—an episode of uncontrolled drinking.

The addict's craving for alcohol becomes marked by several features. The addict thinks about alcohol a lot (obsession), drinks it in spite of resolving not to (broken promises), and then suffers remorse. Someone who exhibits feelings that strong about a substance should suspect addiction. Note, too, that these feelings do not reflect moral degeneracy. The person is simply someone whose internal makeup reacts in a special way to alcohol.

Why is it that all alcohol abusers are considered as risks for poor nutrition status?
Alcohol abusers are at risk for poor nutrition status because alcohol itself can affect the ingestion, digestion, absorption, metabolism, and excretion of nutrients. Since alcohol can affect virtually every organ, other complications frequently develop that also change nutrient requirements. Some of these include

- Accidents (cuts, bruises, or fractures from car accidents, falls, or fights).
- Anemia (Chapter 8).
- Gastritis and ulcers (Chapter 16).
- Pancreatitis (Chapter 20).
- Liver disease (Chapter 22).

I see. What about alcohol's effect on body weight? I had an uncle who abused alcohol, and I remember his getting thinner and thinner. I thought alcohol had a lot of kcalories. Why did he lose weight?
You are right about alcohol's having a lot of kcalories. In some cases, drinking too much alcohol can cause obesity, but chronic alcoholism seems to have the opposite effect. We do not completely understand the reasons for alcohol-induced weight loss, but several factors seem to contribute to it. For one thing, the chronic alcohol abuser loses appetite and has irregular eating habits. For another, alcohol impairs absorption of all nutrients and alcohol abuse often causes diarrhea. Alcohol may also alter metabolism. Researchers have shown that when kcalories from alcohol are substituted for the same number of kcalories from carbohydrate, significant weight loss occurs.

From what you've said, chronic alcohol abusers aren't just losing weight, they are also eating inadequate amounts of other nutrients as well.
Yes, kcalories from alcohol displace kcalories from food. Alcohol is empty kcalories, like pure sugar or pure fat; the more kcalories you spend on it, the fewer you have to spend on nutritious foods. Nutrient deficiencies are an almost inevitable result of alcohol abuse, not only because the person who drinks obtains fewer nutrients from food but also because alcohol interferes with the body's use of nutrients, making them ineffective even if they are present.

What do you mean?
Well, for example, alcohol abuse causes changes in the intestine that result in the malabsorption of thiamin, folacin, and other nutrients. Additionally, major changes also occur

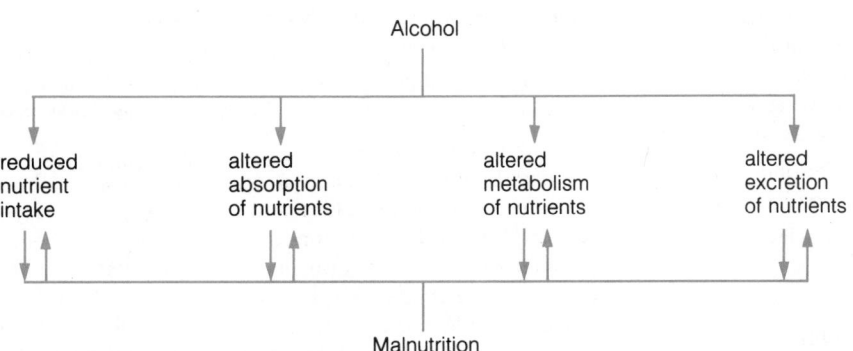

Alcohol and malnutrition interrelationships.

in the way the body metabolizes many nutrients, particularly protein, carbohydrate, and fat. Although we can't discuss all these changes, it is important to mention some of their effects.

Dietary glucose and dietary fat can't be metabolized as they normally are. Instead, they are diverted into making fat, and this fat may accumulate in the liver. Fatty liver, the first stage of liver deterioration in the heavy drinker (which can be reversed by abstinence from alcohol), can progress to cirrhosis (which is irreversible).

Alcohol also interferes with amino acid metabolism. Protein deficiency develops from depression of protein synthesis in the cells and from poor diet. Even the amino acids that a person eats are not used efficiently.

Are other nutrients affected?
Alcohol can also deplete the body's supplies of thiamin and niacin. Not only is thiamin malabsorbed, as mentioned, but also both nutrients are used extensively and preferentially for metabolizing alcohol. This has a profound effect on every cell of the body. There may be abundant glucose going past the cells, but cells need thiamin and niacin to use the glucose to do their work. Brain cells are especially affected because they rely on glucose for their energy.

The metabolism of many other nutrients is altered by chronic alcohol use. Most dramatic is alcohol's effect on folacin. When alcohol is present, the liver, which normally contains enough folacin to meet all needs, leaks folacin into the blood. As blood folacin levels rise, the kidneys are deceived into excreting folacin as if it were in excess. Because alcohol also interferes with the absorption of folacin, the problem is compounded.

Alcohol also causes an increased excretion of water through the kidneys. With it important minerals, such as magnesium, potassium, and zinc, are lost. So you see, alcohol profoundly affects nutrition status.

What are the long-term effects of these nutrient changes caused by alcohol abuse?
The long-term effects of alcohol abuse can cause damage to different organs for different individuals, but alcohol always affects all organs and organ systems to various extents.

The most common damage is to the liver, where the function of affected cells is lost forever. The injury to the liver results in many side effects, such as high blood pressure, which may lead to heart damage and stroke. The protein deficiencies that develop contribute to increased susceptibility to infection. As the synthesis of fat speeds up, fat is deposited in the heart, arteries, and liver. Although alcohol was at one time believed to reduce heart disease risk, the lipoproteins that are elevated by alcohol use are not the same ones that are protective against heart disease.[2]

The central nervous system is particularly sensitive to alcohol. There are mineral alterations in the brain with alcohol consumption.[3] The brain

96 CHAPTER 6

NUTRITION IN PRACTICE 6

shrinks even in people who drink only moderately, but the extent of damage from alcohol is proportional to the amount drunk.[4] The following are a few of the other effects of alcohol:

- Inflammation of the intestines; ulcers of the stomach and intestines.

- Deterioration of the muscles, including the heart muscle.

- Reduced capacity for exercise; heart discomfort sooner during exercise.

- Kidney damage, bladder damage, prostate gland damage.

- Reduced resistance to disease.

- Loss of function of the testicles and damage to the adrenal glands, leading to feminization and sexual impotence in men.

- Failure of the ovaries and early menopause in women.

- Increased susceptibility to lung infections.

The effects of alcohol are frightening. Eating well or even taking supplements of protein, vitamins, and minerals will not protect the drinker. There is no set level of safe drinking where no adverse effects take place. Even just a couple of drinks set in motion the process described, but the next day's abstinence reverses them. Some place between abstinence and alcoholism, there may be alcohol intakes moderate enough not to harm health, but the more a person drinks, the closer to a dangerous extreme that person is.

Notes:

1. U.S. Department of Health and Human Services, *Third Special Report of the U.S. Congress on Alcohol and Health from the Secretary of Health, Education, and Welfare* (Washington, D.C.: Government Printing Office, 1978).
2. D. A. Roe, Alcohol-induced malabsorption, *Nutrition and the MD,* August 1984.
3. C. C. Gibbons, N. Singleton and J. Nyenhuis, Effects of exercise on alcohol-fed rats, *Biochemical Archives,* 3(1987): 23–39.
4. D. W. Walker and coauthors, Neuronal loss in hippocampus induced by prolonged ethanol consumption in rats, *Science* 209 (1980):711–713.

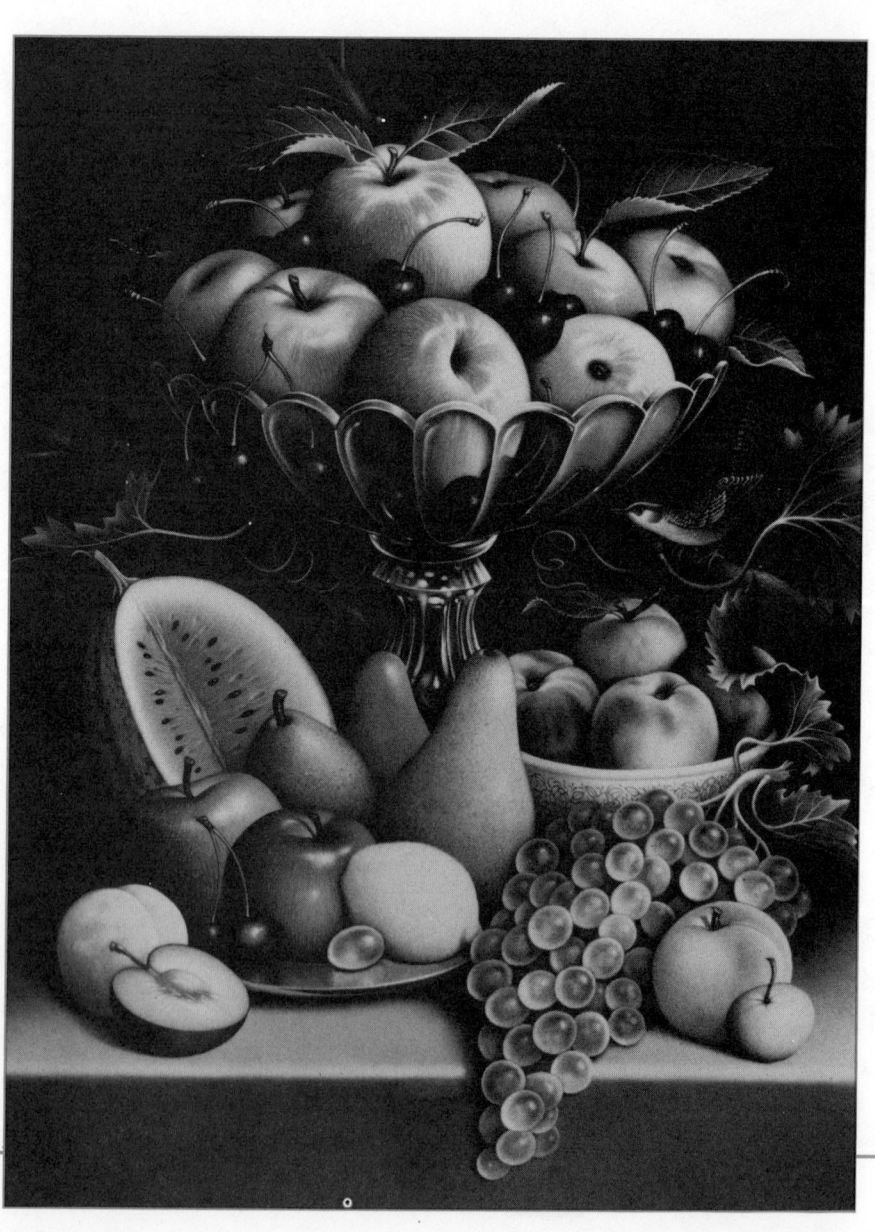

CHAPTER
7
The Vitamins

CONTENTS

Illustration by Braldt Braids with permission to reprint from
Crabtree and Evelyn.

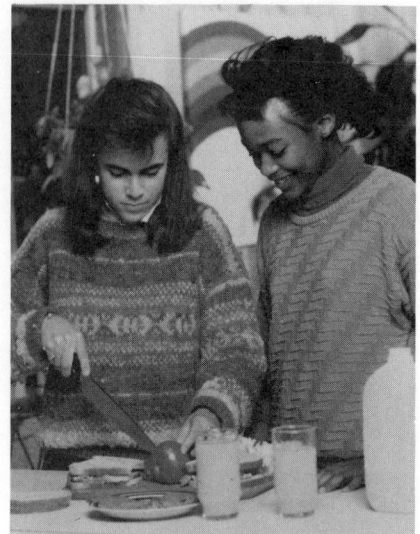

To achieve superb nutritional health, you need much more than a vitamin tablet. You need a variety of nutritious foods.

Television commercials may have you believe that you can transform yourself from a tired, stressed, droopy person to a trim and bouncy picture of health with only a little effort. How? Just take Brand A vitamins. If only life were so simple.

The vitamins themselves make no contribution of energy or even of building materials for the body. Instead, they serve as helpers or facilitators of body processes. It is true that without vitamins, you would certainly feel tired and would lack energy. After all, some of the vitamins serve as helpers to the enzymes that release energy from nutrients. Other vitamins help manufacture red blood cells, which carry oxygen to the tissues. Oxygen must be present for energy release to occur. Still other vitamins play key roles in building and repairing tissues.

Vitamins are key contributors to your physical fitness, but they certainly do not cure all ills. Actually, a vitamin or mineral can cure only the disease caused by a deficiency of that vitamin. To make a magical transformation, you would need much more than a vitamin tablet. You would need adequate amounts of other nutrients—energy nutrients, minerals, and water—as well as adequate sleep and exercise and a positive attitude, to name only a few other elements of lifestyle.

Definition and Classification of Vitamins

A child once defined vitamins as "what, if you don't eat, you get sick." The description is one of the most insightful we've seen, and it is also accurate. A less imaginative definition is that a vitamin is a potent, indispensable, noncaloric organic compound that performs specific and individual functions to promote growth or reproduction or to maintain health and life. Two factors distinguish vitamins from energy nutrients:

1. Vitamins do not provide energy that the body can use.

2. Vitamins are needed in much smaller amounts than the energy nutrients.

Vitamins are often classified on the basis of whether they are soluble in fats or in water. This discussion of vitamins begins with the fat-soluble vitamins.

The Fat-Soluble Vitamins

Vitamins A, D, E, and K are the fat-soluble vitamins. These vitamins are found in the fats and oils of foods. They are absorbed from the GI tract in the same way as lipids. Therefore, any condition that interferes with fat absorption can precipitate a deficiency of the fat-soluble vitamins. Once in the bloodstream, these vitamins are escorted by protein carriers because they are insoluble in water. Because the fat-soluble vitamins can be stored in body tissues, it is possible for them to reach toxic levels.

Vitamin A

Vitamin A has the distinction of being the first fat-soluble vitamin to be recognized. Vitamin A is also one of the most versatile because of its role in several important body processes, one of which is vision.

For a person to see, light reaching the eye must be transformed into nerve impulses that the brain interprets to produce visual images. The transformers are molecules of pigment in the cells of the retina (see Figure 7–1). A portion of each pigment molecule is retinal, a compound the body can synthesize only if vitamin A or certain of its relatives are supplied by the diet. When vitamin A is deficient, the eye has difficulty in adapting to changing light levels. A flash of bright light at night (after the eye has adapted to darkness) might be followed by a prolonged spell of night blindness. Because night blindness is easy to test, it aids in the diagnosis of vitamin A deficiency. Night blindness is only a symptom, however, and may indicate a condition other than vitamin A deficiency.

Although the vital role that vitamin A plays in vision is undeniably important, only one thousandth of the vitamin A in the body is in the retina. Most of the body's vitamin A is involved in maintaining the integrity of the mucous membranes, which are composed of epithelial cells. These cells lining the surfaces of many body tissues secrete a smooth and slippery substance (mucus) that coats and protects them from invasive microorganisms and other harmful particles. The mucous lining of the stomach also shields its cells from digestion by gastric juices.

In vitamin A deficiency, the epithelial cells flatten and harden, losing their protective mucous coating. Instead of staying smooth and well-rounded and producing normal mucus, they secrete keratin in its place. In the eye, this process leads to drying and hardening of the cornea, which may progress to permanent blindness. Damage to the eyes is most pronounced in the young; thousands of cases of blindness result from vitamin A deficiency throughout the world.

In the mouth, a vitamin A deficiency results in drying and hardening of the salivary glands, making them susceptible to infection. Mucous secretion in the

retina (RET-in-uh):
the layer of light-sensitive cells lining the back of the inside of the eye; consists of rods and cones.

pigment:
a molecule capable of absorbing certain wavelengths of light. Pigments in the eye permit us to perceive different colors.

retinal (RET-in-al):
the aldehyde form of vitamin A, active in the pigments of the eye.

night blindness:
slow recovery of vision after flashes of bright light at night; an early symptom of vitamin A deficiency.

The membranes are the **mucosa** (myoo-COH-suh). They are composed of cells that line the surfaces of body tissues. The mucosa include membranes lining the respiratory tract, gastrointestinal tract, urinary tract, uterus, vagina, eyelids, and sinus passageways.

mucus (adjective **mucous**):
a substance secreted by the epithelial cells of the mucosa.

In the eye, the symptoms of vitamin A deficiency are collectively known as **xerophthalmia** (zer-off-THAL-mee-uh).
xero = dry
ophthalm = eye

An early sign is **xerosis** (drying of the cornea); the last and most severe stage is **keratomalacia** (kerr-uh-to-mal-AY-shuh) (total blindness).
malacia = softening, weakening

cornea (KOR-nee-uh):
the transparent membrane covering the outside of the front of the eye.

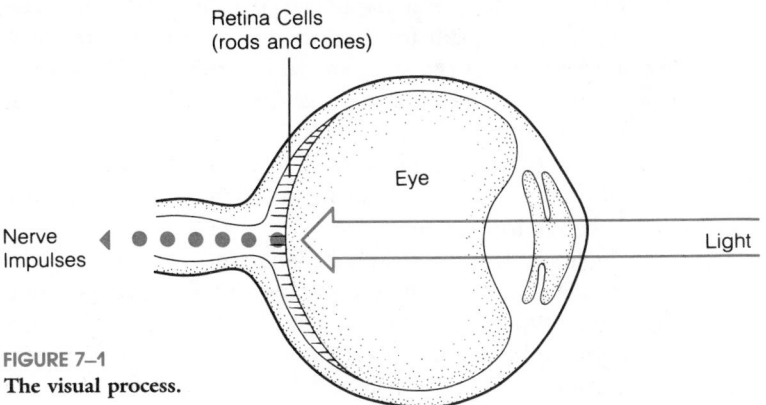

FIGURE 7–1
The visual process.

As light enters the eye, pigments within the cells of the retina absorb the light and generate nerve impulses that travel into the brain.

keratin (KERR-uh-tin):
a water-insoluble protein; the normal protein of hair and nails. Keratin may be produced under abnormal conditions by cells that normally produce mucus. Keratin accumulation is known as *keratinization*. The progression of this condition to the extreme is *hyperkeratosis*. *hyper* = too much

The accumulation of the hard material keratin around each hair follicle is **follicular hyperkeratosis.**

follicle (FOLL-i-cul):
a group of cells in the skin from which a hair grows.

The protein that carries retinol in the blood is **retinol-binding protein (RBP).** Measurement of RBP is a sensitive test of vitamin A status.

preformed vitamin A:
vitamin A in its active form.

precursor:
a compound that can be converted into another compound. For example, carotene is a precursor of vitamin A.

beta-carotene:
an orange pigment found in plants.

RE (retinol equivalent):
a measure of vitamin A activity; the amount of retinol that a vitamin A compound will yield after conversion in the body.

retinol:
one of the active forms of vitamin A, used as the standard for measuring vitamin A activity.

stomach and intestines is reduced, hindering normal digestion and absorption of nutrients. Infections of other mucous membranes are also more likely.

All body surfaces, both inside and out, are maintained with the help of vitamin A. Vitamin A is essential for healthy skin, another epithelial tissue. Cells on the outer body surface harden and flatten, making the skin dry, rough, scaly, and hard when vitamin A is lacking. An accumulation of hard material makes a lump around each hair follicle.

Vitamin A serves many other purposes in the body. It is important for normal bone growth, reproduction, and maintenance of cell membrane stability.

Three different forms of vitamin A are active: retinol, retinal, and retinoic acid. A zinc-containing protein transports vitamin A via the blood from the liver, where it is stored, to sites where it is needed. For this reason, a zinc deficiency can mimic the symptoms of vitamin A deficiency.

Up to a year's supply of vitamin A can be stored in the body, 90 percent of it in the liver. If you stop eating good food sources of vitamin A, deficiency symptoms will not begin to appear until after your stores are depleted. Then, however, the consequences are profound and severe. Table 7–1 itemizes some of them.

Among nutrition problems afflicting the young of the world, vitamin A deficiency is second in extent only to protein-kcalorie malnutrition. In the United States as well, the problem of vitamin A deficiency is all too common. According to recent surveys, about a third of the population has intakes well below the RDA. Spanish Americans and blacks exhibit some outward signs of deficiency.

Because vitamin A is stored in the body, toxicity can also occur. Overdoses damage the same body systems that exhibit symptoms in vitamin A deficiency (see Table 7–1). The availability of breakfast cereals, instant meals, fortified milk, and chewable candylike vitamins, each containing 100 percent of the recommended daily intake of vitamin A, makes it possible for a well-meaning parent to provide several times the daily allowance of the vitamin to a child within a few hours.

Normally, it is possible to suffer toxicity symptoms only when excess amounts of preformed vitamin A from supplements are taken. The precursor, beta-carotene, which is available from plant foods, does not convert to vitamin A rapidly enough to cause toxicity but is instead stored in fat depots as carotene. Being yellow in color, it may accumulate under the skin to such an extent that the overdoser actually turns yellow.

Adults are advised to avoid intakes of more than 5 to 10 times the recommended amounts of preformed vitamin A to ensure safety.[1] It makes sense to get your vitamin A from natural sources.

Vitamin A recommendations have been expressed in retinol equivalents (RE) since 1980, but food contents of vitamin A are sometimes still expressed using an older terminology, international units (IU). Until this discrepancy is corrected in food tables, you will have to convert from one form to the other if you want to compare your vitamin A intake with recommendations. A rule of thumb is that 1 RE = 5 IU on the average, given a diet composed of both animal and plant sources of vitamin A. Thus, for example, 10,000 IU of vitamin A would convert to 2,000 RE.

TABLE 7–1 Key Information About Vitamin A

Vitamin Names and RDA for Healthy Adults	Chief Functions in the Body	Deficiency Disease Name	Deficiency Symptoms	Toxicity Symptoms	Significant Sources
Vitamin A, retinol, retinal, retinoic acid; precursor is provitamin A; carotenoids such as beta carotene RDA: Females: 800 RE Males: 1,000 RE	Maintenance of cornea, epithelial cells, mucous membranes, and skin; bone and tooth growth; reproduction; hormone synthesis and regulation; immunity; cancer protection	Hypovitaminosis A	**Blood/circulatory system** Anemia (small-cell type)[a]	Red blood cell breakage, nosebleeds	Retinal: fortified milk, cheese, cream, butter, fortified margarine, eggs, liver
			Digestive system Diarrhea, general discomfort	Abdominal cramps and pain, nausea, vomiting, diarrhea, weight loss	Beta carotene: spinach and other dark leafy greens, broccoli, deep orange fruits (apricots, peaches, cantaloupe), and vegetables (squash, carrots, sweet potatoes, pumpkin)
			Immune system Depression; frequent respiratory, digestive, bladder, vaginal, and other infections	Overreactivity	
			Mouth, gums, teeth Abnormal tooth and jaw alignment		
			Nervous/muscular systems Night blindness	Blurred vision, pain in calves, fatigue, irritability, loss of appetite, bone pain	
			Skin and cornea Keratinization, corneal degeneration leading to blindness,[b] rashes	Dry skin, rashes, loss of hair	
			Other Kidney stones, impaired growth	Cessation of menstruation, growth retardation, liver and spleen enlargement	

[a]Small-cell anemia is termed *microcycic anemia.*
[b]Corneal degeneration progresses from *keratinization* (hardening) to *xerosis* (drying) to *xerophthalamia* (thickening, opacity, and irreversible blindness).

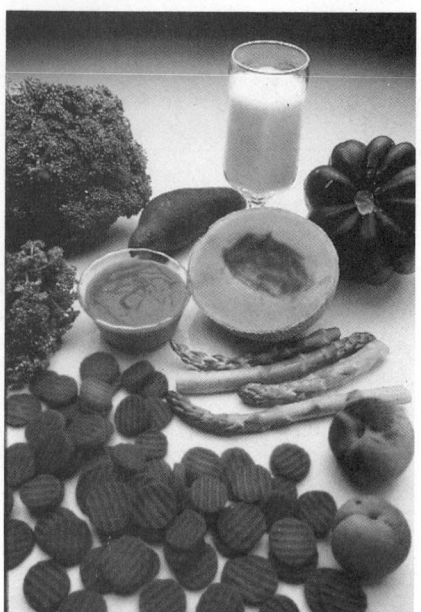

Foods rich in vitamin A.

1 RE = 3.33 IU from animal foods or 10 IU from plant foods. (On the average, 1 RE = about 5 IU.

Vitamin A in Foods

About half of the vitamin A activity in the foods we normally consume comes from fruits and vegetables, and half of this comes from the dark leafy greens (not iceberg lettuce or green beans) and the rich yellow or deep orange vegetables, such as squash, carrots, and sweet potatoes (not corn). The other half comes from milk, cheese, butter, and other dairy products; eggs; and meats. Because vitamin A is fat-soluble, it is lost when milk is skimmed. Nonfat milk is thus often fortified with vitamin A to compensate. The butter substitute, margarine, is usually fortified too.

Fast foods are notable for their *lack* of vitamin A. We advise anyone who dines frequently on fast foods to emphasize vegetables heavily—and not just salads—at other meals.

Liver is an excellent source of vitamin A. In fact, Arctic explorers who have eaten large quantities of polar bear liver have become ill with symptoms suggesting vitamin A toxicity. This problem, however, has never been observed in connection with the frequent use of liver elsewhere.

Certain relatives of vitamin A, available by prescription, have been used to relieve the symptoms of acne when applied directly to the skin surface. Acne sufferers should be warned, however, that taking massive doses of vitamin A supplements will not cure acne and may cause the miseries itemized in Table 7–1.

Some of vitamin A's relatives may have a preventive role with respect to cancer. Retinol itself is not one of them, but this doesn't stop gullible people from taking massive doses of vitamin A in the hope of preventing cancer. Readers of this text are, of course, too sophisticated to make such mistakes.

Vitamin D

Vitamin D is a member of a large and cooperative bone-making and maintenance team composed of nutrients and other compounds, including vitamin C; hormones (parathormone and calcitonin); the protein collagen; and the minerals calcium, phosphorus, magnesium, fluoride, and others. The special function of vitamin D is to help make calcium and phosphorus available in the blood that bathes the bones in order for these minerals to be deposited as the bones harden.

Vitamin D is different from other nutrients in that the body can synthesize the amount it needs with the help of sunlight. In a sense, therefore, vitamin D is not an essential nutrient. Another unique feature of vitamin D is that it acts very much like a hormone—a compound manufactured by one organ of the body that has effects on another.

The precursor of vitamin D made in the liver is 7-dehydrocholesterol, which is made from cholesterol. This is one of the body's many "good" uses for cholesterol.

The liver manufactures a vitamin D precursor, which is converted to vitamin D with the help of the ultraviolet rays from the sun. Regardless of whether your body manufactures vitamin D or obtains it from food, two more steps occur before the vitamin becomes fully active. First the liver alters the molecule, and then the kidneys alter it further to produce the active vitamin. This is why diseases affecting either the liver or the kidneys may lead to bone deterioration.

Active vitamin D promotes the making of several proteins that help with calcium transport into the intestinal cells and assists these proteins in their action.[2] It also has specific attachment sites in the brain, parathyroid glands, bones, and kidneys. At these sites, vitamin D is thought to regulate the production of proteins that manage calcium balance.[3] In the pancreas, vitamin D affects insulin secretion.[4]

The symptoms of an inadequate intake of vitamin D are those of calcium deficiency, shown in Table 7–2. The bones fail to calcify normally and may be so weak that they become bent when they have to support the body's weight. A child with rickets who is old enough to walk characteristically develops bowed legs, often the most obvious sign of the disease. Worldwide, rickets afflict a large number of children.

Adult rickets, or osteomalacia, occurs most often in women who have low calcium intakes and little exposure to sun and who go through repeated pregnancies and periods of lactation. The bones of the legs may soften to such an extent that a girl who grows up tall and straight becomes bent, bowlegged, and stooped by the end of her second or third pregnancy.

The shorthand name for the final, active vitamin is dihydroxy vitamin D.

rickets:
the vitamin D deficiency disease in children.

osteomalacia (os-tee-o-mal-AY-shuh):
the vitamin D deficiency disease in adults.
osteo = bone
mal = bad (soft)

Osteomalacia can also occur in calcium deficiency (see Chapter 8).

TABLE 7–2 Key Information About Vitamin D

Vitamin Name and RDA for Healthy Adults	Chief Functions in the Body	Deficiency Disease Name	Deficiency Symptoms	Toxicity Symptoms	Significant Sources
Vitamin D, calciferol, cholecalciferol, dihydroxy-vitamin D; precursor is the body's own cholesterol RDA: 10 μg	Mineralization of bones (raises calcium and phosphorus blood levels by increasing absorption from digestive tract, withdrawing calcium from bones, and stimulating retention by kidneys)	Rickets Osteomalacia		**Blood/circulatory system** Raised blood calcium	Self-synthesis with sunlight; fortified milk, fortified margarine, eggs, liver, fish
				Digestive system Constipation, weight loss	
				Nervous system Excessive thirst, headaches, irritability, loss of appetite, weakness, nausea	
			Other Abnormal growth, joint pain, soft bones	Kidney stones, stones in arteries, mental and physical retardation	

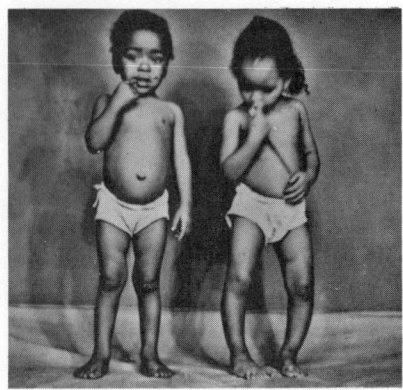

Rickets.
Source: Courtesy of Parke-Davis and Company.

Vitamin D activity was previously expressed in international units (IU), but as of 1980, it is expressed in micrograms of cholecalciferol. To convert, use the following factor:

100 IU = 2.5 μg

400 IU = 10 μg

Exposure to sun should be reasonable. Excessive exposure may cause skin cancer.

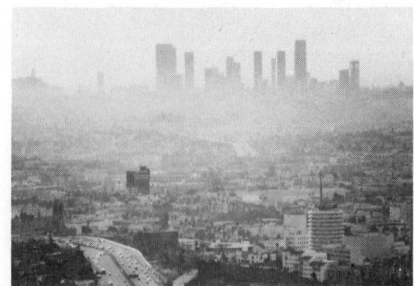

Smog filters out ultraviolet rays of the sun.

Vitamin D deficiency depresses calcium absorption and results in low blood calcium levels and abnormal mineralization of bone. An excess of vitamin D does the opposite, as shown in Table 7–2. It enhances calcium absorption, causing abnormally high concentrations of the mineral in the blood, and promotes return of bone calcium into the blood as well. Excess calcium in the blood tends to precipitate in the soft tissue, forming stones. This is especially likely to happen in the kidneys, which concentrate calcium as they excrete it. Calcification or hardening of the blood vessels may also occur and is especially dangerous in the major arteries of the heart and lungs, where it can cause death.

Vitamin D is the most toxic of all the vitamins. Half the recommended intake is too little, but over a few times the recommended intake may be too much. The amounts of vitamin D found in foods available in the United States and Canada are well within these limits, but pills containing the vitamin in concentrated form should definitely be kept out of the reach of children.

Vitamin D from Sun and Foods

There are two ways to meet your vitamin D needs. You can synthesize the vitamin yourself with the help of sunlight, or you can eat foods containing the preformed vitamin.

Rapidly growing children require a daily intake of close to 10 micrograms of vitamin D; mature adults need half as much. Only a few animal foods supply significant amounts of the vitamin, notably eggs, liver, and some fish. Even the vitamin D content in these foods vary greatly, depending on the animal's exposure to sun and on its consumption of the vitamin in its foods. Neither cow's milk nor human breast milk supplies enough vitamin D to meet human needs reliably; hence, cow's milk must be fortified. Infants must be given either fortified formula or vitamin D supplements. The fortification of milk with vitamin D is the best guarantee that children will meet their vitamin D needs and underscores the importance of milk in children's diets.

Most adults, especially in the sunnier regions, need not make special efforts to obtain vitamin D in food. People who are not outdoors much or who live in northern or predominantly cloudy or smoggy areas, however, are advised to make sure their milk is fortified with vitamin D, to drink at least two cups a day, and to make frequent use of eggs and periodic use of liver in menu planning.

Darker skinned people make vitamin D less rapidly on exposure to the sun. In three hours of sun exposure, however, people with strongly pigmented skin synthesize as much vitamin D as people with very fair skin during 30 minutes of exposure. The difference may account for the fact that darker skinned people in northern, smoggy cities are more prone to rickets. The experiments revealing these findings also suggest that overexposure to sun cannot cause vitamin D toxicity, because synthesis of vitamin D is limited to a fixed maximum at each exposure.[5]

Rapidly growing infants and children need adequate amounts of vitamin D to promote strong bones and teeth. Infant formulas are fortified with vitamin D in adequate amounts for daily intake. Many babies are also given vitamin drops that contain the RDA for vitamin D. These sources, plus any exposure to the sun, provide formula-fed babies with more than enough of this vitamin. Well-meaning parents who give their infants extra vitamin drops are risking vitamin D toxicity symptoms including increased calcium withdrawal from the bones. The effect is just the opposite of the desired outcome of strong bones.

Vitamin E

Many substances found in foods that are important in the body can be destroyed by oxidation. An example is oil, which can turn rancid when exposed to air. Vitamin E is a fat-soluble antioxidant. If there is plenty of vitamin E in the membranes of cells exposed to an oxidant, the chances are that this vitamin will take the brunt of any oxidative attack, thereby protecting the lipids and other vulnerable components of the membranes. Vitamin E is especially effective in preventing the oxidation of the polyunsaturated fatty acids (PUFA), but it protects all other lipids (for example, vitamin A) as well. Table 7–3 summarizes important information about vitamin E.

One of the most important places in the body in which vitamin E exerts its antioxidant effect is in the lungs, because the exposure of cells to oxygen is maximal there. Vitamin E also protects the lungs from oxidizing air pollutants.

When vitamin E intake is deficient and the blood concentration falls below a certain critical level, the red blood cells tend to break open and spill their contents, probably because of oxidation of the PUFA in their membranes. The role of vitamin E in protecting red blood cell membranes has led researchers to ask whether the vitamin might protect white blood cells as well and perhaps participate in the body's immune defenses. Indeed, deficiency of vitamin E suppresses the immune system and supplementation stimulates it in several species of animals.[6]

Abnormal environmental conditions, such as air pollution, can increase human vitamin E needs. Also, a great many diseases can affect people's vitamin E needs. The following individuals can benefit from vitamin E supplementation:

- Premature infants, because the transfer of vitamin E across the placenta becomes maximal only right before full-term delivery.
- Infants, children, or adults who can't absorb fats and oils because of liver, pancreas, or gallbladder disease; GI surgery; or inherited diseases.
- Individuals with certain blood disorders, including sickle-cell anemia, beta thalassemia, and a red blood cell enzyme deficiency (glucose-6-phosphate dehydrogenase deficiency).

Two other conditions seen in human beings appear to respond to vitamin E therapy. One is a nonmalignant breast disease, and the other is an abnormality of blood flow that causes cramping in the legs.

Many extravagant claims have been made for vitamin E. Although researchers have revealed possible roles for vitamin E, they have also shown clearly some things that it does *not* do. During the 1960s and 1970s, vitamin E was said to improve athletic endurance and skill, to increase sexual potency and enhance sexual performance, to prolong the life of the heart, and to reverse the damage caused by atherosclerosis and heart attacks. Vitamin E was also thought to

oxidation:
a type of chemical reaction so named because oxygen is one of the agents that often brings it about.

antioxidant:
a compound that protects other compounds from oxidation by being oxidized itself.

oxidant:
a compound (such as oxygen itself) that oxidizes other compounds.

The breaking open of red blood cells is **erythrocyte** (eh-REETH-ro-cite) **hemolysis** (he-MOLL-uh-sis), the vitamin E deficiency disease in human beings.
erythrocyte: red blood cell
erythro = red
cyte = cell
hemolysis: bursting of red blood cells
hemo = blood
lysis = breaking

Both diseases have unwieldy names. One is **fibrocystic breast disease,** the other is **intermittent claudication.**
fibr = fibrous lumps
cystic = in sacs
intermittent = at intervals
claudicare = to limp
Caution: Other serious conditions can cause lumps in the breast and pain in the legs. Don't self-diagnose; see a doctor.

TABLE 7–3 Key Information About Vitamin E

Vitamin Names and Estimated and Safe Intakes for Healthy Adults	Chief Functions in the Body	Deficiency Disease Name	Deficiency Symptoms	Toxicity Symptoms	Significant Sources
Vitamin E alpha-tocopherol, tocopherol RDA: Females: 8 mg[a] Males: 10 mg	Antioxidant stabilization of cell membranes, regulation of oxidation reactions, protection of PUFA and vitamin A	(No name)	**Blood/circulatory system** Red blood cell breakage, anemia	Interference with anticlotting medication	Plant oils (margarine, salad dressings, shortenings), green and leafy vegetables, wheat germ, whole grain products, butter, liver, egg yolk, milk fat, nuts, seeds
			Digestive system General discomfort		
			Nervous/muscular systems Degeneration, weakness, difficulty walking, intermittent claudication		
			Other Fibrocystic breast disease		

[a]The RDA is expressed in milligrams of D-alpha-tocopherol equivalents. One milligram equivalent has the biological activity of one mg D-alpha-tocopherol. The RNI is expressed in the same units, relative to which beta- and gamma-tocopherol and alpha-tocotrienol have activities of one-half, one-tenth, and one-third the activity, respectively.

muscular dystrophy (DIS-tro-fee): a hereditary disease in which the muscles gradually weaken; its most debilitating effects arise in the lungs. This disease should not be confused with *nutritional muscular dystrophy,* a vitamin E deficiency disease of animals characterized by gradual paralysis of the muscles.

prevent or cure hereditary muscular dystrophy. It was said to slow or prevent other processes of aging, such as graying of the hair, wrinkling of the skin, and reduced activity of body organs. An immense amount of experimentation has discredited these and many other similar claims.

Despite the fact that many vitamin E claims have been discredited, people take vitamin E supplements for a variety of reasons. As a result, signs of toxicity are now known or suspected, including disturbances of the action of many hormones, interference with the action of vitamin K in blood clotting, alteration of the mechanism of blood clotting, alteration of blood lipid levels, impairment of white blood cell activity, GI distress, and many many more.[7] Doses of 100 milligrams, or certainly of 300 milligrams, should be considered megadoses and should be taken only on a physician's advice, with caution, or not at all.[8]

Vitamin E in Foods

Vitamin E is widespread in foods. About 60 percent of the vitamin E in the diet comes directly or indirectly from vegetable oils in the form of margarine, salad dressings, and shortenings. Another 10 percent comes from fruits and vegetables; smaller percentages come from grains and other products. Soybean oil and wheat germ oil have especially high concentrations of vitamin E. Cottonseed, corn, and safflower oils rank second, with a tablespoon of any of these supplying more than 10 milligrams (more than the RDA) of the vitamin. Other oils contain less; for example, peanut oil supplies about half as much per tablespoon. Animal fats, such as butter and milk fat, have negligible amounts of vitamin E. Vitamin E is readily destroyed by heat processing and oxidation, so fresh or lightly processed foods are preferable as sources of this vitamin.

People's needs for vitamin E are higher if the amounts of PUFA they consume are higher. Fortunately, vitamin E and PUFA tend to occur together in the same foods.

On vitamin bottles, vitamin E activity is often expressed as IU. One IU is the same as one milligram of the active form of vitamin E.

There are many reasons for taking vitamin supplements. One of the reasons many give for taking vitamin E is that even if the vitamin does not do all that its advocates claim it will, megadoses won't do any harm. This is false, as we have seen that large amounts of vitamin E may interfere with the action of vitamin K in blood clotting. Fatigue and muscle weakness can also be caused by excess vitamin E.

Vitamin K

Vitamin K seems to act primarily in the blood clotting system. Its presence there can make the difference between life and death. At least 13 different proteins and the mineral calcium are involved in making a blood clot. Vitamin K is essential for the synthesis of at least four of these proteins, among them prothrombin, the precursor of the protein thrombin. As mentioned earlier, vitamin K also participates with vitamin D in synthesizing a bone protein that helps to regulate blood calcium levels.[9] Table 7–4 provides additional information about vitamin K.

When any of the blood-clotting factors is lacking, blood cannot clot and hemorrhagic disease results. If an artery or vein is cut or broken under these circumstances, bleeding goes unchecked. Remember, this is not to say that the cause of hemorrhaging is always a vitamin K deficiency.

Toxicity is not common but can result when water-soluble substitutes for vitamin K are given, especially to infants or to pregnant women. Toxicity symptoms include red cell hemolysis, jaundice, and brain damage.

Bacteria in your intestinal tract can synthesize vitamin K that you can absorb, although you are not dependent on bacterial synthesis for your vitamin K. Many foods contain ample amounts of the vitamin, notably green leafy vegetables, members of the cabbage family, and milk.

K stands for the Danish word *koagulation* (coagulation or clotting).

hemorrhagic (hem-o-RAJ-ik) **disease:** the vitamin K deficiency disease in which blood fails to clot.

hemolysis: see p. 107.

jaundice: yellowing of the skin due to spillover of bile pigments from the liver into the general circulation.

The bacterial inhabitants of the digestive tract are known as the **intestinal flora.** *flora* = plant inhabitants

TABLE 7–4 Key Information About Vitamin K

Vitamin Names and Estimated and Safe Intakes for Healthy Adults	Chief Functions in the Body	Deficiency Disease Name	Deficiency Symptoms	Toxicity Symptoms	Significant Sources
Vitamin K, phylloquinone, naphthoquinone; ESI: 70–140 μg	Synthesis of blood-clotting proteins and a calcium-regulating blood protein	(No name)	Hemorrhaging	Interference with anticlotting medication; vitamin K analogues may cause jaundice	Bacterial synthesis in the digestive tract; liver, green leafy vegetables, cabbage family, milk

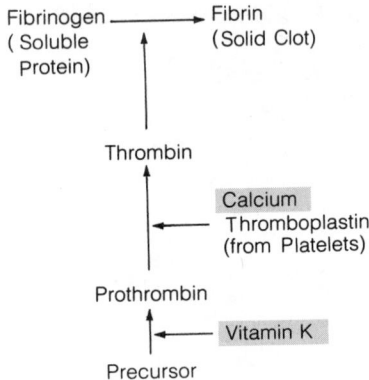

The clotting process.

sterile:
free of microorganisms, such as bacteria.

The synthetic substitute usually given for vitamin K is **menadione** (men-uh-DYE-own).

Vitamin K deficiency is seldom seen except when unusual combinations of circumstances conspire to bring it about. When it does occur, however, it can be fatal. The scenario goes like this: A patient is in the hospital, he has been given antibiotics to prevent or overcome infection, and he is not getting adequate vitamin K from his diet. The antibiotics have killed his intestinal bacteria, and his vitamin K stores are depleted. When he goes into surgery, he bleeds because his blood fails to clot normally. As a result, he may bleed to death. The combination of antibiotics, inadequate vitamin K intake, and surgery raises a warning flag and requires that clotting time be checked before surgery is performed.[10]

New babies are commonly susceptible to vitamin K deficiency for two reasons. First, a baby is born with a sterile digestive tract. Second, a baby may not be fed a good source of vitamin K at the outset. Breast milk is a poorer source of vitamin K than cow's milk. A dose of vitamin K, usually in a water-soluble form, may therefore be given at birth to prevent hemorrhagic disease in the newborn. It must be administered carefully to avoid toxic overdosing. People taking sulfa drugs, which destroy intestinal bacteria, may also become deficient in vitamin K.

On the other hand, a very high intake of vitamin K can reduce the effectiveness of drugs used to prevent the blood from clotting. People taking anticoagulants should use moderation in eating foods high in vitamin K.

The Water-Soluble Vitamins

The water-soluble vitamins include the B vitamins and vitamin C. These vitamins are found in the watery compartment of foods, and they distribute into water-filled compartments of the body. They can easily be excreted if their blood concentration rises too high. As a consequence, the water-soluble vitamins are more easily depleted than the fat-soluble vitamins and are less likely to reach toxic levels. This is not to say they cannot reach such levels because most of them have now been shown to have toxic effects, at least in some people, when taken in large doses.[11]

The B Vitamins

The B vitamins include thiamin, riboflavin, niacin, vitamin B_6, folacin, vitamin B_{12}, pantothenic acid, and biotin. Table 7–5 lists other names used for these vitamins. Each of these eight vitamins is a part of an enzyme helper known as a coenzyme. A coenzyme is a small molecule that can combine with an inactive protein to make an active enzyme. With the coenzyme in place, the substance to be worked on is attracted to the enzyme and the reaction proceeds instantaneously. Figure 7–2 illustrates how a coenzyme works, using niacin as an example.

Thiamin, niacin, riboflavin, and pantothenic acid are each a part of distinct coenzymes necessary for the production of energy from glucose, amino acids, and fats. A coenzyme containing vitamin B_6 is necessary for synthesizing non-essential amino acids. The making of new cells depends on a folacin coenzyme, and the making of this coenzyme depends on vitamin B_{12}. Folacin and vitamin B_{12} together are involved in duplicating genetic material when cells divide. (They serve other functions as well.) Biotin serves as a coenzyme in fatty acid synthesis and in energy metabolism.

These eight B vitamins play many specific roles in helping the enzymes to perform thousands of different molecular conversions in your body. They are found in every cell and must be present continuously for the cells to function as they should.

coenzyme (co-EN-zime):
small molecule that works with an enzyme to promote the enzyme's activity. Many coenzymes have B vitamins as part of their structure.
co = with

B Vitamin Deficiency

Although we know a great deal about their individual molecular functions, we are unable to say precisely why a deficiency of one B vitamin produces the disease beriberi whereas the deficiency of another produces pellagra. We do know, however, that with the deficiency of any B vitamin, many body systems become deranged, and similar symptoms may appear.

TABLE 7–5 B Vitamin Terminology

Correct Name[a]	Other Names Commonly Used
Thiamin	Vitamin B_1
Riboflavin	Vitamin B_2
Niacin	Nicotinic acid, nicotinamide, niacinamide
Vitamin B_6	Pyridoxine, pyridoxal, pyridoxamine
Folacin	Folate, folic acid
Vitamin B_{12}	Cobalamin
Pantothenic acid	(None)
Biotin	(None)

[a]Many of the vitamins have both names and numbers, a mixture of terminology that confuses newcomers to the study of nutrition. As of 1979, a single set of names for the vitamins had been agreed on and was published in Committee on Nomenclature of the American Institute of Nutrition, Generic descriptors and trivial names for vitamins and related compounds. *Journal of Nutrition* 112(1982): 7–14. We use the single set of names agreed on in this book, but the alternative names are still widely used.

FIGURE 7.2.

Coenzyme action.

Each coenzyme is specialized for certain kinds of chemical reactions. NAD (containing niacin), for example, can accept hydrogen atoms removed from other compounds and can lose them to compounds that ultimately pass them to oxygen. In many steps during the breakdown of glucose, hydrogens are removed and NAD participates this way. A model of the way NAD works with an enzyme to remove hydrogens is shown here.

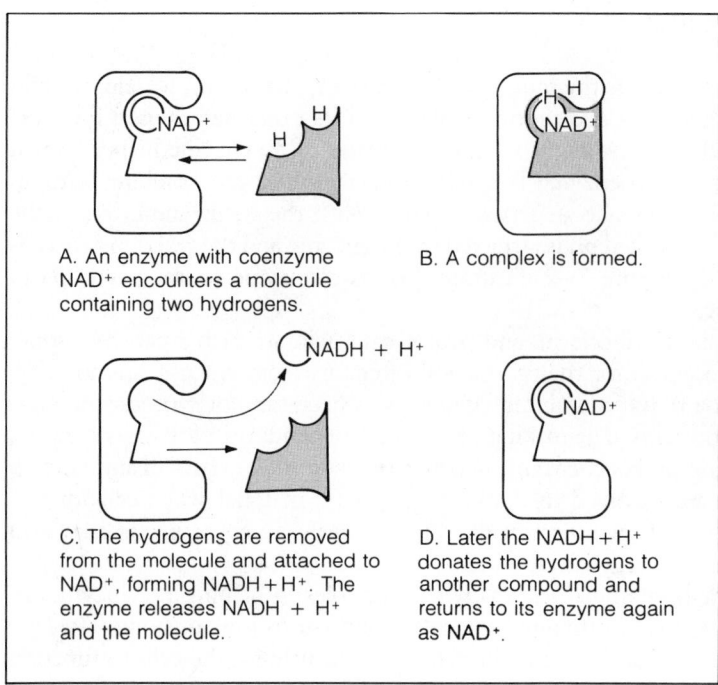

A. An enzyme with coenzyme NAD⁺ encounters a molecule containing two hydrogens.

B. A complex is formed.

C. The hydrogens are removed from the molecule and attached to NAD⁺, forming NADH + H⁺. The enzyme releases NADH + H⁺ and the molecule.

D. Later the NADH + H⁺ donates the hydrogens to another compound and returns to its enzyme again as NAD⁺.

beriberi:
the thiamin-deficiency disease; it pointed the way to the first discovery of a vitamin, thiamin.

pellagra (pell-AY-gra):
the niacin-deficiency disease.
pellis = skin
agra = seizure

A deficiency of a B vitamin seldom shows up in isolation. After all, people do not eat nutrients one by one; they eat foods containing mixtures of nutrients. If a major class of foods is missing from the diet, the nutrients contributed by that class of foods will all be lacking to various extents. In only two cases have dietary deficiencies associated with single B vitamins been observed on a large scale in human populations. Diseases have been named for these deficiency states. One of them, beriberi, was first observed in the Far East when the custom of polishing rice became widespread. Rice contributed 80 percent of the kcalories consumed by the people of those areas, and rice hulls were those people's principal source of thiamin. When the hulls were removed, beriberi spread like wildfire.

The other disease, pellagra, became widespread in the southern United States in the early part of this century. People who subsisted on a low-protein diet with a staple grain of corn were affected by pellagra. This diet was unusual in that it supplied neither enough niacin nor enough of its amino acid precursor tryptophan to make the niacin intake adequate.

Even in cases of beriberi and pellagra, the deficiencies were not pure. When foods were provided containing the one vitamin known to be needed, the other vitamins that may have been in short supply came as part of the package.

Table 7–6 sums up a few of the better established facts about B vitamin deficiencies. A look at the table will make another generalization possible. Different body systems depend to different extents on these vitamins. Processes

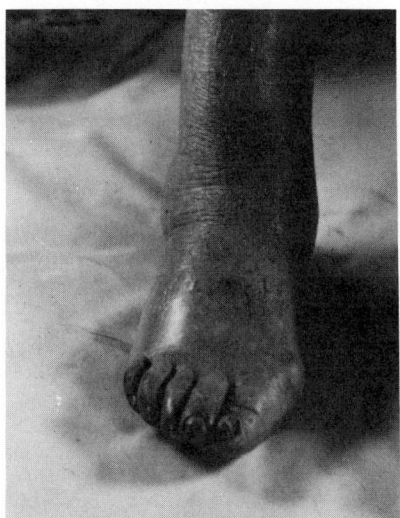

The edema of beriberi. Thiamin deficiency also sometimes produces a "dry" beriberi, without edema, for reasons not well understood. Another marked symptom is inability to walk, manifested by collapse of the lower limbs when the person tries to stand.

Source: Courtesy of Dr. Samuel Dreizen. D.D. S., M.D.

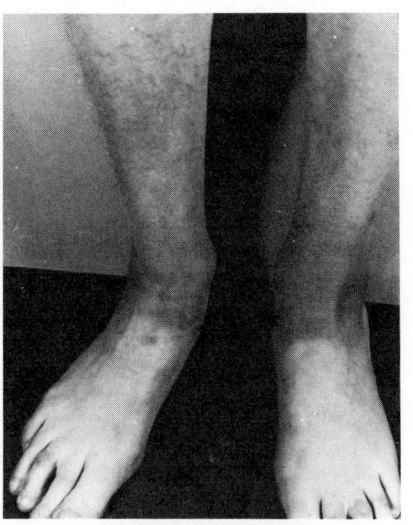

The dermatitis of pellagra. The skin darkens and flakes away as if it were sunburned. In kwashiorkor there is also a "flaky paint" dermatitis but the two are easily distinguishable. The dermatitis of pellagra is bilateral and symmetrical, and occurs only on those parts of the body exposed to the sun.

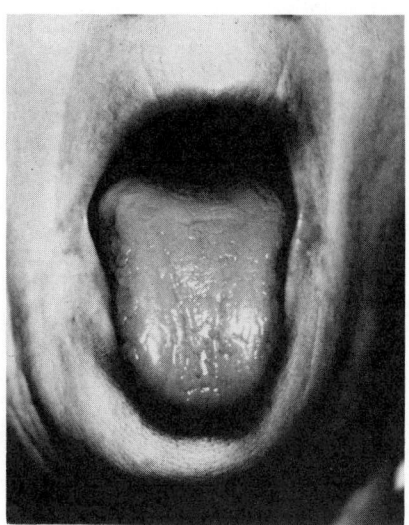

Tongue symptoms of B vitamin deficiency. The tongue is smooth due to atrophy of the tissues (glossitis). This person has a folacin deficiency.

Source: Courtesy of Samuel Dreizen, D.D.S., M.D.

in nerves and in their responding tissues, the muscles, depend heavily on glucose metabolism and hence on thiamin. Thus, paralysis sets in when this nutrient is lacking. Because the replacement of red blood cells and GI tract cells occurs at a rapid pace, two of the first symptoms of a deficiency of either of these nutrients are a type of anemia and GI deterioration. Again, each nutrient is important in all systems, and the list of symptoms in Table 7–6 is far from complete.

Major epidemiclike deficiency diseases, such as pellagra and beriberi, are no longer seen in the United States and Canada, but lesser deficiencies of nutrients, including the B vitamins, sometimes are observed. They occur in people whose food choices are poor because of poverty, ignorance, illness, or health habits such as alcohol abuse. If the staple grain food is refined, vitamin B deficiencies are especially likely. One way to protect these people is to add nutrients to their staple food, a process known as fortification or enrichment. The enrichment of refined breads and cereals, required by law in most eastern states since the late 1940s and in many western states since the early 1970s, has increased many people's iron and B vitamin intakes.

The preceding discussion has shown both the great importance of the B vitamins in promoting normal, healthy functioning of all body systems and the severe consequences of deficiency. Now you may want to know how to be sure you are getting enough of these vital nutrients.

fortification:
the addition of nutrients to a food, often in amounts much larger than might be found naturally in that food.

enrichment:
now considered synonymous with fortification; previously, the addition of four specific nutrients—iron, thiamin, riboflavin, and niacin—to refined breads and cereals in amounts approximately equivalent to those originally present in the whole grain.

More information about vitamin supplements is presented in Nutrition in Practice 7.

TABLE 7–6 Key Information About the Water Soluble Vitamins

Vitamin Names and RDA for Healthy Adults	Chief Functions in the Body	Deficiency Disease Name	Deficiency Symptoms	Toxocity Symptoms	Significant Sources
Thiamin, vitamin B₁; RDA: Females: 0.5 mg/1,000 kcal; Males: 0.6 mg/ 1,000 kcal	Part of a coenzyme used in energy metabolism; supports normal appetite and nervous system function	Beriberi	**Blood/circulatory system** Edema, enlarged heart, abnormal heart rhythms, heart failure **Nervous/muscular systems** Degeneration, wasting, weakness, pain, low morale, difficulty walking, loss of reflexes, mental confusion, paralysis	Rapid pulse Weakness, headaches, insomnia, irritability	Occurs in all nutritious foods in moderate amounts; pork, ham, bacon, liver, whole grains, legumes, nuts
Riboflavin vitamin B₂; RDA: 1.2 mg	Part of a coenzyme used in energy metabolism; supports normal vision and skin health	Ariboflavinosis	**Mouth, gums, tongue** Cracks at corners of mouth,ᵃ magenta tongue **Nervous system and eyes** Hypersensitivity to light,ᵇ reddening of cornea **Other** Skin rash	(No symptoms ordinarily reported) Interference with anticancer medication	Milk, yogurt, cottage cheese, meat, leafy green vegetables, whole-grain or enriched breads and cereals
Niacin, nicotinic acid, nicotinamide, niacinimade; precursor is dietary tryptophan RDA: Males: 18 mg equivalents Females: 13 mg equivalents	Part of a coenzyme used in energy metabolism; supports health of skin, nervous system, and digestive system	Pellagra	**Digestive system** Diarrhea **Mouth, gums, tongue** Black, smooth tongueᶜ	Diarrhea, heartburn, nausea, ulcer irritation, vomiting	Milk, eggs, meat, poultry, fish, whole-grain and enriched breads and cereals, nuts, and all protein-containing foods

ᵃCracks at the corners of the mouth are termed *cheilosis* (kee-LOH-SIS).
ᵇHypersensitivity to light is called *photophobia*.

TABLE 7–6 (continued)

Vitamin Names and RDA for Healthy Adults	Chief Functions in the Body	Deficiency Disease Name	Deficiency Symptoms	Toxocity Symptoms	Significant Sources
			Nervous system		
			Irritability, loss of appetite, weakness, dizziness, mental confusion progressing to psychosis or delirium	Fainting	
			Skin		
			Skin rash on areas exposed to sun	Painful flush and rash	
			Other		
				Abnormal liver function, low blood pressure	
Vitamin B₆, pyridoxine, pyridoxal, pyridoxamine; RDA: Males: 2.2 mg Females: 2.0 mg	Part of a coenzyme used in amino acid and fatty acid metabolism; helps convert tryprophan to niacin; helps make red blood cells	(No name)	**Blood/circulatory system**		Green and leafy vegetables, meats, fish, poultry, shellfish, legumes, fruits, whole grains
			Anemia (small-cell type)ᶜ	Bloating	
			Mouth, gums, tongue		
			Smooth tongueᵈ		
			Nervous/muscular systems		
			Abnormal brain wave pattern, irritability, muscle twitching, convulsions	Depression, fatigue, irratibility, headaches, numbness, damage to nerves, difficulty walking	
			Skin		
			Irritation of sweat glands, rashes		
			Other		
			Kidney stones		
Folacin, folic acid, folate; RDA: 400 μg or 0.4 mg	Part of a coenzyme used in new cell synthesis	(No name)	**Blood/circulatory system**		Leafy green vegetables, legumes seeds, liver
			Anemia (large-cell type)		
			Digestive system		
			Heartburn, diarrhea, constipation	Diarrhea	
			Immune system		
			Frequent infections		

ᶜSmall-cell type anemia is *microcytic anemia*; large-cell type is *macrocytic* or *megalablastic anemia*.
ᵈSmoothness of the tongue is caused by loss of its surface structures and is termed *glossitis* (gloss-EYE-tis).

TABLE 7–6 (continued)

Vitamin Names and RDA for Healthy Adults	Chief Functions in the Body	Deficiency Disease Name	Deficiency Symptoms	Toxocity Symptoms	Significant Sources
Folacin (continued)			**Mouth, gums, tongue** Smooth red tongue[d]		
			Nervous system Depression, mental confusion, fainting	Insomnia, irrability	
			Other	Masking of vitamin B_{12} deficiency symptoms	
Vitamin B_{12}, cyanocobalamin; RDA: 3 µg	Part of a coenzyme used in new cell synthesis; helps maintain nerve cells	(No name)	**Blood/circulatory system** Anemia (large-cell type)[e]	(No toxicity symptoms known)	Animal products (meat, fish, poultry, shellfish, milk, cheese, eggs)
			Mouth, gums, tongue Smooth tongue[d]		
			Nervous system Fatigue, degeneration, progression to paralysis		
			Skin Hypersensitivity		
Pantothenic acid	Part of a coenzyme used in energy metabolism	(No name)	**Digestive system** Vomiting, intenstinal distress	Occasional diarrhea	Widespread in foods
			Nervous system Insomnia, fatigue		
			Other	Water retention (infrequent)	
Biotin Estimated safe and adequate intake: 100–200 mg.	Part of a coenzyme used in energy metabolism, fat synthesis, amino acid metabolism, and glycogen synthesis	(No name)	**Blood/circulatory system** Abnormal heart action	(No toxicity symptoms reported)	Widespread in foods
			Digestive system Loss of appetite, nausea		

[e]The name *pernicious anemia* refers to the vitamin$_{12}$ deficiency caused by lack of intrinsic factor, but not to that caused by inadequate dietary intake.

TABLE 7–6 (continued)

Vitamin Names and RDA for Healthy Adults	Chief Functions in the Body	Deficiency Disease Name	Deficiency Symptoms	Toxocity Symptoms	Significant Sources
			Nervous/muscular systems		
			Depression, muscle pain, weakness, fatigue		
			Skin		
			Drying, rash, loss of hair		
			Blood/circulatory system		
Vitamin C, ascorbic acid; RDA: 60 mg	Collagen synthesis (strengthens blood vessel walls, forms scar tissue, matrix for bone growth), antioxidant, thyroxine synthesis, amino acid metabolism, strengthens resistance to infection, helps in absorption of iron	Scurvy	Anemia (small-cell type),[c] atherosclerotic plaques, pinpoint hemorrhages	Blood cell breakage in certain racial groups[f]	Citrus fruits, cabbage-type vegetables, dark green vegetables, cantaloupe, strawberries, peppers, lettuce, tomatoes, potatoes, papayas, mangos
			Digestive system	Nausea, abdominal cramps, diarrhea	
			Immune system		
			Frequent infections		
			Mouth, gums, tongue		
			Bleeding gums, loosened teeth		
			Muscular/nervous system		
			Muscle degeneration and pain, hysteria, depression		
			Skeletal system		
			Bone fragility, joint pain		
			Skin		
			Rough skin, blotchy bruises		
			Other		
			Failure of wounds to heal	Interference with medical tests; aggravation of gout symptoms; deficiency symptoms may appear at first on withdrawal of high doses	

[f]Groups susceptible to vitamin C toxocity are Sephardic Jews, Africans, and Asians.

Before reading further, keep in mind that foods can provide all the nutrients you need. Some vitamin supplements are inexpensive, while others are absurdly costly. Most people don't need them. If you consume an adequate diet and take a multivitamin supplement, the excess water-soluble vitamins you take will be excreted. Overdosing with water-soluble vitamins has no benefit other than to increase the dollar value of your urine. Besides, overdoses, especially of fat-soluble vitamins, are dangerous due to the risk of toxicity. Nutrition in Practice 7 discusses the use of supplements in more detail.

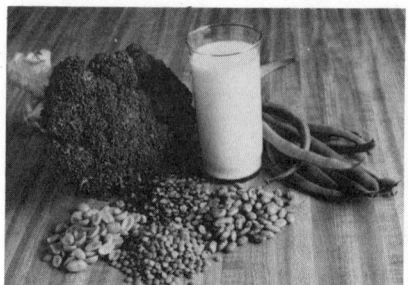

Thiamin. Most nutritious foods contribute about 10 percent of daily needs per serving.

Thiamin

Thiamin is used for energy production; therefore, more is needed when energy expenditure is high. Provided that you are consuming enough kcalories to meet your energy needs—and obtaining those kcalories from thiamin-containing foods—your thiamin intake will adjust automatically to your need. However, people who derive a large proportion of their kcalories from empty-kcalorie items, such as sugar or alcohol, may suffer thiamin deficiency. People who snack heavily on empty-kcalorie foods have been found to have symptoms of thiamin deficiency that disappear when thiamin intake is increased.[12] A person who is fasting or who has adopted a very low-kcalorie diet needs the same amount of thiamin as she did when she was eating more. Needs change little during fasting because they are proportional to energy expenditure, not to energy intake.

No single food eaten daily is notable for its high thiamin content. A useful guideline for meeting your thiamin needs is to eliminate empty-kcalorie foods from your diet and to include ten or more different servings of nutritious foods each day, assuming that each serving will contribute on the average about 10 percent of your needs. Foods chosen from the bread and cereal group should either be made from whole grain or be enriched. Thiamin is not stored in the body to any great extent, so daily intake is best.

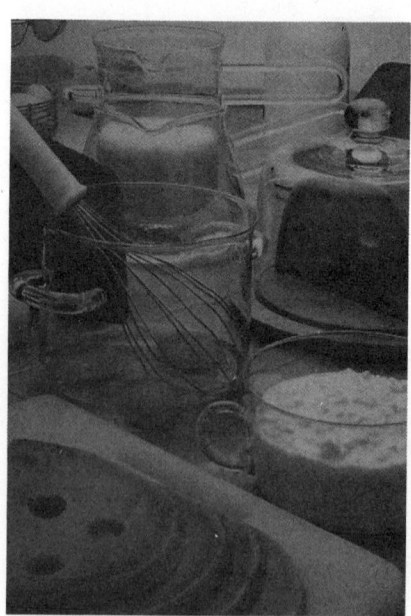

These are among the many dairy foods supplying riboflavin.

Riboflavin

Like thiamin needs, riboflavin needs are related to energy expenditures. Young children's needs rise rapidly during their growing years. Because they are very active, teenagers need more riboflavin than adults. Athletes of any age also need more riboflavin.

Unlike thiamin, riboflavin is not evenly distributed among the food groups. The major contributors of riboflavin in the diet are milk and meat. The need for riboflavin provides a major reason for including milk in some form in everyday meals. No other food that is commonly eaten can make such a substantial contribution. People who don't use milk products can substitute generous servings of dark green leafy vegetables. Among the meats, liver and heart are the richest sources, but all lean meats as well as eggs provide some riboflavin.

Riboflavin is light sensitive; it can be destroyed by the ultraviolet rays of the sun or of fluorescent lamps. For this reason, milk is seldom sold and should not be stored in transparent glass containers. Cardboard or plastic containers protect the riboflavin in the milk from ultraviolet rays.

Riboflavin: Milk contributes about 50 percent, meat about 25 percent, whole-grain or enriched breads and cereals additional amounts. The person who does not drink milk should substitute large amounts of dark green vegetables.

Niacin

Recommended niacin intakes are stated in "equivalents," a term that requires explanation. Niacin is unique among the B vitamins because it can be made in the body from another nutrient source—protein. The amino acid tryptophan can be converted to niacin in the body: 60 milligrams of tryptophan yields 1 milligram of niacin. Protein is usually assumed to be about one percent tryptophan.

Milk, eggs, meat, poultry, and fish contribute about half the niacin equivalents consumed by most people; enriched breads and cereals contribute about a fourth. Vegetarians are advised to emphasize nuts and legumes in their diets, as these are good sources of niacin and protein.

niacin equivalents:
the amount of niacin present in food, including the niacin that can theoretically be made from its precursor tryptophan present in the food.

A food containing 1 milligram of niacin and 60 milligrams of tryptophan contains the equivalent of 2 milligrams of niacin, or 2 milligram equivalents.

Vitamin B$_6$

Because vitamin B$_6$ plays many roles in amino acid metabolism, dietary needs are roughly proportional to protein intake. Data on the amounts of vitamin B$_6$ in foods are not extensive enough to be included in the table of food composition in Appendix C. Averaged amounts of vitamin B$_6$, derived from the available data, reveal that the richest food sources are muscle meats, liver, vegetables, and whole-grain cereals. Large doses of vitamin B$_6$ taken in supplement form are toxic.[13]

Toxic effects of vitamin B$_6$ appeared when a physician reported seven different individuals who had been taking more than two grams a day of vitamin B$_6$ for two months or more. Most were attempting to cure symptoms of premenstrual syndrome (see Nutrition in Practice 8). Their toxicity symptoms started with numb feet; then they lost sensation in their hands and then they became unable to walk. Since then other reports have followed, showing nervous system damage from more moderate doses of vitamin B$_6$.[14]

How vitamin B$_6$ in food is affected by processing is of current interest to researchers. For example, the basic process of cooking increases the availability of vitamin B$_6$ in pinto beans. However, when heat is applied to canned infant formula to sterilize it, vitamin B$_6$ availability is reduced by half. Several decades ago, many infants fed formula treated in this way and not fortified with vitamin B$_6$, suffered convulsions from a deficiency of the vitamin.

Other factors that reduce vitamin B$_6$ availability include some types of fibers and exposure to light, but the effects seem to vary from one food source to the next. Clearly, more research is needed in the area of availability of vitamins from foods.

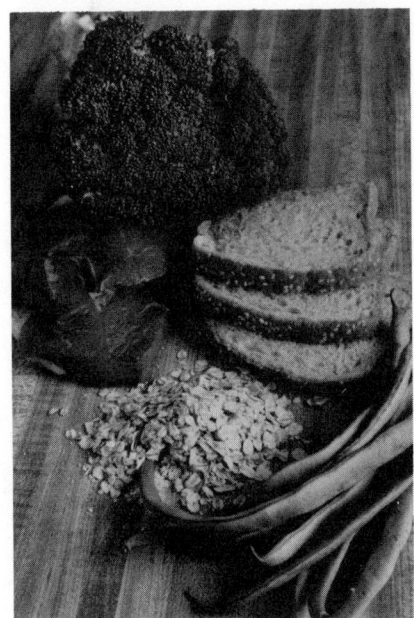

Vitamin B$_6$ is found in meats, vegetables, and whole-grain cereals.

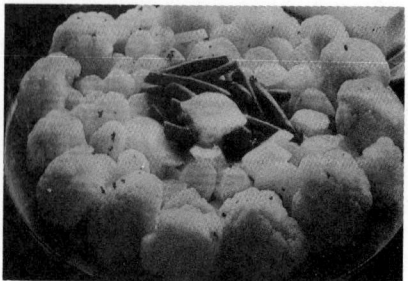

Of these three vegetables, cauliflower is the richest in folacin.

Folacin

Tables of the folacin content of foods, published before 1973, relied on data derived from experiments that are now known to have yielded incorrect, low values. New, more accurate data are now available. The folacin content of foods incorporated into this book's table of food composition is derived from the new method of analysis (see Appendix C). The best food sources of the vitamin are organ meats, such as liver; green leafy vegetables (the name of the vitamin is related to the word *foliage*); beets; and members of the cabbage family, such as cauliflower, broccoli, and Brussels sprouts. Among the fruits, oranges, orange juice, and cantaloupe are the best sources; among the starchy vegetables, corn, lima beans, parsnips, green peas, pumpkin, and sweet potato are good sources. Whole-wheat bread, wheat germ, and milk also supply folacin.

Among the poor and in other parts of the world, folacin deficiency due to inadequate intake is probably the most common of all vitamin deficiencies. Folacin deficiency anemia is especially common among pregnant women. Some authorities recommend that a folacin supplement as well as an iron supplement be given as a preventive measure to pregnant women. The risk of overdosing with folacin is related to vitamin B_{12} discussed next.

Vitamin B_{12}

intrinsic:
inside the system. The intrinsic factor necessary to prevent pernicious anemia is now known to be made in the stomach and to aid in the absorption of vitamin B_{12}. The *extrinsic* factor necessary to prevent pernicious anemia is vitamin B_{12} itself, which must be obtained outside the system from food.

Vitamin B_{12} is unique among the nutrients in being found almost exclusively in animal flesh and animal products. Anyone who eats meat is guaranteed an adequate intake, and lacto-ovo vegetarians (who use milk, cheese, and eggs) are also protected from deficiency. Strict vegetarians must use vitamin B_{12}-fortified soy milk or other such products or take vitamin B_{12} supplements.

A second special characteristic of vitamin B_{12} is that it requires an "intrinsic factor"—a compound inside the body—for absorption from the intestinal tract into the bloodstream. The intrinsic factor is made in the stomach, where it attaches to the vitamin; the complex then passes to the small intestine and is gradually absorbed.

In some cases, intrinsic factor production becomes inadequate or is not produced at all—for example, after surgical removal of the stomach. In such cases, vitamin B_{12} deficiency symptoms will develop if vitamin B_{12} is not supplied by injection.

One of the most obvious vitamin B_{12} deficiency symptoms is the anemia of folacin deficiency, characterized by large, immature red blood cells. Vitamin B_{12} is needed to enable folacin to help manufacture these cells. Either vitamin B_{12} or folacin will clear up this condition. However, vitamin B_{12} also functions in maintaining the sheath that surrounds and protects nerve fibers and in promoting the normal growth of the sheath. Thus, a deficiency causes not only anemia but also a creeping paralysis of the nerves and muscles. This symptom is not detectable from a blood test, and the paralysis cannot be remedied by administering folacin. Early detection and correction are necessary to prevent permanent nerve damage and paralysis.

The name *pernicious* anemia comes from the hidden, sneaky, and frightening way in which vitamin B_{12} deficiency damages nerves without revealing itself in a blood symptom. Because folacin can mask the lack of vitamin B_{12}, the amount of folacin in over-the-counter vitamin preparations is limited by law to 400 micrograms, an amount too low to have this effect.

> The way folacin masks pernicious anemia underlines a point already made several times: it takes a skilled diagnostician to make a correct diagnosis. The risk you take when you diagnose yourself on the basis of a single observed symptom is clearly serious.
>
> A second point should also be underlined here. Because vitamin B_{12} deficiency in the body may be caused either by a lack of the vitamin in the diet or by the body's inability to absorb the vitamin, a change in diet alone might not correct it.

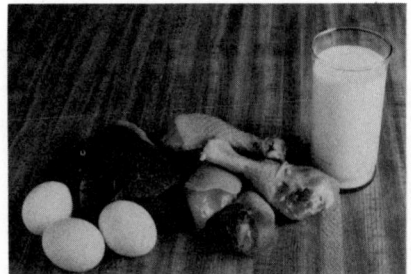

Vitamin B_{12} is adequate in the body if animal foods are included in the diet. Among vegetable products, only a few (those that include microorganisms) contain vitamin B_{12}, most notably yeast and some fermented soy products.

Strict vegetarians are at special risk for undetected vitamin B_{12} deficiency for two reasons: first, because they receive none in their diets and second, because they consume large amounts of folacin from the vegetables they eat. Because the amount of vitamin B_{12} that can be stored in the body is 1,000 times the amount used each day, it may take years for a deficiency to develop in a new vegetarian. When it does, vitamin B_{12} may be masked by the high folacin intake. Sometimes the damage is first seen in the breast-fed infant of a mother who is a strict vegetarian.[15]

Pantothenic Acid and Biotin

The six best known B vitamins have already been discussed. Two others—pantothenic acid and biotin—are needed for the synthesis of coenzymes that are active in a multitude of body systems. Although they are just as important as the vitamins discussed so far, both pantothenic acid and biotin are widespread in foods. No danger of deficiencies will exist, therefore, in people who consume a variety of foods. Claims that pantothenic acid and biotin are needed in pill form to prevent or cure disease conditions are at best unfounded and at worst intentionally misleading.

Biotin deficiencies have been reported in human adults fed artificially by vein. Even then, however, a deficiency is unlikely unless the person is also receiving antibiotics. Otherwise, intestinal bacteria may be able to synthesize enough biotin to meet the host's needs.

Non-B Vitamins

A trio of compounds inappropriately called B vitamins are inositol, choline, and lipoic acid. These are not essential nutrients for human beings. Like the true B vitamins, they serve as coenzymes in metabolism. Even if they were essential, supplements would be unnecessary, because they are abundant in foods.

Numerous false claims have been made about choline and lecithin. Consequently, many people rush to buy and consume bottles of them. As a result, medical practitioners have been able to witness and report on the effects of overdoses of these compounds. Overdoses can cause not only short-term discomforts, such as GI distress, sweating, salivation, and anorexia, but also long-

Remember, lecithin contains choline as part of its structure. See Chapter 3.

When a normal dose of a nutrient clears up a deficiency condition, it is having a **physiological effect.** When a megadose (100 times larger) overwhelms some system and acts like a drug, the nutrient is having a **pharmacological effect.**

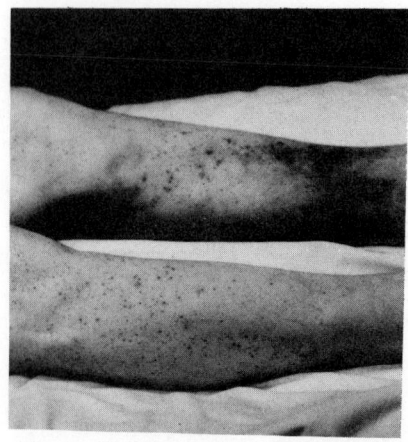

Early skin symptoms of scurvy. There is a tiny hemorrhage around each hair follicle. These pinpoint hemorrhages are called **petechiae** (pet-EEK-ee-eye).

Source: Courtesy of Samuel Dreizen, D.D.S., M.D.

scurvy:
the vitamin C deficiency disease.

antiscorbutic factor:
the original name for vitamin C.
anti = against
scorbutic = causing scurvy

ascorbic acid:
one of the two active forms of vitamin C. Many people consistently and incorrectly refer to all vitamin C by this name.
a = without
scorbic = having scurvy

collagen:
the characteristic protein of connective tissue.
kolla = glue
gennan = to produce

For a definition of antioxidant see p. 107.

term health hazards from disturbance of the nervous and cardiovascular systems.[16]

Other substances have also been mistaken for essential nutrients. They include para-aminobenzoic acid (PABA), bioflavonoids (vitamin P or hesperidin), and ubiquinone. Other names you may hear are "vitamin B_5" (another name for pantothenic acid); "vitamin B_{15}" (a hoax); "vitamin B_{17}" (laetrile, a fake cancer-curing drug and not a vitamin by any stretch of the imagination); "vitamin B_T" (carnitine, an important piece of cell machinery but not a vitamin); and more. There is another water-soluble vitamin of great interest and importance—vitamin C.

Vitamin C

Two hundred years ago, any man who joined the crew of a seagoing ship knew he had only half a chance of returning alive, not because he might be slain by pirates or might die in a storm but because he might contract the dreaded disease scurvy. In 1747, the first nutrition experiment conducted on human beings was devised to find a cure for scurvy. Dr. James Lind, a British physician, found that sailors with scurvy who daily received limes could be cured of the disease within a short time. (This is why British sailors are still called "limeys" today.) The antiscurvy "something" in citrus fruits and other foods was dubbed the antiscorbutic factor. Nearly 200 years later, the factor was isolated from lemon juice and found to be a compound similar to glucose. It was named ascorbic acid. Shortly thereafter, it was synthesized, and today hundreds of millions of vitamin C pills are produced in pharmaceutical laboratories.

Human needs for vitamin C are the subject of much disagreement among experts. There is also a controversy over the risks of taking large doses of vitamin C. We face a difficult task in trying to sort out what is known, what is likely to be shown true, and what claims are clearly unfounded. This section deals with the vitamin's known roles and debunks the obvious myths.

Metabolic Roles of Vitamin C

Vitamin C acts in ways that are imperfectly understood. It plays many different important roles in the body, and the secret may be that its mode of action is different in each case. (see Table 7–6) Investigators studying vitamin C often reach the conclusion that it has to "be present" for certain reactions to occur but that the mechanism of its action will require further research. The best understood metabolic role of vitamin C is the vitamin's function in helping to form the protein collagen, the single most important protein of connective tissue. Collagen serves as the matrix on which bone is formed and is an important part of the tissue that holds cells together.

Vitamin C also acts as an antioxidant. In the intestines, it protects iron from oxidation. In the cells and body fluids, it probably helps to protect other molecules, including the fat-soluble compounds vitamin A, vitamin E, and the polyunsaturated fatty acids.

Vitamin C is also involved in the metabolism of several amino acids. Some of these amino acids may end up being converted to hormones of great importance in body functioning, among them norepinephrine and thyroxin.

During stress, the adrenal glands release large quantities of vitamin C together with the stress hormones epinephrine and norepinephrine. What the vitamin has to do with the stress reaction is unclear, but it is known that stress increases vitamin C needs somewhat.

Eating foods containing vitamin C at the same meal with foods containing iron can double or triple the absorption of the iron from those foods. This strategy is highly recommended for women and for children, whose kcalorie intakes are not large enough to guarantee that they will get enough iron from the foods they eat.

Newspaper headlines touting vitamin C as a cure for colds and cancer have appeared frequently over the years. A review of research suggests that if vitamin C does have an effect on colds, that effect is small.[17] The role of vitamin C as therapy for cancer is still being studied. In one carefully controlled study at the Mayo Clinic in Rochester, Minnesota, the researchers reported that vitamin C is not effective in the treatment of people with advanced cancer who received radiation therapy or chemotherapy.[18] Until the results of further studies can be analyzed, we will not know whether the vitamin C approach to cancer is a hopeful one.

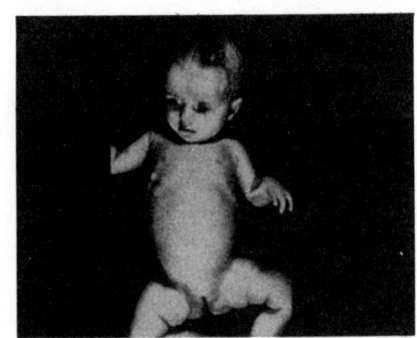

Infant scurvy. This is the characteristic "scorbutic pose," with legs bent and thighs rotated open. The infant's joints are painful, and the infant will cry if made to move.

Source: From C. Conn, *The Specialties in General Practice*, 2nd ed. (Philadelphia: Saunders, 1957).

Vitamin C Deficiency

In both the United States and Canada, vitamin C deficiency is still seen despite the past century's explosion of nutrition knowledge. Surveys have shown intakes well below the RDA for up to one out of every four persons surveyed. Especially in infants, teenagers, and people over 60 years of age, intakes of vitamin C may be less than half the RDA.

The first sign of a developing vitamin C deficiency is a lowered serum or plasma vitamin C concentration. As the vitamin C level continues to fall, latent scurvy appears. Characteristic psychological signs appear early, including hysteria and depression. The gums around teeth begin to bleed easily, and capillaries under the skin break spontaneously, producing pinpoint hemorrhages. If the vitamin level continues to fall, the symptoms of overt scurvy appear. Muscles, including the heart muscle, may degenerate. The skin becomes rough, brown, scaly, and dry. Wounds fail to heal because scar tissue will not form. Bone rebuilding is not maintained; the ends of the long bones become softened, malformed, and painful, and fractures appear. The teeth may become loose in the jawbone and fillings may loosen and fall out. Anemia is frequently seen, and infections are common. Sudden death is likely, perhaps because of massive bleeding into the joints and body cavities.

Once diagnosed, scurvy is readily reversible with intake of vitamin C. Moderate doses in the neighborhood of 100 milligrams per day are all that are needed.

latent:
the period in the course of a disease when the conditions are present but the symptoms have not begun to appear.
latens = lying hidden

overt:
out in the open, full-blown.
ouvrire = to open

Recommended Intakes of Vitamin C

The RDA for vitamin C is 60 milligrams for adults, with an extra 20 to 40 milligrams recommended for pregnant and lactating women. This amount is

Remember the distinction between the *requirement* and the *recommended allowance* or *standard* (see p. 8).

midway between two extremes. At one extreme is the requirement, 10 milligrams per day, which is all you need to prevent the symptoms of scurvy from appearing. At the other extreme is the amount at which the body's pool of vitamin C would be full to overflowing: about 100 milligrams per day.[19]

As is true of all nutrients, unusual circumstances may raise vitamin C needs. Among the stresses known to do so are infections; burns; surgery; extremely high or low temperatures; toxic levels of heavy metals, such as lead, mercury, and cadmium; and the chronic use of certain medications, including aspirin, barbiturates, and oral contraceptives.[20] Smoking may also increase vitamin C needs.[21]

Vitamin C Toxicity

The easy availability of vitamin C in pill form and the publication of books recommending vitamin C to prevent colds and cancer have led thousands of people to take megadoses of vitamin C. Not surprisingly, instances of vitamin C causing harm have surfaced.

Some of the suspected toxic effects of megadoses have not been confirmed. Among these are formation of stones in the kidneys, upset of the body's acid-base balance, destruction of vitamin B_{12} resulting in a deficiency, and interference with the action of vitamin E. Research and reasoning have demonstrated that these effects are theoretically possible, but no cases of their actual occurrence in human beings have yet been seen with intakes as high as 3 grams a day.

Other toxic effects, however, have been seen often enough to warrant concern. Nausea, abdominal cramps, and diarrhea are often reported. Several instances of interference with medical regimens are known. The large amounts of vitamin C excreted in the urine obscure the results of tests used to detect diabetes. People taking anticoagulants may unwittingly abolish the effect of these medicines if they also take massive doses of vitamin C. Vitamin C megadoses can also enhance iron absorption too much, resulting in iron overload (see Chapter 8).

Some black Americans, Sephardic Jews, Orientals, and certain other ethnic groups have an inherited enzyme deficiency that makes them more likely than others to be harmed by vitamin C megadoses. Megadoses of vitamin C can make these people's red blood cells burst, causing hemolytic anemia. Those with sickle cell anemia may also be more vulnerable to megadoses of vitamin C. Those who have a tendency toward gout and those who have a genetic abnormality that alters the way they metabolize vitamin C are more prone to forming stones if they take megadoses of vitamin C.

The body of a person who has taken large doses of vitamin C for a long time adjusts by limiting absorption and destroying and excreting more of the vitamin than usual.[22] If the person then suddenly reduces her intake to normal, the accelerated disposal system can't put on its brakes fast enough to avoid destroying too much of the vitamin. Some case histories have shown that adults who discontinue megadosing develop scurvy on intakes that would protect a normal adult. An innocent victim of this kind of error is the newborn baby of a megadoser, because the baby has adjusted to high levels of vitamin

Doses of 10 to 30 or more times the recommended intake of a nutrient are termed **megadoses.** In the case of vitamin C, any amount over 1 g (1,000 mg) is considered a megadose.

When vitamin C is inactivated and degraded, a product along the way is oxalate, which can form stones in the kidneys (see Chapter 20). People can also have oxalate crystals in their kidneys that are not due to vitamin C overdoses.

The anticoagulants with which vitamin C interferes are warfarin and dicoumarol.

gout: (gowt): a metabolic disease in which crystals of uric acid precipitate in the joints.

The temporary condition manifested by withdrawal symptoms and experienced by the person who stops overdosing is **vitamin C dependency.** The body has adjusted to a high intake and so "needs" a high intake until it can readjust.

withdrawal reaction: a reaction to the withdrawal of a drug revealing in most cases that the user has become dependent.

C in his mother's womb. Once born into an environment providing much smaller amounts, he develops scurvy, a withdrawal reaction.

The experience of a person who stops megadosing and then manifests vitamin C deficiency symptoms on a normal intake may lead her to the wrong conclusion. "I took three grams a day," she may say, "and then when I stopped, my gums started to bleed, and I knew I was vitamin C deficient. That proves I need very high doses."

In reality, this person has deceived herself. To see whether the recommended, moderate intake of vitamin C is sufficient, she will have to taper off, reducing her large intakes gradually and allowing her body to adjust back to the normal condition. The emergence of withdrawal symptoms from drug doses of vitamin C does not prove a need any more than the emergence of withdrawal symptoms in a person giving up heroin or alcohol proves that the person needs heroin or alcohol.

After reviewing the published research on large doses of vitamin C, the National Nutrition Consortium reported in 1978 that there are probably few instances in which taking more than 100 to 300 milligrams a day is beneficial. Adults may not be exposing themselves to severe risks if they choose to dose themselves with one to two grams a day, but above two grams, "genuine caution should be exercised." Amounts above eight grams per day may be "distinctly harmful. It is irresponsible and inexcusable to proclaim that [vitamin C] is safe in any amounts that may be ingested."[23]

Vitamin C in Foods

The inclusion of intelligently selected fruits and vegetables in the daily diet guarantees a generous intake of vitamin C. Even those who wish to ingest amounts well above the recommended 30 to 60 milligrams can easily meet their goals by eating certain foods. Citrus fruits are rightly famous for their vitamin C contents. Certain vegetables and some other fruits are also rich sources: broccoli, Brussels sprouts, cantaloupe, and strawberries. A single serv-

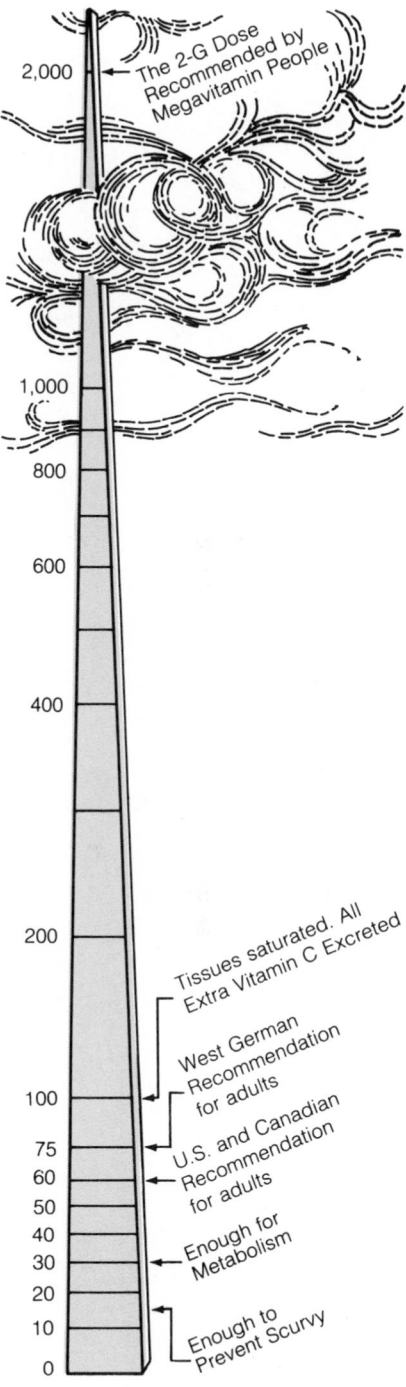

Recommendations for vitamin C intake (mg).

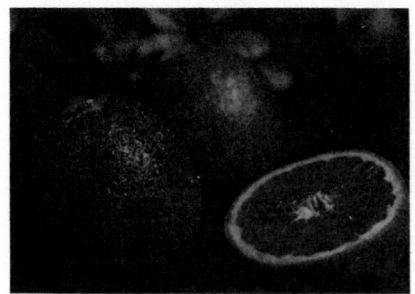

When "vitamin C" is mentioned, people think "oranges" . . .

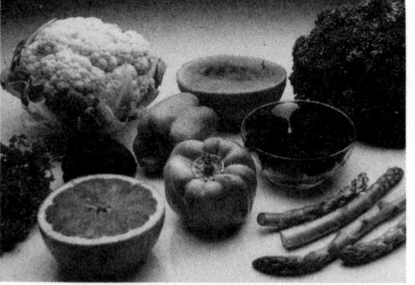

But these foods are actually richer in vitamin C for their kcalorie cost.

ing of any of these provides more than 30 milligrams of the vitamin. No animal foods other than organ meats, such as liver and kidneys, contain vitamin C.

The humble potato is an important source of vitamin C in Western countries because potatoes are eaten so frequently that they make substantial vitamin C contributions overall. They provide about 20 percent of all the vitamin C in the diet.

SELF-STUDY:

How's Your Vitamin Intakes?

Compare your intakes of vitamins with the RDA (inside front cover) or Recommended Nutrient Intakes for Canadians (Appendix A). Express each intake as a percentage of the recommended intake. For example, suppose you ingested 0.9 milligram of thiamin and your RDA is 1.1 milligrams. You ingested (0.9/1.1 × 100), or 82 percent of your RDA. If you had ingested 1.4 milligrams of thiamin, you would have ingested (1.4/1.1 × 100), or 127 percent of your RDA. Use Form 8 to record your findings.

Comment on your intakes. Look closely at any vitamins for which your intakes fell below 80 percent of the recommendations. What are your best food sources of those vitamins? Could you eat more of these foods to bring your intake up to the recommended level? If not, what food or foods could you eat to improve your intake?

Notes

1. Committee on Safety, Toxicity, and Misuse of Vitamins and Trace Minerals, National Nutrition Consortium, *Vitamin-Mineral Safety, Toxicity, and Misuse* (Chicago: American Dietetic Association, 1978).
2. A vitamin D-dependent, membrane-derived intestinal calcium-binding protein, *Nutrition Reviews* 39 (1981): 175–177.
3. Presence of 1,25-dihydroxyvitamin D_3 receptor in rat pituitary, *Nutrition Reviews* 39 (1981): 140–142.
4. A. W. Norman, B. J. Frankel, A. M. Heldt, and G. M. Grodsky, Vitamin D deficiency inhibits pancreatic secretion of insulin, *Science* 209 (1980): 823–825. Vitamin D and insulin, *Nutrition Reviews* 40 (1982): 221–222.
5. M. F. Holick, J. A. MacLaughlin, and S. H. Doppelt, Regulation of cutaneous previtamin D_3 photosynthesis in man: Skin pigment is not an essential regulator, *Science* 211 (1981): 590–593.
6. C. F. Nockels, Protective effects of supplemental vitamin E against infection, *Federation Proceedings* 38 (1979): 2134–2138; B. E. Sheffy and R. D. Schultz, Influence of vitamin E and selenium on immune response mechanisms, *Federation Proceedings* 38 (1979): 2139–2143.
7. H. J. Roberts, Perspective on vitamin E as therapy, *Journal of the American Medical Association* 246 (1981): 129–131.
8. Roberts, 1981.
9. The active form of vitamin D stimulates the synthesis of a vitamin K-dependent bone protein, *Nutrition Review* 39 (1981): 282–283.
10. Intestinal microflora, injury and vitamin K deficiency, *Nutrition Reviews* 38 (1980): 341–343.
11. L. Alhadeff, T. Gualtieri, and M. Lipton, Toxic effects of water-soluble vitamins, *Nutrition Reviews* 42 (1984): 33–40.
12. D. Lonsdale and R.J. Shamberger, Red cell transketolase as an indicator of nutritional deficiency, *American Journal of Clinical Nutrition* 33 (1980): 205–211.

13. More B$_6$ toxicity reported, *Nutrition Forum,* November 1985, p.84.

14. H. Schaumberg and coauthors. Sensory neuropathy from pyridoxine abuse, *New England Journal of Medicine* 309 (1983): 445–448.

15. Vitamin B$_{12}$ deficiency in the breast-fed infant of a strict vegetarian, *Nutrition Reviews* 37 (1979): 142–144.

16. J. L. Wood and R. G. Allison, Effects of consumption of choline and lecithin on neurological and cardiovascular systems, *Federation Proceedings* 41 (1982): 3015–3021.

17. T. C. Chalmers, Effects of ascorbic acid on the common cold, *American Journal of Clinical Medicine* 58 (1975): 532–536.

18. E. T. Creagan and coauthors, Failure of high-dose vitamin C (ascorbic acid) therapy to benefit patients with advanced cancer, *New England Journal of Medicine* 301 (1979): 687–690.

19. A. Kallner, D. Hartmann, and D. Hornig, Steady-state turnover and body pool of ascorbic acid in man, *American Journal of Clinical Nutrition* 32 (1979): 530–539.

20. F. Clark, Drugs and vitamin deficiency, *Journal of Human Nutrition* 30 (1976): 333–337. Committee on Safety, Toxicity, and Misuse of Vitamins and Trace Minerals, National Nutrition Consortium, *Vitamin-Mineral Safety, Toxicity, and Misuse* (Chicago: American Dietetic Association, 1978).

21. A. B. Kallner, D. Hartmann, and D. H. Hornig, On the requirements of ascorbic acid in man: Steady-state turnover and body pool in smokers, *American Journal of Clinical Nutrition* 34 (1981): 1347–1355.

22. Toxicity of vitamin C megadoses, *Nutrition and the MD,* October 1980.

23. Committee on Safety, Toxicity, and Misuse of Vitamins and Trace Minerals, 1978, p. 17.

FORM 8.
Vitamin Intakes Compared with Recommended Intakes

	Vitamin A	Vitamin C	Thiamin	Riboflavin	Niacin	Folacin
My intake						
Recommended intake[a]						
My intake as a percentage of the recommended intake						

[a]RDA or RNI (Appendix A).

NUTRITION IN PRACTICE
7

Vitamin and Mineral Pills and Powders

Billions of dollars are spent on vitamin pills in the United States each year. Two thirds of our citizens use them. You may be one of these users. Or perhaps, after studying nutrition in health and disease, you are wondering if you should be. Nutrition in Practice 7 is intended to help you make that decision and will provide you with some general information about vitamin and mineral pills.

Can anyone really get the nutrients they need from food only?
The answer to this question is an emphatic yes! Foods contain enough vitamins and minerals so that a reasonably careful selection of them will supply all that most people need. The food group plans described in Chapter 1 provide a healthful balance of nutrients, enough to meet the needs of most healthy people.

What if the foods are poor in nutrients? What about nutrients lost in cooking?
The nutrient contents of ordinary grocery store foods were defended in Nutrition and Practice 5. Losses in cooking are moderate if you are careful. The choice of a variety of foods from day to day minimizes your risk of suffering a lack of nutrients in case one item chosen should happen to be nutrient poor.

What if I have unusually high nutrient needs?
Biologically speaking, no two people are exactly alike except identical twins,

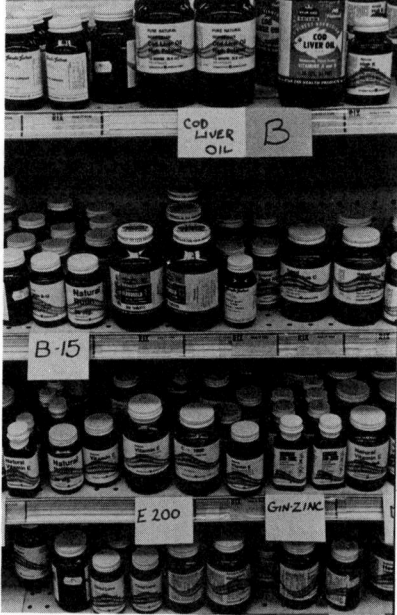

What do you need: an arsenal of supplements, a single daily pill, or just food?

and no two people have exactly the same nutrient needs. You may need a bit more vitamin C than your friend and your friend a bit more protein than you to maintain peak health. Not only are people different biologically, but their different lifestyles affect their nutrient needs. However, rarely (only 1 in 100 cases) are a person's needs above the RDA. These differences between individuals—which are nothing more than normal variations—may make nutrient requirements differ as much as twofold or threefold; that is, you may

need up to twice or three times as much vitamin C as your friend does if her requirement is near the bottom end of the range and yours is near the top. In rare instances, genetic defects may alter nutrient needs considerably; however, only one person in 10,000 has such a defect.

Illness, stress, and prescription and over-the-counter medicines can alter nutrient requirements. But what we are concerned with here are normal variations, and they don't justify the taking of large quantities of vitamins and minerals in concentrated form by the normal, healthy person.

Are there any circumstances under which I should be taking vitamin pills?
Yes, when a doctor prescribes them, when a dietitian recommends them, or when you are at risk for marginal nutrient deficiencies. It has been suggested that all of the following adults are at risk for marginal deficiencies:[1]

• People with low energy intakes, such as habitual dieters.

• The elderly, especially if they are malnourished.

• People who eat bizarre or monotonous diets, such as some food faddists.

• People with illnesses that take away the appetite.

• People with illnesses that impair absorption of nutrients—including diseases of the liver, gallbladder, pancreas, and digestive system.

- People taking medications that interfere with the body's use of specific nutrients (See Appendix B).
- People who have diseases, infections, or injuries, or who have undergone surgery resulting in increased metabolic needs.
- Women who are pregnant or lactating, whose metabolic needs are therefore increased.
- Strict vegetarians.
- Women who bleed excessively during menustration.
- People whose calcium intakes are too low to forestall osteoporosis.

Remember that if vitamins are needed, minerals are needed, too, and a "vitamin pill" is not enough. A vitamin-mineral supplement is called for.

When I do need a vitamin-mineral pill, what kind should I use?
Whenever a physician prescribes one, you should carefully follow directions as to the type and number of pills to take. When you are selecting one yourself, a single, balanced vitamin-mineral pill should suffice. Look for a vitamin-mineral pill in which the nutrient levels are at or slightly below the RDA. Remember, you will still be getting some nutrients from foods. Avoid preparations that are in excess of the RDA. Appendix D lists the nutrients in several vitamin-mineral supplements. The Miniglossary defines a variety of nutrient preparations.

Can taking supplements be dangerous?
Yes. It is a myth that vitamins are nontoxic. You may recall that all of them, not only the well-known vitamins A and D but also the water-soluble B vitamins and vitamin C, have been shown to have toxic effects, at least in some people, when taken in large doses.

Takers of self-prescribed pills need a warning about the risks of overdosing with vitamins, but if they also take minerals, particularly trace minerals, they need a more urgent warning. As discussed in Chapter 7, excessive intakes of fat-soluble vitamins can be toxic—often in quantities not far above the estimated requirement.

A good friend of mine religiously takes several different kinds of vitamin and mineral pills and powders. He says they make him feel better, but I am worried that some of his practices are dangerous. What should I say?
First of all, you have a good reason to worry about a person with a huge

Miniglossary of Nutrient Preparations

cell salts   a mineral preparation sold in health-food stores that is supposed to have been prepared from living, healthy cells. It is not necessary to take such preparations, and it may be dangerous.

desiccated liver   dehydrated liver; a powder sold in health food stores that is supposed to contain all the nutrients found in liver in concentrated form. This supplement has no particular nutritional merit, even though it may not be dangerous, and grocery store liver is considerably less expensive. *Desiccated* means "totally dried."

granola   a cereal made from mixed oats and other grains that is often high in simple sugars and saturated fats.

green pills   pills containing dehydrated, crushed vegetable matter. One pill contains nutrients equal to those in one small forkful of fresh vegetables—minus losses incurred in processing. Sixty pills cost $15.00 and deliver vegetable matter worth about $1.50.

kelp   a kind of seaweed used by the Japanese as a foodstuff. Kelp tablets are made from dehydrated kelp. The urine of people who use kelp has been found to contain raised concentrations of arsenic, a poison and possible carcinogen.

nutritional yeast   a preparation of yeast cells, often praised for its high nutrient content. Yeast is a concentrated source of B vitamins, as are many other foods. The type of yeast used is brewer's, not baker's yeast (see items 992 and 993 in Appendix C).

powdered bone, bone meal   two among many nutrient supplements intended to supply calcium and other bone minerals. Some bone meal has been found to contain high levels of lead.

spirulina   a kind of algae ("blue-green manna") said to contain large amounts of vitamin B_{12} and to suppress appetite. It does neither.

wheat germ   a part of the wheat grain, rich in nutrients.

stockpile of nutrient preparations. Suppose, for example, that this person takes 500 milligrams of vitamin C, 1,000 units of vitamin E, several tablespoons of nutritional yeast, some kelp tablets, capsules of vitamins A and D, a spirulina tablet, some green pills, and assorted other pills containing trace minerals before breakfast, and then sprinkles desiccated liver, powdered bone, bone meal, and wheat germ, and powdered skim milk on his granola. Some people really do such things, and continue with more of the same for lunch and dinner. If your friend is behaving like this, you should be very concerned.

Such a person is trying to obtain all the nutrients he needs. He feels that he can't do this using ordinary foods. This belief is typical of nutritional faddism, which is born of inadequate knowledge applied with sincere interest. Our supplement taker cares profoundly about his health, which is commendable, but unfortunately, he has become a faddist.

To avoid alienating the people we are trying to reach with valid information, we can adopt several strategies. For one thing, we can always acknowledge the validity of the feelings and values that underlie the faddist's practices. Then, we can distinguish between practices that are dangerous and those that are merely neutral. We can ignore the neutral ones and confront only the dangerous ones. Finally, we can make ourselves responsible for learning the facts of the matter as thoroughly as we can, getting them all in perspective, and communicating them clearly.

In counseling the user, you might praise the value system that puts such a high premium on health and express support of the desire to take good care of the body. Then, in the example given, you might reinforce the use of wheat germ and powdered skim milk, agreeing that these foods are nutritious, reasonable in cost, and delicious. When you are sure of your listener's openness to whatever else you might have to say, you might offer a caution about the use of the potent supplements (the A and D capsules and the minerals), but keep your own counsel about the remaining ones unless you are asked. This way you probably won't lose a friend, and you might provide a substantial boost to exactly what he treasures most—his good health.

Notes
1. D. Heber and W. Mertz, Food versus pills versus fortified foods, *Dairy Council Digest*, March-April 1987.

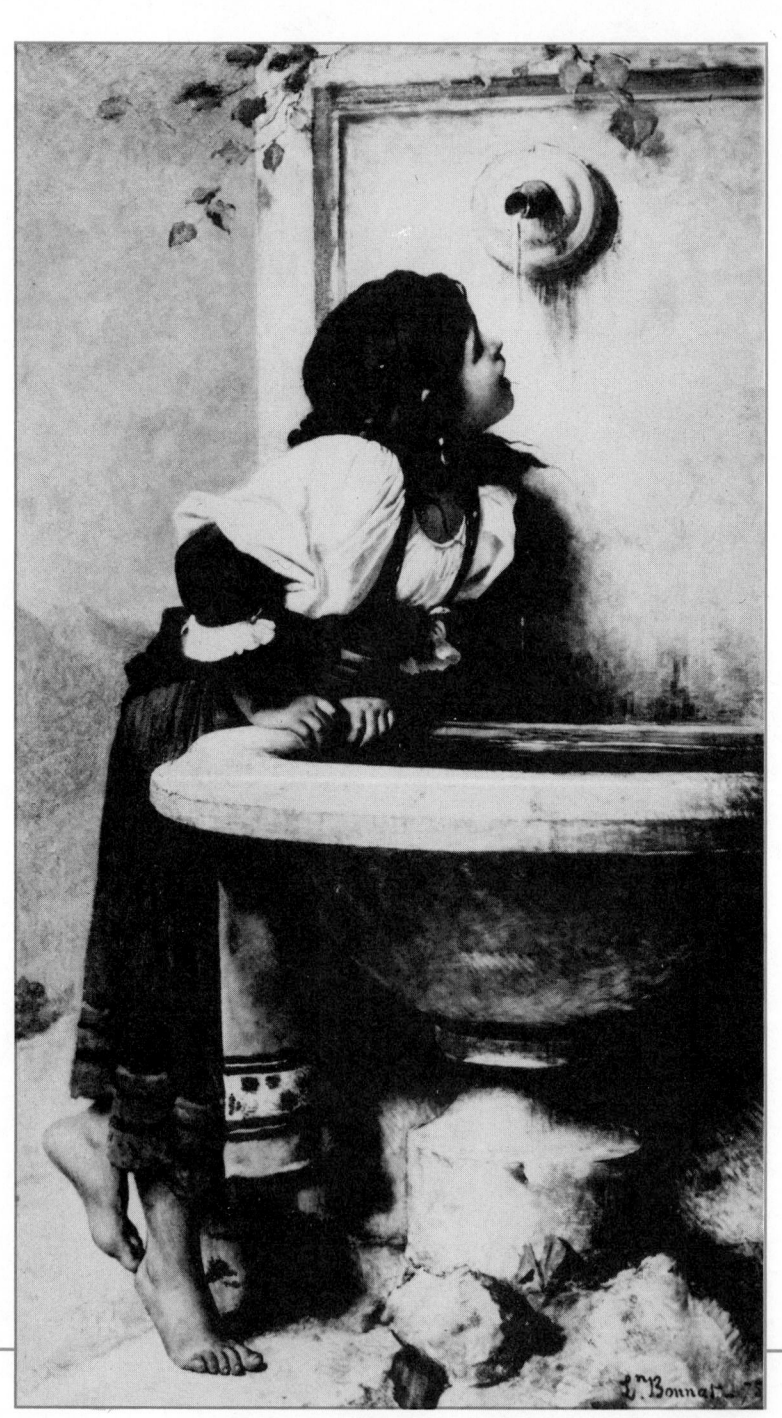

CHAPTER

8

Water and Minerals

CONTENTS

Roman Girl at a Fountain by Leon Bonnat. The Metropolitan
Museum of Art, bequest of Catharine Lorillard Wolfe, 1887.
Catharine Lorillard Wolfe Collection.

The body's water cannot be considered separately from the minerals dissolved in it. One can drink pure water, but in the body, that water mingles with minerals to become fluids in which all life processes take place.

The body fluids provide the medium in which the cells' chemical reactions occur. Every cell in the body is bathed in a fluid with the exact composition that is best for it. These special fluids regulate the functioning of cells. The cells in turn regulate the composition and amount of fluids within and surrounding them. The entire system of cells and fluids remains in a delicate but firmly maintained state of dynamic equilibrium.

Body Fluids

Water brings to each cell the exact ingredients it requires and carries away the end products of the life-sustaining reactions that take place within the cells' boundaries. But water in the body is not simply a river coursing through the arteries, capillaries, and veins. Some of the water is part of the chemical structure of compounds that form the cells, tissues, and organs of the body. Water constitutes about 55 to 60 percent of an adult's body weight.

Water serves many other functions:

- It participates actively in many chemical reactions.
- It serves as the solvent for minerals, vitamins, amino acids, glucose, and a multitude of other small molecules.
- It acts as a lubricant around joints.
- It serves as a shock absorber inside the eyes, spinal cord, and amniotic sac surrounding a fetus in the womb.
- It aids in the body's temperature maintenance.

Our bodies can survive a deficiency of all other nutrients for long periods of time, but they can survive only a few days without water. This is because the body must excrete a minimum amount of water each day—an amount necessary to carry away the waste products generated by a day's metabolic activities. Above this amount (a minimum of about 500 milliliters a day), the amounts of water you excrete can be adjusted to balance your intake. The urine merely becomes more dilute if you drink more water than you need. Hence, drinking plenty of water is one aspect of a balanced diet.

In addition to drinking water itself, nearly all foods contain water. Water is also generated from the energy nutrients in foods during metabolism. Daily water intake from these three sources totals about 2½ liters (about 2½ quarts) on the average. Similarly, in addition to the water excreted via the kidneys, some water is lost from the lungs as vapor, some in feces, and some from the skin. The water loss from these routes also totals about 2½ liters a day on the average. Table 8–1 shows how fluid intake and urine output naturally balance out.

The Body's Salts

Table 8–2 lists the major and trace minerals; Figure 8–1 shows the amounts found in the body. As you can see, the most prevalent minerals are calcium

TABLE 8–1 Fluid Balance

Fluid Intake (ml)	
Liquids	550–1,500
Foods	700–1,000
Metabolic	200– 300
	1,450–2,800

Fluid Output (ml)	
Kidneys	500–1,400
Lungs	350
Feces	150
Skin	450– 900
	1,450–2,800

500 ml = about ½ qt.

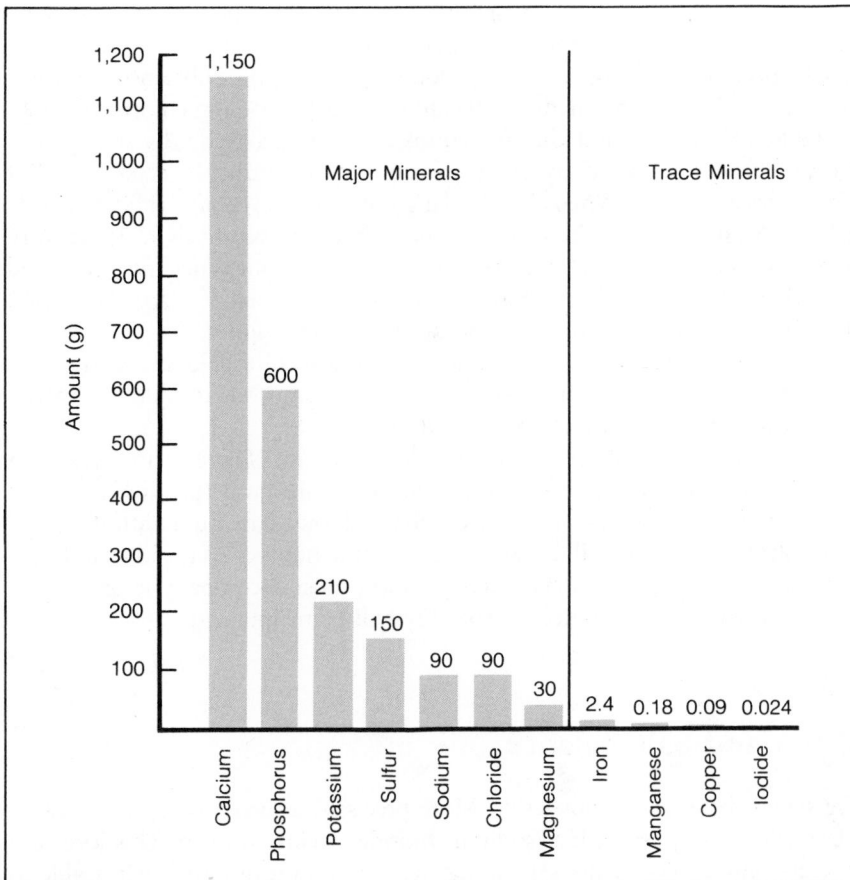

TABLE 8–2 The Minerals

The Major Minerals
Calcium Phosphorus Potassium Sodium Chloride Magnesium Sulfur

The Trace Minerals
Iron Iodine Zinc Chromium Selenium Fluoride Cobalt Molybdenum Copper Manganese Vanadium Tin Silicon Nickel

FIGURE 8–1

The amounts of minerals in a 60-kilogram human body. A vertical line separates the major minerals from the trace minerals. The major minerals are those present in amounts larger than 5 grams (a teaspoon). A pound is about 454 grams; thus only calcium and phosphorus appear in amounts larger than a pound. There are more than a dozen trace minerals, although only four are shown here.

and phosphorus, the chief minerals of bone (discussed later). The distinction between the major and the trace minerals does not mean that one group is more important than the other. A deficiency of the few micrograms of iodine needed daily by the body is just as serious as a deficiency of the several hundred milligrams of calcium. However, the major minerals, because of their larger total quantities, have a larger influence on the body fluids. Four of the major minerals—potassium, sodium, chlorine, and phosphorus—form salts that are abundant in the body fluids.

To understand how cells use salts to regulate the amount of water the cells contain, it is necessary to take a closer look at the minerals as charged particles called ions, the form in which cells use them for water regulation. Cell membranes are freely permeable to water molecules, which are neutral and flow in and out of cells all the time; yet the cells never lose all their water, nor do they

salt:
a compound composed of charged particles (ions). Exceptions: a compound in which the positive ions are hydrogen ions (H+) is an acid; a compound in which the negative ions are hydroxyl ions (OH−) is a base.

cation (CAT-eye-un):
a positively charged ion.

anion (AN-eye-un):
a negatively charged ion.

Na = sodium.
Cl = chlorine.

chloride:
the ionic form of chlorine (Cl⁻).

dissociation:
physical separation of the ions in an ionic compound. A salt that partly dissociates in water is an *electrolyte*.

electrolyte solution:
a solution that can conduct electricity.

This force is known as the **osmotic pressure** of a solution. Water flows *toward* the higher osmotic pressure. The substances that create this pressure are the **solutes** (SOLL-yutes) dissolved in the water.

semipermeable:
more permeable to some substances (such as water) than to others (such as sodium and potassium). This condition is necessary for osmotic pressure to operate.
semi = half

Other terms used to describe electrolyte solutions are **isotonic,** having the same osmotic pressure as a reference solution; **hypertonic,** having a higher osmotic pressure than a reference solution; and **hypotonic,** having a lower osmotic pressure than a reference solution. Standard saline (salt) solutions used in a hospital are made isotonic to human blood.
iso = equal
hyper = too much
hypo = too little

overfill. The water balance is maintained by employing the salts to assist them and by making use of the principle that water follows salt.

Chemists use the term *salt* to include many inorganic substances, not just ordinary table salt. The chemist refers to table salt as sodium chloride (NaCl). In table salt, sodium and chlorine atoms are bound together by strong electrostatic forces in a rigid crystalline structure. Outwardly, the crystals exhibit no electrical charge. When dissolved in water, however, the rigid structure relaxes. Some of the sodium moves about freely as positively charged ions, and some of the chloride also dissociates and moves about as negatively charged ions. The salt thus reveals itself as a compound composed of charged particles. The positive ions are cations, the negative ones are anions.

A salt that partly dissociates in water, as sodium chloride does, is known as an electrolyte. Because the fluids of the body are composed of water and partly dissociated salts, they are electrolyte solutions.

Electrolyte solutions are always electrically neutral. There is no such thing as a test tube filled with sodium ions. Sodium ions are always positively charged and cannot exist apart from negatively charged ions. Any fluid with dissolved electrolytes, therefore, will always have the same number of positive and negative ions. If an anion enters a cell, a cation must accompany it or another anion must leave so that electroneutrality will be maintained.

Water and Salt Balance

We stated that water follows salt. More precisely, a force moves water into a place where a solute, such as sodium chloride, is concentrated. This force can operate only if the divider separating the two fluid solutions is permeable to water but holds the solute back. Figure 8–2 shows this force in operation. In the top compartment, equal amounts of solute on either side of the divider cause the amounts of water also to be equal. In the bottom compartment, the presence of more solute on side Y has drawn water across the divider so that the *concentration* of solute on either side becomes equal. The total *amount* of water is now greater on side Y.

The divider between the water inside and outside a cell is the cell membrane. The cell cannot pump water directly across its membrane, but it does have proteins in its membrane that can attach to sodium ions and move them from one side of the membrane to the other. When these sodium pumps are active, they pump sodium out of the cell faster than the sodium can diffuse into the cell. Water follows the sodium. When potassium pumps are active, they pump potassium into the cell, and water follows the potassium ion. By maintaining a certain amount of sodium outside and potassium inside, the cell can regulate exactly the amount of water it contains.

The Constancy of Total Body Water

In addition to the balance of water and salts within and around the cells, the total amount of water and salt in the body remains delicately balanced. Thirst and satiety govern water intake. We must learn more about the exact

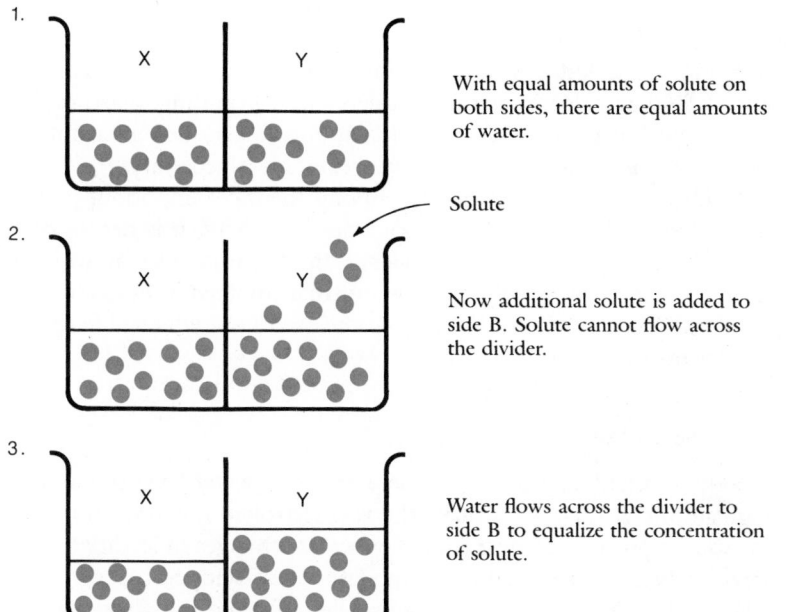

1. With equal amounts of solute on both sides, there are equal amounts of water.

Solute

2. Now additional solute is added to side B. Solute cannot flow across the divider.

3. Water flows across the divider to side B to equalize the concentration of solute.

mechanisms, but it is clear from what we know already that thirst in healthy people is finely adjusted to provide a water intake to meet the body's needs. Thirst itself does not remedy a water deficiency in the body; you have to notice that you are thirsty and take the time to get a drink.[1]

The mechanism of water excretion involves the brain and the kidneys. The cells of the hypothalamus, which monitor salt concentration in the blood, stimulate the pituitary gland to release antidiuretic hormone (ADH) whenever the body's salt concentration is too high. ADH stimulates the kidneys to hold back (actually, reabsorb) water so that the water recirculates rather than being excreted. Thus, the more water you need, the less you excrete. There are also cells in the kidney itself that are responsive to the salt concentration in the blood passing through the kidney. When the cells sense a high salt concentration, they too release a substance. By a roundabout route, this substance also causes the kidneys to retain more water. Again, the effect is that when more water is needed, less is excreted.

The activities of the kidneys in regulating the body's content of sodium as well as water are remarkable. Sodium is absorbed easily from the intestinal tract, then travels in the blood to where it ultimately passes through the kidneys. The kidneys filter all the sodium out; then with great precision, they return to the bloodstream the exact amount needed. Thus, the *body's* total electrolytes remain constant, while the electrolyte composition of the *urine* fluctuates according to what you eat.

The **hypothalamus** (high-poh-THALL-uh-mus) is a part of the brain that helps regulate many body balances, including fluid balance. The **pituitary** (pit-TOO-ih-tary) gland, also in the brain, is the "king gland" that regulates the operation of many other glands.

ADH (antidiuretic hormone): a hormone released by the pituitary gland in response to high osmotic pressure of the blood. The kidney responds by reabsorbing water.

This substance is the enzyme **renin** (REEN-in), released by the kidney in response to a high salt concentration. The mechanism by which renin aids the kidneys in retaining water is the **renin-angiotensin mechanism.**

Technically, these imbalances are known as **fluid** and **electrolyte imbalances.**

Normally, you are well protected from imbalances of water and electrolytes. However, you may be thrown into situations for which your thirst instinct, cell membranes, and kidneys cannot compensate. This is the case when large amounts of fluid and electrolytes are suddenly lost. Vomiting, diarrhea, heavy sweating, fever, burns, wounds, and the like may incur such great fluid and electrolyte losses that emergency medical treatment is necessary.

The details of electrolyte balance are among the most important ones that medical professionals must learn. For our purposes here, it is necessary only to appreciate the importance of this balance and the principles by which it is maintained and to be aware of the situations that threaten it. Water and salts, which we take for granted and usually ignore, are more vital to life than any of the other nutrients considered in this book.

Acid-Base Balance

The body uses its ions not only to help maintain water balance but also to help regulate the acidity (pH) of its fluids. Electrolyte mixtures in the body fluids as well as proteins protect the body against changes in acidity by acting as buffers—substances that can accommodate excess acids or bases.

The body's buffer systems serve as a first line of defense against changes in the fluids' acid-base balance. The lungs, skin, GI tract, and kidneys provide other defenses. Of these organ systems, the kidneys play a primary role in maintaining acid-base balance.

buffer:
a substance or mixture in a solution that is capable of neutralizing both acids and bases and thereby capable of maintaining the original concentration of hydrogen ions (pH) in the solution.

Disorders of the kidney, therefore, impair the body's ability to regulate its fluid and electrolyte and acid-base balances. For a person with renal disease, the physician may order, in addition to many medical procedures, adjustment of the electrolyte intake from food. Chapter 22 gives more information about renal disease.

Up to this point, we have discussed the importance of water and salt and how their concentrations are finely maintained by the body. Now let's turn our attention to the individual minerals.

The Major Minerals

The major minerals are so named because they are the minerals needed in the largest amounts by the body. Calcium, phosphorus, potassium, chloride, sulfur, and magnesium are the major ones. As you will see, they function in many ways in the body.

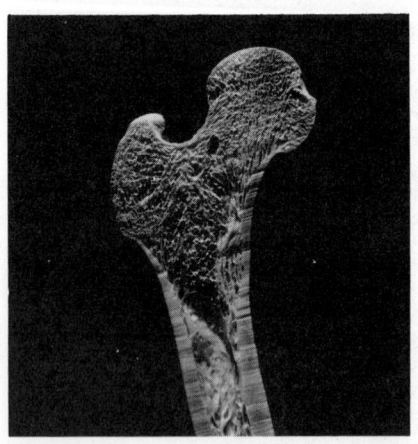

FIGURE 8–3
Cross section of bone. The lacy structural elements are trabeculae (tra-BECK-you-lee), which can be drawn on to replenish blood calcium.

Calcium

Calcium is the most abundant mineral in the body. Ninety-nine percent of the body's calcium is stored in the bones, where it plays two important roles. First, it is an integral part of bone structure. Second, it serves as a calcium bank by providing calcium to the body fluids whenever the supply is running low. Many people have the idea that calcium, once deposited in bone, stays there forever—that once a bone is built, it is inert, like a rock. Not so. Bones are in a state of constant flux, with formation and dissolution taking place every minute of the day and night. Figure 8–3 shows the lacy network of calcium-containing crystals in the bone.

Although only a small part (about one percent) of the body's calcium is in the fluids, circulating calcium is vital to life. Calcium must be present between nerve and nerve and between nerve and muscle for the transmission of nerve impulses. It is essential for muscle action and so helps maintain the heartbeat. Some calcium is found in close association with cell membranes, where it appears to be essential for maintaining the integrity of the membranes. Calcium must also be present if blood clotting is to occur, and it is a cofactor for several enzymes.

Because blood calcium is so important, its concentration is tightly controlled. Whenever the blood calcium concentration rises too high, a system of hormones and vitamin D promote its deposit into bone. Whenever the blood calcium concentration falls too low, the regulatory system acts in three locations to correct the imbalance:

- *Intestine:* enhances calcium absorption.
- *Bone:* increases calcium release.
- *Kidney:* reduces calcium excretion.

Thus, blood calcium rises to normal.

The calcium found in bone provides a nearly inexhaustible source of calcium for the blood. Even in calcium deficiency, blood levels remain normal. But to say that food calcium never affects blood calcium is not to say that blood calcium never changes. In fact, blood calcium sometimes does rise above normal, causing a condition known as calcium rigor. Similarly, calcium levels may fall below normal in the blood, causing calcium tetany. These conditions do not reflect a dietary lack or excess of calcium; they are caused by a lack of vitamin D or by abnormal levels of hormones that regulate calcium homeostasis.

On the other hand, a chronic *dietary* deficiency of calcium or a chronic deficiency due to poor absorption over the course of years can diminish the savings account in the bones. Because this is an important concept, we repeat: It is the bones, not the blood, that are depleted by calcium deficiency.

Calcium deficiencies are widespread in human societies. The price one pays for neglecting to obtain enough calcium throughout early and middle life is extensive degeneration of the skeleton in old age—adult bone loss, which leads to serious fractures in about one of every three people over 65.

The causes of osteoporosis seem to be multiple. A net calcium loss occurs in many adults, especially in women after menopause or hysterectomy, suggesting that hormonal changes are responsible. Many minerals and vitamins are required to form and stabilize the structure of bones, including magnesium, fluoride, and vitamin A. Any or all of these elements may be essential for preventing osteoporosis. One obvious line of defense, however, is to maintain a lifelong adequate intake of calcium.

The disease rickets was mentioned in Chapter 7 in connection with vitamin D deficiency. The amount of calcium in the diet is often adequate in a person with rickets, but the calcium passes through the intestinal tract without being absorbed into the body, leaving the bones undersupplied. Vitamin D

cofactor:
a mineral element that, like a coenzyme, works with an enzyme to facilitate a chemical reaction.

The regulators are hormones from the thyroid and parathyroid glands as well as vitamin D. One, **parathormone,** raises blood calcium. Others, **calcitonin** and **thyrocalcitonin,** lower blood calcium by inhibiting release of calcium from bone. The hormonelike **vitamin D** raises blood calcium by acting at the three sites listed.

calcium rigor:
hardness or stiffness of the muscles caused by high blood calcium.

calcium tetany:
intermittent spasms of the extremities due to nervous and muscular excitability, which is caused by low blood calcium.

Altered composition of the bones is reflected in **osteomalacia,** the condition in which the bones become soft. Osteomalacia is sometimes called **adult rickets.** Reduced density of the bones results in **osteoporosis** (oss-tee-oh-pore-OH-sis)—literally, porous bones. Osteomalacia is related to vitamin D deficiency. The causes of osteoporosis are multiple.
osteo = bone

Chapter 12 addresses in more detail the prevention of osteoporosis.

rickets:
the calcium deficiency (or vitamin D deficiency) disease in children.

deficiency, by depressing the production of the calcium-binding protein, is the most common cause of rickets. (The symptoms of rickets are listed in Table 7–3.) The failure of the body to deposit sufficient calcium in the bones of a child causes growth retardation, bowed legs, and other skeletal abnormalities. In an adult, the disease may set in after a normal childhood during which calcium intake and absorption were adequate and after the skeleton has become fully calcified.

The recommended intake of calcium is currently 800 milligrams (0.8 gram) per day for adults. Authorities are considering raising this recommendation to 1,000 or even 1,200 milligrams a day for women over 50 to guard against bone loss.

Calcium has been implicated in blood pressure regulation. It has been reported that both calcium intake and calcium blood levels are low in people with high blood pressure (see Nutrition in Practice 21B). In fact, the lower the calcium intake, the higher the blood pressure.[2]

Calcium is found almost exclusively in a single class of foods—milk and milk products. For this reason, if for no other, these foods must be included in the diet daily or *wise* substitutions must be made. Because a cup of milk contains almost 300 milligrams of calcium, an intake of two cups of milk provides a good start toward meeting the amount recommended for an adult in a day. Pregnant, lactating, and older women need more. The other dairy food that contains comparable amounts of calcium is cheese. One slice of cheese (one ounce) contains about two-thirds as much calcium as a cup of milk. Cottage cheese, however, is a poor source of calcium.

Some foods appear to be high in calcium but actually provide none or very little. Notably, dark green leafy vegetables and grains have been found to contain great amounts of the mineral, but the calcium seems to be relatively unavailable for absorption.[3] This is because the vegetables and grains contain calcium binders that hold on to the calcium and prevent its absorption. Research presently under way is intended to resolve the many unanswered questions about the availability of calcium from foods.

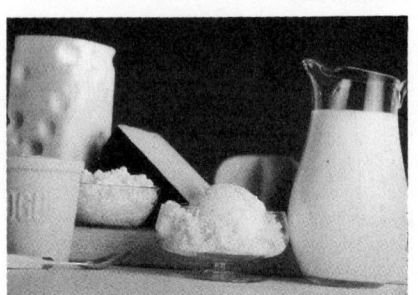

Milk and milk products are rightly famous for their calcium content.

Apparently all fibers in plant foods—cellulose, hemicellulose, pectin, and others—bind calcium to some extent, as do phytic, oxalic, and uronic acids.

People may think that taking a calcium supplement is preferable to getting calcium from food, but there are some important fringe benefits to eating a nutrient in the form of a food. For example, drinking two cups of milk fortified with vitamins A and D would supply the following percentages of the nutrients an adult man needs: calcium, 60 percent; vitamin D, 50 percent; protein, 40 percent; vitamin A, 50 percent; thiamin, 12 percent; riboflavin, 50 percent; plus 24 grams of carbohydrate in the form of lactose. Furthermore, calcium absorption is enhanced by vitamin D, lactose, fat, and possibly other nutrients in the milk. A calcium supplement would supply only calcium—in a less absorbable form.

People who dislike milk may find it helpful to learn how to conceal it in foods. Powdered skim milk, an excellent and inexpensive source of calcium, can be added to many foods (such as baked products and meatloaf) during preparation. Yogurt, kefir (fermented dairy products), and cheese are acceptable substitutes for regular milk. Puddings, custards, and baked goods can be prepared in such a way that they also contain appreciable amounts of milk. For strict vegetarians or people with a milk allergy, a calcium-rich substitute such as calcium-fortified soy milk or tofu (bean curd) must be found.

Many calcium-fortified products such as flour, cereal, ice cream, and orange juice are available in grocery stores. But there is a problem with fortification of products that do not normally contain much calcium. Individuals with an otherwise well-balanced diet may consume too much calcium due to its being added to so many processed foods. Research on the effects of calcium-fortified foods on the normal diet is scant. Calcium-fortified foods may offer calcium but not the other nutrients that are found in calcium-rich foods. For example, people who substitute a glass of calcium-fortified orange juice for a cup of milk receive similar quantities of calcium, but they miss out on important nutrients found in milk—thiamin, riboflavin, phosphorus, vitamin A, vitamin D, and protein.

The word *daily* should be stressed with respect to food sources of calcium. Because of its limited ability to absorb calcium, the body cannot handle massive doses periodically but instead needs frequent opportunities to take in small amounts.

Some factors enhance calcium absorption. The stomach's acidity favors absorption by helping to keep calcium soluble. The body is able to regulate its absorption of calcium by altering its production of the calcium-binding protein aided by vitamin D. More of this protein is made if more calcium is needed. The lactose in milk seems to facilitate calcium absorption by a mechanism as yet unknown. Also, calcium seems to be better absorbed if accompanied by an approximately equal amount of phosphorus.

Phosphorus

Phosphorus is the mineral found in second largest quantity in the body. About 85 percent of it is combined with calcium in the crystals of the bones and teeth.

The concentration of phosphorus in the blood is less than half that of calcium. As part of one of the body's major acids, phosphoric acid, phosphorus is found in all body cells. Phosphorus is a part of DNA and RNA, the genetic code material present in every cell. It also plays many key roles in energy transfers occurring during cellular metabolism. Many enzymes and the B vitamins become active only when a phosphate group is attached. The energy carrier of the cells, ATP, contains three phosphate groups and uses them to do its work.

Lipids containing phosphorus as part of their structure help to transport other lipids in the blood. They also reside in cell membranes, where they affect transport of nutrients into and out of the cells. The phosphate ion also helps in one of the blood's most important buffering systems.

Animal protein is the best source of phosphorus. Deficiencies are unknown.

Sodium

Sodium is the major positively charged ion in the extracellular fluid. Its primary roles, as previously discussed, are in maintaining water and acid-base balance. In addition, sodium is important in normal muscle contraction.

milk allergy:
the most common food allergy; caused by the protein in raw milk. Milk allergy is sometimes overcome by cooking the milk to denature the protein and sometimes "cured" by abstinence from and gradual reintroduction to milk (see Chapter 11). (See also the discussion of lactose intolerance in Chapter 19.)

The Four Food Group Plan recommends daily milk servings:

Children under 9	2–3 cups
Children 9–12	3+ cups
Teenagers	4+ cups
Adults	2 cups
Pregnant women	3+ cups
Lactating women	4+ cups
Older women	3 cups

The RDA for phosphorus: 800 mg.

5 g salt is about 2 g sodium.

1 g salt = ⅕ tsp salt

Certainly no sodium shortage exists in the diet. Foods almost always include more salt than is needed. Other sources of sodium are soft water and many medications. Intakes vary widely; most people in the United States average about 6 to 18 grams of salt per day.

The estimated and adequate level for sodium is 1.1 to 3.3 grams, which is equivalent to about 3 to 8 grams salt per day. The *Dietary Guidelines* recommend that we limit our sodium intake to 5 grams or less of added salt a day—that is, salt added by manufacturers in processing and by consumers in cooking or at the table. This guideline assumes that we normally consume about 3 grams of salt in natural foods.

The guideline is based on inconclusive evidence suggesting that a high sodium intake may contribute to hypertension. It has been seen that a sodium to potassium ratio of 1:1 may be most beneficial in maintaining optimum blood pressure.[4] People are often surprised to learn that as little as one third of the total salt they consume may come from their salt shakers. One fourth to one half comes from processed food, to which salt is added as a preservative and flavoring agent. These same processed foods that are high in sodium are low in potassium and dramatically affect the sodium-to-potassium ratio in individuals whose diets are high in processed foods. Nutrition in Practice 21B presents information regarding this controversial issue, and Chapter 21 offers suggestions on ways to cut down on sodium intake.

Potassium

Potassium is so critical to maintaining the heartbeat that if the cells were to give up only six percent of the potassium they contain, the heart would stop.[5] The sudden deaths that occur in severe diarrhea and in children with kwashiorkor may often be due to heart failure caused by potassium loss. As the most important positively charged ion inside body cells, potassium plays a major role in maintaining water balance and cell integrity. Potassium also assists in carbohydrate and protein metabolism.

A deficiency of potassium caused by insufficient dietary intake is unlikely in healthy people, but diets high in processed (salty) foods and low in fresh fruits and vegetables (good sources of potassium) make it a possibility. In abnormal conditions, such as diabetic acidosis or loss of large volumes of water, potassium deficiency can occur. Furthermore, potassium deficiencies can result from regular use of certain drugs, including some diuretics, steroids, and cathartics. One of the earliest symptoms is muscle weakness.

Potassium toxicity from foods is not a problem because healthy kidneys excrete the excess amounts. Potassium supplements are not advisable, however, except when prescribed, because too much potassium is as dangerous as too little. Even salt substitutes containing potassium should be avoided, especially by people with heart and kidney disorders, except as recommended by a physician.

Other Major Minerals

Magnesium barely qualifies as a major mineral. Only about 1¾ ounces of magnesium are present in the body of a 130-pound person, most of it in the

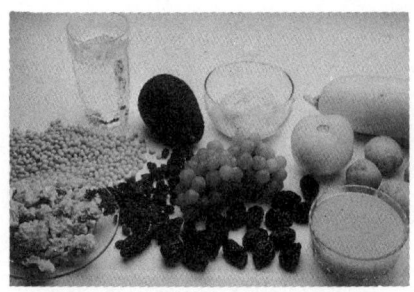

These foods are rich in potassium for the kcalories they contain.

diuretic (dye-yoo-RET-ic):
a drug that promotes the excretion of water through the kidneys. Only some diuretics increase the urinary loss of potassium. Others called *potassium-sparing* diuretics are less likely to result in a potassium deficiency.

steroid (STARE-oid):
a drug used to reduce tissue inflammation, to suppress the immune response, or to replace certain steroid hormones in people who cannot synthesize them.

cathartic (ca-THART-ic):
a strong laxative.
cata = down

bones. Bone magnesium seems to be a reservoir to ensure that some will be on hand for vital reactions regardless of recent dietary intake.

Magnesium acts in all the cells of the soft tissues, where it forms part of the protein-making machinery and where it is necessary for the release of energy. Magnesium also helps relax muscles after contraction and promotes resistance to tooth decay by helping to hold calcium in tooth enamel.

A dietary deficiency of magnesium is not likely but may occur as a result of vomiting, diarrhea, alcohol abuse, or protein malnutrition; after surgery in people who have been fed incomplete fluids into a vein for too long; or in people using diuretics. A severe deficiency causes tetany, an extreme and prolonged contraction of the muscles much like the reaction of the muscles when calcium levels fall. Magnesium deficiencies are also thought to cause the hallucinations experienced during withdrawal from alcohol intoxication.

People whose drinking water has a high magnesium content experience a lower incidence of sudden death from heart failure than other people do. It seems likely that a lack of magnesium makes the heart unable to stop itself from going into spasms once it starts.[6] Good food sources of magnesium include nuts, legumes, cereal grains, dark green vegetables, seafood, chocolate, and cocoa.

The chloride ion is the major negative ion of the fluids outside the cells, where it is found mostly in association with sodium. It has been seen that not just the sodium but also the chloride portion of salt has a role in determining whether the compound will elevate blood pressure.[7] Chloride can move freely across membranes and so is also found inside the cells in association with potassium. In the blood, chloride assists in maintaining acid-base balance. In the stomach, the chloride ion is part of hydrochloric acid, which maintains the strong acidity of the stomach. Salt is a major food source of chloride.

Sulfur is present in all proteins and plays its most important role in helping strands of protein to assume a particular shape and hold it—and thus to do the proteins' specific jobs, such as enzyme work. Skin, hair, and nails contain some of the body's more rigid proteins, and they have a high sulfur content.

There is no recommended intake for sulfur, and no deficiencies are known. Only a person who lacks protein to the point of severe deficiency will lack the sulfur-containing amino acids.

Amino acids containing sulfur are methionine and cysteine. Cysteine in one part of a protein chain can bind to cysteine in another part of the chain by way of a sulfur-sulfur bridge.

The Trace Minerals

If you could remove all the trace minerals from your body, you would have only a bit of dust, hardly enough to fill a teaspoon. Although present in tiny quantities, each of the trace minerals performs some vital role for which no substitute will do. A deficiency of any of them can be fatal, and an excess of many can be equally deadly.

The Committee on RDA has established recommended daily intakes for the best-known trace elements—iron, iodine, and zinc. Tentative ranges for safe and adequate daily intakes of six others are also published. An additional five are known to be essential nutrients, but the amounts needed are so tiny that they have not yet been measured. Many others are presently under study to determine whether they, too, perform indispensable roles in the body, but the eating of a variety of foods in their natural state (not highly processed) should insure adequate intakes.

Iron

Iron is found in every cell, not only of the human body but of all living things, both plant and animal. Most of the iron in the body is a component of the proteins hemoglobin in red blood cells and myoglobin in muscle cells. Both of these proteins carry oxygen and release it.

When a red blood cell dies, the liver saves the iron from its hemoglobin and returns it to the bone marrow to be used for new red blood cells. Thus, only tiny amounts of iron are lost, principally in urine, sweat, and shed skin. If bleeding occurs, iron is lost in blood as well.

Iron losses are greatest whenever blood is lost. Menstruation incurs losses that make a woman's iron needs nearly twice as great as a man's, but anyone who loses blood loses iron.

Iron clearly is the body's gold, a precious mineral to be hoarded and closely guarded. The number of special provisions for its handling shows how vital it is. At the receiving end in the intestines, only about 10 percent of dietary iron is normally absorbed; but if the body's supply is diminished or if the need increases for any reason, absorption increases. This regulation is provided by a blood protein, transferrin, which captures iron from food and carries it to tissues throughout the body. When more iron is needed, more transferrin is produced so that more than the usual amount of iron can be absorbed. Should there be a surplus of iron, special storage proteins in the bone marrow and other organs store it.

If absorption cannot compensate for a reduced supply and stores are used up, the red cells become depleted. The most common tests for iron deficiency are measures of the number and size of the red blood cells and of the cells' hemoglobin content. At the very beginning of an iron deficiency, before these levels fall, the transferrin concentration *rises*. A sensitive test that measures the amount of transferrin in the blood and the amount of iron it is carrying can detect a developing iron deficiency before it is full-blown. Other tests measure iron stores.

If iron stores are exhausted, the body cannot make enough hemoglobin to fill its new red blood cells. A sample of iron-deficient blood examined under the microscope shows smaller cells that are a lighter red than normal (Figure 8–4). The undersized cells can't carry enough oxygen from the lungs to the tissues, so energy release in the cells is hindered. Every cell of the body feels the effect; the result is fatigue, weakness, headaches, and apathy.

Long before the mass of the red blood cells is affected, however, a developing iron deficiency may affect behavior. Even at slightly lowered iron levels, the complete oxidation of pyruvate is impaired, reducing physical work capacity and productivity. Children deprived of iron become irritable and restless due to abnormal levels of the stress hormones in their systems. These symptoms are among the first to appear when the body's iron level begins to fall and among the first to disappear when iron intake is increased again.

A curious symptom seen in some iron-deficient individuals is an appetite for ice, clay, paste, and other nonnutritious substances. Such people have been

---

hemoglobin:
the oxygen-carrying protein of the red blood cells.
hemo = blood
globin = globular protein

myoglobin:
the oxygen-carrying protein of the muscle cells.
myo = muscle

transferrin (trans-FURR-in):
the body's iron-carrying protein.

The storage proteins are **ferritin** (FAIR-i-tin) and **hemosiderin** (heem-oh-SID-er-in).

Transferrin can be measured directly or estimated by measuring the **total iron-binding capacity (TIBC)** and the **transferrin saturation.**

microcytic (my-cro-SIT-ic):
hypochromatic (high-po-KROME-ic)
anemia:
iron-deficiency anemia.
micro = small
cytic = cells
hypo = too little
chrom = color

In all people, including those who are dark skinned, a sign of iron deficiency can be observed by looking in the corner of the eye. The eye lining, normally pink, will be very pale, even white. The skin of a fair person who is anemic may be noticeably pale.

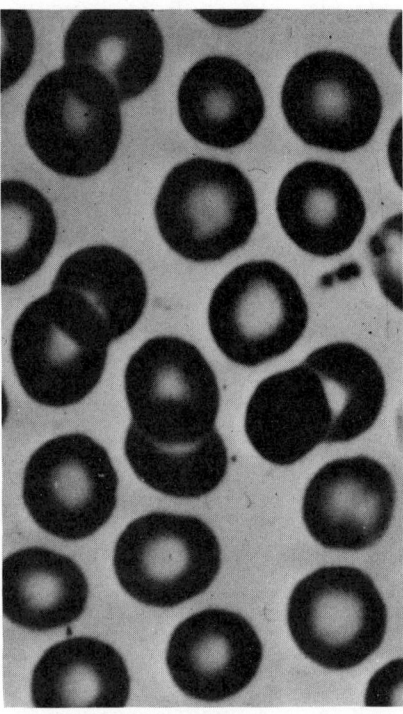

Normal blood cells.

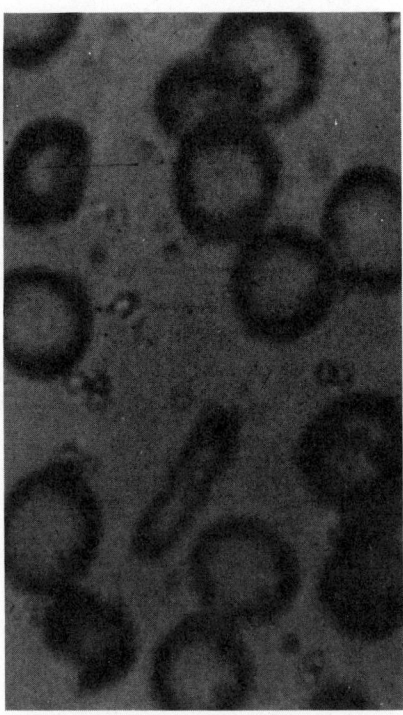

Blood cells in iron-deficiency anemia.

FIGURE 8–4
Normal and anemic cells.

One common test for iron deficiency is measurement of the **hemoglobin concentration** of blood.

Norms for adults:
Men   14–15 g/100 ml
Women   13–14 g/100 ml

Norms for children:
Ages 2–5   11 g/100 ml
Ages 6–12   11.5 g/100 ml

Note that hemoglobin is measured in grams per 100 milliliters, but we often just use the number alone in speaking of it: "hemoglobin, 14."
Another common test, the **hematocrit,** represents the percentage of red blood cells in a whole blood sample.

Norms for adults:
Men   40–54%
Women   37–47%

Norms for children:
Ages 2–5   34%
Ages 6–12   37%

known to eat as many as eight trays of ice in a day, for example. This behavior, which has been named *pica*, has been observed for years, especially in women and children of low-income groups who are deficient in either iron or zinc. Pica clears up dramatically within days after iron is given, long before the red blood cells respond.

A low hemoglobin level may represent a dietary iron deficiency, and if it does, the doctor may prescribe iron supplements. Any nutrient or disease, or any other agent that interferes with hemoglobin synthesis, disrupts hemoglobin function, or causes a loss of red blood cells can precipitate anemia. Nutrient deficiencies other than iron that can cause anemia include, among others, those of protein, vitamin B_6, folacin, vitamin B_{12}, vitamin C, vitamin A, vitamin E, and copper. Nonnutritional causes of anemia include excessive blood loss, infections, and some chronic diseases.

Feeling fatigued, weak, and apathetic is a sign that something is wrong, but it does not indicate that a person should take iron supplements. It means that (you guessed it!) the person should consult a physician. In fact, taking iron supplements may be the worst possible thing a person can do, because such supplements can mask a serious medical condition, such as hidden bleeding from cancer or an ulcer. Furthermore, a person can waste precious time in not seeking treatment. Once again—the caution deserves repeating—don't self-diagnose.

pica (PIE-ka):
a craving for nonfood substances; also known as *geophagia* (jee-oh-FAY-jee-uh) when referring to the clay-eating behavior.
picus = woodpecker or magpie
geo = earth
phagein = to eat

The provision of binding proteins (ferritin and a transferrinlike protein) in the mucosal cells to capture and hold unneeded iron to be shed with the cells is called the **mucosal block** to iron absorption.

iron overload:
toxicity from iron overdose. There are two types, hemochromatosis and hemosiderosis.

hemochromatosis (heem-oh-crome-a-TOCE-iss):
iron overload characterized by deposits of iron-containing pigment in many tissues, with tissue damage. Hemochromatosis is a hereditary defect in iron metabolism.

hemosiderosis (heem-oh-sid-er-OH-sis):
iron overload characterized by excessive iron deposits in hemosiderin, the normal iron-storage protein.

About 40 percent of the iron in meat, fish, and poultry is bound into molecules of **heme** (HEEM), the iron-holding part of the hemoglobin and myoglobin proteins. This **heme iron** is much more absorbable (23 percent) than nonheme iron. Meat, fish, and poultry also contain a factor (MFP factor) other than heme that promotes the absorption of iron, even of the iron from other foods eaten at the same time as meat.

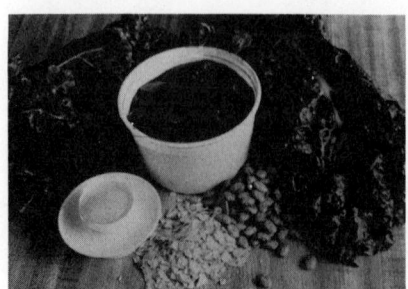

Foods rich in iron.

Iron-deficiency anemia is a major health problem in both the United States and Canada and even more so in the rest of the world. It is especially common in older infants, children, women of childbearing age, and people in low-income and minority groups. But no segment of society is free of iron-deficiency anemia, and the groups mentioned are not the only ones affected.

Iron toxicity is rare but not unknown. Normally the body protects itself against absorbing too much iron by setting up a block in the intestinal cells. The system can be overwhelmed, however, and iron overload is the result.

Two kinds of iron overload are known. One is caused by the excessive absorption of iron from the GI tract. Excessive absorption can occur from hereditary defects, excessive intake, chronic liver disease, and chronic alcoholism and in certain types of nonnutritional anemias. The alcohol abuser is particularly prone to iron overload, because alcohol enhances the absorption of iron. In addition, certain wines contain substantial amounts of iron.

The second type of iron overload occurs when excessive amounts of iron are given by vein. Blood transfusions and iron preparations have been associated with this type of iron overload. Regardless of the cause, tissue damage, especially to the liver, results. Infections are likely, because bacteria thrive in iron-rich blood.

Iron overload is more common in men than in women. An argument against the fortification of foods with iron to protect women is that it might put more men at risk of overload. Indeed, there is some evidence from Sweden, where foods are generously fortified with iron, that this measure has increased the incidence of iron overload in men.

The rapid ingestion of massive amounts of iron can cause sudden death. The second most common cause of accidental poisoning in small children (after aspirin overdose) is ingestion of iron supplements or vitamins with iron. As few as 6 to 12 tablets have caused death in a child.[8] A child suspected of iron poisoning should be rushed to the hospital to have his stomach pumped. Thirty minutes can make a crucial difference.

Most men consuming the usual Western mixed diet can easily meet their iron needs without special effort. But because women have higher iron needs and typically consume fewer than 2,000 kcalories per day, they may have trouble achieving an appropriate iron intake. A woman who wants to meet her iron needs from foods must emphasize the most iron-rich foods in every food group.

Several factors significantly influence the absorption of iron. Although the average amount of iron absorbed is 10 percent, up to 40 percent of the iron in meat, fish, poultry, and soybeans may be absorbed. Less than 10 percent of the iron in eggs, whole grains, nuts, and dried beans is absorbed—fiber, phytates, and other such compounds are probably responsible. At the bottom of the list are spinach and iron supplements; only two percent of the iron from these sources is absorbed. Vitamin C eaten with any iron source doubles or triples the amount of iron absorbed (except heme iron). Tea and coffee interfere with iron absorption.

The following set of guidelines, then, can be used for planning an iron-rich diet:

• *Milk and cheese.* Don't overdo foods from the milk group. They are poor sources of iron; but don't omit them either, because you need them for calcium. Drink skim milk to free kcalories to be invested in iron-rich foods.

- *Meats.* Use liver and other organ meats frequently, perhaps every week or two. Meat, fish, and poultry are excellent iron sources.

- *Meat substitutes.* Don't forget legumes. A cup of peas or beans can supply up to 5 milligrams of iron.

- *Breads and cereals.* Use only whole-grain, enriched, and fortified products (iron is one of the enrichment nutrients).

- *Vegetables.* The dark green leafy vegetables are rich in vitamin C and iron. Eat vitamin C-rich vegetables often to enhance absorption of the iron from foods eaten with them.

- *Fruits.* Dried fruits, such as raisins, apricots, peaches, and prunes, are high in iron. Eat vitamin C-rich fruits often with iron-containing foods.

Table 8–3 shows iron in foods compared to their kcalorie amounts and reveals that some foods are much better choices than others for the person with a limited kcalorie allowance. Additionally, cooking with iron skillets can contribute iron to the diet.

Even after taking all of these precautions, a woman may not accumulate enough storage iron to prepare her for the demands of pregnancy and child-

Overconsumption of milk is a common cause of iron deficiency in children; the resulting anemia is known as **milk anemia.**

Enrichment, fortification; p. 113.

TABLE 8–3 Average Amounts of Iron per 1,000 kCalories in Common Foods

	Iron(mg)/1,000 kCalories		Iron(mg)/1,000 kCalories
Milk and Milk Products		*Grains*	
Milk	0.7	Breads	
Cheddar cheese	1.7	white (enriched)	8.6
		raisin	9.2
Meat and Legumes		whole wheat	12.3
Chicken, broiled	12.5	Cereals	
Chicken, fried	8.1	oatmeal	10.8
Clams, oysters	80.0	fortified wheat cereal, plain	10.9
Eggs	12.5	fortified wheat cereal, sweet	4.3
Frankfurters	4.7	Chocolate cake with icing	4.3
Garbanzo beans (chickpeas)	20.0	Granola bar	7.1
Ground beef, lean	16.2	Popcorn	8.0
Lima beans	22.7	Rice (white, enriched)	8.0
Liver (beef), fried	38.5		
Sirloin steak (with fat)	7.6	*Other*	
Tuna	9.4	Almonds	8.0
		Brewer's yeast	56.0
Fruits and Vegetables		Fats or oils	0.0
Apples	5.0	Peanut butter	3.2
Blueberries	16.7	Minestrone soup	9.5
Broccoli	30.3	Sugar	0.0
Carrots	16.7		
Oranges	7.7		
Orange juice	4.5		
Potatoes	7.6		
Raisins	12.1		
Spinach	100.0		
Strawberries	27.2		
Tomatoes	24.0		
Watermelon	19.1		

Recommended intake of iron (Committee on RDA):

Men	10 mg/day
Women	18 mg/day

How recommended daily intake for iron is calculated, for example, for an adolescent girl:

Losses from urine and shed skin	0.5 to 1.0 mg
Losses through menstruation (about 15 mg total averaged over 30 days)	0.5 mg
Needed for growth	0.5 mg
Average daily need (total)	1.5 to 2.0 mg

Since only 10 percent of ingested iron is absorbed, this girl must ingest 15 to 20 mg per day.

Clay eating: see **pica** p. 145.

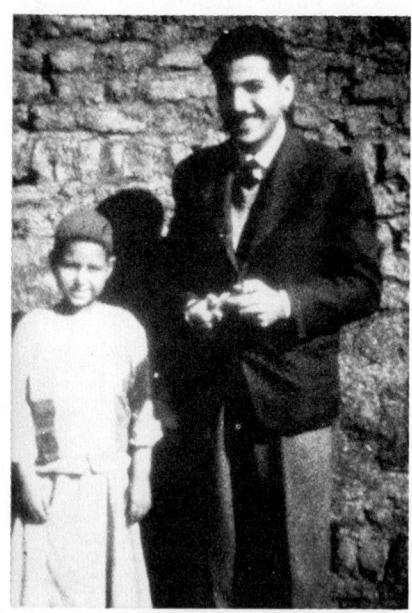

The Egyptian boy in the picture is 17 years old but is only 4 feet tall, the average height of a 7-year-old in the United States. His genitalia are like those of a 6-year-old. The retardation, known as **dwarfism,** is rightly ascribed to zinc deficiency, because it is partially reversible when zinc is restored to the diet.

birth. The Committee on RDA acknowledges that pregnant women may need supplemental iron. Because the iron from supplements is not as well absorbed as that from food, however, the doses have to be as high as 50 milligrams per day. Absorption of iron from supplements is improved when such supplements are taken with meat or with vitamin C-rich foods or juices.

Zinc

Zinc is an incredibly versatile trace element whose roles in metabolism have only recently been elucidated. Over 70 known enzymes require zinc as a cofactor. Each zinc maintains the structural integrity of its protein and may also facilitate the enzyme's catalytic activity by lowering the amount of energy necessary to get the reaction started. Zinc is necessary for normal metabolism of protein, carbohydrate, fat, and alcohol. It is associated with the hormone insulin in the pancreas. It is involved in the synthesis of the genetic materials DNA and RNA, cell replication, immune reactions, the cells' production and disposal of carbon dioxide, utilization of vitamin A, taste perception, wound healing, the making of sperm, and the development of the fetus.

Zinc deficiency is marked by dwarfism or severe growth retardation and arrested sexual maturation—symptoms that are responsive to zinc supplementation. A detailed list of symptoms of zinc deficiency is presented in Table 8–4. Conditions other than poor diet that contribute to development of zinc deficiency include loss of blood due to parasitic infections, climates that increase sweat losses, and clay eating.

Reports of the role of zinc in wound healing are controversial. It appears that in individuals with normal zinc status, zinc has no effect on wound healing. Healing appears to be delayed, however, in persons with zinc deficiency. Similarly, zinc deficiency has been thought to alter taste sensitivity, but research to date has not shown a clear association.

Zinc deficiency also appears to be related to impaired ability of the eyes to adapt to darkness. Zinc is necessary for the reaction that produces the active form of vitamin A (retinal) necessary to form visual pigments.

The members of the population at risk for zinc deficiency are primarily people who are growing—infants, children, teenagers, and pregnant women. Pregnant teenagers are at particular risk, because they need zinc for their own ongoing growth as well as for the developing fetus. Persons on limited food intakes, such as those on weight-control regimens, may also be at risk. A warning to those following very low-kcalorie or starvation diets: Such diets cause not only a low zinc intake but also a loss of zinc from body tissues being broken down as a source of energy. Older people who eat little food may also have limited zinc intakes. People in the hospital with poor appetites or those receiving inadequate nutrition support (Chapter 15) are also at risk. Certain drug therapies can impair zinc absorption (see Appendix B).

Vegetarians, especially pregnant vegetarians, who consume large amounts of fiber, phytate, and dairy foods or low levels of protein, need to have their diets scrutinized for possible zinc deficiency. Populations dependent on food staples or cultural foods high in phytate and fiber content need to be evaluated as well for zinc status.

An average 1,500-kcalorie diet provides about 40 percent of the RDA of zinc.[9] Zinc is highest in foods with high protein content, such as shellfish

TABLE 8–4 Zinc Deficiency

Disease	Area Affected	Main Effects
(No name)	Blood	Tendency to atherosclerosis; elevated ammonia levels; reduced alkaline phosphatase; reduced insulin concentration
	Bones	Growth retardation; abnormal collagen synthesis
	Cells (all)	Reduced DNA synthesis; impaired cell division and protein synthesis
	Digestive system	Lowered taste and smell acuity; weight loss; delayed glucose absorption
	Eyes	Abnormal visual adaptation to darkness
	Glandular system	Delayed onset of puberty; small gonads in males; reduced synthesis and release of testosterone; abnormal gulcose tolerance; reduced synthesis of adrenocortical hormones
	Immune system	Altered skin test responses; reduced cell number in lymph tissue; thymus atrophy; reduced number of antibody-forming cells; altered white blood cell counts; increased susceptibility to infection
	Liver	Enlargement
	Nervous system	Anorexia (poor appetite); mental lethargy; irritability
Acrodermatitis enteropathica (rare inherited disease)	Reproductive system	Impaired reproductive function (rats); low sperm counts; fetal alcohol syndrome
	Skin	Generalized hair loss; lesions; rough dry appearance; slow healing of wounds and burns
	Spleen	Enlargement
	Bones	Retarded growth
	Digestive system	Chronic diarrhea; malabsorption
	Eyes	Inflammation in the corners of the eyes (conjunctivitis); hypersensitivity to light (photophobia); scars on the cornea (corneal opacities)
	Glandular system	Small gonads in males
	Immune system	Frequent infections simultaneous with other diseases
	Nervous system	Emotional disorders; irritability; tremors; inability to coordinate muscular movements (cerebellar ataxia)
	Skin	Loss of hair (alopecia); dermatitis of extremities and of oral, anal, and genital areas, with pus

(especially oysters), meats, and liver. As a rule of thumb, two ordinary servings a day of animal protein will provide most of the zinc a healthy person needs. Milk, eggs, and whole-grain products are good sources of zinc if large quantities are eaten. For the infant, breast milk is a good source of zinc, which is easier to absorb from human milk than from cow's milk. Commercial infant formulas

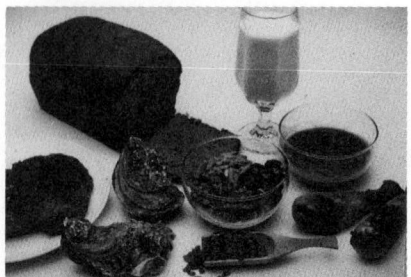

Foods rich in zinc.

are fortified with zinc, of course. Vegetables, fresh or canned, vary in zinc content depending on the soil in which they are grown. The zinc content of cooking water varies from region to region as well. The refining of grains lowers their zinc content.

Whole-grain breads and cereals contain zinc, but they also contain phytate and fiber. Refined breads and cereals are stripped of their phytate and fiber, but they also contain less zinc. Which is a better zinc source, the whole-grain or the refined product? The answer has to do with the numbers of molecules of zinc and zinc binder present in the grain. Whole grains contain phytate and fiber, yes, but they contain relatively more zinc, enough so that the excess zinc is greater per serving of whole-grain bread than the amount available from a comparable serving of refined bread. Even though whole grains do contain some bound, unavailable zinc, they are still preferred to refined products as a zinc source.

This example illustrates a principle that may well have occurred to you many times. Nutrition "facts" are often more complicated than they may at first seem.

Zinc is a relatively nontoxic element; however, it can be toxic if consumed in large enough quantities. A high zinc intake is known to produce copper-deficiency anemia. Accidental consumption of high levels of zinc can cause vomiting, diarrhea, fever, exhaustion, and a host of other symptoms (see Table 8–5).[10] Large doses can even be fatal.

Zinc supplements are not recommended except for an accurately diagnosed zinc deficiency or when needed for use as a drug to displace other ions in unusual medical circumstances. Normally, it should be possible to obtain enough zinc from the diet.

Iodine

Iodine occurs in the body in an infinitesimal quantity, but its principal role in human nutrition is well known and the amount needed is well established. Iodine is part of the thyroid hormones, which regulate body temperature,

TABLE 8–5   Zinc Toxicity

Area Affected	Main Effects
Blood	Anemia, reduced hemoglobin production
Bone	Growth depression
Digestive system	Diarrhea; vomiting; reduced calcium and copper absorption
Immune system	Fever; elevated white blood cell count
Kidney	Renal failure
Muscle	Muscular pain and incoordination
Nervous system	Nausea; exhaustion; dizziness; drowsiness
Reproductive system	Reproductive failure

metabolic rate, reproduction, growth, the making of blood cells, nerve and muscle function, and more.

The amount of iodine in the diet is variable and generally reflects the amount present in the soil in which plants are grown or on which animals graze. Since iodine is plentiful in the ocean, seafood is a dependable source. In areas of the United States where the soil is iodine poor (most notably in the plains states), the use of iodized salt has largely wiped out the iodine deficiency that once was widespread.

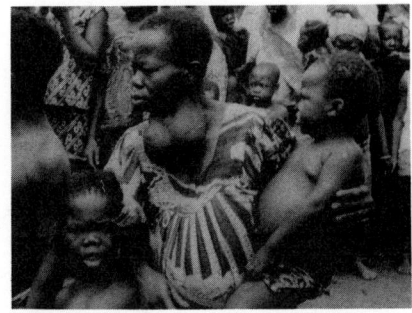

Goiter.

People sometimes wonder whether sea salt, made by drying ocean water, is preferable to purified sodium chloride for use in the salt shaker. Sea salt does contain trace minerals, but it loses its iodine during the drying process. Thus, in a region where goiter is a risk, iodized sodium chloride is the salt to choose.

goiter (GOY-ter):
an iodine-deficiency disease. Goiter caused by iodine deficiency is *simple goiter*.

goitrogen:
a thyroid antagonist found in food that causes toxic goiter.

When the iodine level of the blood is low, the cells of the thyroid gland enlarge in an attempt to trap as many particles of iodine as possible. If the gland enlarges until it is visible, the swelling is called a simple goiter. Goiter is estimated to affect 200 million people the world over. In all but four percent of these cases, the cause is iodine deficiency. As for the four percent (8 million), those people have goiter because they overconsume plants of the cabbage family and others that contain an antithyroid substance whose effect is not counteracted by dietary iodine.

In addition to causing sluggishness and weight gain, an iodine deficiency may have serious effects on the development of an infant in the uterus. Severe thyroid undersecretion during pregnancy causes the extreme and irreversible mental and physical retardation known as cretinism. A cretin has an IQ as low as 20 (100 is normal) and a face and body with many abnormalities. Much of the mental retardation associated with cretinism can be averted with early diagnosis and treatment.

Your need for iodine is easy to meet if you consume seafood, vegetables grown in iodine-rich soil, and (in iodine-poor areas) iodized salt. In the United States, you have to read the label to find out whether salt is iodized.

Excessive intake of iodine can also cause an enlargement of the thyroid gland resembling goiter, which in infants can be so severe as to block the airways and cause suffocation. A dramatic rise in iodine intake in the United States concerns observers. The toxic level at which detectable harm results is thought to be only a few times higher than current average consumption levels.[11] The sudden emergence of this problem points to a need for continued surveillance of the food supply.

cretinism (CREE-tin-ism):
an iodine-deficiency disease characterized by mental and physical retardation.

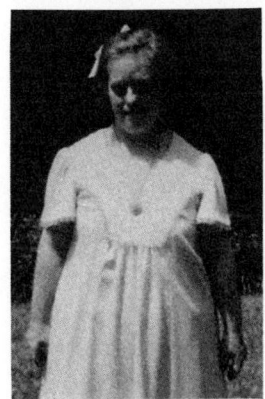

Copper

Copper is part of several enzymes. As a catalyst in the formation of hemoglobin, it helps to make red blood cells. It is involved in the manufacture of the protein collagen, in the healing of wounds, and in the maintenance of sheaths around nerve fibers.

Copper deficiency is rare but not unknown. It has been seen in children with kwashiorkor and with iron-deficiency anemia and can severely disturb growth and metabolism. Excess zinc interferes with copper absorption and can cause deficiency.

The best food sources of copper include grains, shellfish, organ meats, legumes, dried fruits, fresh fruits, and vegetables—a long list showing that copper is available from almost all nutritious foods. About a third of the copper taken in food is absorbed, and the rest is eliminated in feces.

Manganese

Animal studies suggest that manganese cooperates with many enzymes, helping to facilitate dozens of different metabolic processes. Deficiencies of manganese have not been seen in people, but toxicity may be severe. Miners who inhale large quantities of manganese dust on the job over prolonged periods show many symptoms of a brain disease, with frightening abnormalities in appearance and behavior.

The example of manganese underlines the fact that it is as important not to overdose as it is to have an adequate intake. The Committee on RDA underscores this point by adding a special warning to its trace-mineral table: "not to exceed the upper end of the range of recommended intakes." Now that more trace minerals are known, the National Nutrition Consortium also is concerned that these trace minerals will be added to vitamin-mineral pills, making toxic overdoses more likely. Since the FDA is not permitted to enforce limits on the amounts of trace minerals added to supplements, this is an area in which consumers themselves have to be careful. Beware of supplements containing trace minerals. It is a safer bet to consume a diet that provides foods from a variety of sources than to try to put together a combination of pills that will meet all your needs without causing toxicity.

Fluoride

Only a trace of fluoride occurs in the human body, but studies have demonstrated that where diets are high in fluoride, the crystalline deposits in bones and teeth are larger and more perfectly formed. Fluoride built into bones early in life protects the bones later in life from adult bone loss (osteoporosis).

All normal diets include some fluoride, but drinking water is usually the most significant source. Fish and tea may supply substantial amounts. Where fluoride is lacking in the water supply, the incidence of dental decay is high. Dental problems are of great concern, because they can lead to a multitude of other health problems affecting the whole body. Thus, fluoridation of community water where needed is an important public health measure. Despite fluoride's value, violent disagreement often surrounds the introduction of fluoride to a community.

In some areas, the natural fluoride concentration in water is high, and children's teeth develop with mottled enamel. Although this condition, called fluorosis, may not be harmful, it violates some people's prejudice that teeth

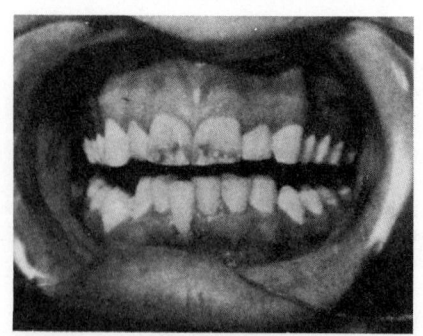

Fluorosis.

fluorosis (floor-OH-sis): mottling of the tooth enamel from ingestion of too much fluoride during tooth development.

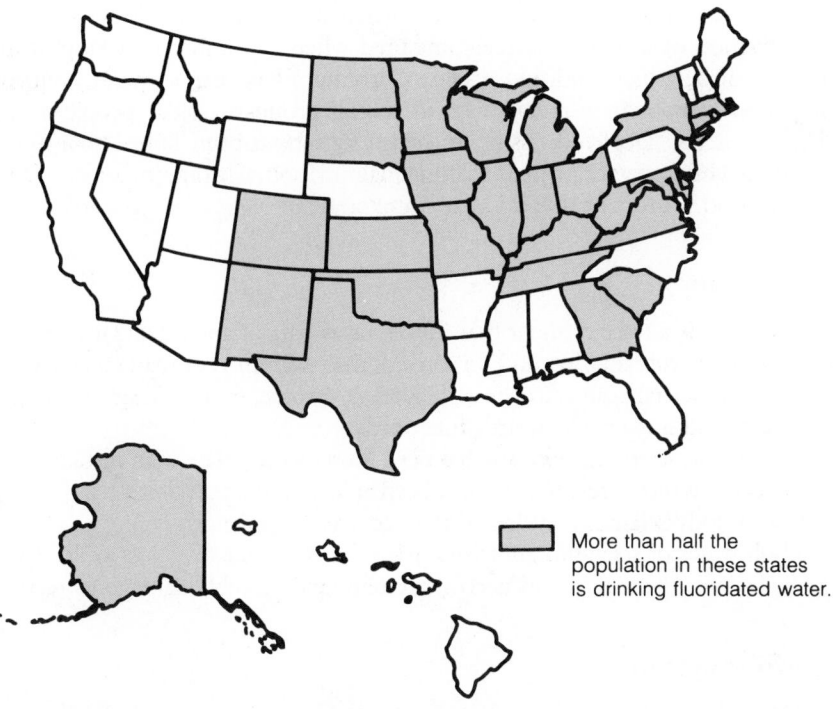

FIGURE 8–5
Fluoridation in the United States.

More than half the population in these states is drinking fluoridated water.

Source: U.S. Department of Health and Human Services, Public Health Service, Centers for Disease Control, Dental Disease Prevention Activity, Fluoridation Census, 1980, Figure 1.

should be white. In fact, such children's teeth may be extraordinarily decay resistant. Fluorosis does not usually occur in communities where fluoride is *added* to the water supply.

In communities where fluoride in the water supply falls short of one part per million, individual consumers who want the protection provided by fluoride can take other measures. They can use fluoride toothpaste or tablets and can make sure their children have fluoride applied directly to their teeth as part of dental care.

Chromium

Experiments on animals have shown that chromium works closely with the hormone insulin. One form of chromium occurs in association with several different complexes in foods. Best absorbed and most active is a small organic compound named the glucose tolerance factor (GTF). This compound has been purified from brewer's yeast and pork kidney and is believed to be present in many other foods. It may be that when more is known, the GTF rather than chromium will be dubbed an essential nutrient and will be classed among the vitamins.

There is some concern that chromium deficiency may become a serious public health problem because of the increased refinement of foods and the resulting

GTF (glucose tolerance factor): a small organic compound containing chromium.

loss of trace minerals.[12] Chromium deficiency is difficult to detect, but the effectiveness of insulin is severely impaired when chromium is lacking in the diet. A diabeteslike condition results. Chromium has been shown to remedy impaired carbohydrate metabolism in several groups of older people in the United States. Depleted tissue concentrations have been linked to growth failure in children with protein-kcalorie malnutrition. Chromium toxicity from eating food sources of this element is unknown.

Selenium

selenium (se-LEEN-ee-um)

The enzyme of which selenium is a part is glutathione peroxidase, which destroys oxidative compounds that could otherwise oxidize other compounds in the cell.

The heart disease caused by selenium deficiency is named **keshan disease,** for one of the provinces of China where it was studied.

molybdenum (mo-LIB-duh-num)

Selenium is a trace element that functions as part of an antioxidant enzyme and can substitute for vitamin E in some of that vitamin's antioxidant activities. A severe deficiency can cause heart failure. A chronic, mild deficiency enlarges the heart and impairs the heart's functions.

In the past, selenium-poor soil has been found to correlate with certain kinds of cancer, but recent research has not been able to find a significant relationship between body selenium levels and the occurrence of cancer.[13]

High doses of selenium are toxic. Selenium toxicity causes loss of hair and nails, lesions of the skin and nervous system, and possible damage to teeth.

Molybdenum

Molybdenum has also been recognized as an important mineral in human and animal physiology. It functions as a working part of several metal-containing enzymes, some of which are giant proteins. Deficiencies or toxicities of molybdenum are unknown in human beings.

Other Trace Minerals

The trace minerals have been known for decades, but their role as nutrients is a recent surprise. Nickel is now recognized as important for the health of many body tissues. Nickel deficiencies harm the liver and other organs. Silicon is known to be involved in bone calcification, at least in animals. Tin is necessary for growth in animals and probably in people also. Vanadium, too, is necessary for growth and bone development and also for normal reproduction; human intakes of vanadium may be close to the minimum needed for health. Cobalt is recognized as the mineral in the large vitamin B_{12} molecule. In the future, we may discover that other trace minerals also play key roles: silver, mercury, lead, barium, cadmium. Even arsenic—famous as the death potion in many murder mysteries and known to be a carcinogen—may turn out to be an essential nutrient in tiny quantities.

As research on the trace minerals continues, many interactions between them are also coming to light. An excess of one may cause a deficiency of another. (A slight manganese overload, for example, may aggravate an iron deficiency.) A deficiency of one may open the way for another to cause a toxic reaction. Good food sources of one are poor food sources of another, and factors that cooperate with some trace elements oppose others. The continuous outpouring of new information about the trace minerals is a sign that we have much more to learn.

The intricate vitamin B_{12} molecule contains one atom of cobalt.

How's Your Mineral Intakes?

1. Compare your intakes of minerals with the RDA (inside front cover) or RNI (Appendix A). Express each intake as a percentage of the recommended intake. For example, suppose you ingested 640 milligrams of calcium and your RDA is 800 milligrams. You ingested 80 percent (640/800 × 100) of your RDA. If you had ingested 1,400 milligrams of calcium, you would have ingested 175 percent (1,400/800 × 100) of your RDA. Use Form 9 to record your findings.

   Comment on your mineral intakes. For any mineral for which your intake fell below 80 percent of the recommendation, what were your best food sources? Could you eat more of them to bring your intake up to the recommended level? If not, what food or foods could you eat to increase your intake?

2. Compute your iron absorption from a meal of your choosing. Three factors go into the calculation—first, how much of the iron in the meal was heme iron and how much was nonheme iron; second, how much vitamin C was in the meal; and third, how much total meat, fish, and poultry (MFP) was consumed. Here's how it works. Begin by answering these six questions:

   1. How much iron was from animal tissues (MFP)? _____ mg

   2. Forty percent of this is heme iron. _____ mg heme iron

   3. How much iron was from other sources? _____ mg

   4. This, plus 60 percent of the iron from animal tissues (MFP), is nonheme iron. _____ mg nonheme iron.

   5. How much vitamin C was in the meal? Less than 25 mg is low; 25 to 75 mg is medium; more than 75 mg is high.

   6. How much MFP was in the meal? Less than 1 oz lean MFP is low; 1 to 3 oz is medium; more than 3 oz is high.

   Now you're ready to calculate. You absorbed 23 percent of the heme iron (see step 2) or _____ mg heme iron. Now take your best response from answer 5 or 6. If either vitamin C or MFP was high, the availability of your nonheme iron was high. If neither was high but either was average, the availability of your nonheme iron was medium. If both were low, your nonheme iron had poor availability. You absorbed:

   • High availability: 8 percent of the nonheme iron.

   • Medium availability: 5 percent of the nonheme iron.

   • Poor availability: 3 percent of the nonheme iron.

   • Your availability: _____ mg nonheme iron absorbed.

   Now compare your iron absorption by adding the two together:
   _____ mg heme iron absorbed.
   _____ mg nonheme iron absorbed.
   Total = _____ mg iron absorbed.

Notes

1. P. H. Baylis, Osmoregulation and control of vasopressin secretion in healthy humans. *American Journal of Physiology* 235 (1987): 671–678.

2. D. A. McCarron, Low serum concentrations of ionized calcium in patients with hypertension, *New England Journal of Medicine* 307 (1982): 226–228; D. A. McCarron and coauthors, Blood pressure and nutrient intake in the United States, *Science* 224 (1984): 1392–1398.

3. L. H. Allen, Calcium bioavailability and absorption: A review, *American Journal of Clinical Nutrition* 35 (1982): 783–808.

4. G. Kolata, Value of low-sodium diets questioned (Research News), *Science* 216 (1982): 38–39.

5. M. J. Fregly, Sodium and potassium, Chapter 31 in *Present Knowledge in Nutrition,* 5th ed. (New York: Nutrition Foundation, 1984), pp. 439–458.

6. P. D. M. V. Turlapaty and B. M. Altura, Magnesium deficiency produces spasms of coronary arteries: Relationship to etiology of sudden death ischemic heart disease, *Science* 208 (1980):198–200.

7. T. W. Kurtz and coauthors, "Salt-sensitive" essential hypertension in men: Is the sodium ion alone important? *New England Journal of Medicine,* 17 (1987): 1043–1048.

8. Committee on Safety, Toxicity, and Misuse of Vitamins and Trace Minerals, National Nutrition Consortium, *Vitamin-Mineral Safety, Toxicity, and Misuse* (Chicago: American Dietetic Association, 1978).

9. M. A. Brown and coauthors, Food poisoning involving zinc contamination, *Archives of Environmental Health* 8 (1964): 657–660. Questions doctors ask, *Nutrition and the MD,* October 1978.

10. J. M. Holden, W. R. Wolf, and W. Mertz, Zinc and copper in self-selected diets, *Journal of the American Dietetic Association* 75 (1979): 23–28.

11. F. Taylor, Iodine—going from hypo to hyper, *FDA Consumer,* April 1981, 15–18.

12. R. A. Anderson and A. S. Kozlovsky. Chromium intake, absorption and excretion of subjects consuming self-selected diets, *American Journal of Clinical Nutrition* 41(1985): 1177–1183.

13. J. Virtamo and coauthors, Serum selenium and risk of cancer: A prospective follow-up of nine years, *Cancer* 60 (1987): 145–148.

FORM 9
Mineral Intakes Compared with Recommended Intakes

	Calcium	Iron	Zinc
My intake			
Recommended intake[a]			
My intake as a percentage of the recommended intake			

[a]RDA or RNI (Appendix A).

Nutrition and Premenstrual Syndrome

Margie has premenstrual syndrome (PMS). Her body feels heavy and sick. Pain invades her, bringing sore breasts, a backache, and a headache. She doesn't want to be touched. She cries easily, is irritated and depressed. She tends to binge on carbohydrates. It comes on predictably every month, stays a week to ten days, then mysteriously disappears like a lifting cloud a few hours after her menstrual period has begun. One of every three women recognizes some of these symptoms.

Is poor nutrition the cause of all this? Some people are tempted to think so; others think not. Research into the relationships between PMS and nutrition has given us few answers to the questions that have been raised, but as research continues we hope to understand this complex syndrome more fully.

Margie sounds a lot like me. But I never really thought nutrition could be involved. How can nutrition be related to menstruation?

The hormones that regulate the menstrual cycle are powerful, and they affect many body organs. Among nutrition-related cyclic rhythms now known are changes in metabolic rate, glucose tolerance, appetite, and food intake. Possible nutrition-related differences in women with PMS involve vitamin B_6 status, blood magnesium concentration, and vitamin E. Researchers have speculated upon the effects of many other nutrients.

Now that you mention it, I have a friend who takes vitamin B_6 supplements for PMS. Why were they prescribed?

Vitamin B_6 has been popularized as a prime candidate for relieving PMS, but trials of vitamin B_6 in PMS have had mixed results. One study in which the researchers attempted to use vitamin B_6 to relieve premenstrual depression found that while vitamin B_6 may improve premenstrual symptoms related to autonomic reactions (such as dizziness and vomiting) and behavioral changes (such as poor performance and less participation in social activities), a significant number of physical symptoms remained during the premenstrual phase.[1] Because of the potentially toxic effect of low doses of vitamin B_6, the benefits derived from this type of therapy must be weighed against the possible detrimental effects of megadoses of this vitamin.

Another pair of researchers tested a particular woman who claimed to be responsive to vitamin B_6 by using a double-blind experiment. The woman experienced relief from her symptoms consistently with the vitamin and not with the placebo, showing clearly that in her case PMS was related to vitamin B_6.[2]

The vitamin B_6-PMS research can be summed up by saying that the vitamin may have real, beneficial effects only if a relative or absolute deficiency of the vitamin has existed. The old lesson of basic nutrition is reinforced here: A vitamin will clear up symptoms caused by a deficiency of that vitamin.

You mentioned that blood magnesium concentrations may be related to PMS. What's the connection?

Magnesium status was studied in "normal" and PMS subjects, and the levels of this mineral in the red blood cells were found to be lower in the PMS group.[3] Unfortunately, the subjects' diets weren't studied, so it's impossible to tell whether the women had a dietary deficiency or were absorbing less or excreting more magnesium. In fact, it's possible that the women's total body contents of magnesium hadn't changed but that there had been a shift of magnesium from the red blood cells into some other body compartment. Clearly, on the basis of the one finding, it is impossible to say whether people with PMS need more or less magnesium or more or less of something else.

What about vitamin E?

Vitamin E deficiency is another candidate for contributor to PMS, and one creditable attempt has demonstrated that vitamin E has some effectiveness in relieving one symptom often experienced in PMS—sore breasts. The research involved 75 women in a double-blind, placebo-controlled study. The results suggested that vitamin E (300 IU) brought relief while the placebo did not.[4] However, some women *without* PMS also have sore breasts that can sometimes be relieved by vitamin E.[5] Possibly the correct logic is that vitamin E deficiency can cause sore breasts and that the menstrual cycle can make them worse, but *not* that vitamin E deficiency causes PMS.

How would you suggest that the person with PMS manage her diet?

All menstruating women can benefit from some findings on nutrition and the menstrual cycle. Many women just plain get hungry during the week or two before their periods. Reliable research shows that two things happen during that time:

• Basal metabolic rate speeds up.[6]

• Appetite and kcalorie intake pick up.[7]

Women report that they crave carbohydrates. When their food intake is actually measured, they eat an average of 500 kcalories a day more during the ten days before their periods than during the ten days after—principally from carbohydrate.[8]

At least one application of these findings seems obvious at first glance. Women need to know that hunger and carbohydrate craving preceding menstruation are natural, probably universal, biological phenomena, and

not signs of their own incompetence, inadequacy, or neuroticism. Rather than attempting to rigidly restrict kcalorie intake to some fixed amount throughout the month, any woman whose appetite is affected by the cyclic rhythm of her hormones would do better to relax and go with it: increase kcalories during the two weeks before her period and reduce them during the two weeks after.

Finally, the same advice holds for women with PMS as for women or men with any other health problem or need. Be sure to get adequate sleep and adequate exercise. Eat well, and be sensible about intakes of sugar, caffeine, salt, alcohol, and any other "abuse-able" substances. If you have reason to think your nutrient intake is inadequate and you *can't* rectify it by eating foods, fall back on a daily supplement for a while. But avoid megadoses. Stay with the moderate amounts available in an ordinary multivitamin-mineral supplement (see Nutrition in Practice 7). And be very skeptical when someone who can pocket your money in return for her goods tells you that her product will relieve your symptoms. Watch out for snake-oil salespeople; there are a lot of them out there.

Notes

1. K. E. Kendall and P. P. Schnurr, The effects of vitamin B$_6$ supplementation on premenstrual symptoms. *Obstetrics and Gynecology* 2 (1987):145–149.

2. J. A. Mattes and D. Martin, Pyridoxine in premenstrual tension, *Human Nutrition: Applied Nutrition* 36A (1982): 131–133.

3. D. Y. Jones and S. K. Kumanyika, Premenstrual syndrome: A review of possible dietary influences, *Journal of the Canadian Dietetic Association* 44 (1983): 195–203.

4. R. S. London and coauthors, The effect of alpha-tocopherol on premenstrual symptomatology, a double-blind study, *Journal of the American College of Nutrition* 2 (1983): 115–122.

5. E. R. Gonzalez, Vitamin E relieves most cystic breast disease; may alter lipids, hormones (medical news), *Journal of the American Medical Association* 244 (1980): 1077–1078.

6. S. J. Solomon, M. S. Kurzer, and D. H. Calloway, Menstrual cycle and basal metabolic rate in women, *American Journal of Clinical Nutrition* 36 (1982): 611–616.

7. S. P. Dalvit, The effect of the menstrual cycle on patterns of food intake, *American Journal of Clinical Nutrition* 34 (1981): 1811–1815.

8. S. P. Dalvit-McPhillips, The effect of the human menstrual cycle on nutrient intake, *Physiology and Behavior* 31 (1983): 209–212.

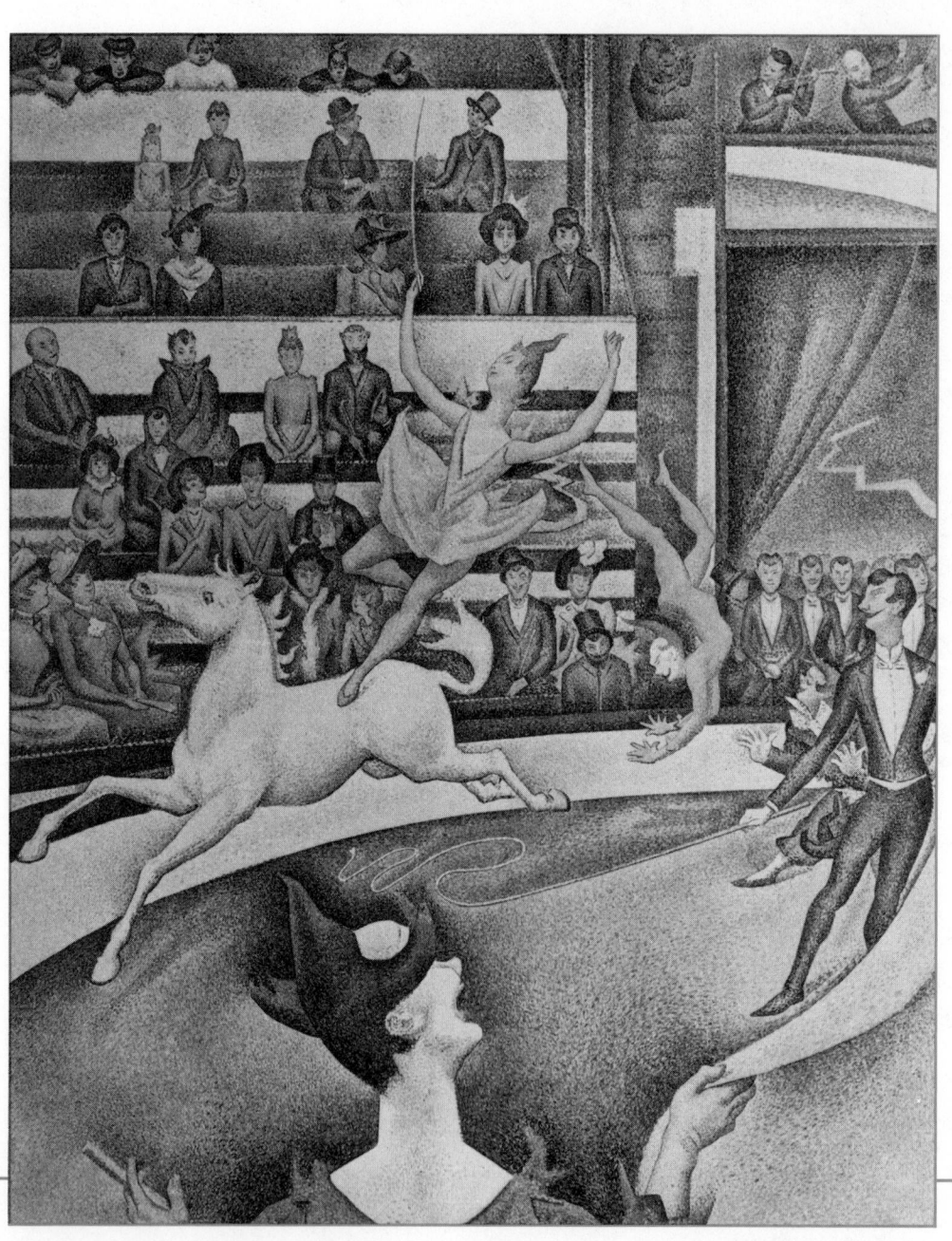

9

Nutrition and Fitness
for Optimal Health

CONTENTS

Le Cirque by Georges Seurat. Reprinted by permission, Paris,
Musée d'Orsay.

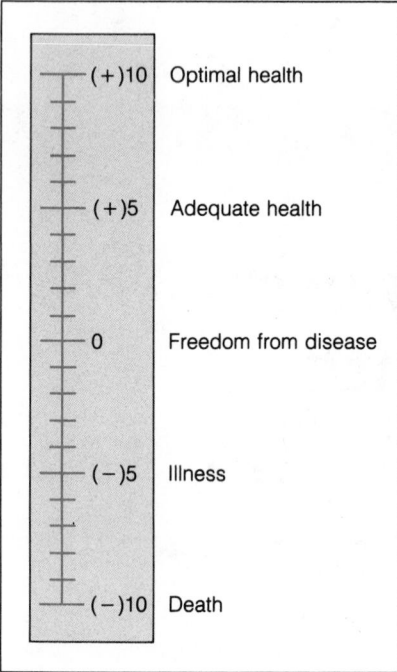

FIGURE 9–1

A wellness scale. You can visualize degrees of health as on a scale. Zero represents the traditional view of health—the person who is not sick but could improve his health status. The negative end of the scale represents varying degrees of illness, ending in death. The positive end of the scale represents optimal health. Positive lifestyle habits that contribute to optimal health include exercise, appropriate diet, stress control, abstinence from cigarette smoking, and moderation in or abstinence from alcohol consumption.

wellness:
the goal of the person who strives to realize his or her full mental, emotional, physical, interpersonal, social, and spiritual potential; this book also uses the term *optimal health.*

calisthenics:
exercise routines for muscular development that use the weight of the body as resistance.

The number of people who are concerned about their health is increasing, and over a third of the population exercise.[1] The fitness boom and subsequent research in the exercise field have expanded the role of nutrition as it relates to the well person. New professional roles and responsibilities for the health care provider have emerged. Health professionals, through training and experience, can prepare themselves for a leading role in the wellness movement. Knowledge of how nutrition promotes health and wellness throughout the life cycle is important in being able to provide people with sound guidelines.

The concept of health has evolved from the goal of mere freedom from disease to the goal of optimal health. Instead of simply treating diseases, people want to achieve a higher level of wellness so that they can not only avoid disease but also feel their best. Figure 9–1 illustrates this concept.

The areas of wellness dealt with in this chapter are the ones that are most closely related to nutrition: fitness, weight control, and modified eating and exercise behaviors. As we look at each one of these topics, we will see that wellness is a balance of many factors.

Exercise and Health

In the early 1900s, fitness was an unknown word. Much of the work performed by both men and women was manual labor that provided adequate exercise. Industrialization and automation eliminated much of the manual work that once existed, and today many jobs are service-oriented jobs that require only light activity. The large muscle groups are not used in such work, and even many leisure activities require little physical effort. Cars, riding lawn mowers, elevators, and escalators are just a few of the labor-saving devices that keep people from physically exerting themselves. The less active people become, the more out of condition they become. The physical consequences of not developing fitness are serious enough that people cannot hope to have optimal health without such fitness.

Total Fitness

The inactivity that is common to most people's workdays needs to be compensated for by daily exercise. The human body is designed to fight enemies; push, pull, and carry heavy objects; and run long distances. The person whose daily routine does not normally involve this type of activity must develop a fitness program that does. A fitness program does not have to be mundane calisthenics or any preset conditioning regimen. In fact it should include activities that are enjoyed, such as walking, jogging, tennis, and others.

When performance is the main reason for fitness, goals for exercise are described in terms of skill, balance, speed, and coordination. The goals are designed for a particular sport instead of for overall wellness. Nutrition in Practice 9 deals with special nutritional concerns of the athlete. This chapter has a broader mission: it aims at overall wellness and recognizes sports as a

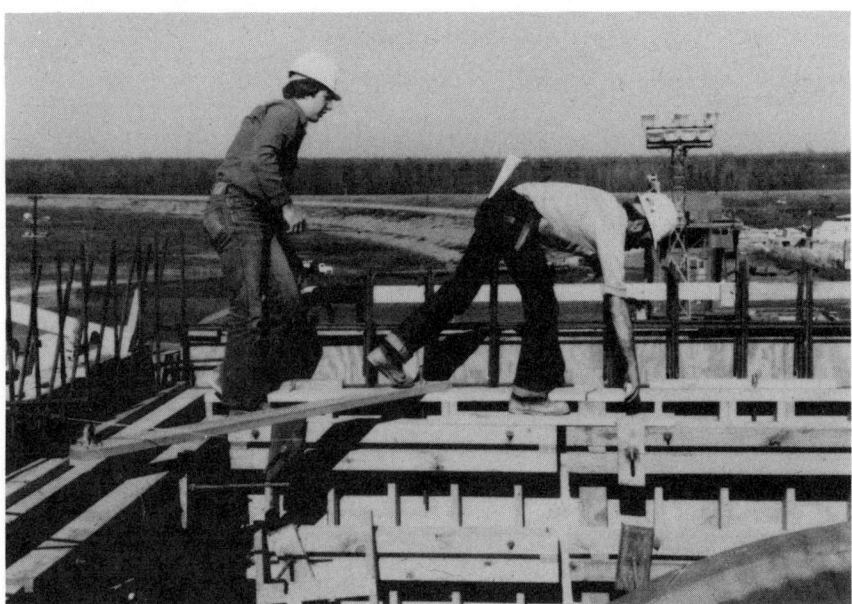

Work that requires physical activity helps build fitness.

flexibility:
a component of fitness, the ability to bend without injury; it depends on the elasticity of muscles, tendons, and ligaments and on the condition of the joints.

muscular strength:
a component of fitness, the ability of a muscle to work against resistance.

muscular endurance:
a component of fitness, the ability of a muscle to contract repeatedly within a given time without becoming exhausted.

cardiovascular endurance:
a component of fitness, the ability of the cardiovascular system to sustain effort over a long time.

use-disuse principle:
the principle that fitness develops in response to demand and diminishes in response to a lack of demand.

hypertrophy (high-PURR-tro-fee):
an increase in size in response to use.

atrophy (AT-tro-fee):
a decrease in size from disuse.

way of making fitness fun and challenging. Intense training for sporting events does not always support optimal health. For example, the elite body builder may not have a well-conditioned heart; the marathon runner may not be flexible.

The requirements of a fitness program are the maintenance of reasonable weight, flexibility, and muscular strength and endurance to meet the everyday demands of life, plus some to spare. Determining reasonable weight for each person is discussed later, but exercise can promote either weight gain or weight loss, depending upon one's activities and diet. A high-kcalorie diet and weight-lifting would help a person gain weight, whereas a lower kcalorie diet coupled with jogging can help a person lose weight.

Fitness is expressed in several ways. With respect to the joints, flexibility is important. With respect to the muscles, muscle strength and endurance are important. Another type of fitness, cardiovascular endurance, is important to the heart and lungs. Table 9–1 describes activities that will help develop these specific types of fitness.

A person's body shape is determined by the physical condition of the muscles. The muscles respond to increased use by gaining strength, size, and ability to endure, a response called hypertrophy. The converse is also true: Muscles, if not called on to perform, atrophy. The same principle is at work internally even though it is more difficult to see. The heart muscle can be strengthened by exercise in much the same way that other more visible muscles are strengthened.

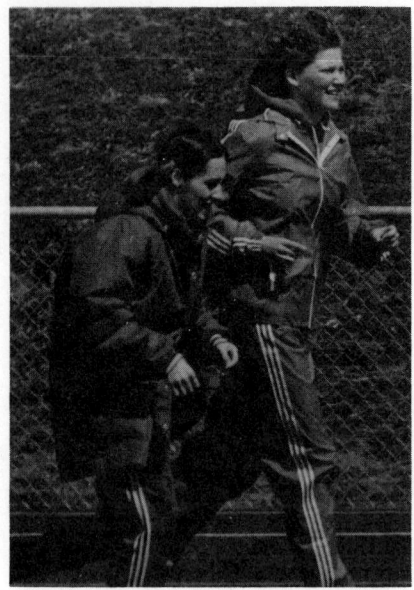

Jogging with a friend can make aerobic workouts enjoyable. All muscles of the body benefit from this type of cardiac conditioning.

TABLE 9–1. Activities to Develop the Four Types of Fitness

Fitness Component	Activity
Flexibility	Stretches will enhance flexibility. They should be long, luxurious, and pleasurable. Hold each stretch for 10 to 15 seconds. Never use bouncy, choppy, or painful stretches that twist or put pressure on joints.
Muscle strength	Calisthenic exercises such as pushups and sit-ups and a few repetitions with heavy weights increase muscle bulk—the key to strength, the ability to exert pressure against a force. Use extreme caution when working with heavy weights or machines; without proper guidance, injury is likely.
Muscle endurance	Repetitive exercises, such as pushups, pull-ups, sit-ups (calisthenics), or many repetitions with light weights will build endurance of the muscle groups worked.
Cardiovascular endurance	Activities include swimming, rowing, fast walking, jogging, fast bicycling, soccer, hockey, basketball, water polo, lacrosse, rugby, and many more. These activities can provide the needed *sustained, submaximal* activity level, because they raise the heart rate for more than 20 minutes and use most of the large muscle groups of the body (legs, buttocks, abdomen).

aerobic:
requiring oxygen.

aerobic metabolism:
that part of energy nutrient breakdown that requires oxygen for completion, such as the metabolism of fat.

Physiology of Exercise

Exercise that places demands on the heart, aerobic exercise, improves not only the heart's condition but also the condition of the lungs and all muscles of the body, whether or not they are directly involved in the exercise.[2] For example, the muscles along the arteries and in the walls of the digestive tract become more fit and able to work more effectively.

In cardiovascular conditioning, the total blood volume increases so that the blood can carry more oxygen. The heart muscle becomes stronger and larger, and each beat empties the heart's chambers more completely so that the heart pumps more blood per beat. This makes fewer beats necessary and the pulse rate falls. The muscles that inflate and deflate the lungs gain strength and endurance, and breathing becomes more efficient. Blood moves easily through the body's arteries and veins, because the muscles of the arteries contract powerfully, and other muscles move more blood through the veins. Blood pressure falls, because vessel resistance is reduced. Figure 9–2 shows major relationships between the heart, circulatory system, and lungs.

When you begin to exercise, the hormones epinephrine and norepinephrine, among others, begin to circulate in the bloodstream, signaling the liver and fat cells to liberate stored energy nutrients. These hormones are also released in response to stress, and the effect on the body is the same, with one important difference. Fuels called forth by stress are not fully used up by muscles but continue cycling around the bloodstream until the stress ceases, hormones diminish, and the fuels are stored once more, perhaps in their original form, or perhaps after conversion to something else—glucose to fat, for example, or

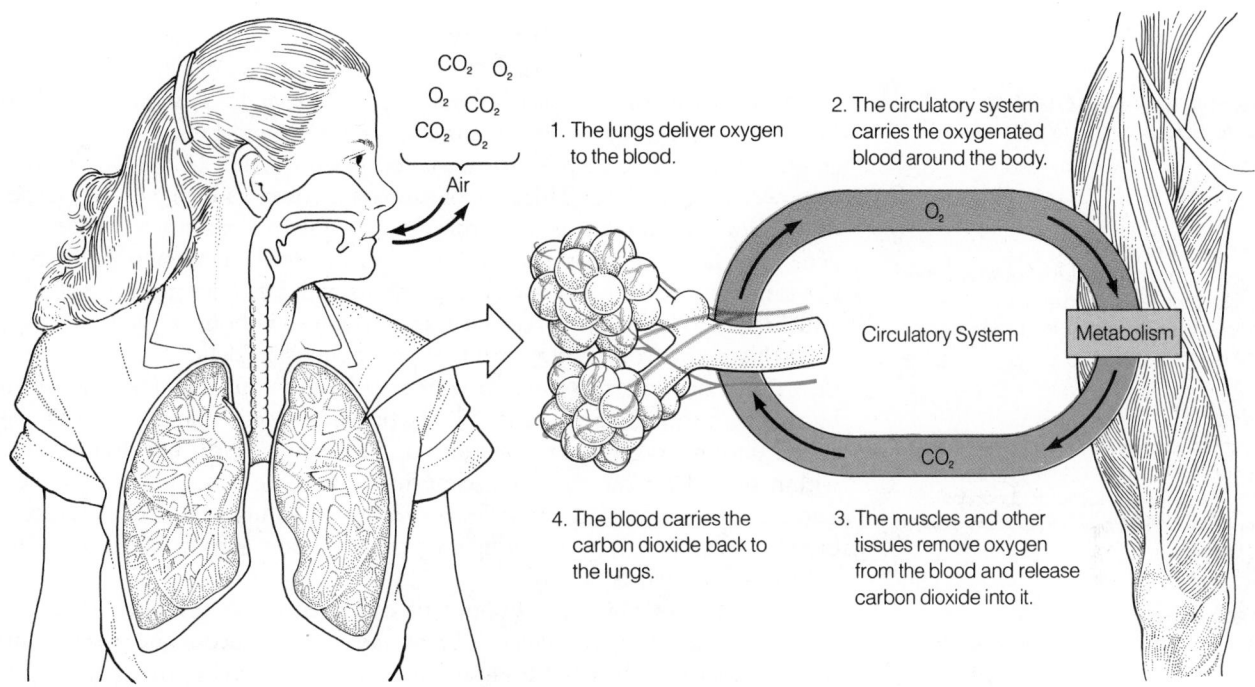

FIGURE 9–2

Delivery of oxygen by the heart and lungs to the muscles. The more fit a muscle is, the more oxygen it draws from the blood. That oxygen is drawn from the lungs, so the person with more fit muscles extracts from the inhaled air more oxygen than a person with less fit muscles. The cardiovascular system responds to the demand for oxygen by building up its capacity to deliver oxygen. Researchers can measure cardiovascular fitness by measuring the amount of oxygen a person consumes per minute while working out, a measure called the VO_2 max.

fat to cholesterol. During exercise, those same hormones cause the muscles to pick up and use the glucose and fatty acids liberated from storage. This is one reason that people under stress often find exercise to be a release—the body is primed for physical action, and action makes use of the fuels in the blood. It may also be a link to understanding how stress is related to heart disease. Perhaps those circulating fuels influence the advancement of plaques that ultimately clog the arteries.

Exercise metabolism requires that the muscles be supplied with three main materials: Oxygen and the two muscle fuels—glucose and fatty acids. As Figure 9–2 showed, the oxygen comes from the lungs, which pass it to the blood, which carries it to the muscles. The glucose is derived chiefly from glycogen stored within the muscle itself; some comes from the liver via the blood. The fatty acids come partly from fat inside the muscles but mostly from fat that is released from the body's fat tissues and delivered by the blood.

During rest, your body uses both fat and glucose for energy. During exercise, though, oxygen availability in the muscles determines which of the two fuels will provide most of the energy to fuel the work. With ample oxygen, muscles can extract all available energy from glucose and fat by means of aerobic

Cardiovascular conditioning is characterized by

- Increased blood volume and oxygen delivery.
- Increased heart strength and stroke volume.
- Slowed resting pulse.
- Increased breathing efficiency.
- Improved circulation.
- Reduced blood pressure.

anaerobic (AN-air-ROE-bic):
refers to processes that do not involve oxygen.
an = without

anaerobic metabolism:
that part of energy nutrient breakdown that can take place without oxygen—for example, the first steps in the breakdown of glucose.

lactic acid:
a fragment produced from glucose during anaerobic metabolism. When oxygen becomes available, lactic acid can be completely broken down to carbon dioxide and water.

oxygen debt:
a deficit of oxygen built up by the body during exercise when the cardiovascular system cannot deliver oxygen fast enough to the muscles to support aerobic metabolism; the debt must be repaid by rapid breathing after the activity slows down or stops.

metabolism. During moderate exercise, your lungs and circulatory system have no trouble keeping up with your muscles' need for oxygen. You breathe deeply and easily, and your heart beats steadily—the exercise is aerobic.

The other kind of exercise, anaerobic exercise, generally does not bring about cardiovascular conditioning but develops strength and bulk of muscles. Examples of anaerobic exercise for a trained person would be a 100-yard dash or power weight lifting. This type of exercise involves sudden, all-out exertion of muscles that far exceeds the cardiovascular system's capacity to deliver oxygen. Since fat requires oxygen for breakdown (aerobic metabolism), the muscles cannot meet their increased energy needs with fat. They must use glucose, a fuel that can be metabolized—at least partially—without oxygen.

At this point, your body is building up an oxygen debt. You may have to slow down or even stop to catch your breath, and your muscles may start to burn. The burning pain is caused by lactic acid—one of the byproducts generated during oxygen debt—building up in the muscles. If not drained away within seconds, it can cause muscle exhaustion. One way to deal with lactic acid buildup is to relax the muscles at every opportunity so that the circulating blood can carry it away and bring oxygen to support aerobic metabolism and reduce the oxygen debt.

The body stores a small amount of carbohydrate as glycogen. The liver contains some glycogen, which it breaks apart into glucose and releases into the bloodstream when the body needs it. During exercise, the muscles pick up and use the glucose donated by the liver, along with glucose from their own private glycogen stores. Compared to fat, the carbohydrate sources of the body are limited and constantly being used and replenished. How much carbohydrate one eats determines how much glycogen is stored and influences the rate at which glycogen will be used in any given exercise. The rate at which a person uses glucose also depends on the duration and intensity of the exercise as well as how well trained the person is. Training helps the body to use its available fuels more efficiently. Low-intensity types of activity such as fast walking burn the greatest amount of fat during exercise.

Compared with glycogen stores, fat stores are almost unlimited. When a person exercises, the fat the muscles burn comes from the fatty deposits all over the body, especially from those with the greatest fat stores. Even after exercise, fat use may continue at an accelerated rate for about a day. The hormones generated during exercise also favor the continued liberation of stored fat.[3]

Nutrition for Fitness

Fitness and nutrition are so closely interwoven that what we eat really does make a difference in how fit we are. The best diet for the exerciser is a nutrient-dense diet as described in Chapter 1.

The more activity a person engages in, the more energy the person will expend and the higher the person's kcalorie requirements will be. Even when kcalories are increased, however, the proportions of nutrients required remain constant. The exerciser who wants to maintain weight should fill extra energy needs with regular whole foods—milk, breads, fruit, and legumes—to provide carbohydrate along with protein, vitamins, and minerals. Only on certain occasions are exceptions recommended. One occasion is during intensive training, when energy needs outstrip the capacity to eat enough kcalories from food, in which case added sugar and fat may be needed. Another special occasion is the pregame meal. Both of these exceptions deal with training for competition rather than fitness.

The optimum diet contains about 55 to 60 percent of its kcalories in the form of carbohydrates, most of which should be complex carbohydrates. This is adequate to ensure glycogen stores sufficient to support moderate exercise lasting not over 1½ hours. Glycogen loading will not benefit moderate exercise but is discussed in Nutrition in Practice 9, as it affects endurance performance.

Glycogen stores can be depleted when an exerciser is on a diet that is high in protein and low in carbohydrates. If glycogen stores are used up during the first few days of exercise and the diet does not provide adequate carbohydrates, the exerciser may start to feel burned out and sluggish. The exerciser may attribute these symptoms to vitamin deficiencies, but they indicate a need not for increased vitamins but for increased energy in the form of glycogen, which comes from a diet adequate in carbohydrates. A low-carbohydrate diet may be responsible for the discouragement and tiredness a person feels a few days after beginning a fitness program.

Protein supplements are often advertised to increase muscle mass. Such supplements would do this only if the diet were deficient in protein. Slightly more protein may be required when a person is exercising more vigorously than usual, but since the average diet is twice as high in protein as necessary, most exercisers do not need to increase their protein intakes even during a strenuous workout.

The human body is designed to work and is healthiest when it is exercised. Adjustment after adjustment is made to accommodate increased activity. An example is in the handling of vitamin B_6, a vitamin critical to building the blood and muscle tissues needed in exercise. The body responds to exercise by conserving vitamin B_6. The livers of those who exercise store more of this vitamin than the livers of those who do not exercise.[4] Hence, exercisers need only the RDA of the vitamin, because their bodies excrete less. This sort of body wisdom has proven to be the case for other nutrients, too. The body conserves what it needs.

Niacin, another B vitamin, may affect exercise performance more directly than do the other vitamins, especially when it is taken in the form of supplements. Niacin taken before exercise suppresses the release of fatty acids, making the body turn to glycogen as its main exercise fuel. Whether or not this impairs performance is unknown, but it probably shortens the time to glycogen depletion and makes the work seem more difficult to the exerciser.[5] Exercisers need no more niacin than that which is supplied by a nutrient-dense diet, and people who take niacin supplements before exercise are probably affecting their workouts for the worse.

Chapter 8 indicated that many people do not get the RDA for iron from their diets, and exercisers are among them. Iron in hemoglobin is essential

sports anemia:
a temporary condition of low hemoglobin in the blood associated with the early stages of sports training or with other strenuous activity.

for carrying oxygen to the working muscles and is therefore critical to physical activity. There are many causes of anemia, dietary causes included. Iron-deficiency anemia hinders exercise performance by limiting the amount of oxygen available to muscles. People who begin exercising develop sports anemia, which is different from iron-deficiency anemia. It is especially likely to develop in teens and women—who have high iron needs and low iron intakes—when they are involved in running and other strenuous sports. Boys and men can also be affected, even though iron intake of this group is usually adequate. Sports anemia is not the same as iron-deficiency anemia in that it does not hinder gains in fitness or the ability to do work.[6] Iron-related anemias do not clear up without treatment, but sports anemia always does. Iron supplements are needed only when athletes or exercisers have iron-deficiency anemia.

Extra vitamins and minerals are rarely needed, even if extra energy is expended in a fitness program. In fact, exercise in some cases improves the way a vitamin or mineral is absorbed or used. Calcium is an example. The body makes more efficient use of the available calcium when exercising. Bones absorb great stresses during exercise, and like the muscles, they respond by growing thicker and stronger along the lines of stress.

The exerciser does need extra fluids, however; in fact, they are critical. The first symptom of dehydration is fatigue, and a rapid water loss equal to 5 percent of the body weight can reduce muscular work capacity by 20 to 30 percent.[7] Water lost via sweat and exhaled vapor needs to be replaced, and thirst is not a sufficient indicator of how much liquid is needed to replace the lost water. Table 9–2 shows the amounts of fluids needed before, during, and after exercise. A person who loses a lot of body water during exercise should weigh before and after the exercise to determine how much body weight has been lost during exercise. The person should then replace each pound of body weight lost with two cups of fluid. Cold water is the best fluid replacement. Even though some electrolytes are lost during exercise, the moderate exerciser does not need to take them in the form of salt tablets or sports drinks. The average diet contains enough sodium to replace losses, and potassium can be replaced through four to eight servings of potassium-rich foods. Fruit and other whole foods whose unbroken cells have not been exposed to too much processing, are rich in potassium.

electrolytes:
charged minerals, such as sodium, potassium, magnesium, and chloride.

Other nutrients besides those mentioned here are important to fitness, but the preceding examples have provided the most important pointers about

TABLE 9–2. Schedule of Hydration Before, During, and After Exercise

When to Drink	Amount of Fluid
2 hours before exercise	About 3 c
10 to 15 minutes before exercise	About 2 c
Every 10 to 20 minutes during exercise	About ½ c or more
After exercise	Replace each pound of body weight lost with 2 c fluid

Source: Adapted from J. W. Marcus, ed., Sports Nutrition (Chicago: American Dietetic Association, 1986), p. 57.

nutrition related to performance. The best diet is derived from whole, minimally processed foods and is high in carbohydrates; adequate in protein, vitamins, and minerals; and low in fat. Another aspect of fitness closely linked to diet is maintaining a reasonable weight, discussed next.

Body Composition and Weight Control

Most people look in the mirror and wish they could change how they look in one way or another. Some feel they are too thin, others would like to rearrange a few pounds, but the overwhelming majority would like to throw away a few pounds altogether. Evaluating body composition can be as easy as looking in the mirror or as complex as determining body density.

Assessment Tools

Stepping on a scale to see what you weigh has become a national habit, but the problem is that weight really says very little about what you want to know. It would be great if that scale could tell you what your weight should be for optimal health or how much fat is too much or too little. All a scale can do is compare your current weight to what you weighed yesterday or to what someone else weighs. In fact, when a person's weight is compared with the weight in a table, it is not being measured against a standard but is simply being compared with the average weight found in other people years ago. Two people of the same sex, height, and age may weigh the same, yet one may be a muscular athlete with well-mineralized bones and the other person may be frail and overweight. (See inside back cover.)

The height-weight tables, therefore, have limited usefulness. Better determinations of appropriate weight are based on measurements of body com-

---

Quick Ways to Assess Body Fatness

These ways to answer the question, What is an appropriate weight for you? are just for fun:

- A crude measure of body fatness is the **pinch test** (this is a fatfold measure without the equipment to make it accurate). Pick up a fold of skin and fat at the back of either arm with the thumb and forefinger of the other hand. Keep your fingers still, so as not to lose the "measurement," and measure the thickness on a ruler. A fatfold over an inch thick reflects obesity.

- Another shortcut method is to measure your waist compared with your chest (not bust). Every inch by which your waist measurement exceeds your chest measurement is said to take two years off your life.

- Another crude measure: lie down, relax, and place a ruler across your abdomen from one hipbone to the other. If it doesn't easily touch both bones while you're relaxing, you're too fat.

fatfold test:
a clinical test of body fatness in which the thickness of a fold of skin on the back of the arm (triceps), below the shoulder blade (subscapular), or in other places is measured with an instrument called a caliper. The older, less preferred, term for this is *skinfold test*. Chapter 13 and Appendix B provide additional information about this test.

hydrostatic weighing:
a clinical test of body fatness, also known as underwater weighing, in which the person is submerged and the displacement of water is measured. It is considered by many to be the most reliable method of determining body composition (see Chapter 13).

bioelectrical impedance:
a clinical test of body fatness based on the electrolyte level and electrical resistance of fat versus lean body tissue. The results at this time are not as accurately reproducible as those obtained by hydrostatic weighing or fatfold measurements (see Chapter 13).

set point:
the point at which controls are set (for example, on a thermostat). In the case of body weight, the set point is that point above which the body tends to lose weight and below which it tends to gain weight.

ratchet effect:
a popular term for the effect that repeated cycles of weight loss and gain without exercise have on body composition, in which the body fat content increases and kcaloric needs fall after each round, making the next round of weight loss harder. Also called the *yoyo effect*.

position such as fatfold tests, hydrostatic (underwater) weighing, and bioelectrical impedance. Each of these measurements requires technical skill and specialized equipment to be reliable and accurate. Even after body composition is accurately determined, we still do not know exactly what weight supports optimal health for each individual.

In 1985, experts reviewed the evidence, and after much discussion, settled on a temporary way to diagnose obesity by estimating body mass. The body mass index (BMI) can be obtained from the following formula:

$$BMI = \frac{Weight\ (kilograms)}{Height^2\ (meters)}$$

A body mass index greater than 27.2 in men or 26.9 in women indicates a need for weight reduction.[8] Both the traditional tables and the body mass index (Figure 9–3) can be used to suggest approximately what people should weigh.

Exercise and Weight Control

The contributions exercise makes to a weight-control program are several. Exercise alters body composition in a desirable direction and thereby alters metabolism, making daily energy needs higher even during rest. Exercise also spends energy directly and helps to control appetite. Exercise offers the psychological benefits of looking and feeling healthy and reduces stress and stress-induced eating. Increased self-esteem accompanies these benefits which tends to support a person's resolve to persist in a weight-control effort—rounding out a beneficial cycle.

Many experiments with both animals and human beings suggest that the body chooses a weight that it wants to be and defends that weight. When below that weight, people tend to gain; when above it, they tend to lose. Circumstances can change that weight, however. For example, people who give up smoking often gain a fixed amount of weight—say, 20 pounds—and then stop gaining and maintain their weight at the newly set level. This illustrates the body's tendency to settle at a weight plateau for long periods of time. The plateau may change occasionally, but the new level then tends to stay as fixed as the old one did. Exercise is thought to be one method for changing the set point of an individual by altering metabolic needs.

A person who diets without exercising loses both lean and fat tissue. Weight gain without exercising mostly reflects addition of fat; the lean is gone forever. Thus, after a round of weight loss and regain, the body may weigh the same as before, but it contains more fat tissue and less lean. More likely, if the person's eating habits haven't changed, the body will wind up weighing more each time than the last, the ratchet or yoyo effect of dieting (see Figure 9–4).

Lean tissue is very active when compared to fat tissue, and its metabolic activity uses up food energy. Therefore, the more lean tissue you develop, the faster your metabolism becomes, the more energy you spend, and the more you can eat and still maintain your weight. The ratchet effect reverses the situation. If you initially weighed 160 pounds, lost 30 pounds, and then returned to your initial weight, all without exercising, you would have less

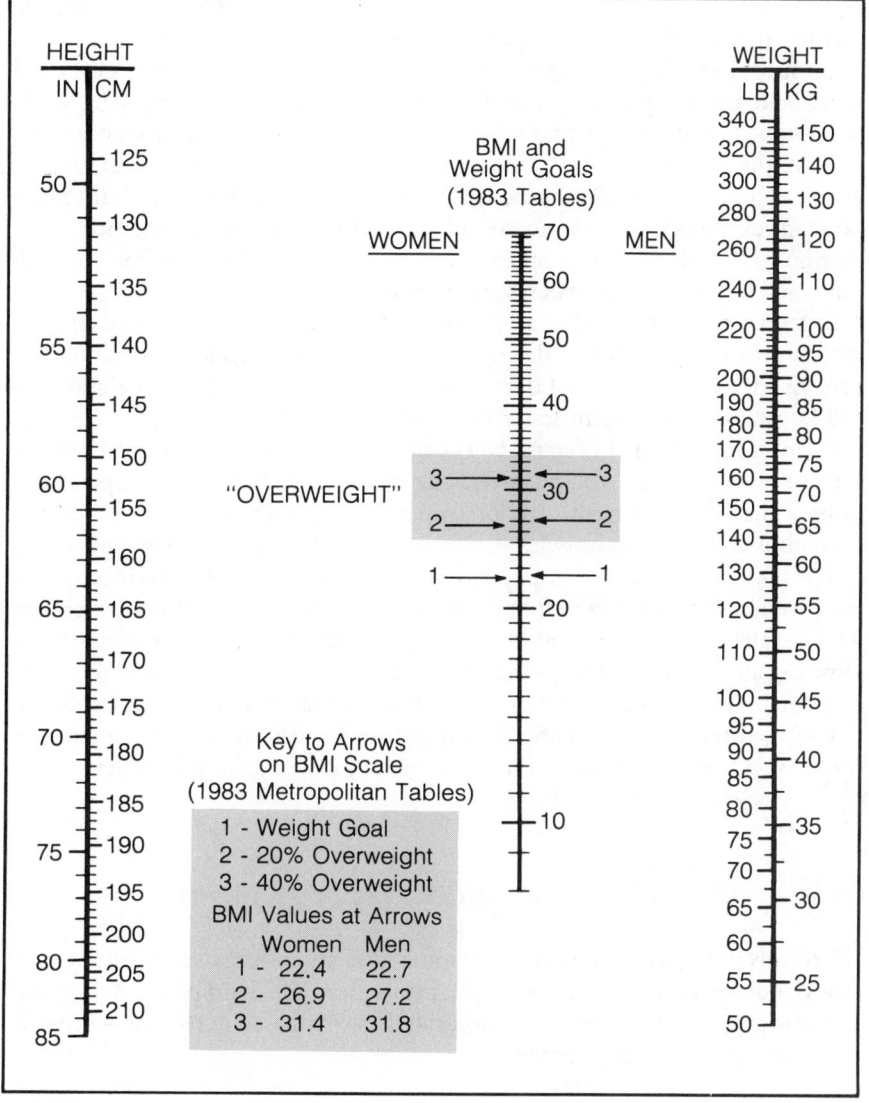

FIGURE 9–3

Nomogram for body mass index. Weights and heights are without clothing. With clothes, add 5 pounds for men or 3 pounds for women, and 1 inch in height for shoes. Draw a straight line from your height (left) to your weight (right). At the point where it crosses the BMI line, read your body mass index. A body mass index greater than 27.2 for men or 26.9 for women indicates obesity.

lean tissue than you did when you weighed 160 the first time. Less lean tissue means that your metabolism is slower. As a result, if you eat as you did at 160 pounds the first time, you will gain fat rather than maintain your weight.

Even when a person follows a medically sound low-kcalorie diet, dieting without exercise causes losses of lean body mass. The only way to avoid lean

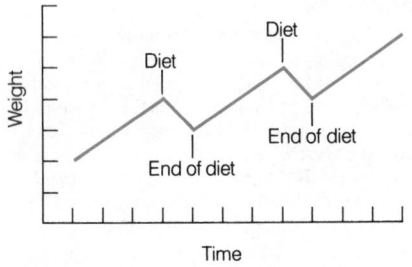

FIGURE 9–4

The ratchet effect of dieting. Each round of dieting without exercise is followed by a rebound of weight to a higher level than before.

body losses while losing fat is to include both vigorous exercise and sensible dieting in your plan. As it happens, this is also the quickest way to lose fat.

It must be clear by now that exercise, by shifting body composition toward more lean tissue, speeds up metabolism for as long as you keep your body conditioned. Exercise has two other beneficial effects we haven't mentioned.

First, the conditioned body is trained to use fatty acids rather than glucose as fuel. Thus, after you have become conditioned, you will tend to burn more body fat during exercise than you did when you were out of condition. Furthermore, the more muscle and lean tissue you have, the more fat you will burn—all day long, even when you are resting.

Second, on any given day, an intensive bout of exercise will speed up metabolism temporarily—for a day or so. Metabolism is stimulated by about 25 percent for as long as three hours after an intensive bout of exercise and may still be running 10 percent faster two days later.

Keep in mind that if exercise is to help with weight loss, it must be *active* exercise, which means voluntary moving of muscles. Being moved passively, as by a machine at a health spa or by a massage, does not increase kcalorie expenditure. The more muscles you move, the more kcalories you spend.

The number of kcalories you spend on specific activities depends more upon your weight than on how fast you can do the exercise. For example, a person who weighs 120 pounds and runs a 6-minute mile burns off 83 kcalories. That same person, ambling along for a mile in 10 minutes, burns almost the same amount—76 kcalories. It should be emphasized that you do not have to work fast to use up energy efficiently. If you choose to walk the distance instead of run it, you will use up about the same energy; it will just take longer.

Modification of Eating and Exercise Behavior

Up to this point we have dealt with some facts about exercise, nutrition, and fitness, but the knowledge must be put into action. The hard part is to develop a fitness program that can be incorporated into your daily routine so that it becomes a part of your lifestyle.

Why Strive for Optimum Fitness?

No matter how fit you are now, making a habit of regular exercise can be one of the best things you can do for your health. Here are some of the benefits of regular exercise:

- More enjoyable, perhaps even longer, life.[9]
- Improved general outlook.[10]
- Improved mental capacity.
- Feeling of vigor.
- Feeling of belonging—the fun and companionship of sports.
- Improved self-image and self-confidence.
- Reduced incidence and severity of personality disorders.[11]

- Reduced fatness and increased lean body tissue.[12]
- Greater bone density (less likelihood of adult bone loss).[13]
- Improved circulation, heart capacity, and lung function.[14]
- Sound, beneficial sleep.
- A youthful appearance, healthy skin, and improved muscle tone.
- Reduced risk of cardiovascular disease.[15]
- Improvement of symptoms in people with diabetes.[16]
- A lower incidence of constipation and colon disorders, including cancer.[17]
- Slowed cardiovascular aging.[18]
- Reduced fat and cholesterol in the blood.
- Reduced blood pressure.
- Slower resting pulse rate.[19]
- Reduced risk of stroke (in oral contraceptive users, too).
- Faster wound healing.
- Possible prevention of arthritis and rheumatism.
- Improvement or elimination of menstrual cramps.
- Improved resistance to colds and infections.[20]

Science cannot promise that you will receive all of these benefits if you exercise, but almost everyone who exercises reaps at least some of them. The health rewards may be enough to motivate you to begin an exercise program, and an added benefit is that exercise can become one of the most enjoyable activities you participate in.

Strategy for Developing a Personal Exercise Program

This section is addressed to you both personally and as a health care professional, because for you to motivate people to change, it is helpful to have good exercise and eating habits yourself. An optimal health goal for everyone is to attain physical conditioning. Conditioning consists of a multitude of adaptations that the body makes to facilitate the work that training demands. We have looked at some of these adaptations and are ready to start a personal exercise program.

First of all, make sure it is safe to begin; a physical examination is the best way to check. Some people have heart disease and do not know it. Sudden, strenuous exercise could bring on the very heart attack you wish to prevent. Start out slowly and gradually, building up to your desired level of fitness. Exercise builds up your body by overloading it in a positive way. Your body's response will be to get itself in shape to meet a greater demand each time you do this.

When you push yourself beyond the normal level of demand, you break down body tissue ever so slightly so that immediately following exercise, your condition is actually at a slightly lower level than before. But not for long: in 24 to 48 hours, nature not only repairs the old tissue but also builds extra tissue to a point that makes the body better conditioned than it was before

overload:
an extra physical demand placed on the body; an increase in the frequency, duration, or intensity of an exercise. A principle of training is that for a body system to improve, it must be worked at frequencies, durations, or intensities that increase by increments over time.

Some aerobic activities that can make a fitness program fun are

Swimming	Soccer
Fast walking	Hockey
Jogging	Basketball
Bicycling	Water polo
Stair walking	Lacrosse
Rope jumping	Rugby
Aerobic dance	

Sample fitness program, 45 minutes a day:

Monday, Wednesday, Friday:
10 minutes of stretching
25 minutes of jogging
10 minutes of calisthenics
Tuesday, Thursday:
10 minutes of stretching
25 minutes of weight training
10 minutes of calisthenics
Saturday or Sunday:
Softball, walking, hiking, biking, or swimming

the workout. This ensures that next time the muscles will meet the more vigorous challenge more easily.

The overload principle can be applied in several different ways. Do the activity more often to increase its frequency, more strenuously to increase its intensity, or for longer periods of time to increase its duration. All three strategies can be used in an exercise program depending upon your preference. If it is difficult to find the time to exercise, try a more intense activity for a shorter time. For those who hate hard work, take it easy and go longer. Some people are better suited to perform different types of activities depending upon heredity and training. You can also choose to develop your body for different kinds of activities by choosing the right exercises.

The factors mentioned will have a bearing on the type of exercise program you choose, but the most important aspect is that you enjoy the activities you choose. Making exercise enjoyable will help you stick with a long-term program.

To improve cardiovascular fitness, you must work up to a point where you can exercise aerobically for 20 minutes or more. The best way to develop cardiovascular fitness is to choose a steady and constant activity that uses the large muscle groups such as the legs, buttocks, and abdomen at an intensity that elevates your heart rate. The heart rate must be considerably faster than the resting rate—fast enough to "push" the heart, but not so fast as to strain it. Your target heart rate can be calculated from your age. As cardiovascular fitness improves, more intense exercise will be required to reach the same target rate. To calculate your target heart rate, follow these three steps:

1. Take your pulse while still lying in bed, before getting up in the morning, to find your resting heart rate.

2. Subtract your age from 220 to estimate the absolute maximum heart rate possible for a person your age. You should never exercise at this rate, of course.

3. Subtract your resting heart rate from your maximum heart rate. Multiply this figure by 60 percent and add it to your resting heart rate to locate your target heart rate.

Here is an example for a person at age 25 whose resting pulse rate is 70 beats per minute. The person's maximum heart rate is $220 - 25$, or 195 beats per minute. The person's target heart rate, then, is 60 percent of $(195 - 70)$, plus 70 (the resting pulse rate), or about 145 beats per minute. Being able to work out at your target heart rate for 20 to 30 minutes is the best indication that you have arrived at your fitness goal.

Whether you spend 2 hours a day or 45 minutes every other day on fitness, you will want to allocate your time to different activities according to your goals. One ambitious person, whose goal is overall fitness, allocates 45 minutes a day as shown in the margin note. Someone wanting more cardiovascular fitness might spend more time in activities at the target heart rate; if more muscle strength is the goal, additional or more intense weight work is in order.

Changing Behavior

Turning your goals into concrete actions may require some lifestyle changes that are not easy. Adopting a fitness program and beginning to eat a more nutritious diet will not be without setbacks. An understanding of behavior modification may help make changing old habits just a little easier.

A part of behavior can be seen to be regulated by environmental factors. In simple terms, the behavior we exhibit is preceded by stimuli and followed by consequences. The more intense the stimuli, the more likely that the behavior is to occur. The more intense the consequences are, the more or less likely the behavior is to occur again. Behavior modification involves manipulating environmental conditions so as to favor the repeated occurrence of a desired behavior and extinguish the occurrence of unwanted behavior.

Behavior modification can be used to change the behaviors of overeating and underexercising that lead to being in less than optimal health. To see the progress you have made, keep track of the types of exercise you are presently doing and record the place, times, and circumstances of what you eat. This will give you a clue to inappropriate behavior. If you are at your desired weight and feel that your eating behavior is usually appropriate, you may just want to focus on starting a fitness program. On the other hand, you may need to change only your eating behavior if you presently exercise regularly.

Once your objectives are defined, start to eliminate cues that keep you from meeting your fitness goals. There probably are several different cues instead of just one, such as watching television, talking on the telephone, passing a vending machine, or being offered food. Resolve to ignore these cues and to respond to cues that are designed by you. For example, instead of skipping a workout because a good television show is on, plan to come home each evening and start getting ready for the workout without even turning on the television. Change your eating habits by resolving to eat in only one particular place.

Set about suppressing those cues that cannot be eliminated. For example, if friends tend to encourage you to do other activities with them when your workout is scheduled, try getting them involved in a fitness program or let them know how they can help you maintain your program. Ask friends and family for positive cues for desired behavior and have them make no comment when you deviate from your desired behavior.

Make sure that positive consequences follow desired behavior. If you reach your goal of working out three times a week for a month, take the time to congratulate yourself and acknowledge that you have made a significant accomplishment.

Magical alterations to the system of hard work to achieve fitness and good health have been offered time and again—ways to shrink the stomach, to gain muscle without work, to eat negative kcalories—but they are born of wishful thinking. They are effective only when they directly affect the kcalorie balance. The rewards of the hard work to reach optimal health will present themselves, and eating poorly and not exercising will become unthinkable.

Evaluating Your Activity Level

All the work you have done to this point will pay off only if you actually take steps to get in shape. Use the following questions to find out just how physically active you are. For each question answered yes, give yourself the number of points indicated. Then total your points to determine your score.

Occupation and Daily Activities

1. I usually walk to and from work or shopping (at least ½ mile each way). 1 point

2. I usually take the stairs rather than use elevators or escalators. 1 point

3. The type of physical activity involved in my job or daily household routine is best described by the following statement (select one):

   a. Most of my day is spent in office work, light physical activity, or household chores. 0 points

   b. Most of my workday is spent in farm activities, moderate physical activity, brisk walking, or comparable activities. 4 points

   c. My typical workday includes several hours of heavy physical activity (shoveling, lifting, etc.). 9 points

Leisure Activities

4. I do several hours of gardening or lawn work each week. 1 point

5. I fish or hunt once a week or more on the average. (Fishing must involve active work, such as rowing a boat. Dock sitting doesn't count.) 1 point

6. At least once a week I participate for an hour or more in vigorous dancing, such as square or folk dancing. 1 point

7. In season, I play golf at least once a week, and I do not use a power cart. 2 points

8. I often walk for exercise or recreation. 1 point

9. When I feel bothered by pressures at work or home, I use exercise as a way to relax. 1 point

10. Two or more times a week I perform calisthenic exercises (sit-ups, push-ups) for at least 10 minutes per session. 3 points

11. I regularly participate in yoga or perform stretching exercises. 2 points

12. I participate in active recreational sports such as tennis or handball:

    a. About once a week. 2 points

    b. About twice a week. 4 points

    c. Three times a week or more. 7 points

13. At least once a week I participate in vigorous fitness activities like jogging or swimming (at least 20 continuous minutes per session).

a. About once a week. 3 points

b. About twice a week. 5 points

c. Three times a week or more. 10 points

Total points earned _____

Scoring:
0 to 5 points—inactive. This amount of exercise leads to a steady deterioration in fitness. Improvement needed.
6 to 11—moderately active. This amount slows fitness loss but will not maintain adequate fitness in most persons.
12 to 20 points—active. This amount will maintain an acceptable level of physical fitness.
21 points or over—very active. This amount of activity will maintain a high state of physical fitness.
Source: Adapted with permission of Russell Pate (University of South Carolina, Human Performance Laboratory).

Notes

1. K. E. Powell and coauthors, Status of the 1990 objectives for physical fitness and exercise, *Public Health Reports* 101 (1986): 15–19.
2. Much of the discussion about fitness is derived from Chapter 7, Fitness, in *Life Choices: Health Concepts and Strategies,* by F. S. Sizer and E. N. Whitney (St. Paul, Minn.: West, 1988).
3. R. Bielinski, Y. Schutz, and E. Jequier, Energy metabolism during the postexercise recovery in man, *American Journal of Clinical Nutrition* 42 (1985): 69–82.
4. C. M. Dreon and G. E. Butterfield, Vitamin B_6 utilization in active and inactive young men, *American Journal of Clinical Nutrition* 43 (1986): 816–824.
5. M. H. Williams, *Nutrition Aspects of Human Physical and Athletic Performance* (Springfield, Ill.: Charles C. Thomas, 1985), pp. 152–155.
6. S. M. Blum, A. R. Sherman, and R. A. Boileau, The effects of fitness-type exercise on iron status in adult women, *American Journal of Clinical Nutrition* 43 (1986): 456–463.
7. J. Bergstrom and E. Hultman, Nutrition for maximal sports performance, *Journal of the American Medical Association* 221 (1972): 999.
8. T. B. Van Itallie, When the frame is part of the picture (editorial), *American Journal of Public Health* 75 (1985): 1054–1055.
9. R. S. Paffenbarger and coauthors, Physical activity, all-cause mortality, and longevity of college alumni, *New England Journal of Medicine* 314 (1986): 605–613.
10. V. Gurley, A. Neuringer, and J. Massee, Dance and sports compared: Effect on psychological well-being, *Journal of Sports Medicine* 24 (1984): 58–68.
11. K. T. Francis and R. Carter, Psychological characteristics of joggers, *Journal of Sports Medicine* 22 (1982): 386–391. R. M. Hayden and G. J. Allen, Relationship between aerobic exercise, anxiety, and depression: Convergent validation by knowledgeable informants, *Journal of Sports Medicine* 24 (1984): 69–74.
12. Quantity and quality of exercise for developing and maintaining fitness in healthy adults, a position paper of The American College of Sports Medicine, *The Physician and Sportsmedicine* 6 (1978): 39–41.
13. N. E. Lane, D. A. Block, and H. H. Jones, Long distance running, bone density, and osteoarthritis, *Journal of the American Medical Association* 255 (1986): 1147–1151.
14. Quantity and quality of exercise for developing and maintaining fitness in healthy adults, a position paper of The American College of Sports Medicine, *The Physician and Sportsmedicine* 6 (1978): 39–41.

15. S. Rainville and P. Vaccaro, Lipoprotein cholesterol levels, coronary artery disease and regular exercise: A review, *American Corrective Therapy Journal* 37 (1983): 161–165. B. Stamford, Improving coronary circulation, *The Physician and Sportsmedicine* 11 (1983): 163.

16. K. Jung, Physical exercise therapy in juvenile diabetes mellitus, *Journal of Sports Medicine* 22 (1982): 23–31.

17. D. H. Garabrant and coauthors, Job activity and colon cancer risk, *American Journal of Epidemiology* 119 (1984): 1005–1014.

18. N. B. Belloc and L. Breslow, Relationship of physical health status and health practices, *Preventive Medicine* 1 (1972): 409–421.

19. C. M. Tipton, Exercise, training, and hypertension, *Exercise and Sports Sciences Reviews* 12 (1984): 245–306.

20. J. G. Cannon and M. J. Kluger, Exercise enhances survival rate in mice infected with *Salmonella typhimurium, Proceedings of the Society for Experimental Biology and Medicine* 175 (1984): 518–521. H. B. Simon, The immunology of exercise, *Journal of the American Medical Association* 252 (1984): 2735–2738. A. Viti and coauthors, Effect of exercise on plasma interferon levels, *Journal of Applied Physiology,* August 1985, pp. 426–428.

Nutrition for the Athlete

Athletes are one of the most susceptible groups for nutrition promotions. They have invested much time and effort in training and many are open to trying any product if it could possibly give them an edge in competition. The desire to win is strong, but that doesn't change the fact that an overwhelming majority of supplements sold for athletes are frauds. If the products that are tried have no effect and are harmless, they are only a waste of money; when the products are harmful or actually impair performance, they are a waste of athletic potential.

On the positive side, athletes should know that nutrition affects their performance. Unfortunately, much of what the athlete learns about nutrition is locker-room rumors by those with little, incorrect, or no nutrition education. This Nutrition in Practice summarizes the minimum knowledge that a trainer, athlete, or nutrition teacher should have.

My coach told me to take protein supplements. Should I take them?
You don't need them. Extra protein cannot be forced into the muscles to make them grow. Cells don't respond to what's given to them by helplessly accepting it. They respond to the hormones that regulate them and to the demands put upon them, and they select the nutrients they need from what is offered. The way to make muscle cells grow is to put a demand on them—that is, to make them work.

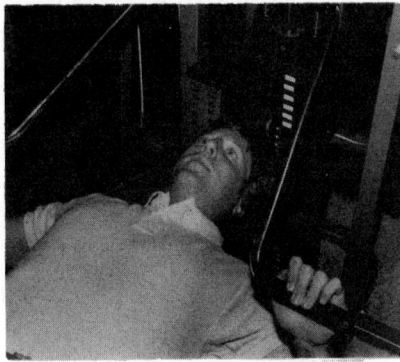

Exercise, not excess protein, increases muscle mass.

They will respond by taking up nutrients—amino acids included—so that they can grow. The idea is not to *push* protein at the muscles, but to exercise in order to demand that the muscles *pull* protein in for themselves. One needs to then make sure that protein is available by eating a diet adequate in protein. The margin of safety built into the protein recommendation for all people is high enough to cover the athlete's need, so the recommended protein intake is not higher for the athlete than for anyone else. There's no advantage to eating excess protein.

Oh, come on now, I'm sure I need more protein.
No, you really don't; it's food *energy* that athletes need more of. Depending on the sport, an athlete in active training and competition may have extraordinarily high energy needs.

Football players, for example, seem to average close to 6,000 kcalories a day during the season, with some days' intakes topping 10,000 kcalories.[1] With the high kcalorie intake goes a high need for the B vitamins, especially thiamin, used to generate energy during metabolism.

That's a lot of kcalories! I guess I need a vitamin supplement, then, don't I?
No, a vitamin supplement isn't necessary. Just eat foods rich in B vitamins—breads, cereals, fruits, and vegetables. This is easy with a food energy allowance of 5,000 kcalories or more.

My coach recommended that I gain some weight. What is the best way to do this?
The healthful way to gain weight is to build yourself up by patient and consistent training while eating enough kcalories (of nutritious foods) to support a gain of 1 to 1½ pounds per week. To gain a pound of muscle mass requires 2,500 kcalories, which is fewer than the kcalories needed to gain a pound of fat.[2] This is because muscle tissue is less dense kcalorically than fat tissue. An athlete who adds a big snack—for example, a quarter-pound hamburger on a bun, french fries, and a milk shake—between meals can eat 700 to 800 extra kcalories a day this way, thus achieving a healthful weight gain of about two pounds a week. If body fat rather than muscle accumulates, however, it is necessary to reduce food

energy intake and raise energy expenditure.

A word of caution: Don't go on a high-fat diet to gain weight. This technique is said to be one of the most widespread nutrition-related abuses in sports. A high-fat diet worsens the risk of heart disease to which athletes are not immune.

Remember to cut *down* on kcalories between and after training periods. Muscles respond to reduced demand by losing mass. The mass cannot simply disappear. Instead, it is converted to fat unless it is expended in activity. It should be no surprise, then, that a heavily muscled individual of 20 who stops working out but keeps on eating like a football player in training can become an oversized, flabby, and obese person at 30.

The coach told my friend to lose several pounds. What is an appropriate weight-loss plan for an athlete?
To achieve ideal body composition—the optimum ratio of muscle strength to body mass—people must reduce only body fat, which they can't do for more than a very few weeks at a rate faster than about two pounds a week. Hurry-up techniques, such as sauna bathing, exercising in a plastic suit to sweat fat off, using diuretics or cathartics, or inducing vomiting, achieve faster weight loss only by causing dehydration, and dehydration seriously impairs athletic performance. What is achieved by quick weight loss dieting is loss of lean tissue, glycogen, bone minerals, and fluids—all materials vital to healthy body functioning.

Even if it is achieved by healthful methods, extreme weight loss can be

hazardous to the athlete, as to any person. Occasionally you hear that an elite runner—in superb physical condition and at the peak of his career—has died suddenly at the end of an intensive exercise session. Such deaths were a mystery at first, but now a reason for them seems to be emerging. In many cases, a person had been severely restricting kcalories and had reached a new, all-time low weight while breaking his own previous records for distance or time. Exactly what causes the deaths is still not known, but severe kcalorie restriction and weight loss combined with hard training seem to be contributing factors.[3]

I have heard of a technique for improving endurance called glycogen loading. What is glycogen loading?
The fuel for intense muscular activity is carbohydrate, stored in the muscle as glycogen. Athletes who compete in long-distance endurance events naturally want to have as much stored energy in their muscles as they can. Glycogen loading is a technique of tricking the muscles into storing more glycogen than normal. When the technique was first introduced, athletes were taught to reduce their carbohydrate intake for several days by eating meals high in protein and fat. Simultaneously, they were to exercise heavily to deplete the muscle glycogen stores. The next step was to reduce exercise intensity and switch abruptly to a diet high in carbohydrate. Muscle glycogen stores rebounded to about two to four times the normal level and thus provided fuel that would last longer in an endurance event.

Glycogen loading practiced this way can have side effects, including abnormal heartbeat; swollen, painful muscles; and weight gain immediately before competition. Most exercise physiologists recommend a modified plan whereby the athlete exercises intensely without restricting carbohydrates, then during the week before competition gradually cuts back on exercise, rests completely the day before, and eats a very high carbohydrate diet.

What should I eat right before an athletic event?
A light, carbohydrate-rich meal eaten at least two to four hours before an event is a recommended pregame meal. There's no need to avoid milk; the idea that it causes cotton mouth is pure superstition.

The notion is widespread that it is smart to eat a candy bar or a few teaspoons of honey right before the event for quick energy. This practice probably confers a disadvantage physically, at least for aerobic exercise, if it has any effect at all. The body's response is to secrete insulin, which retards fat use at a time when fat use should be maximal. Other foods athletes may choose to eat before events may have special, personal meanings associated with them, but none has any special power to promote speed, coordination, or endurance.

My coach told me not to drink fluids during competition. Do you agree?
Dehydration can disable the athlete more seriously than any other nutritional factor and can cause fatigue and cramps. It is important to

promptly replace the fluids lost through sweating.

The best drink to replace lost fluid is water, because it is rapidly absorbed. Salt tablets are unnecessary. When the event is over, eating regular foods can make up for the salt loss. Many athletes mistakenly believe that drinking water during an event will cause cramps. On the contrary, it is dehydration that causes cramps. We recommend drinking water before, during, and after the event. (See Table 9–2).

Are sugar and the electrolytes found in Gatorade and other sports drinks beneficial before or during competition?
Because the electrolytes lost during a sporting event can be replenished by eating regular foods, they are not needed in a sports drink and can actually be detrimental. The fluid you choose should have a lower concentration of dissolved solids, such as electrolytes, than the body does, so that the fluids will be absorbed rapidly. If the solution has too much dissolved solid, as most sports drinks do, it will demand dilution in the digestive tract, pulling still more fluid from the tissues instead of replenishing them. Sports drinks that are diluted with twice as much water as normal will reduce the concentration of electrolytes to the point that it will not hinder absorption.

Sugar should not be taken within about three hours before beginning to exercise for an athlete to perform her best. However, some sugar may improve performance during critical moments late in endurance

competition. Small amounts of glucose from slightly sweetened drinks taken during exercise slowly make their way from the digestive tract to the muscles and augment the body's supply of glucose enough to postpone exhaustion.[4] Sugar taken during exercise helps only athletes who are exercising so strenuously and long that they are about to run out of glycogen, such as triathletes or marathoners. Once again, sports drinks are too concentrated and need to be diluted with equal amounts of water. Diluted fruit juice or other solutions containing not over two percent glucose are good fluid replacements during endurance events.

I have heard that steroids are dangerous, but my father is a doctor and constantly monitors my blood pressure while I am taking steroids that he gives me. Are they safe in my case?
Steroids have serious side effects and are illegal. They are not safe in your case or for other athletes. Whether steroids boost athletic performance is still unproven, but the risks associated with steroid use are certain.[5] You are sure to develop side effects no matter how closely a trainer or doctor monitors you. All steroid users experience a sharp change in their blood lipid content, the type associated with high risk of heart disease.[6] Some steroid users suffer impairment of liver function, cancerous liver tumors, liver rupture and hemorrhage, permanent changes in the reproductive system, and altered facial appearance.

The recommendations for athletes provided here are simple, common-

sense suggestions. To sum up, a normal, balanced diet is best for the athlete, as for anyone else. Wise food choices and adequate fluid intake can ensure that athletes will get all the nutrients they need.

Notes

1. S. Short and W. R. Short, Four-year study of university athletes' dietary intake, *Journal of the American Dietetic Association* 82 (1983): 632–645.
2. N. J. Smith, Nutrition and the athlete, in *Sports Medicine and Physiology,* ed. R. H. Strauss (Philadelphia: Saunders, 1979).
3. T. J. Bassler, Body build and mortality (letter to the editor), *Journal of the American Medical Association* 244 (1980): 1437. Sometimes, however, an athlete obviously has heart disease, either hereditary or acquired. Diet can't always be blamed for sudden deaths in athletes.
4. J. L. Ivy and coauthors, Enhanced performance with carbohydrate supplements during endurance exercise, *Report of the Ross Symposium on Nutrient Utilization During Exercise* (Columbus, Ohio: Ross Laboratories, 1983), pp. 54–60.
5. H. Haupt and G. D. Rovere, Anabolic steroids: A review of the literature, *American Journal of Sports Medicine* 12 (1984): 469–484. D. R. Lamb, Anabolic steroids in athletics: How well do they work and how dangerous are they?: *American Journal of Sports Medicine* 12 (1984): 31–38.
6. O. L. Webb, P. M. Laskarzewski, and C. J. Glueck, Severe depression of high-density lipoprotein cholesterol levels in weight lifters and body builders by self-administered exogenous testosterone and anabolic-androgenic steroids, *Metabolism* 33 (1984): 971–975. M. Alen and P. Rakhila, Reduced high-density lipoprotein-cholesterol in power athletes: Use of male sex hormone derivatives, an atherogenic factor, *International Journal of Sports Medicine* 5 (1984): 341–342.

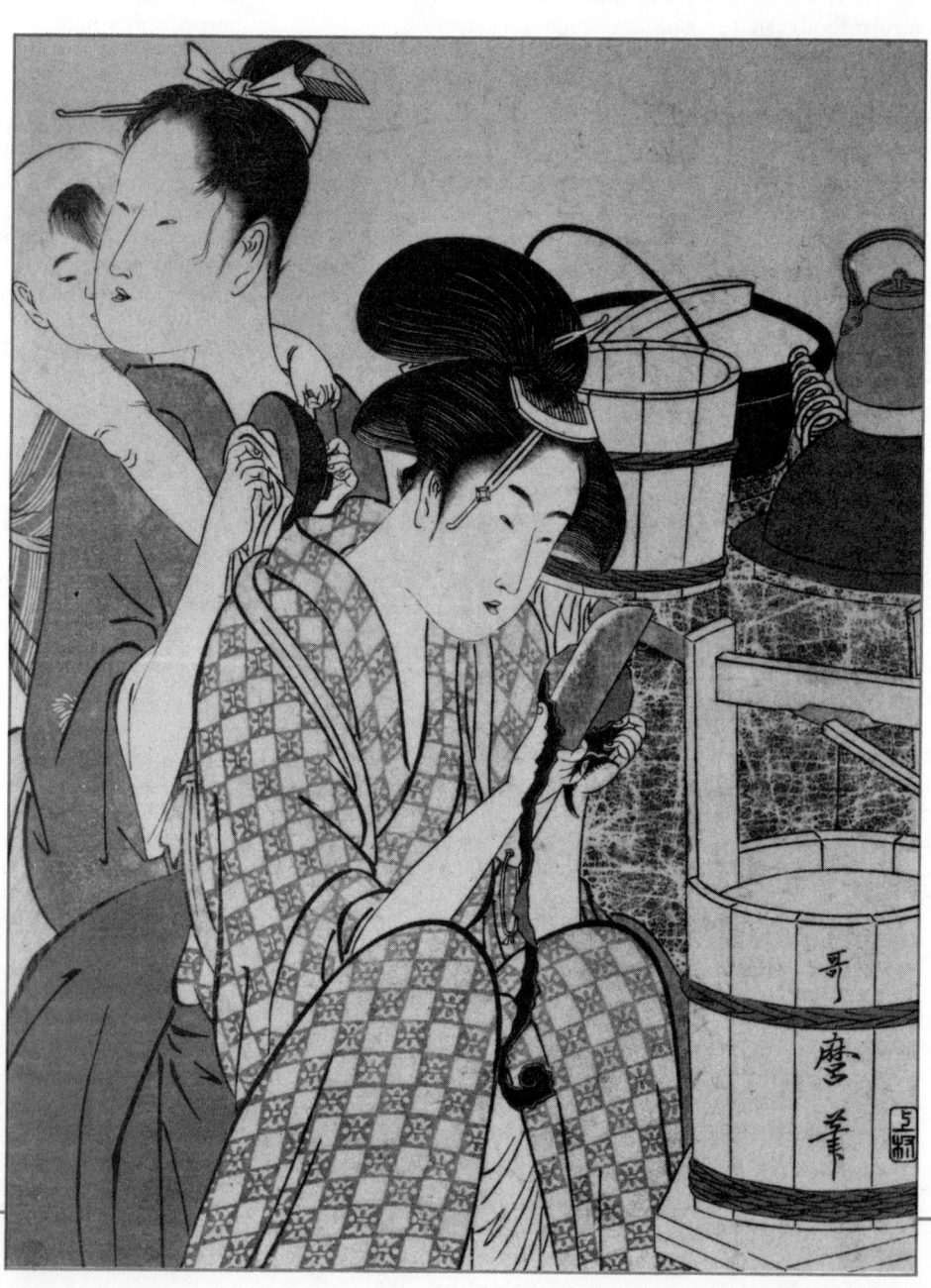

CHAPTER

10

Mother and Infant

CONTENTS

Nutrient Needs During Pregnancy

Complications

Breastfeeding

Formula Feeding

Vitamin-Mineral Supplements for the Infant

Nutrition of the Infant

Case Study: Overweight Pregnant Woman

Nutrition in Practice: Nutrition
and Behavioral Problems in Children

Detail of *Kitchen Scene* by Utamaro, Spaulding Collection,
courtesy of Museum of Fine Arts, Boston.

We normally think of nutrition as affecting us here and now. You feel good this afternoon because you ate a good breakfast this morning. But the effects of nutrition also extend over years. The woman who is expecting a baby and the health professional advising such a woman will be strongly motivated to attend to the woman's nutrition needs if they both understand how critical the nutrients are to the normal course of events in prenatal and postnatal development.

Nutrient Needs During Pregnancy

The organ inside the uterus in which the mother's and fetus's circulatory systems intertwine and in which exchange of materials between maternal and fetal blood takes place is the **placenta** (pla-SEN-tuh). The fetus receives nutrients and oxygen across the placenta; the mother's blood picks up carbon dioxide and other waste materials to be excreted via her lungs and kidneys.

A finite period occurs during development in which the events that take place will have irreversible, determining effects on later developmental stages. This is a **critical period,** usually a period of cell division in a body organ.

Recommended energy intake: 40 kcal/kg (18 kcal/lb).

Minimum energy intake: 36 kcal/kg (17 kcal/lb).

For a 120-lb woman, this represents at least 2,000 kcal and preferably 2,200 kcal/day.

Recommended protein intake: 75–100 g/day.

Recommended carbohydrate intake: about 50% of energy intake. In a 2,000-kcal/day intake, this represents 1,000 kcal of carbohydrate, or about 250 g. Four cups of milk will contribute about 50 g carbohydrate. An apple provides 10 g carbohydrate and a slice of bread provides 15 g, so this recommendation implies generous intakes of fruit and bread exchanges.

Foods containing folacin:
   Green leafy vegetables.
   Legumes.
   Liver.
   Orange juice and cantaloupe.
   Other vegetables.
   Whole-wheat products.

Human life begins at the time of conception with a single fertilized egg cell that grows to a 7½-pound baby by delivery. During that time, each organ and tissue must be assembled according to its own unique pattern and timing. Each organ needs nutrients most during its own intensive growth period. A nutrient deficiency during one stage of development might affect the heart, and during another stage, the developing limbs.

If the mother's nutrient stores are inadequate early in pregnancy, the early development of the infant will be adversely affected. Poor nutrition of a woman during her early pregnancy can theoretically have an impact on the health of her grandchild, even after that child has become an adult.[1]

Nutrient needs during such periods of intensive growth as pregnancy are greater than at any other time. Some nutrients are in greater demand than others during pregnancy, as shown in Figure 10–1. A study of the figure reveals some of the key nutrient needs of the pregnant woman.

During pregnancy, one of the smallest increases is in the need for food energy. An increase of only 15 percent (mostly in the latter half of pregnancy) is recommended, but many women may need much more. In each case, enough kcalories are needed to spare protein for its all-important tissue-building work. A recommended average energy intake is 40 kcalories per kilogram of body weight. Energy intake should never fall below 36 kcalories per kilogram. The increased need for protein is more dramatic—from about 56 grams to about 75 grams per day or more and there is no harm in a pregnant woman's taking up to 100 grams of protein or even more. In fact, if the woman has been poorly nourished before pregnancy, this may be an ideal intake. Generous amounts of carbohydrate are needed to spare the protein.

The pregnant woman's extraordinary need for folacin is due to the great increase in her blood volume. Folacin-deficiency anemia is more often seen in pregnant women than iron-deficiency anemia. It is often advisable for the physician to prescribe folacin as a supplement. As you might expect, the vitamin needed in the next highest amount is the other B vitamin associated with the manufacture of red blood cells—vitamin B_{12}.

Among the minerals, those involved in building the skeleton—calcium, phosphorus, and magnesium—are in great demand during pregnancy, and increases of about 50 percent are recommended. Intestinal absorption of calcium doubles early in pregnancy, and the mineral is stored in the mother's bones. Later, as the fetal bones begin to calcify, there is a dramatic shift of calcium across the

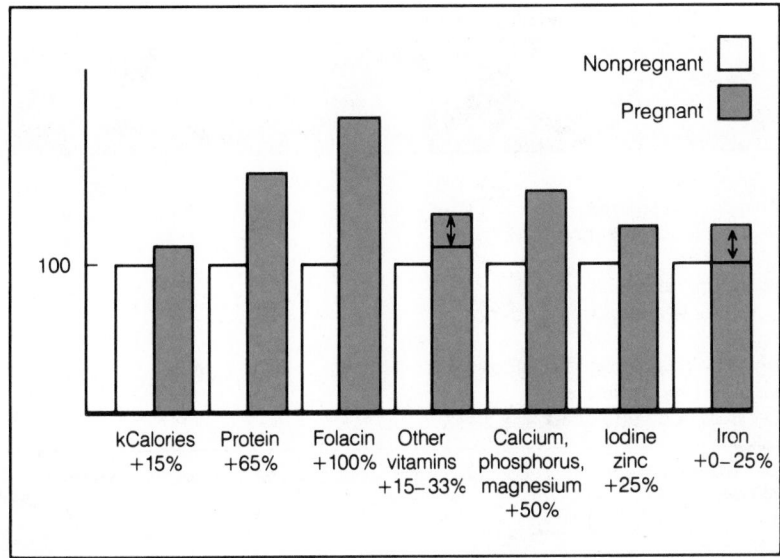

FIGURE 10–1

Comparison of the nutrient needs of nonpregnant and pregnant women (over 23 years old). The nonpregnant woman's needs are set at 100 percent, the pregnant woman's needs are shown as increases over 100 percent.
Source: Calculated from the RDA table, inside front cover.

placenta, and the mother's bone stores are drawn upon. Most mothers' calcium intakes have to be raised well above their prepregnancy intakes. If a mother's intake is less than 1.2 grams per day, she will pay by losing more calcium from her bones than she has stored for this purpose.

Calcification of the baby's teeth begins in the fifth month after conception. Fluoride may be needed for teeth and bones to form properly. It is not clear from research whether supplemental fluoride crosses the placenta, but some evidence suggests that it does. Children whose mothers received one milligram of fluoride daily in addition to using fluoridated water have been observed to have more decay-free teeth at five to nine years of age compared with children whose mothers only used fluoridated water.[2] If water is not fluoridated, a prescribed supplement may be desirable.

The body conserves iron even more than usual during pregnancy. Menstruation ceases, iron absorption increases, and the hormones of pregnancy raise the concentration of iron in the blood. Thus, a woman *theoretically* needs no more iron during pregnancy than she has needed all along. Her RDA for iron is not higher than for the nonpregnant woman. Most women, however, have minimal iron stores, and the demands of pregnancy deplete them to the deficiency point. Even if a woman makes it to the end of pregnancy without developing anemia, she may bleed excessively at delivery. Furthermore, a newborn should have enough stored iron to last three to six months; this iron must also come from the mother's iron stores. Thus, almost all pregnant women are advised to take an iron supplement throughout pregnancy and for two to three months after delivery.

Foods containing calcium:
Four cups of milk a day will supply 1.2 g calcium. For other food sources, see Chapter 8. The milk should be fortified with vitamin D; if it is not, a vitamin D supplement may be needed.

Ordinarily, a hemoglobin level below 13 g/100 ml is considered low for a woman (see Chapter 8). In pregnancy, values of 12 g are not unusual, and 11 g is where the line defining "too low" is often drawn.

Food sources of iron:
  Liver, oysters.
  Red meat, fish, other meat.
  Dried fruits.
  Legumes (dried beans, peas, lima beans).
  Dark-green vegetables.

TABLE 10–1. Daily Food Guide for Women

| Food | Number of Servings | | |
	Nonpregnant Woman	Pregnant Woman	Lactating Woman
Protein foods			
Animal (2-oz serving)	2	2	2
Vegetable (at least one serving of legumes)	2	2	2
Milk and milk products	2	4	5
Enriched or whole-grain breads and cereals	4	4	4
Vitamin C-rich fruits and vegetables	1	1	1
Dark-green vegetables	1	1	1
Other fruits and vegetables	1	1	1

Source: California Department of Health, as cited in Nutrition and the pregnant obese woman, *Nutrition and the MD,* January 1978.

Eating Pattern and Weight Gain

During pregnancy, the nutrients needing the greatest emphasis in a woman's diet are protein, calcium, phosphorus, magnesium, and folacin. The foods selected to supply these nutrients are therefore normally those in the milk, meat, and vegetable categories.

Because food energy needs increase less than nutrient needs, the pregnant woman must select foods of high nutrient density. For most women, appropriate choices include foods like nonfat milk, nonfat plain yogurt, lean meats, eggs, liver, dark-green vegetables, and whole-grain breads and cereals. For vitamin C, the woman should either increase the size of her one daily serving of a vitamin C-rich food, such as broccoli, or add a second, fair vitamin C source, such as tomatoes. A suggested food pattern is shown in Table 10–1.

The pregnant woman must gain weight. Ideally, she will have begun her pregnancy at the appropriate weight for her height and will gain about 25 to 30 pounds, most of it in the second half of pregnancy. The ideal pattern is thought to be about two to four pounds during the first three months and a pound per week thereafter. A woman who is underweight to begin with should gain more—perhaps 30 pounds. The teenager who needs to support her own growth as well as her baby's should also gain more. A woman who is obese at the start of pregnancy could perhaps gain less but still should gain between 16 and 24 pounds.

Twenty-five pounds for a normal-weight woman sounds like a lot, but if you look at the components of the pregnant woman's weight gain (Table 10–2), you will see that she needs all these pounds—from *nutritious* kcalories—to provide for the growth of her placenta, uterus, blood, and breasts as well as for a strong 7½-pound baby. Much of the weight she gains is lost at delivery. The remainder is generally lost within a few weeks or months as her blood volume returns to normal and as she loses the fluids and fat she has accumulated.

TABLE 10–2. Overall Weight Gain During Pregnancy

Development	Weight Gain (lb)
Infant at birth	7½
Placenta	1
Increase in mother's blood volume to supply placenta	4
Increase in size of mother's uterus and muscles to support it	2½
Increase in size of mother's breasts	3
Fluid to surround infant in amniotic sac	2
Mother's fat stores	4
Total	24

If a woman has gained more than the expected amount of weight early in pregnancy, she should not try to diet in the last weeks. Women have been known to gain up to 60 pounds in pregnancy without ill effects. A *sudden* large weight gain, however, is a danger signal that may indicate the onset of a complication known as pregnancy-induced hypertension (discussed later in the chapter).

A mother who does not gain the full amount of weight recommended may give birth to an underweight baby. To the uninitiated, this may not seem like a catastrophe, and in some instances it is not. A small mother may give birth to a small, normal, alert, and healthy baby. On the other hand, a baby with a low birthweight may be a malnourished baby, who is likely to get sick. Nutritionists seeking to find a measure by which they can evaluate the outcome of pregnancy have found that birthweight is the most potent single indicator of the infant's future health status. Statistically, a baby with a low birthweight has a greater than average chance of contracting diseases and of dying early in life. About one in every 15 infants born in the United States has a low birthweight, and about a quarter of them die within the first month of life. The infant's birth is more likely to be complicated by problems during delivery than that of a normal size baby. Furthermore, low birthweight is often associated with mental retardation.

low birthweight (LBW): a birthweight of 5 ½ lb (2,500 g) or less, used as a predictor of poor health in the newborn and as a probable indicator of poor nutrition status of the mother during and/or before pregnancy. Normal birthweight is 6 ½ lb (3,000 g) or more. Low-birthweight infants are of two different types. Some are *premature;* they are born early and are the right size for their gestational age. Others have suffered growth failure in the uterus; they may or may not be born early but they are *small for gestational age (small for date).*

Practices to Avoid

The potential impact of harmful practices during pregnancy cannot be overestimated. Some of these practices are

- *Smoking.* Smoking restricts the blood supply to the fetus, limiting the delivery of nutrients and the removal of wastes.

- *Drug use.* Misuse of drugs during pregnancy can result in grotesque malformations and addiction and withdrawal symptoms in the infant.

- *Excessive alcohol consumption.* As few as two drinks a day can lead to irreversible brain damage and mental and physical retardation (fetal alcohol syndrome).

- *Dieting.* Low-carbohydrate diets or fasts that cause ketosis during pregnancy can cause congenital deformity, permanently defective carbohydrate metabolism, or brain damage in the infant.

- *Protein deprivation.* Inadequate protein intake during pregnancy can lead to irreversibly diminished height and head circumference in the offspring. Excessive caffeine consumption (more than eight cups of coffee a day) has also been thought to cause complications in delivery, but a review of the evidence suggests that this may have been a false alarm. One or two cups of coffee or tea a day or the equivalent are well within safe limits. Some questions exist about the overuse of aspartame and saccharin as well as sugar. A general guideline can be offered: Don't feel obligated to avoid sugar and sugar substitutes altogether, but use them and similar substances in moderation.

fetal alcohol syndrome: the cluster of symptoms seen in an infant or child whose mother consumed excess alcohol during her pregnancy; includes mental and physical retardation with facial and other body deformities.

A table of the caffeine amounts in beverages and medications is provided in Chapter 12.

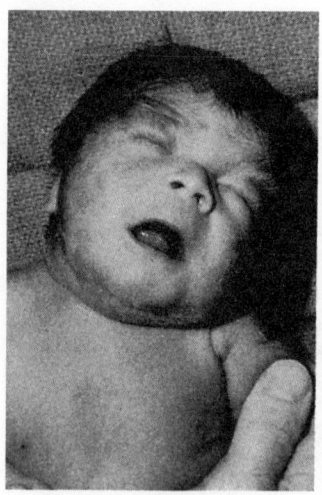
1 day

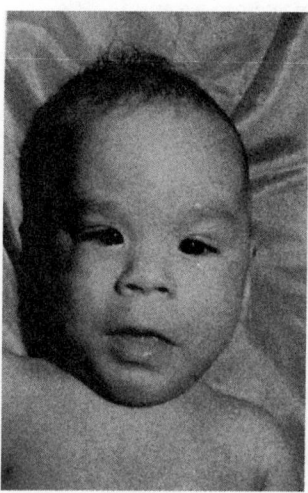
9 months

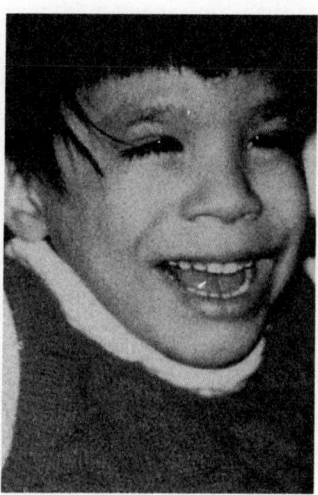
4½ years

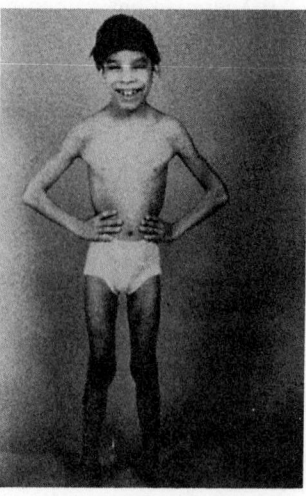
8 years

These facial traits reflect fetal alcohol syndrome caused by a woman's drinking early in pregnancy. Brain damage and irreversible mental and physical retardation accompany these surface features.

glycosuria (GLIGH-cose-YOUR-ee-uh):
sugar in the urine.
glyco = sweet

ketonuria (KEE-tone-YOUR-ee-uh):
ketones in the urine.

pregnancy-induced hypertension (PIH), formerly known as **toxemia** (tox-EEM-ee-uh):
a cluster of symptoms seen in pregnancy, including edema and often hypertension and kidney complications (*tox* = poison; *emia* = in the blood). A variety of terms are associated with PIH. Most common is *eclampsia*; its symptoms include convulsions and coma associated with high blood pressure, edema, and protein in the urine. Eclampsia may be preceded by *preeclampsia*, from mild to severe. High blood pressure can also exist throughout pregnancy without toxemia developing.

The normal edema of pregnancy responds to gravity; blood pools in the ankles. The edema of PIH is a generalized edema. The distinction helps with diagnosis.

Complications

Some common problems encountered during pregnancy can be avoided or corrected. Pregnancy precipitates many changes in the normal, healthy woman that the body handles very well. However, there are a few instances when medical attention is warranted so as to not allow these changes to become serious problems.

Diabetes can make pregnancy more difficult than usual. Gestational diabetes is the type of diabetes that develops only during pregnancy, usually in the later part of gestation when the tissues become insulin resistant. Concern for this type of diabetes has arisen because it occurs in up to three percent of all pregnancies in the United States.[3]

Pregnant women should be screened for diabetes in about the sixth month. Thereafter, their urine should be tested for sugar and ketones at every checkup. Glycosuria and ketonuria are suggestive of diabetes. Ketonuria can also indicate starvation ketosis in a woman following an ill-advised diet. Permanent brain damage to the fetus may result. Chapter 19 provides additional information about gestational diabetes.

Although a certain degree of edema is to be expected in late pregnancy, in a poorly nourished woman, it is often part of the larger cluster of symptoms known as pregnancy-induced hypertension (PIH), a condition involving high blood pressure and kidney problems that requires medical attention. PIH causes thousands of infant deaths every year; and babies born to mothers with PIH are likely to have retarded growth, lung problems, and other, even more severe birth defects.

Treatment of PIH is medical, and salt restriction is not a part of treatment until and unless the kidneys prove unable to handle a normal sodium load. A normal salt intake is necessary for good health.

Other common problems of pregnancy include anemia, nausea and vomiting, constipation, and emotional changes. Iron-deficiency anemia and folacin-deficiency anemia are both common during pregnancy. It is important to detect and correct both types of anemia. Iron and folacin supplements are often prescribed as a preventive measure against developing a deficiency.

The nausea of what is known as morning sickness—which can happen at any time of the day—seems unavoidable, because it arises from the hormonal changes taking place early in pregnancy. It can, however, sometimes be alleviated. A strategy some expectant mothers have found effective in quelling nausea is to start the day, before they get out of bed, with a few nibbles of a soda cracker or other bland carbohydrate food. The note in the margin offers additional suggestions for relieving nausea. Nausea often subsides after the first trimester but in some cases may continue to be a problem until the end of pregnancy.

Don't be fooled into thinking that the nausea many pregnant women experience is always a minor complaint. True, nausea is not health threatening. And true, nausea may not be a problem for the woman with a small touch of it that subsides after a short time. But for the woman who has nausea all day long (sometimes accompanied by vomiting), the problem can be depressing.

Comments like "Don't worry, nausea usually subsides after the first trimester" may actually make things worse. The woman may be thinking, "You mean I'm going to feel like this for TWO MORE MONTHS?" Think of how much worse the woman who is nauseated for a longer time may feel.

How can you help? For one thing, don't ignore the problem or treat it as unimportant. Let your client know that you understand what she is going through. Offer the suggestions given here for dealing with nausea. If appropriate (if the woman is happy about having a baby), it may help to focus her attention on the end result of her efforts—the beautiful baby she has been waiting for.

As the hormones of pregnancy alter muscle tone and the thriving infant crowds intestinal organs, an expectant mother might complain of constipation. A high-fiber diet, exercise, and a plentiful fluid intake will help to relieve this condition. Also, responding promptly to the urge to defecate can help. Laxatives should be used only as prescribed by the doctor. Mineral oil should not be used, because it robs the body of fat-soluble vitamins. Chapter 16 provides more details about constipation.

Pregnancy for many women is a time of adjustment to major changes. The woman who is expecting a baby is a growing person in more ways than one. Her needs are changing, not only physically but also emotionally. If it is her first baby, she senses that her lifestyle will have to change as she takes on the

Hints for controlling nausea and vomiting:
· Eat soda crackers before getting out of bed.
· Eat frequent, small meals. Keep something in your stomach.
· Drink liquids before or after meals rather than during meals. Carbonated drinks may help.
· Avoid fried foods and limit the fat you use in foods.
· Avoid using foods with strong odors if the odors make you feel nauseated.
· Everybody is different. Keep track of what you eat and when you feel nauseated, and do what's best for you.
· Take prenatal vitamin and iron supplements on a full stomach or at a time of day when you are not nauseated.
· Allow for some quiet time after eating. Rushing around after meals increases nausea.

Risk factors for malnutrition in pregnancy:
Age 15 or under.
Unwanted pregnancy.
Many pregnancies close together.
History of poor outcomes.
Poverty.
Food faddism.
Heavy smoking.
Drug addiction.
Alcohol abuse.
Chronic disease requiring special diet.
More than 15% underweight.
More than 15% overweight.
These factors at the start of pregnancy indicate that poor nutrition is very likely to be present and may adversely affect the pregnancy.

new responsibility of caring for a child. Ideally, she will be encouraged to develop this sense of responsibility by caring for herself during pregnancy. The expectant mother needs support in thinking of herself as a thoroughly worthwhile and important person with a new and challenging task that she can and will perform well.

A woman's cravings during pregnancy do not seem to reflect real physiological needs. Yet a woman going through this major experience should not be laughed at, and the validity of her feelings should be recognized. Through her cravings she may be expressing a need—for support, understanding, and love—as important as her need for nutrients.

A pregnant woman may crave and eat clay, ice, cornstarch, and other nonnutritious substances. This is *pica* (recall Chapter 8) and reflects a need for iron or zinc. The behavior is not adaptive; however, the substances she craves do not deliver the nutrients she needs.

Breastfeeding

Breast milk is a thin, watery substance, but its looks are deceiving, to say the least. Breast milk is tailor-made to meet the nutrient needs of the human infant. Its carbohydrate is lactose; its fat is a mixture with a generous proportion of the essential fatty acid, linoleic acid; and its protein is largely lactalbumin, a protein the human infant can easily digest. Its vitamin and mineral content is ample and easily absorbed. Even vitamin C, for which milk is not normally a good source, is adequately supplied by breast milk.

Powerful agents against bacterial infection also occur in breast milk. White blood cells are present which help protect the infant's GI tract. Lactoferrin, an iron-grabbing compound, keeps bacteria from getting the iron they need to grow on, helps absorb iron into the infant's bloodstream, and works directly to kill some bacteria.

Antibodies are present in breast milk and are especially abundant in colostrum, the premilk secreted in the first few days of lactation. These antibodies protect specifically against the intestinal diseases most likely to threaten the infant's life. Some of the antibodies also find their way into the infant's bloodstream, where they provide additional protection against such diseases as polio. Breast milk also contains the bifidus factor that favors the growth of normal bacterial flora in the infant's digestive tract so that harmful bacteria cannot grow there. Another factor present in breast milk stimulates the development of the infant's GI tract. Other factors help the infant to absorb zinc, manganese, and folacin. In addition, there are indications that breastfeeding may provide other benefits:

lactalbumin (lact-AL-byoo-min): the chief protein in human breast milk, as opposed to *casein* (CAY-seen), the chief protein in cow's milk.
lac = milk

lactoferrin (lak-toe-FERR-in): a factor in breast milk that binds iron and keeps it from supporting the growth of the infant's intestinal bacteria, helps absorb iron, and helps kill bacteria.
fer = iron

colostrum (co-LAHS-trum): a yellowish, milklike secretion from the breast, rich in protective factors; present for up to two weeks before milk appears.

bifidus (BIFF-id-us or by-FEED-us) **factor:** a factor in breast milk that favors growth of the "friendly" bacteria *lactobacillus* (lack-toh-ba-SILL-us) *bifidus* in the infant's intestinal tract so that other, less desirable intestinal inhabitants will not flourish.

bonding: the forming of a bond between mother and infant. A critical event in bonding, thought to be mediated by chemical messengers in breast milk, occurs in the first 45 minutes after birth, so this is an especially important time for mother and infant to be close, if possible. However, emotional bonding is facilitated by many other events and behaviors of mother and infant during the early months and years, so that bonding can be successful even if the mother does not breastfeed.

- It may be less likely to produce an obese child.
- It promotes better tooth and jaw alignment.
- It protects against allergy development during the vulnerable first few weeks.
- It may favor optimum bonding between mother and child.

Many other factors in breast milk are currently being identified and characterized. Much remains to be learned about the composition and characteristics of human milk, but clearly it is a very special substance.

Preparing to Breastfeed

Toward the end of her pregnancy, a woman who plans to breastfeed her baby should begin to prepare. Many handbooks are available to breastfeeding mothers. Talking with women who have breastfed their babies successfully is helpful, as is having a family and medical team support system.

Before the birth time, a mother should acquire at least two nursing bras that provide good support and have drop-flaps so that either breast can be freed for nursing. A woman with flat or inverted nipples should ask a health care professional for solutions to this problem.

You can tell if a nipple is inverted by pressing the areola between two fingers. An inverted nipple folds inward toward the breast. A nipple shield can be used to correct this problem.

Nutrient Needs

If a mother chooses to breastfeed, her nutrient supplies will continue to support the infant's development as well as her own even after birth. Adequate nutrition of the mother makes a highly significant contribution to successful lactation. Without it, lactation is likely to falter or fail.

The energy allowance for a lactating woman is a generous 750 kcalories per day above her ordinary need. The RDA table suggests that 500 kcalories come from added food, assuming the rest will come from the stores of fat her body accumulated during pregnancy for that purpose. Calcium, phosphorus, magnesium, and protein needs continue to be high because these nutrients are secreted into the milk for the baby. Since little iron is secreted in milk, no increase in iron intake is needed as long as the mother's iron nutrition has been good all along. Iron nutrition is often a problem, however, so it may be wise for a lactating mother to continue taking an iron supplement after delivery. The folacin requirement is lower in lactation than in pregnancy because the mother's blood volume declines.

Eating Pattern

Logically, because the mother is making milk, she needs to consume something that resembles it in composition. The obvious choice is cow's milk. The nursing mother who can't drink milk needs to find nutritionally similar substitutes, such as cheese or soy milk and greens. As stated before, nutritious foods should make up the remainder of the needed kcalories. Because breast milk is a fluid, the mother's fluid intake should be liberal. A busy new mother often forgets to drink fluids. She should drink between six and eight glasses of liquids daily.

The question is often raised whether a mother's milk may lack a nutrient if she is not getting enough in her diet. The answer differs from one nutrient to the next, but in general the effect of nutritional deprivation of the mother reduces the quantity, not the quality, of her milk.

The period of lactation is the natural time for a woman to lose the extra body fat she accumulated during pregnancy. If her choice of foods is judicious, a kcalorie deficit and a gradual loss of weight (one pound per week) can easily be supported without any effect on her milk output. Fat can only be mobilized slowly, however, and too large a kcalorie deficit will inhibit lactation. On the other hand, if a mother does not breastfeed, she may find it difficult to lose the fat she gained during pregnancy.

Suggestions for Successful Breastfeeding

To save space, the most important pointers for the breastfeeding mother are presented here in list form. To help follow these pointers, the team present at the baby's birth ideally will provide the necessary support. Thereafter, whoever attends the mother should make sure the mother learns these things. A home visit after a week or 10 days is advisable for followup.

1. The sucking reflex of the healthy, full-term infant is especially strong within the first 30 minutes after birth. During this same period, a critical event in bonding is thought to be mediated by chemical messengers in breast milk. Nursing the baby right away will therefore get breastfeeding off to a good start. If the baby cannot take the breast during this time the mother should *not* give him a bottle, for he can develop an attachment to it and then resist the breast later.

2. Beginning at the first feeding, the mother should learn how to *relax* and position herself so that she and the baby will both be comfortable. The baby needs to be able to suck without having his breathing obstructed. A mother needs to learn how to squeeze the areola between two fingers so that she can slip enough of it into the baby's mouth to promote good pumping action. She also needs to learn how to make the baby let go. The mother should not pull but should break the suction by slipping a finger between the baby's gums or holding the baby's nose for a second.

3. The infant's sucking is the stimulus for the release of a hormone that promotes the making of more milk. Therefore, if the infant is hungry, he should be allowed to suck longer. This will ensure a greater milk supply at the next nursing. The same hormone promotes the contraction of the uterus, enabling it to stop bleeding and return to normal size as quickly as possible after birth. Initially, it may be helpful to keep nursing sessions short enough to prevent sore nipples.

4. The rooting reflex makes the infant turn his mouth toward whichever side of his face is touched. The mother should touch the baby's cheek with the nipple so that the baby will turn and take the nipple.

5. The letdown reflex makes the milk flow when the mother perceives the need. Letdown has to occur for the baby to obtain milk easily. The mother must learn to relax and go with the let-down reflex; it may take several weeks for this habit to become established. A glass of water before nursing can help.

6. The draught reflex, which occurs later during a nursing session, draws the milk from the hindmost milk-producing glands of the breast after the foremilk has been released. The mother can feel this as a tingly sensation within the breast. The baby should be allowed and encouraged to nurse after the draught has begun. Hindmilk is richer in fat than foremilk and so provides satiety after the baby has sucked enough to satisfy his sucking need.

We're calling the baby *he* most of the time, because we have to call the mother *she*. But we like girl babies, too.

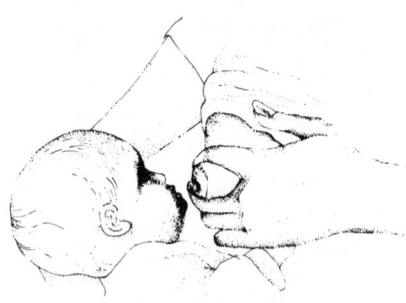

The mother should gently squeeze the areola between two fingers to insert the nipple far enough into the baby's mouth.

areola (a-REE-uh-luh):
the colored halo around the nipple. Beneath the areola lie the ducts that bring milk from the mammary glands. Pumping action on the areola promotes flow of milk from the glands through the ducts.
areola = a small space

The hormone that promotes milk production is **prolactin;** the one that initiates letdown is **oxytocin** (ox-ee-TOE-sin).

rooting reflex:
the reflex that makes a newborn turn toward whichever cheek is touched and search for the nipple.

letdown reflex:
the reflex that forces milk to the front of the breast when the infant begins to nurse.

draught reflex (DRAFT reflex):
the reflex that moves the hindmilk toward the nipple after the infant has drawn off the foremilk.

satiety (sat-EYE-uh-tee):
a feeling of fullness or satisfaction from eating or drinking.

7. The sucking and swallowing reflexes work together so that the baby's tongue and jaw pump milk from the breast and the swallow follows. The nipple has to rest well back on the baby's tongue, and the baby's lips and gums have to be pressing on the areola if the baby is to successfully stimulate milk release and then swallow the milk.

8. Although the baby can suck half the milk from the breast within two minutes and 80 percent to 90 percent of it within four minutes, he should continue sucking for ten minutes or more on one breast. The sucking itself as well as the removal of milk from the breast is believed to stimulate lactation. After the baby has put in his ten minutes or so on one breast—his share of the work—he can be given the other breast to finish satisfying his hunger. Nursing sessions should normally start on alternate breasts so that each breast is emptied regularly. When the baby seems full, the mother should hold him upright to let him expel any swallowed air (burping), and then give him another chance to nurse.

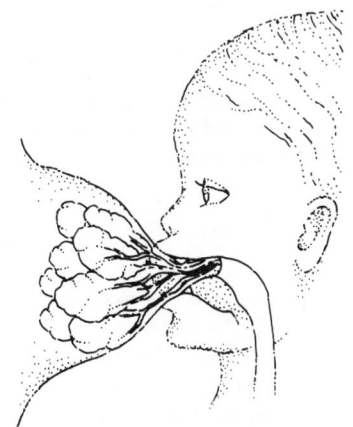

The baby's gums are milking the mammary glands by pressing on the milk ducts; the milk is squirting into the baby's throat.

9. Even if everything is going smoothly at home, the nursing mother should ideally have enough help and support so that she can rest in bed for several hours a day for the first 10 days. Rest and plentiful fluid intake are indispensable to successful lactation.

10. Demand feeds, no fewer than six a day, are most likely to promote optimal milk production and infant growth. The infant should be encouraged to nurse, or the milk should be manually pumped out at intervals to keep the supply going. A mother who nurses her baby even 12 times a day during the first two weeks will ensure that supply keeps up with demand. The midnight feeding should not be skipped, even if the baby is inclined to sleep through it.

11. Supplemental water can be offered if the baby seems to be thirsty after a long feeding, but offering sugar-water or other supplemental feedings in the first few weeks is not advised. The full extent of the baby's kcalorie demand should be communicated to the mother's body by way of sucking, so that the milk supply will increase to meet this demand.

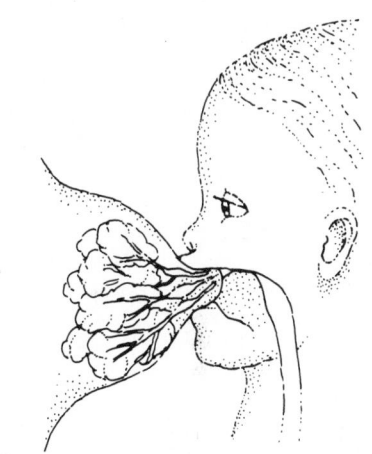

This baby hasn't got an adequate grasp on the nipple and will not get enough milk.

12. Mothers often want to know if they can skip an occasional feeding, substituting a bottle of formula. To be sure not to suppress lactation, the mother can express milk from the breast and store it in the refrigerator for her infant to drink. In this way, the breast gets the message to keep on producing the proper amount of milk. The mother who is confident that lactation is well established, however, may not bother to do this; she can substitute a bottle of formula and will experience no noticeable diminution of her milk supply.

A mother who wants to skip one or two feedings daily—for example, if she goes to work outside the home—can substitute formula for those feedings and continue to breastfeed morning and evening. She will probably find that her milk is not adequate to restore the missed feedings easily on weekends, for example, although she and her baby can continue to enjoy the morning and evening feedings for as long as desired.

Solutions can be found for most of the problems that arise in connection with breastfeeding. Breastfeeding manuals and breastfeeding support groups can give additional information.

Several problems may cause concern for breastfeeding mothers, including engorgement, sore nipples, inverted nipples, (see p. 191), and breast infections. All of these problems are minor and are *not* indications to discontinue breastfeeding.

engorgement:
overfilling of the breasts with milk so that they become swollen and hard. Manually expressing some milk before feeding time will make it easier for the baby to suck and will relieve pressure in the breasts.

Sore nipples are treated by allowing the infant to suck on the less sore nipple first—when he sucks hardest—and then switch to the sorer nipple.

Infection of a breast is **mastitis.** Continuing to breastfeed is the best management of this problem.

When Not to Breastfeed

If a woman has a communicable disease that could threaten the infant's health, then of course she cannot breastfeed, because mother and infant have to be separated. Similarly, if she must take medication that is secreted in breast milk and is known to affect the infant, she must not breastfeed. Drug addicts, including alcohol abusers, are capable of taking such high doses of drugs that their infants can become addicts by way of breast milk, in which case breastfeeding is also contraindicated.

Most prescription drugs do not reach nursing infants in sufficiently large quantities to affect them adversely. Moderate use of alcohol and moderate smoking are compatible with breastfeeding. Coffee drinking is fine, in moderation, as is the eating of foods such as garlic and spices. A particular food may affect the baby's liking for the mother's milk, which is a matter that requires individual detective work. If a woman has an ordinary cold, she can go on nursing without worry. The infant will catch it from her anyway if he is susceptible, and he may be less susceptible than a bottle-fed baby, thanks to immunologic protection.

A woman sometimes hesitates to breastfeed because she has heard that environmental contaminants, such as DDT or PCB, may enter her milk and harm her baby. The decision whether to breastfeed on this basis might best be made after consultation with a physician or dietitian familiar with the local environment.

Formula Feeding

Because breastfeeding has so many advantages for both mother and infant, it should be encouraged whenever possible. However, the mother who has decided to formula feed her infant should be supported in her choice just as the breastfeeding mother should be. The mother who offers formula to her baby has valid reasons for making her choice, and she and her baby can benefit in many ways from the supportive approval of those around them.

Formulas can be prepared from cow's milk in such a way that they do not differ significantly from human milk in nutrient content. Although formulas do not contain protective antibodies for human babies, the high level of preventive medical care (vaccinations) and public health measures achieved in the developed countries make these considerations less important than they were in the past. Safety and sanitation can be achieved with either mode of feeding by the educated mother whose water supply is reliable.

The mother who feeds formula can offer the same closeness, warmth, and stimulation during feedings as the breastfeeding mother can. Furthermore, other family members can help with feedings and thus develop a warm relationship with the baby and allow the new mother additional time to rest. Formula feeding may enable a mother to contribute to the family's income by returning to work sooner.

Another advantage of formula feeding is that gained by the mother whose attempts at breastfeeding have met with frustration. If the mother truly doesn't want to breastfeed or, worse, if she earnestly does want to but can't, continuing to try is an agonizing course, as hard on the baby as on the mother. When the mother finally accepts the necessity of formula feeding and weans the baby to the bottle, a period of anguish for both may be followed by the onset of peace and the first real opportunity to develop the important mother-child love.

The attendant who is asked to advise a mother on breastfeeding versus bottle-feeding should remember the advantages of both. In fact, when addressing any audience, you should remember that some members will be women who bottle-fed their babies. To praise breastfeeding out of proportion or without qualification can only make these women feel guilty or angry.

Many mothers choose to breastfeed at first but wean their children within the first one to six months. Even a few weeks of breastfeeding will significantly reduce the likelihood of the baby's developing an allergy to cow's milk. This advantage alone is important if such an allergy is likely. Furthermore, the baby gets the immunologic protection and all the special advantages of breastfeeding during the most critical first few weeks or months. Then the mother can choose to shift to the bottle and can know she has already given the baby those benefits. When the mother does shift, it is imperative that she wean the baby onto *formula*, not onto cow's milk of any kind—whole, low-fat, or nonfat. Only formula contains enough iron (to name but one of many factors) to support normal development in the baby's first year.

How to Feed Formula

A few pointers are important to all mothers who choose to feed formula from the start, those who bottle feed later, and those who will need to substitute occasional bottles of formula for breast milk:

1. National and international standards have been set for the nutrient contents of infant formulas. The Infant Formula Act of 1980 requires that formulas meet nutrient standards based on the American Academy of Pediatrics (AAP) recommendations, and in 1982 the FDA adopted quality control procedures to be sure that the formulas do. Formulas that meet the standard are nutritionally similar; small differences in nutrient content are sometimes confusing but not usually important. For the allergic or ill baby, or for the one with a metabolic disorder, however, special formulas are necessary (see Figure 10–2). The formula should be chosen according to the health of the infant. Soy-based formula is correctly given when an allergy to milk protein is present but is not the correct choice for a healthy infant with no allergy, since it lacks sufficient kcalories and requires vitamin A and D supplementation.

2. Formula is often purchased premixed and sterile in cans from the store. Prepackaged formula is easy to feed in disposable bottles, but the mother who mixes or bottles her own must learn the rules of safe formula preparation and administration. Until the baby is strong and clearly resistant to infection (at two to three months), formula should be prepared with great care and with safe, pure water. It must be sterilized and kept sterile until it is given to the baby. These rules can be relaxed if the total environment is clean and the water

FIGURE 10–2

Choosing a formula.

Source: E. N. Whitney and C. B. Cataldo, Highlight 15: Choosing formulas and milk substitutes, in *Understanding Normal and Clinical Nutrition* (St. Paul, Minn.: West, 1983), pp. 559–568.

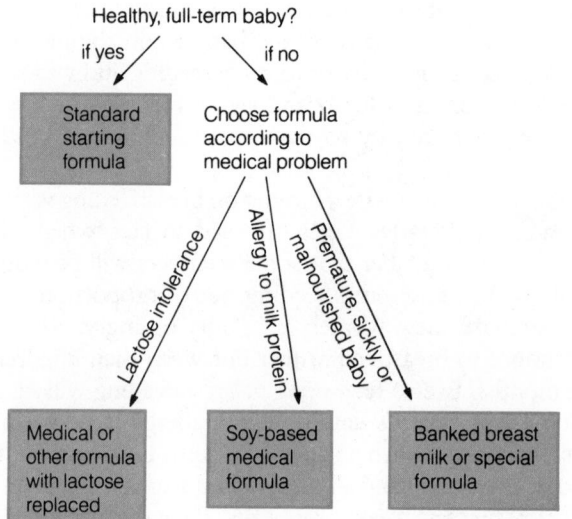

Healthy, full-term baby?

if yes / if no

Standard starting formula

Choose formula according to medical problem

Lactose intolerance

Allergy to milk protein

Premature, sickly, or malnourished baby

Medical or other formula with lactose replaced

Soy-based medical formula

Banked breast milk or special formula

Review infant's needs periodically and alter choice of formula as appropriate.

Formula preparation:

Liquid concentrate (moderately expensive, relatively easy)—mix with equal part water.

Powdered formula (least expensive, lightest for travel)—read label directions.

Ready-to-feed (easiest, most expensive)—pour directly into clean bottles.

Whole milk—do not use until the baby is 8 to 12 months.

supply is pure. All that is necessary, then, is to wash the bottles and nipples well with soapy water and rinse them thoroughly before preparing a fresh batch of formula. When half a bottle is left after a feeding, it should be resterilized immediately if it is to be used again. Using leftover formula shouldn't be a regular practice, however, because nutrient losses are incurred by high temperature treatment. Unsterile formula should never stand at room temperature.

The mother should be trained in formula preparation by an experienced person and should be observed and guided at least once as she goes through the steps herself. These safeguards are more important if the mother is inexperienced, not well educated, or if the baby is not strong and healthy. In poor areas, especially where a sanitary water supply is not dependable, these rules and training are crucial.

3. Formula can be offered warm or cool. The baby may prefer warm formula if accustomed to it, but no harm is done by feeding it cool unless he refuses it. Mothers should be cautioned about heating formula in the microwave. Even though the bottle feels cool, the milk may be unevenly heated and may burn the child. After the bottle is heated in a microwave, the mother should shake it and test a drop on the wrist to be sure it is warm and not hot.

4. Close contact during feeding is important. Infant and mother should both be comfortable and relaxed. The infant should be positioned so that he can drink easily. His head should be higher than his body so that he will be drinking "downhill." This position may help prevent fluid from going into the inner ear canal, which can lead to ear infections. The nipple hole should be large enough to allow one swallow of milk to flow each time the baby sucks. If it is too small, it should be enlarged; if it is too large, it should be replaced. The

nipple should be checked to make sure the formula is flowing. The bottle should be tilted so that the nipple is full of formula, not air, while the baby is sucking. Bottles should never be propped, because the infant might choke if left unattended and will be deprived of the warm and intimate contact that makes feeding time pleasurable.

5. When the baby stops drinking or after 1 to 2 ounces in the young infant, position him upright and gently burp him to help him bring up any bubbles of air he may have swallowed. After he has burped, the mother should offer him more formula but should not try to force him to finish the bottle. Like making children clean their plates, this promotes obesity.

6. The feeding schedule can vary, but it promotes development best if adjusted to the baby's expressed hunger needs at first. Some babies need to feed much more frequently than others. One should keep in mind that a dehydrated baby (feverish, hot) may be thirsty for water, which can be offered in place of formula if the baby cries soon after a feeding.

7. Sterilized formula can be replaced by regular, clean, fresh formula and then by milk as the baby grows older. Some authorities say the switch to milk can be made at six months; others say to wait until a year. The pediatrician should be consulted in each individual case.

8. Babies love their bottles; the sucking provides needed stimulation as well as nutrients. Babies should never be allowed to sleep with their bottle, however, because of the potential damage to developing teeth. The bedtime bottle may be the most cherished, but it should be firmly removed. At weaning time (sometime around nine months when the baby can sit up and begin to manage a cup), one of the daily bottles at a time can be taken away and replaced by milk in a drinking cup. The last bottle to go may be the one at bedtime, which could be given up at about a year of age at the discretion of the parents and pediatrician.

9. Most importantly, we repeat, the mother who bottle-feeds should hold the baby as closely and lovingly as a breastfeeding mother does. Much more occurs during a feeding than the mere transfer of nutrients into the baby's body. The human warmth and stimulation delivered with the formula do as much as the formula itself to promote normal, healthy development.

Vitamin-Mineral Supplements for the Infant

It is unnecessary to give vitamin-mineral supplements to a newborn infant. If he is breastfed, breast milk and his own internal stores will meet most of his nutrient needs until he is well into the second half of his first year. At that time, the introduction of intelligently chosen juices and foods will keep up with his changing requirements. The only exceptions to this statement have to do with vitamin D, fluoride, and possibly iron.

Breast milk does not provide adequate vitamin D; therefore, the infant who has little exposure to sunlight is at risk for developing rickets (see Chapter 7).

TABLE 10–3. Transitions in Milk Feeding Before 6 Months

Breastfed infant should receive:
· Breast milk.
· Vitamin D.
· Fluoride and iron at pediatrician's discretion.

Formula-fed infant should receive:
· Vitamins A and D in formula or separately.
· Vitamin C in formula or separately.
· Fluoride at pediatrician's discretion.

If weaning from breast milk before 6 months, wean to formula as above. Wait to wean from formula until at least 6 months.

Source: Adapted from recommendations made in *Pediatrics* 62 (1978): 733, and *Nutrition and the MD,* March 1980.

Exposure of a small amount of skin to the sun at midday each day would provide a protective dose of vitamin D for most babies in most circumstances.

The fluoride content of breast milk may be somewhat unreliable. If the infant is not drinking fluoridated water, the baby's pediatrician may prescribe appropriate supplementation. Iron-deficiency anemia occurs when iron stores are reduced and dietary iron is limited. This is uncommon in breastfed infants before age 6–9 months because of the high bioavailability of the small amounts of iron found in human milk. However, an iron supplement may be desirable for the breastfed infant when he is about four months old.[4]

If the baby is formula fed, the makeup of the formula determines what further supplementation might be necessary. Commercially prepared formulas contain adequate amounts of vitamins and minerals, and further supplementation is unnecessary. Homemade formulas may lack some nutrients. The pediatrician is the expert to consult when such formulas are used. Table 10–3 shows what supplements are needed as the transitions are made from breastfeeding to formula and from formula to milk.

Nutrition of the Infant

A baby grows faster during the first year than ever again, as Figure 10–3 shows. The growth of infants and children directly reflects their nutritional well-being and is the most important parameter used in assessing their nutrition status. The birthweight doubles in four months from 7 to 14 pounds, and another 7 pounds is added in the next eight months. If a ten-year-old child

FIGURE 10–3

Weight gain of human infants (boys) in the first five years.

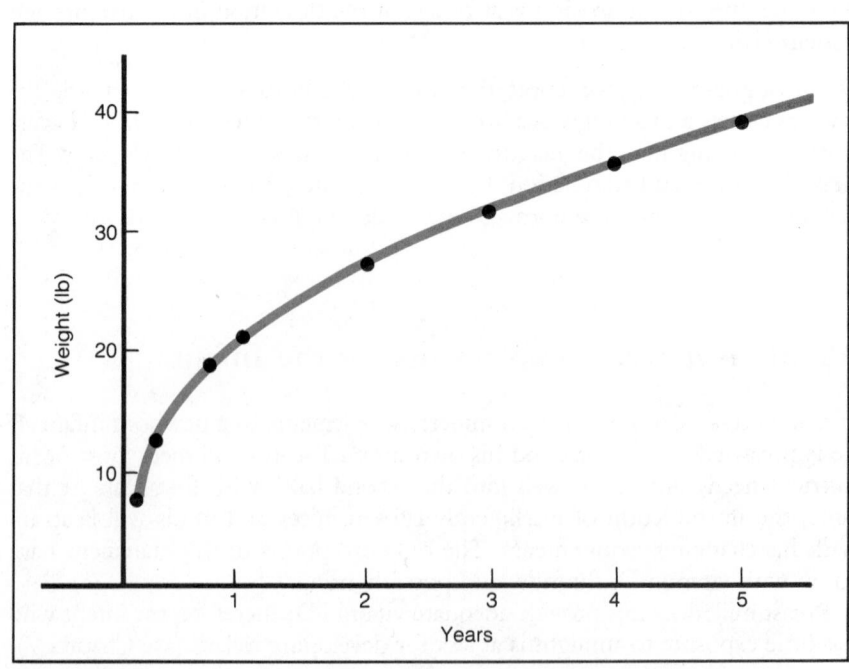

were to grow at this rate, the child's weight would increase from 70 to 210 pounds in a single year. This tremendous growth is a composite of the differing growth patterns of all the internal organs. For example, brain development continues through the tenth month after birth. Many critical periods occur early. By the end of the first year, the growth rate has slowed down. The weight a child gains between the first and second birthdays amounts to only about five pounds.

The rapid growth and metabolism of the infant demand ample supplies of the growth and energy nutrients. Because they are small, babies need smaller total amounts of these nutrients than adults do; but as a percentage of body weight, babies need over twice as much of most nutrients. Figure 10–4 compares a three-month-old baby's needs with those of an adult man. As you can see, some of the differences are extraordinary. After three months, energy needs continue to increase even though the growth rate slows down. As a baby nears the first birthday, the kcalories saved by slower growth are spent in greatly increased activity. Babies are now known to require fewer kcalories in the middle of their first year than was believed in the past.

Iron is the nutrient hardest to provide for infants, because it doesn't occur in adequate amounts in milk (except breast milk or iron-fortified formula). Iron is probably the nutrient that most needs attention in infant nutrition.

The baby's kidneys are unable to concentrate waste efficiently, so a baby must excrete relatively more water than an adult to carry off a comparable amount of waste. This means that dehydration, which can be dangerous, occurs more easily in an infant than in an adult. Because infants can communicate their needs only by crying, it is important to remember that they may be crying for fluid.

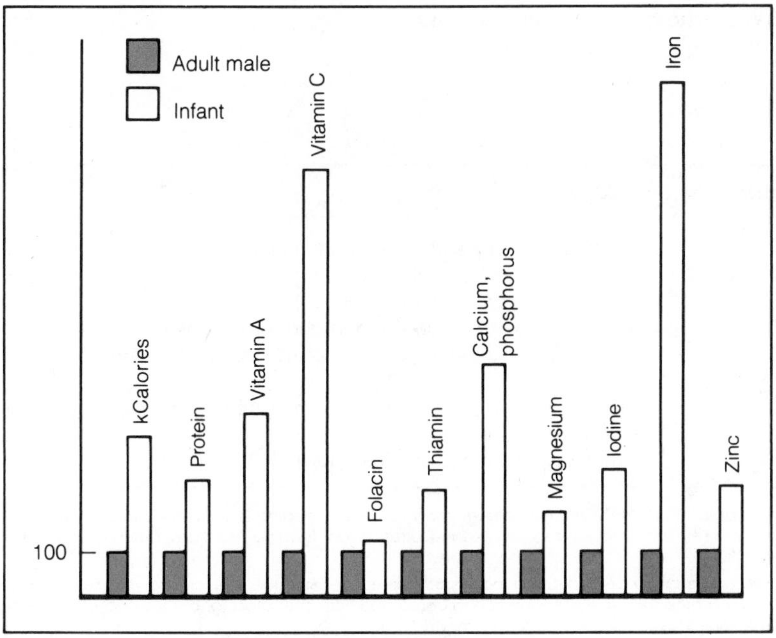

Baby's metabolism:
  Heart rate: 120–140 beats/min.
  Respiration rate: 20/min.

Adult's metabolism:
  Heart rate: 70–80 beats/min.
Respiration rate: 12–14/min.

FIGURE 10–4

Comparison of the nutrient needs of three-month-old infants with those of adult males (23 years old and up) per pound of body weight. Adult males' needs are set at 100 percent.

Source: Calculated from the RDA tables, inside front cover.

A term used by many authorities to mean supplemental or weaning foods is **belkost** (BYE-cost).

First Foods

The baby's most important food is milk: breast milk or formula at first, cow's milk or a substitute later. Recommended transitions from one form of milk to another are shown in Table 10−3.

The timing for adding solid foods to a baby's diet depends on several factors. If the baby is breastfed, additions to the diet can wait until four to six months. Babies not fed solid foods before the end of the first year suffer delayed growth. A reasonable pattern for adding foods to the diet is shown in Table 10−4. The following are some potential disadvantages of early introduction of solid foods:

* Increased risk of allergies.
* Poor oral motor coordination.
* Insufficient energy and nutrient replacement for breast milk and infant formula.
* Increased renal solute load and hyperosmolality.
* Disturbance of appetite regulation may encourage overfeeding.
* Possible increase in the infant's desire for sugar and salt intake later in adult life.[5]

Remember that babies are all different, and the program of additions should depend on the individual baby's readiness and not on any rigid schedule. Indications of readiness are any of the following:

* When the infant has doubled its birth weight.
* When the infant can consume eight ounces of formula and still is hungry in less than three to four hours.
* When the infant is consuming 32 ounces a day and wanting more.
* When the baby reaches six months.

TABLE 10−4. First Foods for the Formula-Fed Baby

Age (Months)	Addition
0−4	Supplement (depending on what's in the formula)
4−6	Iron-fortified rice cereal followed by other cereals (for iron; baby can now swallow and can digest starch)[a]
5−7	Mashed vegetables and/or fruits and their juices, one by one
6−8	Protein foods (cheese, yogurt, cooked beans, meat, fish, chicken, egg yolk)
9	Finely chopped meat (baby can chew now), toast, teething crackers (for emerging teeth)
10−12	Whole egg (allergies less likely now)

Source: Adapted from the 1979 *Recommendations for Infant Feeding Practices of the California Department of Health Services* as presented in Current infant feeding practices, *Nutrition and the MD*, January 1980.

[a]Later you can change cereals, but don't forget to keep on using the iron-fortified varieties. According to *Nutrition and the MD*, April 1981, the iron in cereal specially prepared for babies is so bioavailable that three level teaspoons a day is all they need.

The addition of foods to a baby's diet should be governed by three considerations: The baby's nutrient needs, the baby's physical readiness to handle different forms of foods, and the need to detect and control allergic reactions. The nutrients needed early are iron and vitamin C. Juices and fruits that contain vitamin C are usually among the first foods introduced. Commercially prepared infant formulas contain adequate vitamin C to meet the infant's need, and it is recommended that juices be given only when the baby can drink from a cup.[6] Since a baby's stored iron supply from before birth runs out after the birthweight doubles, formula with iron, iron-fortified cereals, and later meat are recommended.

It has been suggested that the early introduction of sweet fruits to babies' diets might favor babies' developing a preference for sweets and lessen their liking for vegetables introduced later. To prevent this, the order should perhaps be changed: vegetables first, fruits later. This practice now has a wide following.

Physical readiness develops in many small steps. For example, the ability to swallow solid food develops at around four to six months. Later, as a baby learns to sit up and handle finger foods and starts teething, hard crackers and other hard finger foods should be introduced, because they promote the development of manual dexterity and control of the jaw muscles.

It is a myth that feeding solids at an early age will help the baby to sleep through the night. On the average, babies start to sleep through the night when they are ready to do so, regardless of when solid foods are introduced.

Perhaps one out of every five to ten people may have an allergy of one kind or another. About half of these allergies are caused by foods—most commonly, nuts, eggs, milk, and wheat. If parents detect allergies in their infant's early life, they can spare the whole family much grief. New foods should be introduced singly so that allergies can be detected. For example, when cereals are introduced, try rice cereal first for several days, because it causes allergy least often. Try wheat cereal last, because it is the most common offender. If a cereal causes an allergic reaction (irritability, misery) in an infant, discontinue its use before going on to the next food. See Chapter 11 for more about food allergies in children.

Commercial baby foods are heavily advertised but are not necessary for a healthy infant. They are generally safe and nutritious and have a high nutrient density with the exception of mixed dinners (which contain little meat) and desserts (which are heavily sweetened). Commercial baby foods are convenient but do not teach chewing skills, which is one advantage of giving infants table foods mashed to a consistency that they are able to handle. However, infants fed table foods can easily overconsume sodium and energy from fat and sugar. Feeding an infant table foods requires more knowledge of nutrition than using commercial baby foods and necessitates cooking without salt or added fat or sugar and avoiding the use of canned vegetables, which are often salted. One should take precautions against food poisoning and avoid the use of vegetables in which nitrites are likely to form—notably, home-prepared carrots, beets, celery, and spinach—for the young infant. Low stomach acidity in the young infant may convert nitrate to nitrite, which can displace oxygen in hemoglobin. Stomach acidity increases by age six months, and nitrate overload becomes less of a problem. Honey should never be fed to infants under one year of age because of the risk of botulism.

Babies develop sensitivity to their own satiety at about ten months, another example of developmental readiness.

TABLE 10–5. Meal Plan for a One-Year-Old

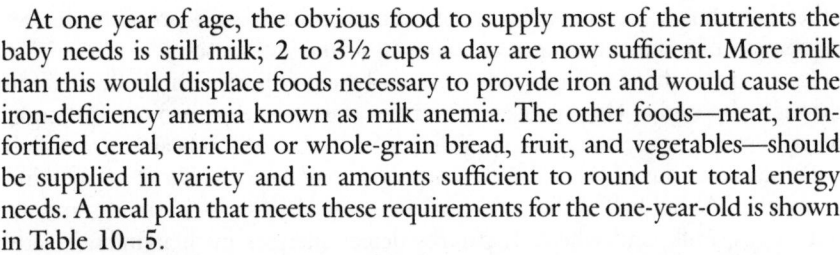

Breakfast	Lunch
1 cup milk	1 cup milk
½ cup cereal	3 tbs. vegetables
5 tbs. fruit	5 tbs. chopped meat
Teething crackers or dry toast	¼ cup rice, potato, cereal, or macaroni

Dinner	Snack
1 cup milk	½ cup milk
1 egg	Teething crackers or dry toast
½ cup rice, potato, cereal, or macaroni	
2 tbs. vegetables	
Teething crackers or dry toast	

milk anemia:
iron-deficiency anemia caused by drinking so much milk that iron-rich foods are displaced from the diet.

At one year of age, the obvious food to supply most of the nutrients the baby needs is still milk; 2 to 3½ cups a day are now sufficient. More milk than this would displace foods necessary to provide iron and would cause the iron-deficiency anemia known as milk anemia. The other foods—meat, iron-fortified cereal, enriched or whole-grain bread, fruit, and vegetables—should be supplied in variety and in amounts sufficient to round out total energy needs. A meal plan that meets these requirements for the one-year-old is shown in Table 10–5.

The wise parent of a one-year-old child offers nutrition and love together. Both promote growth. The person feeding a one-year-old has to be aware that this is a period in the child's life when exploring and experimenting are normal and desirable behaviors. The child is developing a sense of autonomy that if allowed to flower will provide the foundation for later confidence and effectiveness as an individual.

Looking Ahead

The first year of a baby's life is the time to lay the foundation for future health. From the nutrition standpoint, the relevant problems most common in later years are obesity and dental disease. Prevention of obesity should also help avert the development of the obesity-related diseases—atherosclerosis, diabetes, and cancer.

Probably the most important single measure to undertake during the infant's first year is to encourage eating habits that will support continued normal weight as the child grows. Primarily, this means introducing nutritious foods in an inviting way. A baby should not be forced to finish the bottle or the baby food jar. Concentrated sweets and empty-kcalorie foods should be avoided. Parents should encourage vigorous physical activity. To discourage the development of behaviors and attitudes that plague the obese, parents should avoid teaching babies to seek food as a reward, to expect food as comfort for unhappiness, or to associate food deprivation with punishment.

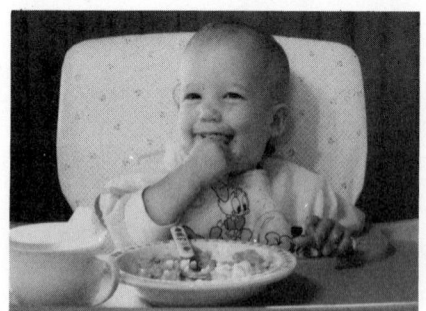

Ideally, the one-year-old eats many of the same foods the rest of the family eats.

Beyond these recommendations, some thought is being given to the idea that infants should be started on a "prudent diet" like that recommended to prevent heart disease: Restrict fat, increase the ratio of polyunsaturated to saturated fat, and reduce cholesterol intake. The Committee on Nutrition of the American Academy of Pediatrics has investigated this type of diet and reports, ". . . there is insufficient evidence to warrant nutritional manipulation to reduce serum cholesterol in the first year of life."[7] Babies need the kcalories and fat of milk, and most experts agree that they should be fed whole milk until they are over a year old. The exception might be the seriously obese baby or a child over two years old with a positive family history of heart disease.

Normal dental development is promoted by the same strategies as those outlined previously: Supplying nutritious foods, avoiding sweets, and discouraging association of food with reward or comfort. In addition, the practice of giving a baby a bottle as a pacifier is strongly discouraged by dentists on the grounds that sucking for long periods of time pushes the normal jawline out of shape and causes the bucktooth profile: protruding upper and receding lower teeth. Further, prolonged sucking on a bottle of milk or juice bathes the upper teeth in a carbohydrate-rich fluid that favors the growth of decay-producing bacteria. Babies permitted to do this are sometimes seen with decayed upper teeth all the way to the gum line.

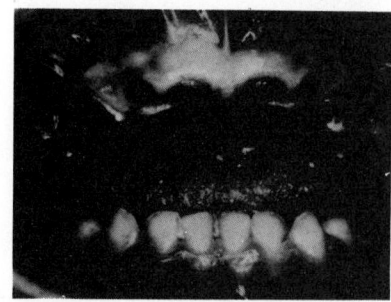

A baby that goes to sleep sucking on a bottle of juice, formula, or milk may lose his teeth to decay before he is two years old. This is called the **nursing bottle syndrome.**

CASE STUDY:

Overweight Pregnant Women

Ellen is a 24-year-old housewife who is four months pregnant. It is her first pregnancy, and she is eager to know how to feed herself during pregnancy as well as her infant after birth. She is five feet three inches tall and currently weighs 150 pounds. Her prepregnancy weight was 148 pounds. Ellen is very concerned about her two-pound weight gain.

1. Assess Ellen's weight. What would her ideal weight be if she were not pregnant? Should she be concerned about her two-pound weight gain? Why? What advice should you give Ellen about her weight gain during pregnancy? What other dietary advice would you give her?

2. Discuss methods of infant feeding with Ellen. What advantages would breastfeeding offer her? What are the advantages of formula feeding? What advice will you give Ellen if she decides to breastfeed? What information should she have about formula feeding?

Notes

1. E. Hackman and coauthors, Maternal birth weight and subsequent pregnancy outcome, *Journal of the American Medical Association* 250 (1983): 2016–2019.

2. F. B. Glenn, W. D. Glenn, and R. C. Duncan, Fluoride tablet supplementation during pregnancy for caries immunity: A study of the offspring produced, *American Journal of Obstetrics and Gynecology* 143 (1982): 560–564.

3. R. K. Kalkhoff, Medical management of diabetes in pregnancy, in *Clinical Diabetes Mellitus: A Problem Oriented Approach,* ed. J. K. Davison (New York: Thieme, 1986), pp. 472–484.

4. D. W. Thomas, Milk feeding in infancy, Special Report on Pediatric Eating Disorders, Nutrition and the MD, (1987), ed. R. J. Merritt.

5. P. M. Queen and S. E. Wilson, Growth and nutrient requirements of infants, *Pediatric Nutrition,* ed R. J. Grand, J. L. Sutphen, and W. H. Dietz (Boston: Butterworths, 1987), p. 336.

6. Queen and Wilson, 1987.

7. A 'prudent diet' for infants? Special Report on Pediatric Eating Disorders, *Nutrition and* the MD (1987).

Nutrition and Hyperactive Behavior

One of the most common misconceptions about children's nutrition today is that sugar causes hyperactivity. This Nutrition in Practice is intended to dispel that illusion and to show the real connecting link between children's high sugar intake and disturbed behavior: malnutrition.

It's clear from what you just said that sugar doesn't cause hyperactivity. Why do so many people think that it does?

Probably because they think they've seen the evidence with their own eyes. They've seen children who have eaten a lot of sugar and have also had behavior disturbances, and they've seen children who have eaten high-nutrient-density foods with little or no sugar who seemed to be better behaved. If there's a correlation, though, it's probably between disturbed behavior and malnutrition, not between disturbed behavior and sugar.

What do you mean by malnutrition? How can malnutrition cause disturbed behavior?

Practically every nutrient deficiency you can name has effects on behavior. Look at Table NP10–1. Although we can't say which nutrient deficiencies might be involved in a particular child's case, it's obvious that any child who eats a lot of sugar might have some nutrient deficiencies that will adversely affect behavior.

It's not obvious to me. Show me how badly a child has to eat to have nutrient deficiencies.

Okay. Take a look at the food intake of a hypothetical five-year-old child we'll call Freddie. Freddie eats in a way most people would agree is not unusual for a child who hasn't learned to like vegetables:

- *Breakfast:* 1 cup of cornflakes with ½ cup of milk and fresh apple slices.
- *Lunch:* Bologna sandwich with 1 ounce bologna and 2 slices of whole-wheat bread; 1 bag of pretzels; 1 cup of milk.
- *Supper:* 2 fried chicken drumsticks; about 20 french fries; 1 roll; a carbonated beverage; and ½ cup of gelatin with nondairy topping (from fast-food restaurant).
- *Snack:* 4 chocolate sandwich cookies.

Freddie didn't do too badly on the day we've shown you. He ate three meals and a snack, including milk at two of his meals. But look at his nutrient intakes, shown in Table NP 10–2. You can see that he received less than the RDA for seven of the nine nutrients listed. Then think how much worse he would fare on days when he missed meals or when he ate more sugary foods in place of nourishing ones. Clearly, he's at risk for malnutrition.

I see. But this is all theoretical. Has it ever actually been shown that nutrient deficiencies caused disturbed behavior in children?

Behavioral changes are difficult to measure. At least one study suggests that iron deficiency causes behavioral changes. The implications of these findings are staggering when you consider that actual anemia occurs in about one out of every twenty children nationwide. Iron deficiency shy of frank anemia must be more common still. A child's *brain* is sensitive to slightly lowered iron levels long before anemia appears.

Although the effects of iron deficiency are hard to distinguish from the effects of other factors in children's lives, it is likely that iron deficiency in children manifests itself in a lowering of the motivation to persist in intellectually challenging tasks, a shortening of the attention span, and a reduction of overall intellectual performance. Anemic children perform less well on tests and have more conduct disturbances than their nonanemic classmates. This is similar to a description of hyperactivity, but sugar isn't the cause. Before blaming sugar for these problems, it makes sense to check for the absence of iron.

That's interesting. Do we know how iron exerts these effects?

Iron carries oxygen in the blood and then helps transport that oxygen into the cells, where it is needed for essential processes, like energy production. A lack of iron not only causes an energy crisis but also directly affects behavior, mood, attention span,

TABLE NP10—1. Nutrient Deficiencies and Behavior

Deficiency	Behavioral Symptoms[a]
Protein-Energy	Apathy; fretfulness; lack of energy; lack of interest in food
Thiamin	Confusion; uncoordinated movements; depressed appetite; irritability; insomnia; fatigue; general misery[b]
Riboflavin	Depression; hysteria; psychopathic behavior; lethargy; hypochondrias—all evident before onset of clinical deficiency[c]
Niacin	Irritability, agitated depression, headaches, sleeplessness, memory loss, emotional instability—early signs of pellagra; mental confusion progressing to psychosis or delirium
Vitamin B_6	Irritability; insomnia; weakness; mental depression; abnormal brain wave pattern; convulsions; mental symptoms of anemia; fatigue, headache[d]
Folacin	Mental symptoms of anemia; tiredness; apathy; weakness; forgetfulness; mild depression; abnormal nerve function; irritability; headache, disorientation, confusion; inability to perform simple calculations[e]
Vitamin B_{12}	Degeneration of peripheral nervous system; mental symptoms of anemia
Vitamin C	Hysteria; depression; listlessness; lassitude; weakness; aversion to work; hypochondria; social introversion; possible iron-deficiency anemia with resulting mental symptoms; fatigue
Vitamin A	Mental symptoms of anemia
Iron	Fatigue; weakness; headaches; pallor; listlessness; irritability; mental symptoms of anemia
Magnesium	Apathy; personality changes; hyperirritability
Copper	Mental symptoms of iron-deficiency anemia
Zinc	Poor appetite; mental symptoms of iron-deficiency anemia; irritability; emotional disorders; mental lethargy[f]
Anemia[g]	Anorexia; apathy; listlessness; clumsiness; conduct disturbances; decreased attentiveness; hyperactivity; irritability; learning disorders; lowered IQ; low scores on vocabulary tests and on latency and associative reactions; perceptual restriction; reduced physical work capacity; repetitive hand and foot movements.

[a]Unless otherwise noted, all deficiency symptoms can be found in R. S. Goodhart and M. E. Shils, eds., *Modern Nutrition in Health and Disease,* 6th ed. (Philadelphia: Lea and Febiger, 1980).

[b]Marginal vitamin deficiency, *Nutrition and the MD,* July 1983, p. 3.

[c]R. Sterner and W. Price, Restricted riboflavin: Within-subject behavioral effects in humans, *American Journal of Clinical Nutrition* 26 (1973): 150–160.

[d]Marginal vitamin deficiency, 1983.

[e]J. H. Pincus, E. H. Reynolds, and G. H. Glaser, Subacute combined system degeneration with folate deficiency, *Journal of the American Medical Association* 221 (1972): 496–497. Possibly, because folacin is required for many steps in amino acid metabolism, its lack causes altered amino acid levels in the blood, and therefore altered neurotransmitter levels in the brain. Neurological disease in folic acid deficiency. *Nutrition Reviews* 39 (1981): 337–338.

[f]A. S. Prasad, Clinical, biochemical and nutritional spectrum of zinc deficiency in human subjects: An update, *Nutrition Reviews* 41 (1983): 197–206.

[g]Anemia is included here because it produces mental symptoms of its own and many of the nutrient deficiencies listed here include anemia. These symptoms are not caused by anemia itself, but by iron deficiency in the brain. Children with more severe anemias from other causes, such as sickle cell anemia and thalassemia, show no reduction in IQ when compared with other children.

and learning ability. Iron has a vital effect on the functioning of many molecules in the brain and nervous system. Deficiencies of iron produced experimentally in animals have caused abnormal synthesis and degradation of chemical messengers in the nervous system that help regulate a child's ability to pay attention, which is crucial to learning.[1]

It seems that people concerned with children should make every effort to ensure that the children they care about get enough iron.

Yes, but that measure alone isn't nearly enough to protect children from the ill effects of malnutrition on behavior. In fact, it isn't even enough to make sure they get all their nutrients! We have to be concerned with protection against environmental

TABLE NP10–2 Freddie's Nutrient Intakes

Nutrient[a]	RDA for Five-Year-Old	One Day's Meals Provided	% of RDA
Protein	30 g	58 g	193—higher than necessary
Vitamin A	500 RE	177 RE	35—too low
Thiamin	0.9 mg	0.7 mg	78—marginal
Riboflavin	1.0 mg	1.2 mg	120—adequate
Folacin	200 μg	179 μg	90—probably adequate
Vitamin C	45 mg	42 mg	93—probably adequate
Calcium	800 mg	544 mg	68—too low
Iron	10 mg	7.6 mg	76—marginal
Zinc	10 mg	5.8 mg	58—too low

[a]A key point to remember: The nutrients that are noted here are just a representation. This child's diet probably lacks others, too.

contaminants, too—lead poisoning, for example, can cause iron-deficiency anemia. Iron deficiency impairs the body's defenses against absorption of lead. The anemia brought on by lead poisoning might be mistaken for a simple iron deficiency. Lead toxicity symptoms are widespread among children—one out of every fifty children in rural areas and more than one out of every ten inner-city children are affected by lead poisoning.[2]

Interestingly, lead poisoning also presents the classic symptoms of hyperactivity in children, as does iron deficiency. Hyperactivity has been blamed on additives, allergies, and sugar, as you know, but the evidence hasn't supported these claims. On the other hand, evidence has supported the connection of both iron deficiency and lead poisoning with hyperactivity.

You've told me how iron deficiency leads to symptoms of hyperactivity. What's the evidence on lead?

An experiment was performed in which lead-affected hyperactive children were treated either with a drug that would remove lead from their bodies or with a fake medicine that would not. Their behavior was scored by observers who didn't know which child was which. The children whose lead poisoning was relieved also became less hyperactive.[3]

I am impressed. I see that nutrition has a lot to do with children's behavior. That puts sugar in a different perspective for me.
Yes. Sugar isn't a poison, but it does displace nutrients. That's why there's very little room for it in a child's diet.

How can I be alert to nutrient deficiencies in children?
Keep things in perspective. Remember that poor nutrition may be one cause of disturbed behavior in children. Use that fact in performing a nutrition assessment. If a child—or, in fact, if any person—looks abnormal and acts

abnormally, she *may* be malnourished. Find out if she has a good breakfast daily. See if she obtains wholesome foods of all kinds on a regular basis. If she doesn't, do what you can to see that she does.

Figure NP10–1 compares characteristics of well-nourished and malnourished children. Imagine a child in class or at home with any of these constellations of symptoms of malnutrition. The child may be irritable, aggressive, disagreeable, or sad and withdrawn. You might label such a child "hyperactive," "depressed," or "unlikable," when in fact he may be suffering from simple, albeit marginal, malnutrition. In any such case, inspection of the child's diet by someone knowledgeable about children's nutrient needs is clearly in order. Should suspicion of dietary inadequacies be raised, *no matter what other causes may be implicated,* the people responsible for feeding the child should take steps to correct those inadequacies promptly.

Notes

1. D. M. Tucker and H. H. Sandstead, Body iron stores and cortical arousal, in *Iron Deficiency: Brain Biochemistry and Behavior,* eds. E. Pollitt and R. L. Leibel (New York: Raven Press, 1982), pp. 161–182.
2. These figures were obtained from the *Journal of the American Dietetic Association* 80 (1982): 591, 594. A complete discussion of lead and other contaminants in foods is found in E. N. Whitney with M. A. Boyle Highlight 11: Contaminants in foods, in *Understanding Nutrition,* 3rd ed. (St Paul, Minn.: West, 1984).
3. O. J. David and coauthors, The relationship of hyperactivity to moderately elevated lead levels, *Archives of Environmental Health* 38 (1983): 341–346.

FIGURE NP10–1

The well-nourished versus the malnourished child

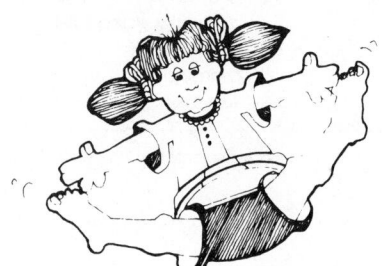

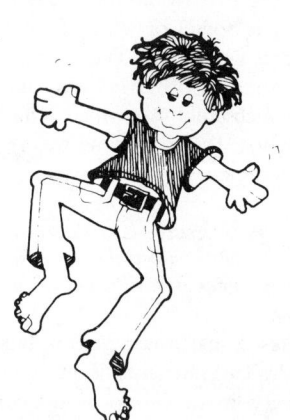

Normal hair: shiny, firm in the scalp.
Malnourished hair: dull, brittle, dry, loose and falls out.

Normal face: good complexion.
Malnourished face: off color; scaly, flaky, cracked skin.

Normal glands: no lumps.
Malnourished galnds: swollen at front of neck, cheeks.

Normal skin: smooth, firm, good color.
Malnourished skin: dry, rough, "sandpaper" feel, spotty, or sores; lack of fat under the skin.

Normal nails: firm, pink.
Malnourished nails: spoon-shaped, brittle, ridged.

Normal internal systems: heart rate, rhythm, and blood pressure normal; normal GI function; reflexes, psychological development normal.
Malnourished internal systems: heart rate, rhythm, or blood pressure abnormal; liver, spleen enlarged, GI dysfunction; mental irritability, confusion; burning, tingling of hands, feet; loss of balance, coordination.

Normal eyes: bright, clear, membranes pink, adjust easily to darkness.

Malnourished eyes: pale membranes, spots, redness, slow adjustment to dark.

Normal lips: smooth, good color.
Malnourished lips: red, swollen, cracks at corners of mouth.

Normal tongue: red, rough, bumpy.
Malnourished tongue: sore, smooth, purplish, swollen.

Normal teeth and gums: no pain or cavities; gums firm, teeth bright.
Malnourished teeth and gums: missing, discolored, decayed teeth; gums bleed easily, swollen, spongy.

Normal behavior: alert, attentive, cheerful.
Malnourished behavior: irritable, apathetic, inattentive, hyperactive.

Normal muscles and bones: good muscle tone, posture, long bones straight.
Malnourished muscles and bones: "wasted" appearance of muscles, swollen bumps on skull or ends of bones; small bumps on ribs; bowed legs or knock-knees; pain.

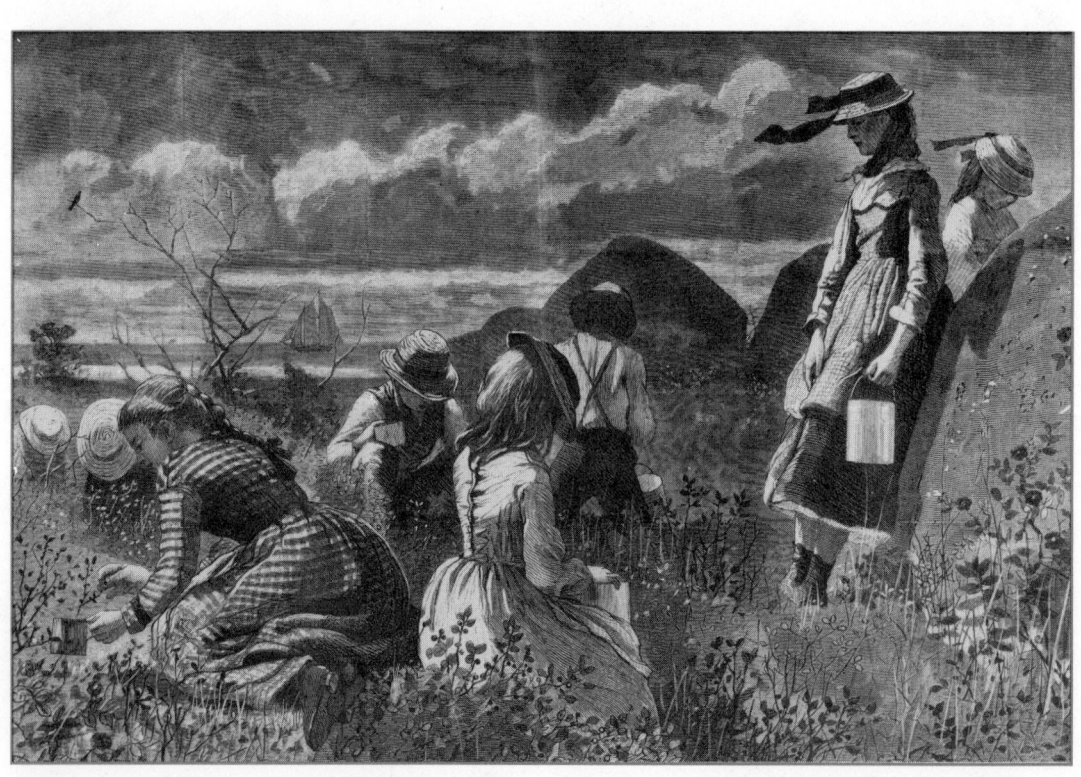

11
Child and Teen

CONTENTS

Gathering Berries by Winslow Homer, published in Harper's Weekly, July 11, 1874.

The years of life described in this chapter are often called "the growing years," although, as we have seen, the year before and the first year after birth may be the most growing years of all. Still, there is more to come. From age one to twenty or thereabouts, height more than triples and weight increases six to tenfold. Optimal nutrition permits children to develop to their full potential.

Early and Middle Childhood

Nutrient needs change steadily throughout life and vary from individual to individual, depending on such factors as rate of growth, sex, and previous nutrition and health history. This section takes a general look at preschool and school-age children's needs. Later sections are devoted to the special concerns of teenagers.

After the age of one, a child's growth rate slows, but the body continues to change dramatically. At one, babies have just learned to stand and toddle; by two, they can take long strides with solid confidence and are learning to run, jump, and climb. The internal change that makes these new accomplishments possible is the accumulation of a larger mass and greater density of bone and muscle tissue. The changes are obvious if you compare the bodies of a one-year-old and a two-year-old. The two-year-old has lost much of his baby fat. His muscles, especially in the back, buttocks, and legs, have firmed and strengthened, and his leg bones have lengthened and increased in density.

Thereafter, the same trend—lengthening of the long bones and increase in musculature—continues, unevenly and more slowly, until adolescence. Growth comes in spurts. A six-year-old child may wear the same pair of shoes for a year, then need new shoes twice in the next four months. Figure 11−1 is an example of the growth charts used to monitor the smoothed average of height and weight changes as children grow.

Just before adolescence, the growth patterns of girls and boys begin to become distinct. In girls, fat becomes a larger percentage of the total body weight, and in boys the lean body mass—muscle and bone—becomes much greater. Around this time, growth in height may seem to stop altogether for a while. This is the calm before the storm.

Nutrition Needs and Feeding

According to the RDA a one-year-old child needs perhaps 1,000 kcalories a day; a three-year-old needs only 300 to 500 kcalories more. Appetite wanes markedly around the age of one year, corresponding to the great reduction in growth rate. Thereafter, the appetite fluctuates; a child will need and demand much more food during periods of rapid growth than during slow periods. Protein, calcium, phosphorus, magnesium, and zinc continue to need emphasis, and milk is still the most important single food in the diet.

The preadolescent period is the last one in which parental food choices have much influence. As children gather their forces for the adolescent growth spurt,

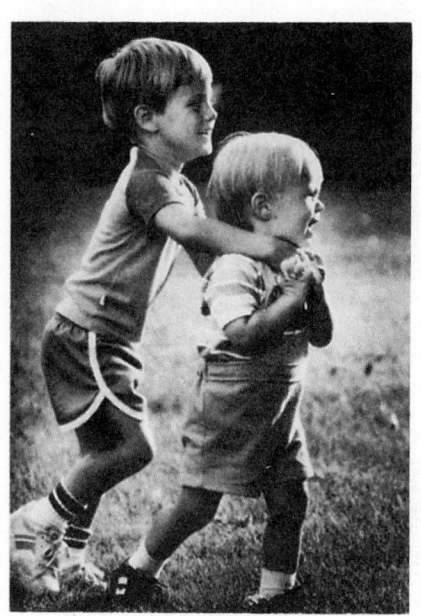

As a child grows, body shape changes. Body fat is lost and the muscles and bones become longer and stronger.

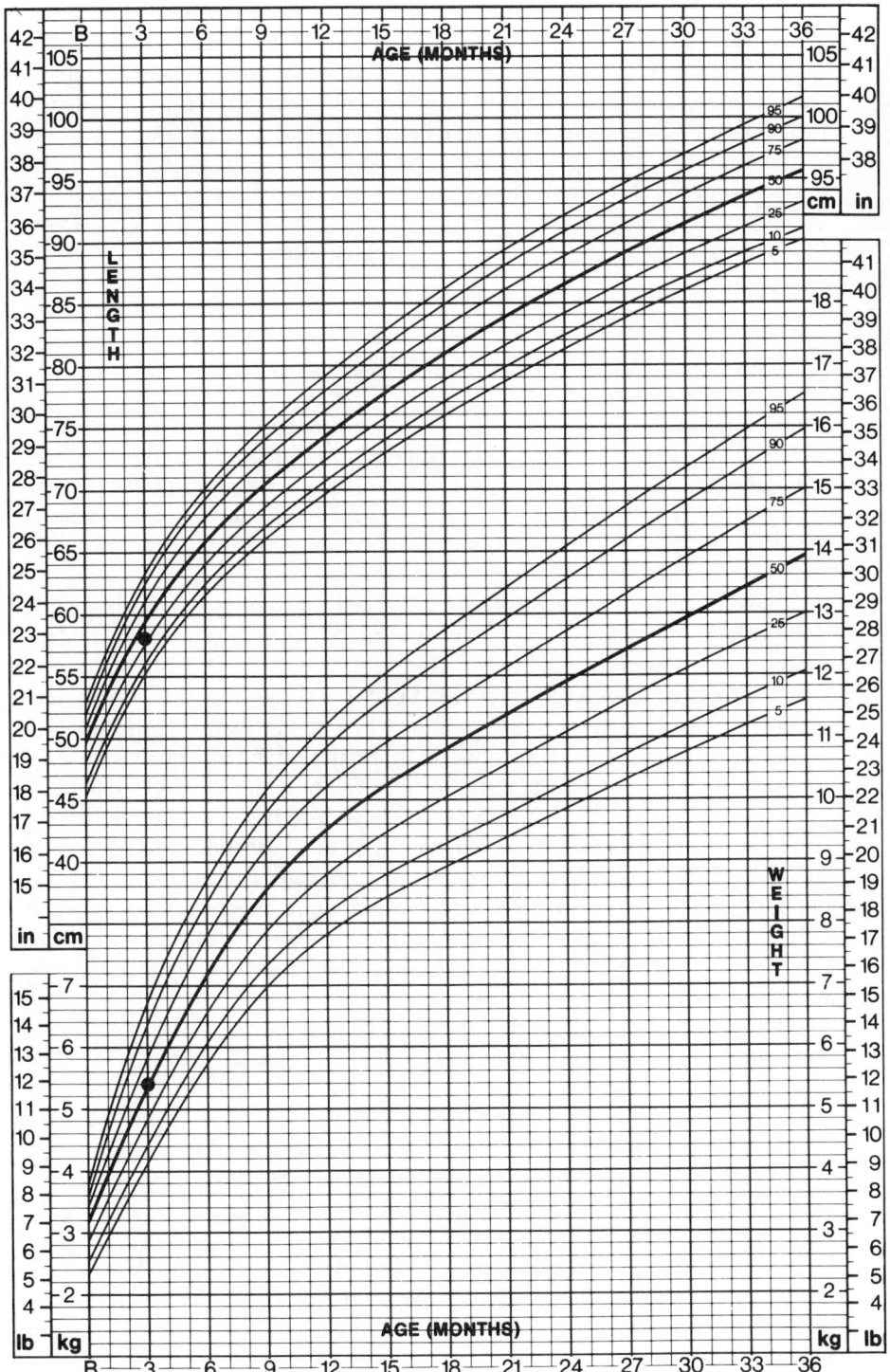

Figure 11–1
Girls, birth to 36 months, length and weight for age. Percentiles are from the National Center for Health Statistics (NCHS). Example: A three-month-old baby girl is 23 inches long and weighs 12 pounds. Dots on the 3-month line opposite this length and weight show that she is at the 50th percentile in both measures for her age.

Source: Adapted from P. V. V. Hamill and coauthors, Physical growth: National Center for Health Statistics percentiles, *American Medical Journal of Clinical Nutrition* 32 (1979): 607–629. Data from the Fels Research Institute, Wright State University School of Medicine, Yellow Springs, Ohio. Provided as a service of Ross Laboratories. © 1980 Ross Laboratories.

they are accumulating stores of nutrients that will be needed in the coming years. When they take off on that growth spurt, there will be a period during which their nutrient intake, especially of calcium, cannot meet the demands of rapidly growing bones. They will draw on their nutrient stores at this time. The denser their bones are before this occurs, the better prepared they will be.

The gradual increasing needs for all nutrients during the growing years are evident from the RDA table (inside front cover), which lists separate averages for each span of three years. To provide these nutrients, the Four Food Group Plan recommends the following for growing children:

- Three servings of milk or milk products.
- Two servings of meat or meat substitutes.
- Four or more servings of fruits and vegetables.
- Four or more servings of breads and cereals.

For meats, fruits, and vegetables, a serving is loosely defined as one tablespoon per year of the child's age. Thus, at four years of age, a serving of any of these foods would be four tablespoons ($\frac{1}{4}$ cup). Because the serving sizes adjust as the child grows older, these recommendations are good from age two to the teen years.

After the crucial first year, there is still much a parent can do to foster the development of healthy eating habits in a child. The goal is to teach children to like nutritious foods in all four categories.

Experimentation with children's food patterns shows that candy, cola, and other concentrated sweets must be limited in a child's diet if the needed nutrients are to be supplied. If such foods are permitted in large quantities, only two possible outcomes exist: nutrient deficiencies and/or obesity. The child can't be trusted to choose nutritious foods on the basis of taste alone; the preference for sweets is innate. On the other hand, an underweight, active child can enjoy the higher-kcalorie nutritious foods in each category: ice cream or pudding in the milk group and pancakes or crackers (whole-grain or enriched only, however) in the bread group. These foods, made from milk and grain, carry valuable nutrients and encourage a child to learn appropriately that eating is fun.

Children sometimes lose their appetites when they are sick with colds or flu and sometimes for no apparent reason at all. This is usually nothing to worry about. What they don't eat today they will make up for tomorrow. The child who is sick should be encouraged to drink plenty of fluids. Chapter 14 gives suggestions to improve the appetite of the hospitalized child.

The perfection of appetite regulation in children of normal weight guarantees that such children's food energy intakes will be right for each stage of growth. As long as the kcalories they do consume are from nutritious foods, they are well provided for. (One caution, however: wandering school-age children may be spending pocket money at the nearby candy store.) Unfortunately, many people mistakenly believe it is necessary to control children's portion sizes. An innovative study showed otherwise. Researchers wanted to determine how much lunch children would eat if given snacks of different energy value before lunch. The children ate puddings that contained either 40 kcalories or 150 kcalories but were otherwise identical. The children were then given lunch.

They compensated for the kcaloric difference: those who had eaten the high-calorie pudding ate less lunch than those who had eaten the low-kcalorie pudding. Overweight children, however, may eat in response to external cues, disregarding appetite regulation signals.[1]

Mealtimes with Children

Feeding children requires not only providing a variety of nutritious foods but also nurturing growing children's self-esteem and well-being.[2] Parents face a number of challenges in preparing meals that appeal to their children's tastes as well as providing needed nutrients. The interactions between parents and children regarding food intake set the stage for lifetime attitudes and habits.

It is not surprising that feeding problems often arise during the second or third year when children are asserting their independence. Many of these problems arise from the conflict between children's developmental stages and capabilities and parents who, in attempting to do what they think is best for their children, try to control every aspect of eating. Such conflict can cause harm to the children. It can disrupt their ability to regulate their own food intakes or to determine their own likes and dislikes. The end result is usually far from the desired one. For example, many people share the misconception that children must be persuaded or coerced to try new foods. Research with children indicates the opposite. When children are forced to try new foods, even by way of rewards, they are less likely to try those foods again than are children who are left to decide for themselves. The parent is responsible for *what* the child is offered to eat and the child is responsible for *how much* and even *whether* to eat.

When introducing new foods at the table, parents are advised to offer them one at a time and only in small amounts at first. Whenever possible, the new food should be presented at the beginning of the meal, because the child is hungriest then. If the child is cross, irritable, or feeling sick, one should not insist but should withdraw the new food and try it again a few days later. Parents have inclinations and dislikes to which they feel entitled; children should be accorded the same privilege. One should never make an issue of food acceptance. A power struggle almost invariably results in a confirmed pattern of resistance and a permanently closed mind on the child's part.

Food dislikes in childhood consistently include cooked vegetables, mixed dishes, and liver. Why children respond negatively to these foods that look "off" or "messy" to them is a matter for conjecture. Parents need only be aware that this is how many children feel and then honor those feelings. Children prefer vegetables that are slightly undercooked and crunchy, attractive in shape, and easy to eat. The vegetables should be warm, not hot, because a child's mouth is much more sensitive than an adult's. Smooth foods, such as mashed potatoes or pea soup, should have no lumps in them, because a child may wonder, with some disgust, what the lumps might be. Irrational as the fear of strangeness may seem, the parent must realize that this fear is practically universal among children.

Small children like to eat at little tables and to be served little portions of food. They also love to eat with other children and have been observed to stay

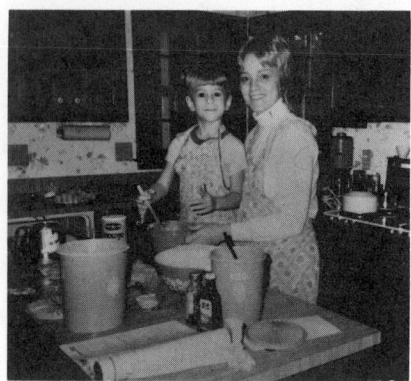

Children enjoy helping in the kitchen.

at the table longer and eat much more when in the company of their peers. Parents who serve the food in a relaxed and casual manner, without anxiety, provide the emotional climate in which a child's negative emotions will be minimized.

Ideally, each meal is preceded, not followed, by the activity the child looks forward to the most. In a number of schools, it has been discovered that children eat a much better lunch if recess occurs before, rather than after, the meal. Before sitting down to eat, small children should be helped to clean themselves thoroughly, washing their hands and faces so that they can enjoy their meal with "that clean feeling."

Many little children, both boys and girls, enjoy helping in the kitchen. Their participation provides many opportunities to encourage good food habits. Vegetables are pretty, especially when fresh, and provide opportunities for children to learn about color, about growing things and their seeds, about shapes and textures—all of which are fascinating to young children. Measuring, stirring, decorating, cutting, and arranging vegetables are skills even a very small child can practice with enjoyment and pride.

The key word during a child's first year is *trust;* the parental behavior best suited to promote it is affectionate holding. At two years, the key word is *autonomy;* parents should allow children to help make family choices, including sometimes giving them the right to say their favorite word—NO! At the same time, of course, parents should sensibly prevent children from dominating the family. At four, when the development of *initiative* is their proudest achievement, children can be encouraged to participate in the planning and preparation of meals. At each age, food can be given and enjoyed in the context of encouraging emotional as well as physical growth. If the beginnings are right, children will grow with a positive attitude that will foster good eating habits throughout life.

Nutrition at School

While parents are doing what they can to establish favorable eating behavior in their children during the transition from infancy to childhood, other factors are entering the picture. At five or so, the child goes to school and encounters foods prepared and served by outsiders. The U.S. government funds several programs to provide nutritious, high-quality meals for children at school. School lunches are designed to meet certain requirements and must include specified servings of milk, protein-rich food (meat, cheese, eggs, legumes, or peanut butter), vegetables, fruits, bread or other grain foods, and butter or margarine. The design is intended to provide at least a third of the RDA for each of the nutrients. Different school lunch patterns exist for children of different ages (see Table 11–1).

Along with the school lunch program is the nutrition education and training (NET) program in all the public schools. Originally allocated 50 cents per year per child, this program was cut in 1980 to 9 cents per child. Highly motivated program administrators are credited with maintaining a high-quality program by using ingenious and creative techniques to accomplish the program's highest priority objectives despite the cuts.

TABLE 11–1. School Lunch Patterns for Different Ages

| Food Group | Preschool | | Grades | | |
	Ages 1–2	Ages 3–4	K–3	4–12	7–12
Meat or meat alternate					
One serving					
Lean meat, poultry, or fish	1 oz	1½ oz	1½ oz	2 oz	3 oz
Cheese	1 oz	1½ oz	1½ oz	2 oz	3 oz
Large egg(s)	1	1½	1½	2	3
Cooked dry beans or peas	½ c	¾ c	¾ c	1 c	1½ c
Peanut butter	2 tbsp	3 tbsp	3 tbsp	4 tbsp	6 tbsp
Vegetable and/or fruit					
Two or more servings,					
both to total	½ c	½ c	½ c	¾ c	¾ c
Bread or bread alternate					
Servingsᵃ	5 per week	8 per week	8 per week	8 per week	10 per week
Milk					
A serving of fluid milk	¾ c	¾ c	1 c	1 c	1 c

Source: Adapted from School lunch patterns: Ready, set, go! *School Food Service Journal* (August 1980), p. 31.

ᵃA serving is 1 slice of whole-grain or enriched bread; a whole-grain or enriched biscuit, roll, muffin, etc.; ½ c cooked pasta or other cereal grain, such as bulgur or grits.

Television and Vending Machines

For the most part, children learn nutrition from parents or teachers who know little about it. Meanwhile, they hear a great deal about foods from the television set. Many authorities are concerned that television commercials may have a less than desirable impact. According to estimates, the average child sees more than 10,000 commercials a year, of which many more than half are for sugary foods. Hundreds of millions of dollars are spent in the effort to sell these foods to children. Most of the concern centers on the issue of sugar. You may recall that not all the public disapproval of sugar is based on scientific findings. However, there is widespread agreement on one point: Sticky, sugary foods left on the teeth provide an ideal environment for the growth of mouth bacteria and for the formation of cavities. Also, sugary foods may displace needed nutrients in the diet (see Nutrition in Practice 2 and 10). No regulations to prevent the promotion of sticky, sugary foods are in force, however. A model eating plan that favors dental health is shown in Table 11–2.

Television is not the only environmental force affecting children's food choices. Another is vending machines, especially those in schools. Children choose more nutritious snacks if offered them side by side with sugary foods. When milk is made available, soft-drink use drops.

The Teen Years

Teenagers are not fed, they eat. They make their own food choices. At the same time, they are intensely involved in day-to-day life with their peers and

TABLE 11–2. Eating Habits to Favor Good Dental Health

Food Group	Foods to Eat	Foods to Avoid
Milk and milk products	Milk Cheese Plain yogurt	All dairy products with added sugar
Fruit	Fresh fruit Water-packed canned fruit	Dried fruit Sugar-packed canned fruit Jams and jellies
Juice	Unsweetened juice	Sweetened juice
Vegetables	Most vegetables	Candied sweet potatoes Glazed carrots
Grains	Most grain products	Grain products with added sugar[a]

Source: L. P. DiOrio, What should we eat? A dentist's perspective (address presented at the American Dental Association annual meeting, 11 October 1977).

[a]Note that granola bars are among the "bad guys" singled out by dentists. They are a grain food but so sticky that dentists consider them akin to candy bars. Similarly, dentists see fruit yogurt as the equivalent of ice cream.

in preparation for their future lives as adults. Social pressures thrust choices at them: to drink or not to drink, to develop their bodies to meet sometimes extreme ideals of slimness or athletic prowess. The next few sections highlight the factors that affect teenagers' health for good or for ill and the information that teenagers need in order to develop and maintain food habits conducive to good health throughout adulthood.

Growth and Nutrient Needs

The adolescent growth spurt begins in girls at 10 or 11 years of age and reaches its peak at 12, being completed at about 15. In boys, it begins at 12 or 13 years of age and peaks at 14, ending at about 19. This intensive growth period brings not only a dramatic increase in height but also hormonal changes that profoundly affect every organ of the body, including the brain, and culminate in the emergence of physically mature adults within two or three years. The same nutrition principles apply to this period as to the growth periods previously discussed.

During adolescence, the growth nutrients are needed in higher quantities than before. An added need for iron is caused by the onset of menstruation in girls and by the great increase in lean body mass in boys. These changes, which are taking place in nearly adult-size people, may make total nutrient needs higher at adolescence than at any other time in life. A rapidly growing, active boy of 15 may need 4,000 kcalories or more a day just to maintain his weight. At the same time, an inactive girl of the same age whose growth is nearly at a standstill may need fewer than 2,000 kcalories if she is to avoid becoming overweight. Thus, adolescents vary tremendously in their nutrient needs.

Teenagers also vary tremendously in the timing and patterns of their growth. No two are alike. A teenager who wants to know what he or she should weigh should be reassured that any of a wide range of weights is considered normal at this time in life. The weights given on the inside back cover can be modified for teenage girls of age 18 or 19. These can be considered weights at which to aim, but weights well above or below these are normal, too. Teenage boys can be told that when they have finished growing, they should expect to weigh what the adult charts show but that while they are growing, it is not unusual for their weights to be quite different from the standards. Growth charts in Appendix B show patterns of growth that are acceptable for teenagers, but patterns that differ widely from these may be normal, too.

Teenagers have some characteristic nutrition problems. Nearly every nutrient can be found lacking in one or another group: Iron in young women; kcalories in young men, especially in blacks; vitamin A in young women, especially in Mexican and Hispanic Americans; calcium, riboflavin, vitamin C, and even protein in many teenagers. The insidious problem of obesity becomes apparent, mostly in females, especially in blacks. Serious nutrient deficiencies often arise in pregnant teenagers.

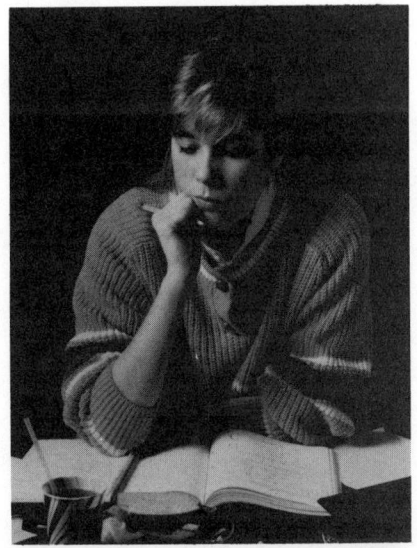

Teenagers' Food Choices

Teenagers come and go as they choose and eat what they want when they have time. With a multitude of after-school, social, and job activities, they almost inevitably fall into irregular eating habits. The adult becomes a gatekeeper, controlling the availability but not the consumption of food in the teenager's environment. The adult can't nag, scold, or pressure teenagers into eating as they should, because teens typically turn a deaf ear to coercion and often to persuasion. The gatekeeper must make every effort to allow these young people independence while providing an emotional climate that encourages adaptive choices.

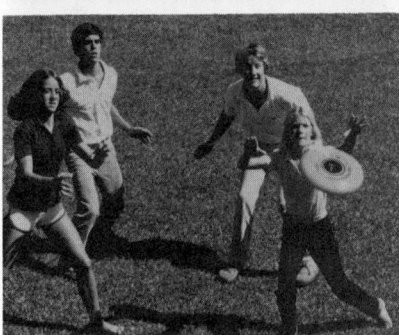

The kcalorie needs of teenagers vary widely depending on their activity level.

In the home, a wise maneuver is to provide access to nutritious and economical energy foods that are low in sugar and fat and discourage tooth decay. A well-established characteristic of teenagers is that they are snackers. The snacker who finds only nutritious foods around the house is well provided for.

Inevitably, teenagers will do a lot of eating away from home, where—as well as at home—their nutritional welfare can be favored or hindered by the choices they make. Nutrition in Practice 11 discusses some of the better choices teenagers can make when eating on the run. On the average, about a fourth of a teenager's total daily food energy intake comes from snacks. Irregular schedules may worry adults who think their teenagers are feeding themselves poorly, but usually the foods teens eat are quite nutritious. Teenagers receive substantial amounts of protein, thiamin, riboflavin, vitamin B_6, iron, magnesium, zinc, and even calcium if they snack on dairy products. Protein usually need not be stressed, but some teenagers should be encouraged to recognize and consume more dairy products for calcium and more good vitamin A and folacin sources.

Independence is especially valued during the teen years, and food selection is one way to express it. The choice of what to eat is up to teenagers themselves. Access points already mentioned include the kitchen, the school lunch, and vending machines. Other than controlling the contents of these, adults can expect to have little impact on the nutrient intakes of adolescents—especially by such conventional means as education. Still, most young adults in this country are well fed, for reasons perceptively stated long ago: They get hungry; they like to eat; they want energy, vigor, and the means to compete and excel in whatever they do; and they have many good habits, which are just as hard to break as the bad ones.

The parent or teacher concerned about a teenager's food habits should be aware of how teenagers feel about themselves. If you reflect upon your own past, you may recall vivid memories in this connection. Teenagers crave acceptance, especially from their peers. They need to fit in. In many cases, they are greatly dissatisfied with themselves. One of the most important aspects of their self-images is their body images. Young men want larger biceps, shoulders, chest, and forearms; young women want smaller hips, thighs, and waists. Young men often want to gain weight, even though they may not need to. Conversely, young women may want to lose weight, even if weight loss is not necessary.

Words to the effect that "you look fine as you are" fall on deaf ears. (The same can be said of adults in some cases, up to the age of about 99.) To be conveyed effectively, nutrition information can be sold as part of a package that will bring about these desired changes. Fortunately, it happens to be true that nutrient-dense, low-kcalorie foods favor the development of strong biceps in men and trim figures in women. (Additional nutrition information for the aspiring athlete appears in Nutrition in Practice 9.)

When the young person who is the target of your campaign possesses and cherishes nutrition misinformation, one of the first questions to ask is whether the practice is beneficial, neutral, or harmful. Opposing a loved ideal is more likely to polarize than to convert the opposition. A practice, such as vegetarianism, dieting, or consuming a "muscle-building diet," can be encouraged with modifications rather than condemned. Only the most hazardous nutrition practices should be singled out for attention; silence is an option that can be taken toward the others.

One of the most effective ways to teach nutrition is by example. The athletic coach and gym teacher, the friendly English teacher, the admired city recreation director—those who enthusiastically maintain their own health—can have a great impact on teenagers. Remember, this is the period of identity formation, the time of seeking and emulating models.

Health professionals communicating nutrition information need to be sure that they have the facts straight. Teachers of nutrition have little credibility when they admonish students to follow restrictive patterns when the students' choices are already as good as or better than their own. There may be no harm in using candy bars to meet part of the kcalorie allowance of an active young adult who is eating an otherwise nutritious diet. It may not be necessary for a teenager to drink milk if cheese and other foods are meeting his calcium, vitamin D, and riboflavin needs. Satisfactory diets can be designed on a great variety of foundations. It is the nutrient content and balance of foods, not the specific foods consumed, that make the differences among diets.

Among the best materials prepared to teach teenagers the importance of good nutrition are those made by teenagers themselves. Those who are interested and motivated can be guided to reliable sources and allowed to indulge their own desire to benefit their friends and classmates.

Finally, remember that teenagers have the right to make their own decisions, even if they are ones you disagree with. You can set up the environment so that the foods available are those you favor, and you can stand by with reliable nutrition information and advice, but you will have to leave the rest to them. Ultimately, they make the choices.

Nutrition Problems

The childhood and teen years are times when nutrition problems begin to arise. Foremost among those problems are those discussed in the following sections.

Obesity

Childhood obesity is a major nutrition problem that follows many children into adulthood. To avoid obesity, the preschool child should be trained to "eat thin." Mealtimes should be relaxed and leisurely. Children should learn to eat slowly, pause and enjoy their table companions, and stop eating when they are full. Instead of teaching children to clean their plates, parents should help children learn to satisfy their hunger and not to eat for other reasons, such as just because the food is in front of them. Parents who wish to avoid wasting food can learn to serve smaller portions or teach their children to serve themselves the actual amounts they want to eat. Physical activity should be encouraged on a daily basis to promote strong skeletal and muscular development and to establish habits that will undergird good health throughout life.

The child who has already become obese needs careful handling. Weight loss may easily have a harmful effect on growth. Those who work with obese children should feed the children so as to maintain a constant weight while they grow. The object is to restrict the accumulation of body fat while promoting normal lean body development. Thus, obese children can "grow out of" their obesity.

Iron-Deficiency Anemia

Of all nutrition disorders, other than obesity, found in U.S. children, the most common is iron-deficiency anemia. Iron status is most likely to be poor during four times of life: In infancy, during growth spurts, during the female reproductive years, and in pregnancy.

The diets of infants should be monitored to ensure an iron intake of 7 milligrams a day. Food intakes must be modified as infants grow so that they will receive 5.5 milligrams of iron or more per 1,000 kcalories. To achieve this goal, milk must not be overemphasized in the diet, because it is a poor iron source. Dairy products should be consumed only in the amounts needed to ensure adequate calcium and riboflavin intakes. For children over age 2, the use of nonfat or low-fat milk instead of whole milk leaves kcalories free for investment in such iron-rich foods as lean meats, fish, poultry, eggs, and legumes. Grain products should be whole-grain or enriched only. Candies, soft drinks, and bakery goods unfortified with iron should be discouraged.

Poor iron status in teenagers is a special problem caused by several factors. Two already mentioned are the teenagers' greatly increased needs and the lack of iron in traditional snack foods. Other factors are the overemphasis on dairy products by some teenagers, vegetarianism, and the minimal contribution made by fast foods to iron intakes. A National Academy of Sciences committee recommends that physicians and clinics screen all teenagers for low levels of iron in the blood. Their report stresses the fact that the best dietary source of absorbable iron is meats of all varieties, a point that should in turn be stressed in the nutrition education of teenagers.[3] No doubt teenagers should also learn to enjoy iron-rich plant foods, such as legumes and whole grains.

Food Allergies

Another nutrition problem encountered in children is food allergies. A true food allergy occurs when the body's immune system reacts to a food protein or other large molecule as it does to an antigen—by producing antibodies, histamines, or other defensive agents. This reaction occurs whenever an antigen penetrates the body's tissues far enough to encounter cells of the immune system, which can happen anywhere: in the skin, the lungs, or the GI tract.

The term *food allergy* has been much misused, and allergies have been wrongly blamed for many problems seen in children that in fact do not involve true immune-system-mediated reactions to food. Notable among the problems incorrectly attributed to allergy is the hyperactivity syndrome in children. In 1973, Dr. Benjamin Feingold proposed that this syndrome was caused by allergic reactions to certain foods or to the additives in them. Feingold suggested, in a book written for the public, that hyperactive children be placed on a diet of natural foods totally free of additives and claimed a great success rate with this diet.[4] By 1978, his theory was so well received that more than 20,000 children were on his diet.[5]

Since 1978, many careful, extensive studies of the Feingold hypothesis have discredited allergies to foods as a cause of behavioral problems in children except in rare cases. Some studies have shown, however, that hyperactive children do benefit from the attention and care they receive when their families work together to alter their lifestyles, as they must do when they make major changes in their eating habits. If there is a connection between a child's nutrition and his behavior, it may be because of malnutrition rather than allergies, a possibility explored in Nutrition in Practice 10.

The symptoms of a true allergic reaction to food include swelling and irritation, especially of the mouth, eyes, and mucous membranes; stomach pain; sometimes nausea or headaches; and general misery. Allergic reactions to foods can be immediate or delayed. In either case, the interaction of the antigen with the immune system is immediate, although symptoms may appear within minutes or take up to 24 hours to appear. Not all allergy researchers agree on the existence of delayed allergic reactions, because such reactions are hard to identify and assess. Immediate food allergy reactions are known not to occur in more than one percent of all individuals; delayed reactions have been reported to occur in from 0.3 percent to 25 percent or more of all individuals, reflecting the uncertainty that surrounds them.

---

allergy:
an immune reaction to a foreign substance, such as some component of food, in which antibodies are produced. An immune reaction involving only histamine production but not antibodies is termed *sensitivity* by some researchers; some prefer the term *hypersensitivity* instead of *allergy*. Allergies can be *symptomatic* or *asymptomatic*, but they always involve antibody protection. Symptoms without antibody production are *not* caused by allergy.

antibody:
a large protein produced in response to an antigen, which inactivates the antigen. An *antigen* is a molecule foreign or unfamiliar to the body.

histamine:
a substance produced by cells of the immune system in reaction to an antigen. Histamine participates in causing the redness and swelling known as *inflammation*.

hyperactivity syndrome:
in children, a cluster of symptoms including developmentally inappropriate inattention, impulsivity, and hyperactivity. Other important features are onset before age seven, duration of six months or more, and proven absence of mental illness or mental retardation. Other names associated with hyperactivity: *attention deficit disorder, hyperkinesis, minimal brain damage, minimal brain dysfunction, minor cerebral dysfunction.*

Testing for immediate allergic reactions can be attempted by any of about 14 different methods, including histories, diaries, challenges with the suspected food, skin tests, blood tests, and tests of other tissue samples. Performed correctly, many of these tests can lead to accurate diagnosis. The foods that most often cause immediate allergic reactions are listed in Table 11–3. About 90 percent of all allergic reactions are caused by nuts, eggs, milk, and soy. Reactions to multiple foods are the exception, not the rule.

The identification of delayed allergic reactions is difficult and time consuming. One way to obtain a valid diagnosis is to do a double-blind challenge study. In such a study, the suspected food or foods are eliminated from the diet until all symptoms have subsided. Then coded capsules are given containing either the suspected food in concentrated, dehydrated form or a fake substitute, and records of reactions are kept. Parents are often surprised to see that about half the time or more their children do *not* react to the suspected foods under these conditions.

Another means of testing for food allergies is to initiate an elimination diet: First feed a restricted diet, then introduce groups of suspected foods until symptoms appear. Removal of the guilty foods correlates consistently with relief—and reintroduction with reappearance—of symptoms. A suspected group of foods can be split into subgroups for further testing until the individual offending foods have been identified.

Dental Caries

Poor dental health is a preventable condition. The measures recommended for its prevention center around two objectives. First, adequate nutrition is needed to help the mouth and teeth develop properly. This means providing an adequate diet, especially in terms of protein; calcium; vitamins A, C, and D; and fluoride. Where local water supplies are not fluoridated, fluoride supplements and direct application of fluoride to the teeth at intervals may be necessary. Second, it is important to restrict the supply of carbohydrate foods to the bacteria that causes tooth decay. This means brushing the teeth or rinsing the mouth after meals, especially after meals high in carbohydrate; avoiding snacks that contain sticky carbohydrate (see Table 11–2); and dislodging persistent particles with dental floss or other devices. Regular dental checkups can be invaluable in preventing serious problems with dental caries.

Alcohol, Drugs, and Smoking

The teen years bring exposure to factors not encountered before. Some complicate the nutrition picture: use and abuse of alcohol, use and abuse of drugs, use of caffeine, use of oral contraceptives, and many more. Alcohol is by far the most widely used of all drugs in the United States.

The nutrition implications of alcohol use and the consequences of its abuse are described in Nutrition in Practice 6. To sum them all up, alcohol is an empty-kcalorie beverage that can displace needed nutrients from the diet while simultaneously altering absorption and metabolism of nutrients. Thus, even if nutrient intake is adequate, imbalances result from altered nutrient absorption and

TABLE 11–3. Foods That Most Often Cause Immediate Hypersensitivity Reactions (Type I Allergy)

Nuts	Peanuts
Eggs	Chicken
Milk	Fish
Soybeans	Shellfish
Wheat	Mollusks

Source: F. M. Atkins, The basis of immediate hypersensitivity reactions to foods, *Nutrition Reviews* 41 (1983): 229–234.

marijuana: alternative spelling, *marihuana*.

metabolism. Those who are unable to use alcohol with moderation must abstain completely from its use if they are to maintain good health.

As for the nutrition implications of drugs, smoking marijuana has characteristic effects on taste and smell. Among the taste changes apparently induced is an increase in appetite ("the munchies"), especially for sweets, but it is not known how this effect occurs. Prolonged use of the drug does not seem to bring about a weight gain, however. Despite much current research, little is known about the possible nutritional risks of regular marijuana smoking.

When marijuana use escalates into the use of other drugs, however, the nutrition and health effects become pronounced. Among the drugs in most common use today are heroin, morphine, LSD, amphetamines, PCP, and cocaine. Users of these drugs face multiple nutrition problems:

- They spend their money for drugs rather than for food.
- They lose interest in food during "high" periods.
- Their lifestyle lacks the regularity and routine that would promote good eating habits.
- They often have hepatitis, a liver disease that they are likely to contract by using contaminated needles. Hepatitis causes taste changes and loss of appetite.
- They often depend on alcohol, especially when withdrawing from drug use.
- They often become ill with infectious diseases that increase their needs for nutrients.

One of the most important aspects of treatment is to identify and correct these nutrition problems while teaching and supporting adaptive eating habits in addicts who are withdrawing from drugs.

Chronic Diseases

Many experts seem to agree that early childhood is the time to begin taking measures to prevent cardiovascular disease. Parents can steer children away from high-fat, high-sugar, and high-salt foods; support their children in forming habits that will help keep them free of atherosclerosis and hypertension; and emphasize foods with high nutrient density. These suggestions might also help to prevent or retard the onset of diabetes in children who have a genetic tendency toward it. Similarly, those who have been studying the effects of nutrition on cancer have suggested that children over the age of two who have positive family histories of cancer may benefit by following a prudent diet. The prudent diet was originally developed to prevent heart disease, but its outlines are the same as those recommended by nutritionists interested in the prevention of cancer.

The prudent diet is described in Chapter 21.

Special emphasis on wise eating habits is particularly important for a child with a family history of chronic disease. Thus, the child of a parent with high blood pressure should be raised on a diet relatively low in salt; the child of a diabetic parent should avoid sugar and be encouraged to eat foods high in complex carbohydrate; and the child of a parent with coronary artery disease should eat foods low in fat—especially saturated fat—and possibly cholesterol. In all these situations, the greatest success is likely to be achieved if the whole family, and not just the child, follows the recommended dietary guidelines.

Teenage Pregnancy

A special case is that of the pregnant teenage girl. Even if she were not pregnant, she would be hard put to meet her own nutrient needs at this time of maximal growth. Nourishing the baby doubles her burden. For a girl who begins pregnancy with inadequate nutrient stores or who lacks the education, resources, and support she needs, these problems are compounded.

The complications of pregnancy are discussed in Chapter 10, where it is shown that the consequences of poor nutrition are acute and long lasting. Sickness is common in pregnant teenagers, with pregnancy-induced hypertension occurring in about one of every five girls under the age of 15. One pregnancy following another can precipitate irreversible kidney damage and hypertensive heart disease.

Teenage pregnancy has become common. Faced with her parents' and classmates' often insensitive reactions, a pregnant teenager is likely to wind up alone, with little or no money to buy food and with no motivation to seek prenatal care. She urgently needs programs, including medical attention, nutritional guidance, emotional support, and continued schooling, that address all her problems. A model program for helping teenage and other mothers is the Women's, Infants', and Children's (WIC) program, a federally funded program that provides nutrition information and nutritious foods to low-income pregnant women and their children. This program has produced measurable improvements in maternal and infant health.

The nutrition advisor consulting with a pregnant girl should make special efforts to evaluate the girl's nutrition status and eating habits and counsel her appropriately. Is she gaining weight as she should? (See Chapter 10 and Appendix B.) Even if she is obese to begin with, she should gain weight. Is she eating enough foods and choosing them intelligently so as to support her own and her infant's growth? The pregnant teenager needs

- Four to five cups of milk or the equivalent.
- Two or more servings of protein-rich food each day.
- Five, six, or more servings of breads and cereals, preferably whole-grain.
- Four or more servings of fruits and vegetables, at least one each rich in vitamins A and C.

If her nutrient intake is less than desirable, it is important to make sure she is taking a prenatal multivitamin-mineral supplement supplying RDA levels, not megadoses, of the nutrients and preferably prescribed by a physician. Remember, such a supplement cannot supply enough protein, calcium, or fiber to meet recommendations.

Among concrete items of advice acceptable to the teenager are these:

- Eat at least one serving every day of a vitamin C-rich food.
- Restrict soft drinks to one each day.
- Try a breakfast shake made with milk, egg, and fruit.

A model program for giving nutrition help to teenage mothers, among others, is the WIC (Women's, Infants' and Children's) program, a federally funded program that provides nutrition information and low-cost nutritious foods to low-income pregnant women and their children.

Nearly 10 percent of teenage girls become pregnant each year—that's nearly one million teenage pregnancies annually.

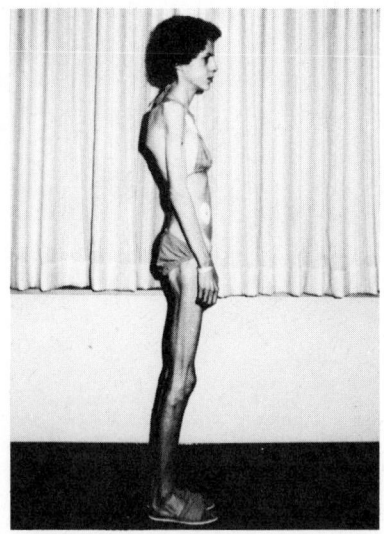

Anorexia nervosa

Right now I weigh 58 lbs., which isn't too bad for 5'2", though I want to lose a few more pounds—my hips are still fat. Lately I've got it down to no breakfast, a can of mushrooms for lunch, and a can of wax beans for dinner with lots of iced tea. I reward myself with a big, green apple at the end of the day, if I've stuck to The Plan.

A. Ciseaux

anorexia nervosa:
literally, "nervous lack of appetite," a disorder (usually seen in teenage girls) involving self-starvation to the extreme.

Eating Disorders

Attitudes about personal appearances dictate many of the behaviors of adolescents. The adolescent's physical appearance is changing, and sensitivity to peer opinions and media impressions is heightened. Attitudes are forming, and behaviors are being established.

To teenagers, growing means getting taller and heavier. For some female teenagers, this is not a welcome occurrence. Such girls do not want to grow bigger, and they become dissatisfied with their appearance. Thinness has become the sociocultural ideal. Most teenage girls are "on diets" and are terrified of being fat.[6] Such an attitude can lead to weight goals that are not always healthy or obtainable for most teenagers.

Attitudes about body weight and physical appearance have profound effects on a person's self-image. Distorted attitudes and self-perceptions can lead to such eating disorders as anorexia nervosa and bulimia.

Anorexia Nervosa

Anorexia nervosa is an extreme preoccupation with weight loss that seriously endangers the health and even the life of the dieter. It arises only in developed countries where food is abundant, suggesting that it is a societal problem. Although no two persons with anorexia nervosa are alike, certain features are considered typical of the condition. The anorexic is almost always female and in her midteens. She is usually from an educated, middle-class, success-oriented, weight-conscious family that is proud of her and is surprised to see her develop a problem. She strives to achieve and chooses weight loss as one means of becoming successful. Being highly competitive and perfectionistic, she carries the weight-loss effort to an extreme: She will have the slimmest, most perfect body of anyone in her high-school class.

So far this description probably fits many young women you know; but unlike most of them, this girl develops anorexia nervosa. When she has lost weight to well below the average for her height and is no longer slim but too slim, she still doesn't stop. Weight loss has become an obsession. She is afraid of losing control, and she allows her self-imposed starvation regimen to rule her life.

At this point, starvation has begun to affect her physiology, thinking patterns, and personality, and physical symptoms are emerging. Although they are the symptoms of starvation, the girl sees them as desirable and prides herself on holding out against her extreme hunger. When the anorexic has reached an absolute minimum body weight, 65 to 70 pounds for a woman of average height, she is on the verge of incurring permanent brain damage and chronic invalidism or death.

A typical psychological profile of a female with anorexia includes depression, early developmental failure, and family dysfunction. She strives for perfection, finds fat disgusting and thin admirable, and believes gaining weight means being out of control. For a teenager in a growth phase, gaining weight is normal. Thus, part of recovery for the teenager with anorexia is an understanding of growth and its relationship to food.

Before 1950, the condition was very rare, one in 2,000, and only one out of four such girls could be expected to recover. Since that time, the incidence has been increasing while the success rate in treatment has steadily improved. Still, of every five anorexics, one dies.

The specific causes of anorexia are difficult to define, because they are often interwoven and the symptoms show themselves in a variety of physical and psychological ways. Treatment must artfully combine medical and dietary intervention to initiate and sustain weight gain with psychological techniques to resolve personal and family problems.

Bulimia

A distinct eating disorder that shares some characteristics with anorexia is bulimia. Bulimia is characterized by periodic binge eating alternating with intervals of dieting or self-starvation. Bulimia usually starts with a diet and may accompany anorexia or may occur separately. Bulimia was officially recognized only in 1980, although it had existed long before that. The binge ends when it would hurt to eat any more or when the person goes to sleep, induces vomiting, or is interrupted.

Since 1980, bulimia has attracted much media attention, especially the variety in which the person binges and then vomits, takes laxatives, or takes diuretics to undo the "damage." Most bulimics are within 10 pounds of their ideal weight. Although binge eating is seldom life threatening, at the extreme it can be physically damaging, causing lacerations of the stomach, irritation of the esophagus, electrolyte imbalances in those who vomit frequently, and malnutrition in those who vomit and take laxatives. It is highly desirable that binge eaters should learn to see food and themselves in a more positive light and should come to accept a realistic weight goal for themselves. An effective measure in the treatment of bulimia is psychological counseling to teach subjects to eat well and not to restrict kcalories too severely.[7]

Anorexia and bulimia often arise in young people, but the problems don't always resolve in adolescence. People with anorexia and bulimia may retain abnormal eating behaviors and fearful attitudes toward food throughout their adult lives.

bulimia, bulimarexia:
binge eating (literally, eating like an ox). Known popularly as "pigging out" or "blind munchies." When followed by self-induced vomiting or the taking of laxatives, this form of eating behavior has been called the *binge-purge syndrome.*
buli = ox
orex = mouth

Diuretics are drugs that promote the loss of water and some minerals from the body. Because water is lost, the person taking diuretics may temporarily lose weight.

CASE STUDY:

Girl with Anorexia Nervosa and Bulimia

Sally is an energetic 14-year-old who seems to be involved in everything from the French club to gymnastics. At five feet two inches tall, she weighs 90 pounds and looks slim. During Sally's last physical examination, her mother expressed concern over Sally's diet: "Lately, she barely eats at all and she has been losing too much weight." Sally shrugs off her mother's comments and says, "I don't know why you say that, Mom. Look how fat I am." When Sally's mother is alone with the doctor, she discusses some other concerns. She states that on occasion, when Sally is home alone, she returns to find many foods missing. At first, Sally's mother thought nothing of it, but as it happened more frequently, she became worried. She also thought she heard her daughter vomiting several times, but Sally always said that she was fine.

1. What factors in Sally's history suggest that she may be a victim of anorexia nervosa or bulimia? What are the dangers of anorexia nervosa? What are the dangers of bulimia?

2. If Sally is found to be anorexic and/or bulimic, what steps will be important in her treatment?

Notes

1. *Nutrition News,* February 1987.
2. Much of the discussion about child and teen is derived from Chapters 5 and 6 in *Maternal and Child Nutrition,* by (St. Paul, Minn.: West, 1988).
3. Committee on Nutrition of the Mother and Preschool Child, Food and Nutrition Board, National Academy of Sciences, *Iron Nutriture in Adolescence,* DHEW publication no. (HSA) 5100 (Washington, D.C.: Government Printing Office, 1977).
4. B. F. Feingold, *Why Your Child Is Hyperactive* (New York: Random House, 1975).
5. M. Morrison, The Feingold diet (letter to the editor), *Science* 199 (1978): 840.
6. N. S. Moses, M. Banilivy, and F. Liftshitzy, Fear of obesity among adolescent females (abstract), *American Journal of Clinical Nutrition* 43 (1986): 664.
7. S. Dalvit-McPhillips, A dietary approach to bulimia treatment, *Physiology and Behavior* 33 (1984): 769–775.

11

The Best Choices for Fast Food

Fast-food establishments are so popular that there is usually one just around every corner. They are frequented by every age group and have started to become the mainstay of many people's diets, but the meals are often low in or devoid of fruits, vegetables, complex carbohydrates, and milk. Any diet that excludes even one of the food groups can easily cause deficiencies of many of the more than 40 vitamins and minerals needed. The answers to the following questions can help you make wise decisions about food choices in fast-food establishments.

I really like fast foods but am wondering, how nutritious are they?
Fast foods are really tempting and not just because they are convenient. The flavors and types of foods appeal to many people. Part of their appeal comes from high salt and fat contents, two ingredients that make foods smell and taste delicious.

Salt is one of the cheapest ingredients that processors can add to foods to enhance flavor. Frying foods in fat adds flavor and crispiness that many people enjoy. In fact, population surveys show that we enjoy these foods a little too much. If you remember back to the dietary guidelines given in Chapter 1, you know that reducing fat and sodium are both important goals.

Salt and fat are associated with high blood pressure; fat is associated with obesity, cardiovascular disease, cancer, and other conditions. That is the negative side of salt and fat, but remember that salt and fat also contribute necessary nutrients to the diet, although not in the quantities in which they are found in the average diet. Since other nutrients found in fast foods include protein, carbohydrate, and some vitamins and minerals, fast foods can be a part of a healthy diet. The key is what fast foods one is eating and how often one is eating them.

An underweight person eating one meal a week that consists of a hamburger, a shake, and french fries is getting needed kcalories. Table NP11–1 shows the nutrients in this meal. Depending upon the food choices for the other two meals, this type of meal occasionally is acceptable. The next meal that is eaten can make up for the

TABLE NP11–1. Nutrients in a Hamburger, Chocolate Shake and Fries

Nutrient	% of RDA[a]
Protein	45
Calcium	48
Iron	21
Zinc	25
Vitamin A	13
Thiamin	33
Riboflavin	38
Niacin	36
Folacin	15
Vitamin C	28

[a]RDA for an 18-year-old young man, except for iron, where the RDA for a young woman is used.

lack of fiber, vitamins, and minerals by including extra whole grains, fruits, and vegetables.

Let's consider a different scenario. Joe is slightly overweight and eats most of his meals at one of his two favorite fast-food places. He almost always orders a double hamburger, large fries, and a large soft drink. This is definitely not a nutritious diet. It is too high in kcalories, especially for an overweight person. Fat, salt, and protein are also too high; and vitamins, minerals, and complex carbohydrates are low.

In previous chapters we have seen what vitamin and mineral deficiencies can do to a person's body. A steady diet of hamburgers, fries, and soft drinks could lead to scurvy from a lack of vitamin C, eye problems from a deficiency of vitamin A, rickets in children from a deficiency of vitamin D and calcium, and skin disorders from a lack of the B vitamins, to name but a few. In the remaining chapters in this book, you will see yet more reasons to have a balanced diet. Many of the diseases discussed there may be forestalled by good nutrition throughout life.

How about if I just keep a close tab on the kcalories I eat and get the vitamins and minerals I need from a supplement?
A supplement can be made that has all the known vitamins and minerals in it, but our bodies still require specific trace elements. These elements are needed in such small quantities that some of the necessary elements have

not even been identified. A person on a diet of hamburgers and supplements could still be lacking some valuable nutrients including fiber. The nutrients in foods enhance the absorption of other nutrients. When a diet is very restrictive, even some of the nutrients present in it might be so poorly absorbed that deficiencies would occur.

That does remind me of many of the things I have learned about needing a balanced diet, but fast foods are so convenient. Do you have any suggestions for eating a balanced diet at fast-food places?

When fast foods are a major part of your diet, it is important to choose them wisely. Asian fast-food restaurants often include vegetables with their main dishes. Instead of choosing sweet and sour breaded chicken, try chicken stir-fried with several vegetables and a side dish of rice. At Mexican fast-food places, a bean burrito with cheese is a better choice than fried tortillas. When it's a hamburger you are craving, a salad and milk can make it a complete meal.

To improve a fast-food diet, you may need to start ordering milk in place of soft drinks, depending upon how often you eat out. A shake can add some calcium to your diet but at a great kcaloric expense that few people can afford. Even processed cheeses that are usually used for cheeseburgers are much less nutrient dense than milk. Side dishes that are a better nutritional choice than french fries are a baked potato, beans, rice, coleslaw, or a roll.

The method used in preparing foods can make a big difference in the nutrient contributions of those foods to your diet. Although many fast foods are fried, they are not all equal in fat content. For instance, chicken that is fried in an open fryer using animal fat is higher in cholesterol, saturated fat, and total fat than chicken pressure-fried in vegetable oil.[1] Whole pieces of white meat are usually lower in fat than chicken nuggets that contain more breading and fried surface in proportion to meat. Some fast-food outlets have baked or broiled chicken breasts that are lower in fat than fried chicken. A roll usually has less fat than a biscuit, and an even better choice is a whole-grain bun that is offered at a few national chains.

Be aware of what you load on that hamburger, chicken sandwich, or baked potato. In place of catsup and mayonnaise, choose lettuce, tomato, and raw onion. An alternative to sour cream and butter for a baked potato is broccoli and cheese.

I can really use those suggestions, but what about the times when I have to eat food from a vending machine?

Even when your lunch is from a vending machine, you have more and less nutritious choices.[2] A few ideas:

- Choose cracker sandwiches in place of chips or fried snacks.
- Choose peanuts, pretzels, and popcorn over cookies.
- Choose milk and juices over soft drinks.

- Choose fresh fruit and yogurt over candy.
- Choose sandwiches or soups when they are offered.

When we think of fast foods, the vending machine or the hamburger stand down the street is what usually comes to mind, but your own kitchen can produce fast foods that are good choices nutritionally. Prepare ahead for busy times by freezing whole-wheat sandwiches so that they are available at a moment's notice. Have the butcher thinly slice turkey breast to have on hand. Add tomatoes, lettuce, cheese, and sprouts to the sliced turkey for a gourmet sandwich.

Keep a stock of oranges, apples, bananas and vegetables that can be eaten raw as fast foods to reach for when you get hungry. Crackers and cheese, yogurt with fresh fruit, and oatmeal and peanut butter bars are a few foods that can be packed for meals away from home. When eating on the run, you can make yourself feel a lot better by giving a little thought to nutrition.

Notes

1. J. A. Bowers and coauthors, Vitamin and proximate composition of fast-food fried chicken, *Journal of the American Dietetic Association* 6 (1987): 736–739.
2. Tips about vending machine foods are derived from Chapter 5, Nutrition, in *Life Choices: Health Concepts and Strategies,* by F. S. Sizer and E. N. Whitney (St. Paul, Minn.: West, 1988).

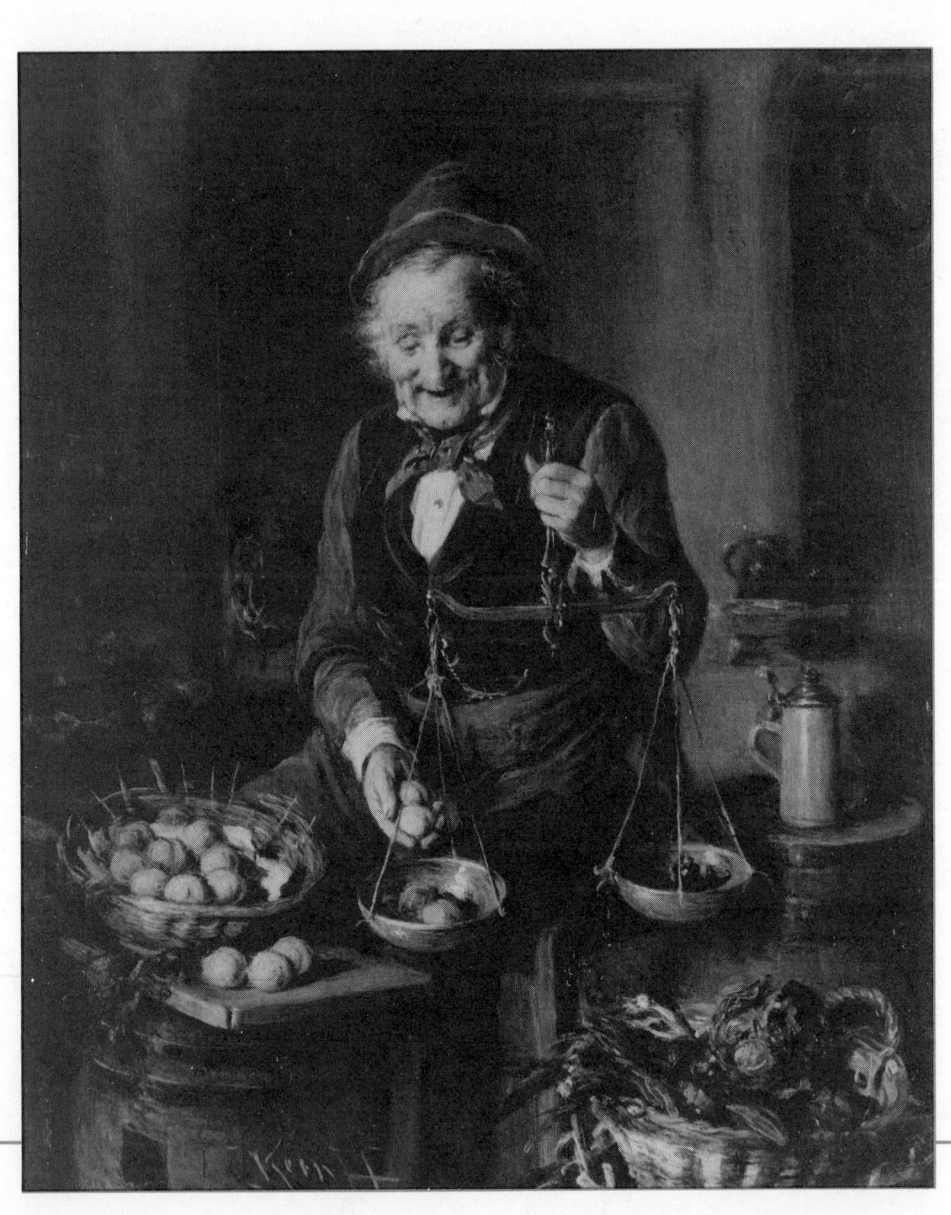

12

Adulthood and the Later Years

CONTENTS

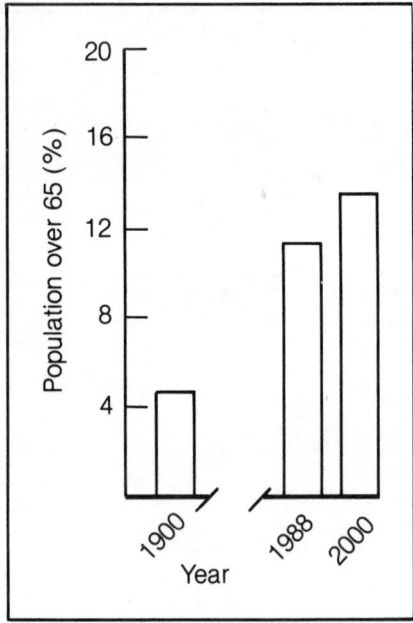

FIGURE 12–1

The aging of the population. (In 1900, 4 percent of the U.S. population was over 65; 11 percent is over 65 today; 12.5 percent (30,500,000 people) will be over 65 in the year 2000.

Chapter 16 gives more information about diverticulosis.

The bulk of the U.S. population may not be old yet, but it is aging. The ratio of old people to young grows steadily larger (see Figure 12–1). In fact, the fastest growing age group in the U.S. is people over 65. This fact is evident everywhere. Retirement villages are springing up, especially in the warmer climates. Senior citizen centers are being established for congregate meals and leisure activities. Older adults can be heard on political matters at "silver-haired legislatures."

The later years aren't characterized by physical growth, but changes take place in the adult mind and body. Even though it is true that some of these changes are degenerative, we also find that some of the world's greatest works are accomplished by people in their 70s and 80s.

Older people are an incredibly diverse group, and for the most part they are self-sufficient, socially sophisticated, mentally lucid, fully participating members of society who report themselves to be happy and healthy. About 60 percent of the elderly are women, and only 5 percent live in nursing homes.[1] Most live in the community, either alone or with nonrelatives, and thus remain independent. As we will see, this very independence can sometimes foster nutrition problems that the health care professional should be aware of. Two-thirds of the elderly are relatively free of major problems. The one-third who live at or below the poverty line deserve our attention. Clearly, these people need help in many areas, one of them being nutrition.

Effects of Aging on Nutrition

The unique nutrient needs of older people are influenced by the changes in organ function that often occur with aging. Some of the most significant changes occur in the digestive system. One such change is painful deterioration of the gums and subsequent loss of teeth. Peridontal disease may affect as many as 9 out of every 10 people by age 65. The senses of taste and smell may also be altered, reducing the pleasure of eating. The stomach's secretion of hydrochloric acid and enzymes decreases, as do the secretions of digestive juices by the pancreas and small intestine. Muscles of the GI tract weaken with reduced use so that pressure in the large intestine may cause the outpocketings of diverticulosis. Food moves slowly through the GI tract, and constipation becomes a problem.

The heart and blood vessels also age, becoming weaker and, in the case of the arteries, less flexible. Since all organs and tissues depend on the circulation of nutrients and oxygen, degenerative changes in the cardiovascular system critically affect all other systems. Reduced blood flow through the kidneys makes the kidneys gradually less efficient at removing wastes and maintaining the blood's normal composition. As the heart pumps blood less forcefully, the capillary networks in the kidneys deteriorate, and some kidney cells die. This degenerative process can be retarded by regular exercising, which ensures that an ample volume of blood is pumped into the kidneys, keeping the capillaries open.

Visual impairment that occurs with aging can make it difficult for the older person to shop for and prepare foods. Hearing loss is also common. Poor vision and hearing can lead to depression and thus interfere with the desire to eat.

As the metabolic rate slows with age, the older person may not have the same strength and energy he had when he was younger. Purchasing and preparing foods may become a difficult task. In his mind, these tasks may not be worth the effort they require, another reason for poor food intake.

Chronic diseases become increasingly common in later life, and older people often have to take prescription drugs over long periods of time. Although the elderly comprise 12 percent of our population, they consume about 30 percent of all over-the-counter and prescription drugs.[2] Drugs—from aspirin and laxatives to prescription drugs of all types—interact with nutrients in several ways, usually resulting in higher needs for specific nutrients. Older people are especially vulnerable to the negative physical impacts of these drugs. And like the effects of illnesses, the effects of drugs are cumulative over time. The risk of drug-related malnutrition increases both with the number of drugs the individual takes and with the length of time over which the drugs are used.

Since the aged are at a time in life when friends and family may be chronically ill or have died, their own mortality takes on an immediate presence, and the desire for a longer life becomes an urgent quest. What can we do to avoid growing old? Is there a magic potion we can drink, a food we can eat, a pill we can swallow? Or, on a more down-to-earth level, are there any lifestyle habits we can adopt to prolong our youth?

As far as potions, foods, and pills go, the answer seems to be no. However, the claims of quacks give false hope to many intelligent people by leading them to believe that a specific product will help them live longer.

A recent product promoted to prevent aging is superoxide dismutase (SOD). Superoxide dismutase is an enzyme that occurs naturally in the cells of animals, including humans. It acts as an antioxidant, as do vitamin C, vitamin E, and a selenium-containing enzyme. Animal species that live the longest, such as human beings, have the highest concentrations of SOD in their tissues, and it has been hoped that the concentration of this enzyme in the human body could be raised and would prolong life.

It does not work.[3] Like any other enzyme taken orally, SOD is digested in the stomach and intestine to fragments that the body uses to make its own proteins. If it were injected, it would still be external to cells and could cause irritation and allergic reactions but not longer life. The trick would be to induce the cells to make more of it themselves (genetic engineering), but who is to say that the higher levels would have a beneficial effect? The body tends to make the right amount of what it needs, as this book has shown in countless examples. More SOD would probably not be better. Still, many health-food stores and other establishments are doing a brisk business selling it.

Good health habits, including good nutrition throughout life, are the best guarantee of healthy and enjoyable later years. Some of the degenerative changes associated with aging can be retarded by maintaining a strong cardiovascular

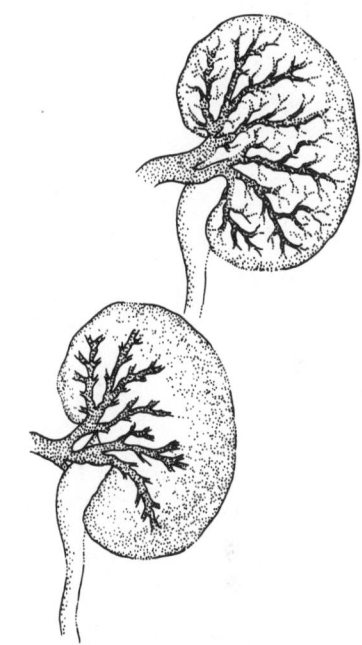

As the heart pumps less blood into an organ, the capillary trees within that organ recede, leaving some of the cells without nourishment. Exercise promotes maintenance and even growth of capillaries.

superoxide dismutase (SOD): an antioxidant enzyme. Purified from animal tissues and sold in powder form, it is one of many fraudulent antiaging products on the market.

and respiratory system. Exercise, regular and active enough to increase heart-beat and respiration rate, is one of the keys to good health in later years.

Nutrition, Aging, and Disease

Some diseases are much more responsive to nutrition than others. Some, such as the vitamin-deficiency diseases, can be entirely prevented by good nutrition. Others are hereditary, and no amount or combination of nutrients has any effect on them at all, even over many years. A compelling question of great interest to nutritionists studying aging today is, To what extent are the so-called diseases of old age the result of undetected nutrient deficiencies, excesses, or imbalances?

We have already discussed some of the better known relationships between foods or nutrients and diseases. One example is the connection between sugar and dental disease. Others to be taken up in the chapters to come are the relationships between sodium, potassium, calcium, and high blood pressure; between dietary fat, atherosclerosis, and cancer; and between fiber and diseases of the GI tract, such as constipation, diverticulosis, and possibly colon cancer. Here, it seems appropriate to devote a few paragraphs to three diseases of aging: arthritis, adult bone loss, and brain disease.

Hardly a food item exists that has not been promoted as a cure for arthritis at one time or another. The only conclusive relationship research has shown between nutrition and arthritis is that weight loss of the obese person relieves pressure on the weight-bearing joints.[4] A list of quack remedies and fraudulent diet "cures" for arthritis appears in the margin. Actually, no known diet prevents, relieves, or cures arthritis, but as long as the public keeps buying books that make these claims, such books will keep being published.

Researchers have found that the diets of people with arthritis are marginal with respect to several nutrients—especially vitamin E and zinc. These two nutrients, among others, are important for normal function of the body's immune system, and an abnormal response may contribute to arthritis. It seems advisable to obtain an adequate, balanced diet.[5]

One nutrient link that may prove significant in the future is EPA, the fatty acid found in fish oil. Chapter 3 discussed EPA in relation to heart health, and research is beginning to show that the same diet recommended for the heart—a diet low in saturated fat from red meats and dairy products and high in the fish oil EPA—might have potential to reduce the suffering of people with arthritis. Researchers theorize that EPA could interfere with the action of prostaglandins involved in the inflammatory response that causes pain in arthritis.[6]

Adult bone loss is another major disease of the elderly. After 40, bone loss becomes more rapid than bone building. Bone loss occurs in both sexes, although severe bone loss is more prevalent in women than in men after 50. No one knows for sure what the causes are, but the result is osteoporosis—thinning and weakening of the bones so severe as to produce fractures in many older people. By the time a person realizes there has been bone loss, the damage has already been done.

Not effective against arthritis:
  Watercress
  Burdock root
  Vitamin D
  Celery juice
  Calcium
  Megadoses of vitamins
  Fasting
  Fresh fruit
  Honey
  Lecithin
  Yeast
  Kelp
  Raw liver
  Fish liver oil
  Alfalfa tea
  Aloe vera liquid
  Superoxide dismutase (SOD)

FIGURE 12–2

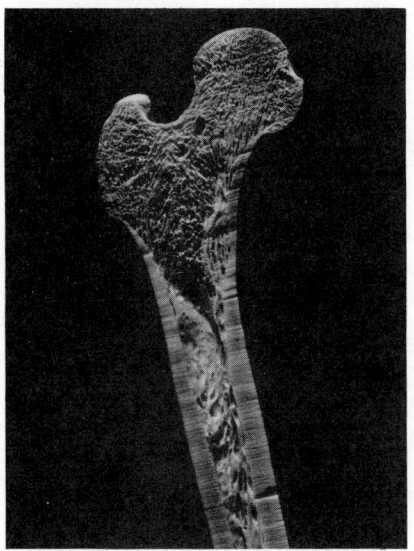

A. Cross section of bone. The lacy rural elements are **trabeculae** (tra-BECK-you-lee), which can be drawn on to furnish blood calcium.

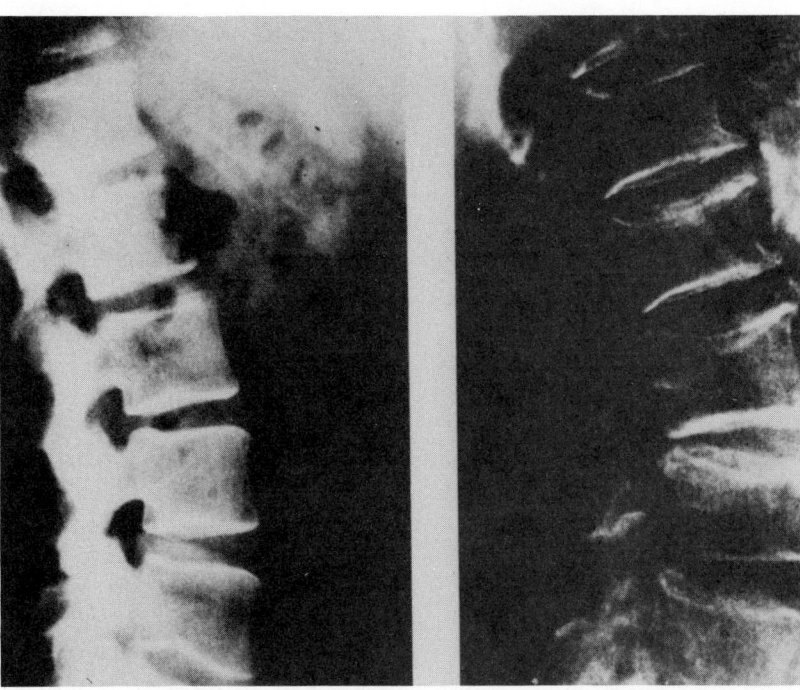

B. A healthy spine and one that has deteriorated from adult bone loss (osteoporosis). Notice how the vertebrae are crumbling.

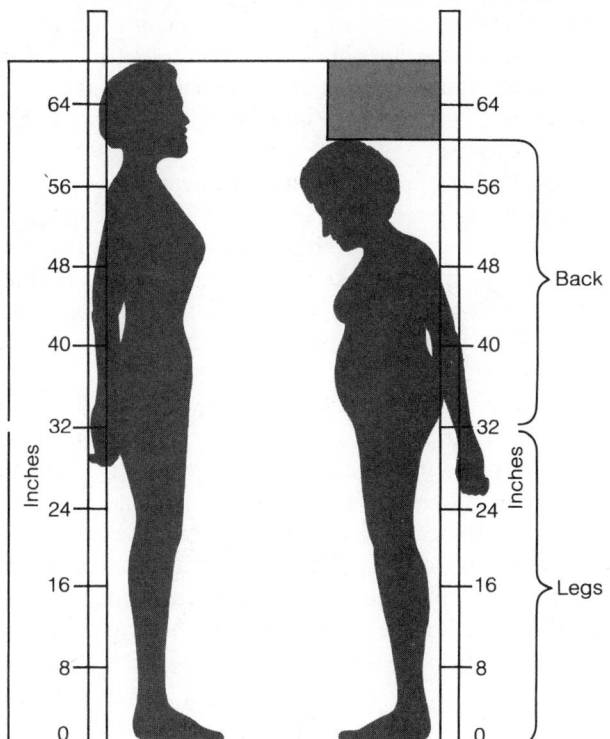

C. Normal and osteoporotic bone.
Effects of osteoporosis on a woman's height. On the left is a women at menopause and on the right, the same woman 30 years later. Notice that collapse of her vertebrae has shortened her back; the length of her legs has not changed.

Among the factors suspected of causing or contributing to osteoporosis are these:

- Too low an intake, reduced absorption, or increased excretion of calcium.
- Hormonal changes.
- Reduced physical activity.

The person who wants to prevent or delay the process of bone loss should be aware of all these factors.

A too-low calcium intake is, of course, any intake that does not completely compensate for total calcium losses. For most men, the minimum intake to ensure calcium balance appears to be above 400 milligrams; and for women after menopause, calcium intake should be much higher. By 1980, in the light of several research findings confirming the high calcium need of older women, many authorities were recommending that women maintain a daily intake of 1 to 1 ½ grams of calcium, the amount available from five cups of milk a day. Nutrition in Practice 12 offers suggestions for incorporating milk in the diet.

The second factor named in contributing to osteoporosis is hormonal changes. Estrogen and other hormones are implicated in bone loss, and knowledge now being gathered may lead some day to effective therapy for osteoporosis. Women should consider estrogen therapy at menopause, and possibly even before, so as to catch the early, accelerated loss of calcium from bone that begins at menopause. No matter how high a woman's calcium intake, it cannot override the influence of estrogen lack that accelerates bone loss.

The third factor, physical exercise, deserves strong emphasis. Bones lose material at a dramatic rate when they are inactive or immobilized. No matter how many glasses of milk a woman drinks in a day, the calcium will not be maximally deposited in bone unless she *works* her bones. Bones are like muscles; it takes regular exercise to make them strong and keep them that way. Accumulating evidence indicates that bone loss can indeed be slowed, prevented, or even reversed by physical exercise.

Perhaps the factors that promote or prevent the development of osteoporosis can be traced back to the growing years at the beginning of life. The higher the density of the bones at maturity, the more bone can be lost before osteoporosis becomes debilitating. Adequate intake of both calcium and fluoride throughout life doubtless protect against osteoporosis. The condition is not usually seen in a person who has had a consistently high calcium intake. Heredity also plays some part.

No one of middle age or over can, however, revisit her childhood, obtain the calcium and other nutrients she needs to build bone, and exercise them into place. It is important for the younger person to plan positively to obtain the needed nutrients and schedule physical workouts as part of a regular routine.

Another disorder associated with aging is brain disease. Brain disease actually involves many processes, some of which may be the result of gradual, insidious nutrient deficits. Among the nutrients implicated have been vitamins C, B_6, and B_{12}, riboflavin, thiamin, niacin, and the mineral copper. Among the effects have been inability to think clearly and poor memory as well as structural alterations in brain cells.[7]

The many factors affecting the body's handling of calcium are discussed in Chapter 8.

Other degenerative changes seen in aging may also be nutrition related. After all, while a day or so of inadequate nutrient intake may have only a passing, negligible effect on the body, the accumulation of repeated small insults over years and decades must have a major impact. By the time you are 65, you will have eaten about 100,000 pounds of food. If you haven't chosen well, the price of neglect will begin to show.

Nutrition Implications of Aging

Many of the nutrient needs of the elderly are the same as for younger persons, but some special needs deserve emphasis. As you read the following discussions about particular elements of the diet, remember that older adults who over-emphasize one food group to the exclusion of others are most at risk nutritionally. The best dietary guideline is to eat a balanced and varied selection of foods.

Energy and Energy Nutrients

Energy needs decrease with advancing age. For one thing, the number of active cells in each organ decreases, bringing about a reduction in the body's overall metabolic rate. For another, older people become less and less active physically, although they need not be. In 1980, the RDA tables presented recommended energy intakes for older people for the first time. These recommendations reflect an estimated reduction of about five percent per decade in energy output. Average figures for people 75 and older are 2,050 kcalories per day for the man and 1,600 for the woman.

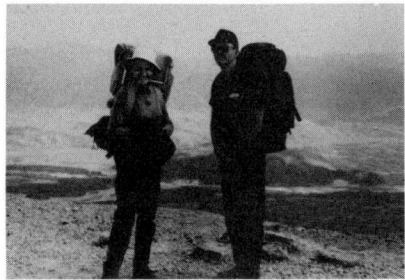
People spending energy in physical activity can afford to eat more food.

On such a limited kcalorie allowance, all foods eaten must be nutrient dense. There is less leeway for empty-calorie foods such as sugar, sweets, fats, oils, and alcohol.

Older adults should be encouraged to increase their activity levels to help maintain an optimal energy balance. Ideally, the exercise should be intense enough to speed the heartbeat and respiration rate and to prevent the atrophy of all muscles that normally occurs with aging. The aerobic capacity of sedentary older people is so low that just getting dressed or making beds may take 50 percent of their maximal capacity. Even mild exercise, like a 10-minute walk taken daily, can greatly improve this work capacity.

One study on exercise for the elderly suggests that individuals aged 65 to 75 begin with a three-day-a-week program of walking, cycling, or other activity. One could alternate two to three minutes of increased activity with two or three minutes of rest over 15 minutes. Increase the activity by 5 to 10 minutes per week until 30 minutes per week is reached. For those over 75, the emphasis should be on walking and range-of-motion exercises to maintain strength, balance, flexibility, and coordination.[8]

The nutritional needs of older athletes are similar to those of younger athletes. Both characteristically consume more kcalories than their sedentary counterparts. Any additional requirements for specific nutrients in the older athlete would likely be obtained by increased food intake. Modest endurance training can improve cardiovascular and respiratory function and promote good muscle tone while controlling the accumulation of body fat.

You may have heard of some experiments in which just-weaned young rats were fed diets extremely restricted in kcalories for a short period early in life and then lived much longer than rats of the same age that had enjoyed ample kcalories throughout life. The first of these experiments was performed long ago, but recent reviews of them have inspired articles in the popular press with titles like "EAT LESS—LIVE LONGER."

These experiments, however, do *not* suggest any direct applications to human nutrition. One thing often overlooked in discussing them is the disadvantages incurred in the animals given restricted feedings. For example, half of the restricted animals died *very* early (before 300 days). The average length of life was long, because the few survivors lived a very long time. The food restriction was also very severe. Furthermore, the restricted animals that survived were retarded and malformed in a number of ways. Old people, then, need not conclude on the basis of this evidence that their parents should have starved them when they were younger.

Because the older person needs to get the same amount of essential amino acids from less food, protein sources should be of high quality. Protein-kcalorie malnutrition (PCM) is common in older people and often goes unnoticed. An observer seeing the wasted muscle, weakness, and sometimes swelling of protein deficiency may think, "That person looks old," when in fact, what he sees are the symptoms of PCM. Older people who have been trying to lose weight or who have been eating monotonous or bizarre diets are most likely to be affected.

Emphasis in the older person's diet should be on securing a wide variety of complex carbohydrate foods to provide the vitamins and minerals such foods contain and to spare protein. As people age, they tend to omit fruits and vegetables from their diets, possibly because they find fruits and vegetables too expensive or too difficult to store and prepare or because raw fruits and vegetables may be difficult to chew. Any educational campaign conducted to improve diets of the elderly should emphasize the great amounts of vitamins, minerals, and fiber contributed by complex carbohydrate foods.

Fat should be limited to no more than 30 percent of the total kcalories in the older person's diet. Limiting fat helps cut kcalories. It would be difficult to obtain the many vitamins and minerals that come from foods rich in protein and complex carbohydrates if too much of the energy came from the relatively empty kcalories of fat. On the other hand, enough fat is needed to supply the fat-soluble vitamins and essential fatty acids.

Vitamins and Minerals

Adequate vitamin intake can be ensured by including foods from each of the food groups. As previously stated, foods from the fruit and vegetable groups are often omitted. Some men and women do not eat whole-grain breads and cereals. These foods are significant sources of many vitamins and several minerals. Their omission from the diet can lead to vitamin deficiencies.

Conditions other than the omission of certain food groups can contribute to vitamin deficiency in the elderly. Older people who are housebound or hospital-bound are thus deprived of the vitamin D they would get from sunshine on their skin. If they do not drink milk, they increase their risk of vitamin D deficiency. Many older people take laxatives regularly, causing such a rapid transit of nutrients through the intestines that many vitamins do not get absorbed. The use of mineral oil as a laxative especially robs a person of the fat-soluble vitamins.

Among the minerals, iron deserves first mention. Iron-deficiency anemia is not as common in older adults as has been believed in the past, but it still occurs in some, especially in those with low kcalorie intakes. Any diet that is low in kcalories and lacks color (and therefore lacks iron-containing red meats as well as fruits and vegetables rich in vitamin C to aid in iron absorption) suggests risk of iron deficiency.

Aside from diet, other factors in many older people's lives increase the likelihood of iron deficiency:

- Chronic blood loss from ulcers, hemorrhoids, or other disease conditions.
- Poor iron absorption due to reduced stomach acid secretion.
- Antacid use, which interferes with iron absorption.
- Medicines that cause blood loss, including arthritis medicines, anticoagulants, and aspirin.

The person counseling an older client on health and nutrition should not forget to ask about these possibilities.

Zinc deficiencies are probably common in older people. Most often associated with zinc deficiencies are loss of taste and slowed wound healing. Loss of taste is often not responsive to zinc supplementation, but when wounds—for example, bed sores in the sick—are slow to heal, a zinc deficiency should be suspected. Wound healing often responds to zinc therapy.

Another mineral often lacking in older people's diets is calcium, the need for which increases with advancing age. As already mentioned, bone loss may be alarmingly extensive and severe before a person realizes there is any problem at all. The recommendation that an older adult ingest the equivalent of five cups of milk a day is difficult to meet, especially for the person who is unaccustomed to using much milk at all. However, many alternative strategies for obtaining the needed calcium are offered in Nutrition in Practice 12.

The use of some medications severly impairs calcium absorption. So does the use of alcohol. Older people who use both are especially prone to calcium deficiency.

The older person may be wise to curtail her intake of salt. Sodium promotes fluid retention in susceptible people which can result in raised blood pressure.

To obtain the needed minerals, the older person should follow the same recommendation as for vitamins. Every food group—milk and milk products, meat and meat alternates, fruits and vegetables, and grains—should be represented in the diet every day.

More information about fiber can be found in Nutrition in Practice 16A.

Fiber and Water

Fiber recommendations for the general population should be stressed to older citizens as well: Increased intake of fruits, vegetables, legumes, and whole-grain cereals. The fiber content of these food groups is important to prevent constipation and diverticulosis and to bind cholesterol and carry it out of the body.

Perhaps the most important nutrient of all is water. A thirst deficit is common in elderly persons and is often the cause of dehydration.[9] The elderly need to be reminded to drink fluids, because they are likely to be somewhat insensitive to their own thirst signals. They should drink six to eight glasses a day, enough to bring their urine output to about 1,500 milliliters (six cups) per day. A large percentage of foster home operators note that one of the biggest problems with their elderly clients is getting them to consume more water and fruit juices.

Caffeine

Older people often find they cannot tolerate caffeine as well as they could when they were younger. Caffeine is a stimulant drug, increasing respiration rate, heart rate, blood pressure, and secretion of the stress and other hormones. An overdose of caffeine produces actions in the body that are indistinguishable from those of an anxiety attack. Older people should be aware of these signs, which indicate that they need to reduce their customary caffeine intakes. Moderation in the use of caffeine-containing foods and beverages is advisable for all ages. The amounts of caffeine in different items are listed in Table 12–1.

Alcohol

A recent estimate sets the incidence of alcoholism in people over 60 in our society at 2 to 10 percent. Alcohol use has its most profound effects on the vitamins thiamin and folacin and on the minerals calcium and zinc, but it affects nearly every nutrient to some extent. The problem in elderly people must be recognized before it can be dealt with. (More about alcoholism is discussed in Nutrition In Practice 6).

Vitamin-Mineral Supplements

The RDA for vitamins for the elderly are currently under study and probably will change. It seems likely that the RDA for some vitamins will decrease while the RDA for others will increase. Among those likely to decrease are vitamin A and folacin; among those that may increase are vitamins B_6, B_{12}, and D. Vitamin C and E requirements may remain the same.[10] While work progresses, it still seems likely that adequate vitamin intake can, in general, best be ensured by improving the diet.

Although many older people use vitamin and mineral supplements, many do not know why they are taking vitamins, and most do not even know what vitamins they are taking. The most widely used supplement of the elderly is

TABLE 12–1. Caffeine Content of Beverages, Foods and OTC Drugs

Drinks and Foods	Average (mg)	Range (mg)
Coffee (5-oz cup)		
Brewed, drip method	130	110–150
Brewed, percolator	94	64–124
Instant	74	40–108
Decaffeinated, brewed or instant	3	1–5
Tea (5-oz cup)		
Brewed, major U.S. brands	40	20–90
Brewed, imported brands	60	25–110
Instant	30	25–50
Iced (12-oz glass)	70	67–76
Soft drinks (12-oz can)		
Dr. Pepper		40
Colas and cherry colas		
regular		30–46
diet		2–58
caffeine-free		0–trace
Jolt		72
Mountain Dew, Mello Yello		52
Big Red		38
Fresca, Hires Root Beer, 7-Up, Sprite,		0
Squirt, Sunkist Orange		0
Cocoa beverage (5-oz cup)	4	2–20
Chocolate milk beverage (8 oz)	5	2–7
Milk chocolate candy (1 oz)	6	1–15
Dark chocolate, semisweet (1 oz)	20	5–35
Baker's chocolate (1 oz)	26	26
Chocolate-flavored syrup (1 oz)	4	4

Drugs[a]		
Cold remedies (standard dose)		
Dristan		0
Coryban-D, Triaminicin		30
Diuretics (standard dose)		
Aqua-ban, Permathene H_2Off		200
Pre-Mens Forte		100
Pain relievers (standard dose)		
Excedrin		130
Midol, Anacin		65
Aspirin, plain (any brand)		0
Stimulants		
Caffedrin, NoDoz, Vivarin		200
Weight-control aids (daily dose)		
Prolamine		280
Dexatrim, Dietac		200

[a]Because products change, contact the manufacturer for an update on products you use regularly.

Source: Data from C. Lecos, The latest caffeine scoreboard, *FDA Consumer,* March 1984, p. 14; Measuring your life with coffee spoons. *Tufts University Diet and Nutrition Letter,* April 1984, pp. 3–6; Institute of Food Technologists, Expert Panel on Food Safety and Nutrition, *Evaluation of Caffeine Safety,* a publication (1986) available from the Institute of Food Technologists, 221 N. LaSalle St., Chicago, IL 60601.

vitamin E, which has been shown to have little influence on the health or clinical disorders of this group.[11] It is apparent that the supplements taken are not always the nutrients most likely to be deficient in the diet. In light of this and what is known about nutrient needs, older people should first be encouraged to eat a balanced diet that is low in fat, high in fiber, and rich in vitamins and minerals. However, it may be appropriate to supplement the diet with a balanced, once-daily multivitamin-mineral preparation. The older person would probably be wise to follow the rule of thumb that if the energy intake is below about 1500 kcalories per day, a vitamin-mineral supplement—not a megavitamin—is recommended.

Mealtime Alone

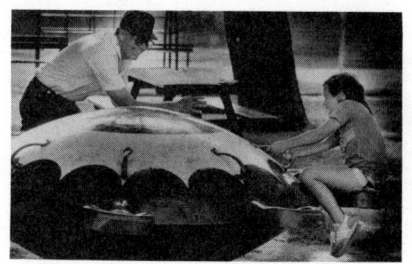

Involvement of the old with the young benefits both.

Many authorities believe that malnutrition among the elderly is most often due to loneliness. The lack of social interaction is no respector of income. It is equally important in the lives of the financially secure and in the lives of the poverty stricken. For the six million adults over 65 who live alone, the pressing need seems to be for companionship first, then for food. Without companionship, appetite decreases. Much of the social life of the adult is built around food. Most invitations into adults' homes are accompanied by an offer of food or drink. We must admit that eating to human beings is as much a social and psychological event as a biological one.

Jack Weinberg, professor of psychiatry at the University of Illinois, wrote perceptively of this problem:

> In our efforts to provide the aged with a proper diet, we often fail to perceive it is not *what* the older person eats but *with whom* that will be the deciding factor in proper care for him. The oft-repeated complaint of the older patient that he has little incentive to prepare food for only himself is not merely a statement of fact but also a rebuke to the questioner for failing to perceive his isolation and aloneness and to realize that food . . . for one's self lacks the condiment of another's presence which can transform the simplest fare to the ceremonial act with all its shared meaning.[12]

Let's look at what happens when a person receives too little food. With malnutrition from lack of food added to apathy from loneliness, there is even less energy with which to make the effort to secure nourishment. If the confusion of vitamin or mineral deficiency is diagnosed as senility, the elderly person may be wrongly confined to a nursing home.

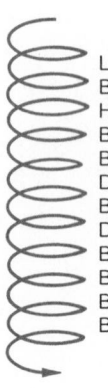

Lonely people:
Become apathetic.
Have no energy to seek food.
Become tired.
Become more apathetic.
Don't reach out to others.
Become more lonely.
Do not eat.
Become malnourished.
Become mentally confused.
Become more isolated.
Become more lonely.

The story is told of a woman who exhibited the classic signs of senility—mental confusion, inability to make decisions, forgetting to perform important tasks, such as turning off a stove burner. The woman's family decided to move her into a nursing home. While she was waiting for a place there, her family took her into their own home. After several weeks of eating good meals and enjoying social stimulation, the woman became her old self again and was able to return to her home. This story has been repeated with many variations and serves to remind us to think about loneliness and nutrition before concluding that a person is senile and needs institutional care. What harm could there be in first trying good, balanced meals served with plenty of tender, loving care?

Money and Other Worries

To add anxiety to their problems, most retired persons have a loss of income that occurs because the retirement check is fixed while all other expenses rise. This has a direct effect on the amount of money spent on food. Forced to practice economy, the older person usually first eliminates so-called luxury items, such as citrus fruits, juices, and vegetables. In some cases, up to 17 percent of the elderly surveyed rarely ate foods from these food groups. Instead of eating several servings a day, they were eating these foods once a week or less. A quarter of the same group had fewer than seven hot meals a week.[13]

Those at the greatest nutritional risk are the frail elderly and those with the very lowest incomes. People who are homebound and living alone may go for days without meals. In less extreme cases, older people may still find transportation to and from the market both expensive and difficult, so shopping is done at a nearby convenience store. The foods offered there are limited in variety and are, for the most part, more expensive than the same items in the larger markets. The amount of food that can be purchased is thus curtailed even further, and eating, which should be a pleasure, becomes another reminder of reduced status.

Sometimes older persons fall prey to food fads and fallacies. Led by false claims to believe that health can be improved, aging forestalled, and illness cured by magical food and nutrient preparations, they spend money needlessly on fraudulent health-food products, thus depleting their already limited funds.

Two programs are helpful with older people's money problems, although they are not designed specifically for the elderly but for the poor of all ages. The Food Stamp program enables people who qualify to obtain stamps with which to buy food. The Supplemental Security Income (SSI) program is aimed at directly improving the financial plight of the very poor by increasing a person's or family's income to the defined poverty level. This sometimes helps older people retain their independence.

A self-help effort aimed at enabling older people on limited incomes to buy good food for less money is the establishment of food banks in several areas. A food bank project buys industry's "irregulars"—perfectly good products that have been mislabeled, underweighted, redesigned, or mispackaged and would ordinarily be thrown away. The food can be purchased for a small handling fee and can be made available for a greatly reduced price or at no charge.

Independence is rated high by those over 65 and is usually equated with staying in the home where these people have lived for many years. But this aloneness may not be a wise choice from a nutrition standpoint. Suggestions for alternatives that would enhance elderly people's health without threatening their independence are given in the margin.

There are several alternatives to living alone for older people who seek companionship. **Covenant living** is a lifestyle in which a number of people agree to live together in a family group. **Retirement communities** offer another alternative. For the sake of companionship at mealtimes, groups of senior citizens can form **diners' clubs** that meet regularly for meals, either at a participant's home or at a restaurant.

Assistance Programs

In recent years, we have come to recognize that the responsibility for support in old age cannot be left entirely to the individual. Two programs arising from this awareness have already been mentioned (the Food Stamp and Supplemental

Security Income programs). A third program is Social Security: employees and employers pay into a fund from which the employee collects benefits at retirement.

Another major political move to benefit the elderly is the Older Americans Act. Title III C (formerly title VII) of this act is an amendment, "Nutrition Program for the Elderly." The major goals of this amendment are to provide

- Low-cost nutritious meals.
- Opportunity for social interaction.
- Auxiliary nutrition, homemaker education, and shopping assistance.
- Counseling and referral to other social and rehabilitative services.
- Transportation services.

The nutrition program of Title III C is based on the belief that people living alone are apt to be poorly nourished. If their nutrition status could be improved, they might avoid medical problems, continue living in communities of their own choice, and stay out of institutions.

Sites chosen for congregate meals under this program must be accessible to most of the target population. Every effort should be made to persuade the elderly person to come to the congregate meal site for the social interaction. Providing transportation increases the cost of meals by 20 to 30 percent, but it often is indispensable to the existence of a project. Volunteers may help with transportation or may deliver meals to those who are homebound (home-delivered meals are known as Meals on Wheels). Despite these programs, many eligible people are still missing meals and are malnourished simply because they don't know of the available programs.

People who need constant medical care have to surrender their independence. For these people, nursing homes provide a less expensive facility than hospitals. Unfavorable publicity surrounding some substandard homes has frightened many older people and their families, but investigation by relatives can identify a home that provides the kind of service the individual needs.

The relative inquiring into nursing homes should find out some things about the food service:

- Can the residents choose their food?
- How often are the menus repeated? Is the cycle monotonous or is a wide variety of menus offered?
- How often are fresh fruits and vegetables served?
- Is a plate check conducted regularly, at least once a week, to discover what and how much the resident is consuming?
- Does the staff keep track of each person's weight?
- Is there good communication between the nursing staff and the dietitian so that the dietitian will know if someone is not eating?
- Is the resident encouraged and helped to the dining room for meals in order to enjoy other people's company?
- Is the dining room attractive?
- Is help available for those who can't manage feeding themselves?

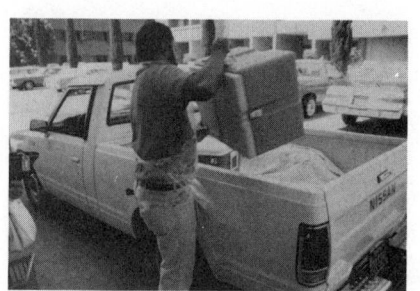

Meals on Wheels.

- Are minced meats offered to those who have problems with their dentures?
- Are religious and ethnic dietary requests honored?
- How high a proportion of the foods are prepackaged? (No guide can be given for what proportion is desirable, but it should be remembered that processed foods may be low in vitamin content and high in salt.)

Other questions that the investigator will want to ask have to do with the general atmosphere of the nursing home, because the social climate of a place affects a person's appetite. A nursing home that views residents as persons, not as patients, gets a mark in its favor.

In the nursing home, the dietitian, nutritionist, or nurse responsible for the residents' care should keep in mind the special needs associated with such people's time in life. The average age of a nursing home resident is 81, and many residents have problems that can affect nutrition status:

- At least one chronic disease.
- Chronic use of prescription drugs; often several drugs are used regularly.
- Confusion due to change in environment.
- Poor eyesight or hearing.
- Ill-fitting or missing dentures.
- Inability to feed themselves because of arthritis or stroke.
- Psychological problems, especially depression.
- Anorexia and loss of interest in eating.
- Lack of opportunity to socialize at mealtime.
- Long-established food preferences.
- Slowed reactions in seeing, holding utensils, chewing, swallowing.

Table B–1 in Appendix B lists the effects of prescription drugs on nutrients. The effects of various diseases on nutrient needs are discussed in Chapters 16 through 22.

Suggestions for helping people in institutions to eat are given in Chapter 14.

On admission to a nursing home, a person should have his nutrition status assessed immediately, and the staff responsible for his nutrition care should make every effort to rectify any problems promptly. Thereafter, he should be reassessed at regular, frequent intervals, and adjustments in his care should be made as needed.

Psychological and nutritional preparation for the later years begins early in life. Everyone knows older people who have gathered around themselves many contacts—through relatives, church, synagogue, social groups or fraternal orders—and have not allowed themselves to drift into isolation. Upon analysis, you will see that their favorable environment came through a lifetime effort that is also required for good nutrition status in the later years. A person who has eaten a wide variety of foods, has stayed trim, and has remained physically and socially active will be most able to withstand the assaults of change. The health care professional working with the elderly may be most effective by emphasizing these aspects and keeping a positive outlook on aging.

CASE STUDY

Elderly Man with a Poor Diet

Mr. Hawkins is a 75-year-old man who lives alone. He has been losing weight slowly since he lost his wife a year ago. At 5 feet 8 inches tall, he currently weighs 135 pounds. His previous weight was 150 pounds. In talking with Mr. Hawkins, you realize that he doesn't even like to talk about food, let alone eat it. "My wife always did the cooking before, and I ate well. Now I just don't feel like eating." You manage to find out that he skips breakfast, has soup and bread for lunch, and sometimes eats a cold-cut sandwich or a TV dinner for supper. He seldom sees friends or relatives. Mr. Hawkins has also lost several teeth and doesn't eat any raw fruits or vegetables that he feels are hard to chew. He lives on a meager but adequate income.

1. What percent is Mr. Hawkins' weight in relationship to the ideal body weight of a 75-year-old man of his size (% IBW)? What is his percent usual body weight (% UBW)? Is his weight loss significant? What factors are contributing to his poor food intake? What nutrients are probably deficient in his diet?

2. Look at Mr. Hawkins as an individual. Suggest ways he can improve his diet that fits his lifestyle. What other aspects of Mr. Hawkins' physical and mental health should you consider in helping him to improve his food intake?

Notes

1. A. E. Harper, Nutrition, aging, and longevity, *American Journal of Clinical Nutrition* 36 (Supplement, October 1982): 737–749.
2. Drug-induced malnutrition in the geriatric patient, *Nutrition and the MD,* August 1987, p. 1.
3. Life extension with SOD and other dietary antioxidants, *Nutrition and the MD,* December 1985, p. 3.
4. P. G. Wolman, Management of patients using unproven regimens for arthritis, *Journal of the American Dietetic Association* 9 (1987): 1211–1214.
5. Questions readers ask, *Nutrition and the MD,* August 1985, p. 6.
6. J. M. Kremer and coauthors, Fish-oil fatty acid supplementation in active rheumatoid arthritis: A double-blinded, controlled crossover study, *Annuals of Internal Medicine* 106 (1987): 497–503.
7. J. S. Goodwin and P. J. Garry, Association between nutrition status and cognitive functioning in a healthy elderly population, *Journal of American Medical Association* 298 (1983): 2917–2921; E. J. Root and J. B. Longenecker, Brain cell alterations suggesting premature aging induced by dietary deficiency of vitamin B and/or copper, *American Journal of Clinical Nutrition* 37 (1983): 540–552.
8. M. E. Wheat, Exercise: Advice for the aging, *Western Journal of Medicine* 147 (1987), p. 477.
9. P. H. Baylis, Osmoregulation and control of vasopressin secretion in healthy humans, *American Journal of Physiology,* 253 (1987): 671–678.
10. P. M. Suter and R. M. Russell, Vitamin requirements of the elderly, *American Journal of Clinical Nutrition* 45 (1987):501–512.
11. W. E. Hale and coauthors, Vitamin E effect on symptoms and laboratory values in the elderly, *Journal of the American Dietetic Association* 5 (1985): 625–629.
12. J. Weinberg, Psychological implications of the nutritional needs of the elderly, *Journal of the American Dietetic Association* 60 (1972): 293–296.
13. Many frail elderly get inadequate food, according to Cornell study, *Journal of the American Dietetic Association* 86 (1986): p. 647.

Buying and Preparing Food for Singles

Many people living alone have difficulty buying and preparing foods. Some of the same problems that plague senior citizens affect young singles and others living alone. Each group can benefit from these suggestions that make food preparation easier and more economical.

My grandmother is on a fixed income and doesn't have much money for groceries once the rent, utilities and other bills are paid. Do you have any advice I could give her?

Yes. We understand the problem, and it is possible to lower a food bill just by being a wise shopper. The first decision an elderly shopper must make is where to shop. Large supermarkets are usually less expensive than independent stores, but the cost of transportation to the market must be considered.

Once a person knows where he or she will be shopping, a grocery list taking into account specials and coupons will help reduce impulse buying. Specials and coupons are a bargain only when they are items that are needed and are in appropriate quantities that can be used without any waste or spoilage. Some foods that are almost always a good buy are nonfat dry milk in place of fluid milk, whole pieces of cheese in place of sliced or shredded, fresh produce that is in season, variety meats such as

chicken livers, cereals that require cooking in place of ready-to-serve cereals, and homebaked goods instead of storebought goods of the same type.

The foods to be purchased should be dependent upon the ability, interest, and desire the individual has for cooking. If a person enjoys cooking, homebaked foods could be both good therapy and economical. However, if a person would just as soon skip a meal as prepare it, convenience foods may be worth the extra cost.

The biggest money saver when it comes to purchasing foods is to buy only what will be used. Turkey may be on sale and is one of the most economical meats for its nutritional value, but a single person living alone could hardly make use of even a small turkey. The savings thus could easily be lost by the waste of such a large amount of meat.

That's a big problem for my grandmother. How can she buy small quantities when so many foods are packaged for families?

This is a problem not only for the elderly but for all singles as well. Packages of meat and fresh vegetables often come already wrapped in large servings. Even a head of lettuce can perish before one person can use it all. Try these hints:

- *Milk group.* Buy fresh milk in the size best suited for you. If your grocer doesn't carry pints or half-pints, try a nearby service station or convenience store. Pint-size and even cup-size boxes of heat-treated milk are also available and can be stored unopened on a shelf for up to three months without refrigeration. Dry powdered milk can be stored for months before it is reconstituted. You can use only the amount you need and store the rest.

- *Meat group.* Buy only what you will use. Ask the grocer to break open a package of wrapped meat and rewrap the portion that you need. Eggs can be purchased by the half-dozen—usually a dozen carton can be broken in half. However, eggs keep for long periods in the refrigerator and are such a good source of high-quality protein that you will probably use a dozen before they lose their freshness.

  If you have ample freezing space, you can buy large packages of meat, such as pork chops, ground meat, or chicken, when they are on sale. Immediately divide the package into individual servings. Wrap in aluminum foil, not freezer paper: the foil can become the liner for the pan in which you bake or broil the meat, thus saving work over the sink. Don't label these individually, but put them all in a brown bag marked "hamburger" or "chicken thighs" or whatever, along with the date. The bag is easy to locate in the freezer, and you'll know when your supply is running low.

- *Fruits and vegetables.* Purchase fresh fruits and vegetables individually. Buy only three pieces of each kind of fresh fruit: a ripe one, a semiripe one, and a green one. Eat the first right away, the second soon after, and let the last one ripen on your windowsill. If vegetables are packaged in large quantities, ask the grocer to break open the package so that you can buy what you need. Buy small cans of fruits and vegetables even though they are more expensive per unit. Remember, it is expensive to buy a regular-size can and let the unused portion spoil in the refrigerator. If you have space in your freezing compartment, buy frozen vegetables in large bags rather than in small boxes. You can take out the exact amount you need and close the bag tightly with a rubber band. If you return the package quickly to the freezer each time, the vegetables will stay fresh for a long time.

- *Grains.* Breads and cereals usually must be purchased in larger quantities. When you buy bread, take out the amount you will use in a few days and freeze the rest. Cereal grains generally have a long shelf life if you keep them sealed in jars.

Those are great suggestions! I know my grandmother can use them, and so can I. But sometimes you just can't purchase foods in the needed amounts. Do you have hints for what to do then?

One thing you can do is to make mixtures of what you have on hand. A thick stew prepared from leftover green beans, carrots, cauliflower, broccoli, and any meat with added onion, pepper, celery, and potatoes makes a complete and balanced meal—except for milk. But see the uses of powdered milk that follow: you could add some to your stew.

You can also set aside a place in your kitchen for rows of glass jars containing shelf staple items that you can't buy in single-serving quantities—rice, tapioca, lentils or other dry beans, flour, cornmeal, nonfat dry milk, macaroni, cereal, or coconut, to name only a few possibilities. Freeze each filled jar for one night first, to kill any insect eggs that might be in it. The jars will then keep bugs out of the food indefinitely. They make an attractive display and will remind you of different choices you can make to vary your menus. Cut the directions-for-use labels from the package and store them in the jars.

Think up a variety of ways to use a vegetable when you must buy it in a quantity larger than you can use. For example, you can divide a head of cauliflower into thirds. Cook one third and eat it as a hot vegetable. Put the other two thirds into a vinegar and oil marinade for use as an appetizer or in a salad. You can keep half a package of frozen vegetables with other vegetables to be used in soup or stew.

Another problem my grandmother has is with preparing foods. Sometimes she doesn't feel like cooking a meal, other times she does. I'm worried that she may not be getting the nutrients she needs.

When your grandmother does feel like cooking, she can cook several meals at a time. For example, she can boil three potatoes with skins. She can eat one hot with margarine and chives. When the others have cooled, she can use one to make a potato-cheese casserole ready to be put into the oven for the next evening's meal. The third one can be sliced into a covered bowl and the juice from pickles poured over it. The pickled potato will keep several days in the refrigerator and can be used in a salad.

Depending on her freezer space, she can make double or even six portions of a dish that takes time to prepare: a casserole, vegetable pie, or meatloaf. Save the little aluminum trays from frozen foods and freeze the extra servings in labeled trays. She needs to be sure to date them and use the oldest first. Somehow the work seems worthwhile when several meals are prepared at once.

Finally, an occasional frozen TV dinner can be useful—although expensive—when it makes the difference between a person's eating and not eating. Many such dinners that are now available are low in kcalories and nutritious. Adding a fresh salad, a whole-wheat roll, and a glass of milk can make quite a nice meal.

You just reminded me of something else. My grandmother never drinks milk. What can I suggest?

She can try using nonfat dry milk. It is the greatest convenience food there is. Dry milk can be used in just about everything: hamburgers, gravies, soups, casseroles, sauces, and beverages, such as iced coffee. The taste is negligible, but five heaping tablespoons would be the equivalent of a cup of fresh milk. Ask a friend who is a member of Weight Watchers to give you some recipes for delicious milk shakes and "ice cream" using nonfat dry milk. Their recipes are for single servings. (See also Chapter 7 for more ideas for people who don't or can't use milk.)

Your grandmother can also increase her calcium intake by making soup stock from pork and chicken bones soaked in vinegar. The bones release their calcium into the acid medium, and the vinegar boils off when the stock is boiled. One *tablespoon* of such stock may contain over 100 milligrams of calcium.[1] Something can then be cooked in this stock every day: vegetables, rice, and stews. And of course, this stock can be used as a soup base.

Recommending a nutritious diet does no good if the individual feels that such a diet would be too difficult to live with. Offering the person suggestions such as the ones provided here can go a long way in helping people incorporate nutritious foods into their diets.

Note

1. A. Rosanoff and D. H. Calloway, Calcium source in Indochinese immigrants (correspondence), *New England Journal of Medicine* 306 (1982): 239–240.

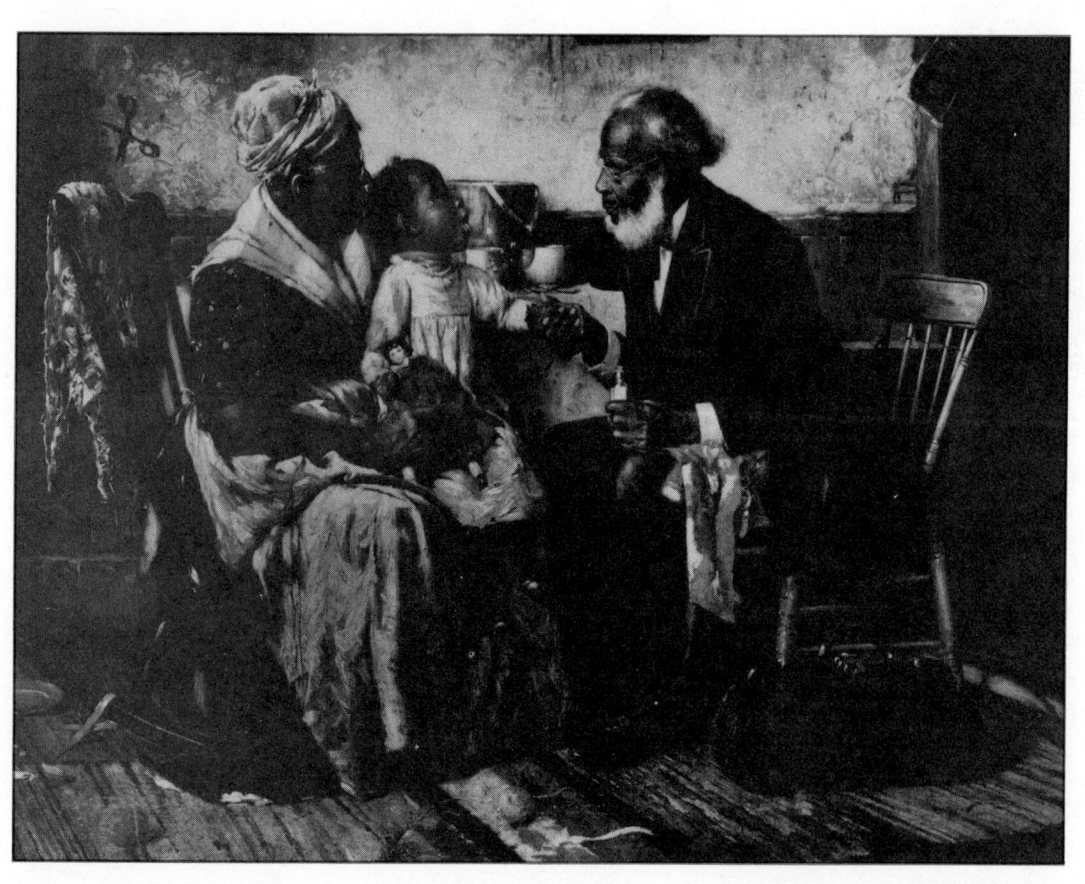

13

Nutrition Assessment and Care Plans

CONTENTS

Visit from the Doctor—*A Serious Case*, 1898, by Harry Roseland
(1868–1950). Oil on canvas, 25 × 35 inches. Courtesy
Demosthenes D. Dasco, M.D.

Throughout the earlier chapters of this book you have discovered nutrients and seen how they are handled by the body. You have also learned of the body's dependence on nutrients for optimal physical and mental health and have seen how these needs change throughout the life cycle. In this chapter, the focus shifts to the question of how well an individual's nutrient needs are being met. You will learn how you can use a nutrition assessment to define a plan for maintaining optimal nutrition status or correcting nutrition problems.

The Nutrition Care Process

In consideration of the unique needs of each individual, how can successful nutrition intervention be effectively provided? A systematic and logical approach must be used. The nutrition care process is such an approach. To identify and solve nutrition problems, follow these five steps:

nutrition care process:
an organized approach to problem solving that consists of five steps (assessing, analyzing, planning, implementing, and evaluating).

1. Assess nutrition status.

2. Analyze assessment data to determine nutrient requirements.

3. Develop a plan of action, including client education, for meeting nutrition needs.

nutrition care plan:
a strategy for translating nutrition assessment data into a plan for meeting the client's nutrient and nutrition education needs.

4. Implement the nutrition care plan.

5. Evaluate the effectiveness of the nutrition care plan through ongoing assessment and make appropriate changes.

Responsibility for developing and implementing nutrition care plans is shared by all members of the health care team, although the dietitian, physician, nurse, and client assume the primary roles. The dietetic technician, social worker, pharmacist, and physical therapist can also make valuable contributions to nutrition assessment and care (see Nutrition and Practice 1). The principles and techniques of nutrition assessment described here apply to people seen in hospitals, outpatient clinics, community centers, nursing homes, private practices, personal residences, and other health care settings.

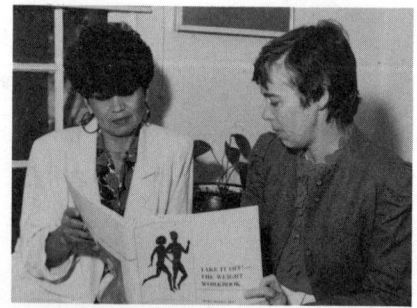

Successful nutrition intervention requires logical and systematic planning.

Nutrition Assessment

To learn whether a person's nutrient needs are being met, the dietitian or other health professional performs a nutrition assessment. To give the details of such a procedure would go beyond the scope of this book (graduate courses are taught in the subject). Any student of nutrition, however, should know the basics of a typical nutrition assessment procedure, because competent medical care includes attention to nutrition. For the person who is healthy, a nutrition assessment can identify aspects of the diet that can be improved to achieve optimal health. For the person who is ill, a nutrition assessment can alert the health care team to nutrition factors that could hinder the response to medical treatment and recovery from illness.

Nutrition assessments performed on the same individual at regular intervals provide a method of monitoring changes in nutrition status to see if the nutrition care plan is working. Nutrition assessment involves making an inventory of an individual's nutrition assets and liabilities. These techniques are used to assemble such an inventory:

- History taking.
- Anthropometric measures.
- Physical examination.
- Biochemical analysis (clinical or lab tests).

Each of these techniques involves collecting data by a number of means and interpreting the findings in relation to the total picture.

Historical Data

A person's history reveals many clues about nutrition status. The person making a nutrition assessment explores the history of the subject from a number of different angles: medical, social, and drug history as well as diet. Table 13–1 shows how each of these angles contributes to nutrition assessment. Table 13–2 lists the historical information that might indicate poor nutrition status, and Form 13–1 shows how such information might be collected.

Medical and Social Histories

As you can see, many circumstances of a person's life, including the environment he lives in, his cooking facilities, previous illnesses, ability to ingest food, persons he associates with, religious and cultural food practices, and many other factors, have an impact on his nutrition status and provide the assessor with clues to likely problems. Medical and social histories are often obtained in a nutrition assessment by reference to charts already filled out by the attending physician, nurse, or other worker. Conversations with the client

TABLE 13–1 The Use of Historical Data in Nutrition Assessment

Histories	Identifies
Medical	Disorders or conditions that affect nutrition status
Social/economic	Environmental influences that affect nutrient intakes
Drug	Medications that affect nutrition status
Diet	Nutrient intake excesses or deficiencies
24-hour recall	
food diary	
food frequency record	

TABLE 13–2 Historical Data of Significance to Nutrition Status

Medical History	Diet History	Social/Economic History	Drug History
Recent major illness	Chewing or swallowing difficulties (including poorly fitted dentures, dental caries, and missing teeth)	Inadequate food budget	Antibiotics
Recent major surgery		Inadequate food preparation facilities	Anticancer agents
Surgery of the GI tract		Inadequate food storage facilities	Anticonvulsants
Overweight	Inadequate food intake	Age (elderly)	Antihypertensive agents
Underweight	Restricted or fad diets	Living (eating) alone	Catabolic steroids
Recent weight loss or gain	Frequent eating out	Poor education	Oral contraceptives
Anorexia	No intake for 10 or more days		Vitamin and other nutrient preparations
Nausea	Intravenous fluids (other than total parenteral nutrition) for 10 or more days		
Vomiting			
Diarrhea			
Alcoholism			
Cancer			
Circulatory problems			
Liver disease			
Lung disease			
Kidney disease			
Diabetes			
Heart disease			
Heavy smoking			
Hormonal imbalance			
Hyperlipidemia			
Hypertension			
Mental retardation			
Multiple pregnancies[a]			
Neurologic disorders			
Pancreatic insufficiency			
Paralysis			
Physical disability			
Radiation therapy			
Teenage pregnancies[a]			

[a]See also Risk Factors for Poor Nutrition Status in Pregnancy, p. 189.

can uncover valuable medical information that was not recorded because "no one asked" or because the client was too upset on admission to think clearly.

The purpose of establishing a sound medical history when assessing nutrition status is to uncover any conditions that place a client at risk for nutrient deficiencies. Of particular concern are significant weight change, anorexia, vomiting, diarrhea, edema, and the presence of chronic diseases (see Table 13–1). Remember that disease can have either long-term or short-term effects on nutrition status. An illness can:

edema (eh-DEEM-uh): accumulation of fluid in the spaces beween the cells.

- Lead to a loss of appetite.
- Interfere with a person's ability to chew or swallow food.
- Alter the way food is digested or interfere with the way nutrients are absorbed.
- Alter the way nutrients are metabolized.
- Alter the way nutrients are excreted.

One, several, or all of these effects can occur during illness and alter nutrition status.

FORM 13–1.
History

Name _____   Today's date _____
Address _____   Age _____
_____   Sex _____
_____   Phone _____
Date of last medical checkup _____   Height _____
Reason for coming in _____   Weight _____
                                                         Usual Weight _____

PERSONAL DATA

1. Last grade of school completed _____ Still in school? _____
2. Are you employed? _____ Occupation _____
3. Does someone else live at your home? _____ Who? _____
4. Do you smoke in any way? _____ How much? _____
5. Have you recently lost or gained more than 10 lb? _____ If yes, please explain how _____
6. Are you pregnant? _____ How many months? _____
7. How many pregnancies have you carried to term? _____
8. Are your menstrual periods normal? _____ If not, please explain _____
_____

9. Have you been told that you have (check any that apply):
   Diabetes _____ High blood pressure _____ Hardening of the arteries _____
   Lung disease _____ Kidney disease _____ Liver disease _____ Ulcers _____
   Cancer _____ Other _____
10. Do you eat at regular times each day? _____ How many times per day? _____
11. Do you usually eat snacks? _____ When? _____
12. Where do you usually eat your meal?
    Morning _____ Noon _____ Night _____
    With whom?
    Morning _____ Noon _____ Night _____
13. Would you say your appetite is good? _____ Fair? _____ Poor? _____
    If poor, please explain _____
14. What foods do you particularly dislike? _____
15. Are there foods you don't eat for other reasons? _____
16. Do you have any difficulty eating? _____
17. How would you describe your feelings about food? _____
_____
_____
18. Who prepares your meals? _____
19. Are you, or is any member of your family, on a special diet? _____
    If yes, who and what kind? _____
20. Do you drink alcohol? _____ How many drinks per day? _____
    Do you ever drink alcohol excessively? _____ How often? _____
21. Do you take any kind of medication, either described by a doctor or over the counter, for any condition? _____
22. How would you describe your exercise habits?
    Kind of exercise _____ How intense? _____
    How long at a time? _____ How often? _____
23. Are there any other facts about your lifestyle that you think might be related to your nutritional health? _____ Explain _____

Drug History

Hundreds of drugs interact with nutrients, creating the possibility of imbalances or deficiencies. Medicines can profoundly affect nutrition status, and nutrients can affect the way the body responds to drugs. Not all drug-nutrient interactions occur each time a person takes a drug. The chances that an adverse

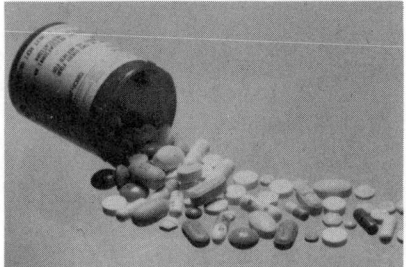

Nutrients and drugs interact in many ways.

Significant drug nutrient interactions are
more likely if:
• Many drugs are taken simultaneously.
• Drugs are taken over long periods of time.
• The user of the drug is in poor nutrition
  status or is at risk for poor nutrition status.
• Nutrient needs are high.

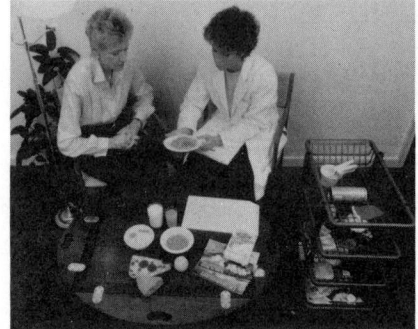

The dietitian uses food models to help a
client accurately report portion sizes.

interaction will result in nutrient deficiencies multiply if the drug is taken over long periods of time, if the person is taking several drugs simultaneously, or if the person is at risk of, or has, poor nutrition status to begin with. Understandably, the elderly and people with serious illnesses that increase nutrient requirements are most likely to develop problems. In these groups of people, you are likely to find several risk factors: Poor nutrition status, chronic disorders, use of many drugs, and the long-term use of drugs.

Drugs and nutrients can interact in many ways, producing one or more of the following effects:

• Drugs can alter food intake by depressing or stimulating the appetite.
• Nutrients and foods can change the way a drug is absorbed; drugs can change the way nutrients are absorbed.
• Nutrients can interfere with the intended action of drugs.
• Nutrients can alter the metabolism and excretion of drugs; drugs can alter the metabolism and excretion of nutrients.

Table 13–3 summarizes the mechanisms by which several nutrient-drug interactions occur. Table B–1 in Appendix B provides a listing of numerous drug-nutrient interactions. Interactions of many drugs used in the treatment of specific disorders are described in the appropriate chapters.

Diet History

Food intake data can be obtained in several ways: the 24-hour recall, the usual intake record, the food frequency checklist, and the food diary. Regardless of the method used, a word of caution is in order. People may respond to your questions with answers they think you want to hear, they may be truly unaware of their eating habits or the amounts of foods they eat, or they may be embarrassed by what they eat. Many of these problems can be overcome by a skilled interviewer. Questions asked regarding food intake must always be nonjudgmental to elicit accurate information. Food models and measuring devices help clients visualize the serving sizes of foods they eat.

The most common method of obtaining food intake data is the 24-hour recall. To use this method, you ask the person to recount all solids and liquids consumed in the past 24 hours or on the previous day. Form 13–2 shows a typical 24-hour recall form. Seldom does this method give enough accurate information about an individual's food intake to be valid, however. It is more often used in nutrition surveys to obtain estimates of the typical food intakes of large numbers of people in given populations.

An advantage of the 24-hour recall is that it is easy to obtain. To elicit information from the past 24 hours is also less frustrating than to require a person to estimate his intake over a long period of time. The previous day's intake, however, may not be the usual intake. In such a case, obtaining a usual intake pattern may be more meaningful.

An inquiry on usual intake might begin with, What is the first thing you usually eat or drink during the day? Similar questions follow until a typical intake pattern is obtained. Use the same form as the 24-hour recall to record the information (Form 13–2). A skilled and patient interviewer can obtain

TABLE 13–3. Mechanisms of Food/Drug Interations

Drugs Can Change Food Intake by

Altering the appetite.
Interfering with taste or smell.
Inducing nausea or vomiting.
Causing sores or inflammation of the mouth.

Foods Can Change Drug Absorption by

Changing the acidity of the digestive tract.
Stimulating secretion of digestive juices.
Altering motility of the digestive tract.
Binding to drugs.

Drugs Can Change Nutrient Absorption by

Changing the acidity of the digestive tract.
Altering digestive juices.
Altering motility of the digestive tract.
Inactivating enzyme systems.
Damaging mucosal cells.

Foods Can Change Drug Metabolism by

Interfering with a drug's action.
Contributing pharmacologically active substances (example: tyramine).

Drugs Can Change Nutrient Metabolism by

Acting as structural analogs.
Interfering with metabolic enzyme systems.
Binding to nutrients.

Foods Can Change Drug Excretion by

Changing the acidity of the urine.

Drugs Can Change Nutrient Excretion by

Altering reabsorption in the kidneys.
Displacing nutrients from their plasma protein carriers.

much useful information from it. For a person whose intake varies widely from day to day, however, the questions may be hard to answer, and the data obtained may be useful only for giving a general impression of a person's eating habits and not for estimating nutrient intake.

Another approach is to use a food frequency checklist. The purpose of this record is to ascertain how often an individual eats a specific type of food per day, week, month, or year. Subjects are asked to state how often they eat a certain food or food type. A long list of foods is used to cover all possibilities.

FORM 13–2.
Food Intake for a 24-Hour Recall

Name and address _____   Date _____

_____

_____

_____

Did you take a vitamin/mineral supplement? _____

If yes, what kind? _____   Dose _____

Please record the amount and type of foods and beverages consumed today. [Or: Please record the amount and type of foods and beverages you typically consume each day.]

FOOD	AMOUNT (c, tbsp, or piece)	DESCRIPTION (how cooked, how served)

(etc.)

The information obtained can help pinpoint nutrients that may be excessive or deficient in the diet. If used in conjunction with the usual intake or 24-hour recall, the food frequency record permits the user to double-check the accuracy of the information obtained. Form 13–3 is a food frequency checklist.

Still another alternative is the food diary, an example of which is provided in Form 13–4. Completion of a diary often helps to determine factors associated with food intake (time of day, place eaten, mood, others present). The person keeping the diary is instructed to write down the required information immediately after eating. Food diaries work well with cooperative people but require considerable time and effort on their part.

The advantages of the food diary are several:

• The diary keeper must assume an active role.

• The person may for the first time begin to see and understand her own food habits.

• The assessor obtains an accurate picture of the diary keeper's lifestyle and factors that affect food intake.

outpatient:
a client seen in a setting outside of the hospital, extended care facility, or rehabilitation center.

Food diaries are particularly useful in outpatient counseling for such nutrition problems as weight reduction and food allergy. The major disadvantages stem from a client's poor compliance in recording the data or from conscious or unconscious changes in eating habits that may occur while a food diary is being kept.

FORM 13.3.
Food Frequency Checklist

The following information will help us to understand your regular eating habits so that we may offer you the best service possible. If you have any doubt about some items, be sure to underestimate the "goodness" of your habits rather than to overestimate.

1. How many timer *per week* do you eat the following foods? Circle the appropriate number:

PER WEEK

Poultry	0 <1 1 2 3 4 5 6 7 8 9 >9	_____
Fish	0 <1 1 2 3 4 5 6 7 8 9 >9	_____
Hot dogs	0 <1 1 2 3 4 5 6 7 8 9 >9	_____
Bacon	0 <1 1 2 3 4 5 6 7 8 9 >9	_____
Lunch meat	0 <1 1 2 3 4 5 6 7 8 9 >9	_____
Sausage	0 <1 1 2 3 4 5 6 7 8 9 >9	_____
Pork or ham	0 <1 1 2 3 4 5 6 7 8 9 >9	_____
Salt pork	0 <1 1 2 3 4 5 6 7 8 9 >9	_____
Liver	0 <1 1 2 3 4 5 6 7 8 9 >9	_____
Beef or veal	0 <1 1 2 3 4 5 6 7 8 9 >9	_____
Other meats (which?) _____	0 <1 1 2 3 4 5 6 7 8 9 >9	_____
Eggs	0 <1 1 2 3 4 5 6 7 8 9 >9	_____
Fast foods	0 <1 1 2 3 4 5 6 7 8 9 >9	_____

2. How many timer *per day* do you eat the following foods? Circle the appropriate number:

PER DAY

Bread, toast, rolls, muffins	0 <1 1 2 3 4 5 6 7 8 9 >9	_____
Milk (including on cereal)	0 <1 1 2 3 4 5 6 7 8 9 >9	_____
Yogurt or tofu	0 <1 1 2 3 4 5 6 7 8 9 >9	_____
Cheese or cheese dishes	0 <1 1 2 3 4 5 6 7 8 9 >9	_____
Sugar, jam, jelly, syrup, honey	0 <1 1 2 3 4 5 6 7 8 9 >9	_____
Butter or margarine	0 <1 1 2 3 4 5 6 7 8 9 >9	_____

3. How many times *per week* do you eat the following foods? Circle the appropriate number:

PER WEEK

Fruit or fruit juice	0 <1 1 2 3 4 5 6 7 8 9 >9	_____
Vegetables other than potato	0 <1 1 2 3 4 5 6 7 8 9 >9	_____
Potatoes and other starchy vegetables	0 <1 1 2 3 4 5 6 7 8 9 >9	_____
Salads or raw vegetables	0 <1 1 2 3 4 5 6 7 8 9 >9	_____
Cereal (which kind?)	0 <1 1 2 3 4 5 6 7 8 9 >9	_____
Pancakes or waffles	0 <1 1 2 3 4 5 6 7 8 9 >9	_____
Rice or other cooked grains	0 <1 1 2 3 4 5 6 7 8 9 >9	_____
Noodles (macaroni, spaghetti)	0 <1 1 2 3 4 5 6 7 8 9 >9	_____
Crackers or pretzels	0 <1 1 2 3 4 5 6 7 8 9 >9	_____
Sweet rolls or doughnuts	0 <1 1 2 3 4 5 6 7 8 9 >9	_____
Cooked dry beans or peas	0 <1 1 2 3 4 5 6 7 8 9 >9	_____
Peanut butter or nuts	0 <1 1 2 3 4 5 6 7 8 9 >9	_____
Milk or milk products	0 <1 1 2 3 4 5 6 7 8 9 >9	_____
TV dinners, pot pies, other prepared meals	0 <1 1 2 3 4 5 6 7 8 9 >9	_____
Sweet bakery goods (cake, cookies)	0 <1 1 2 3 4 5 6 7 8 9 >9	_____
Snack foods (potato or corn chips)	0 <1 1 2 3 4 5 6 7 8 9 >9	_____
Candy	0 <1 1 2 3 4 5 6 7 8 9 >9	_____
Soft drinks (which?) _____	0 <1 1 2 3 4 5 6 7 8 9 >9	_____
Coffee or tea	0 <1 1 2 3 4 5 6 7 8 9 >9	_____
Frozen sweets (which?) _____	0 <1 1 2 3 4 5 6 7 8 9 >9	_____
Instant meals such as breakfast bars or diet meal beverages (which?)	0 <1 1 2 3 4 5 6 7 8 9 >9	_____
Wine	0 <1 1 2 3 4 5 6 7 8 9 >9	_____
Beer	0 <1 1 2 3 4 5 6 7 8 9 >9	_____
Whiskey, vodka, rum, etc.	0 <1 1 2 3 4 5 6 7 8 9 >9	_____

(form continued on next page)

FORM 13.3. **(continued)**
Food Frequency Checklist

4. What specific kinds of the following foods do you eat most often? Include the name of the food; whether it is fresh, canned, or frozen; and how it is prepared.

Fruits and fruit juices _____

Vegetables _____

Milk and milk products _____

Meats _____

Breads and cereals _____

Desserts _____

Snack foods _____

5. Please list the names of any liquid, powder, or pill form of vitamin or mineral product you take, and state how often you take it. Please list also any diet supplement you use (such as protein milk shakes or brewer's yeast), how much you use, and how often you use it. _____

6. Is there anything else we should know about your food/nutrient intake? _____
_____
_____

Remember that diet analyses provide only *estimates* of actual nutrient intakes.

primary deficiency:
a nutrient deficiency caused directly by lack of that nutrient in the diet.

secondary deficiency:
a deficiency caused by the body's inability to digest, absorb, or utilize a nutrient in the normal fashion, or by excess destruction or excretion of the nutrient.

anthropometric:
relating to measurement of the physical characteristics of the body, such as height and weight.
anthropos = human
metric = measuring

The collection of food intake data allows the assessor to determine nutrient intakes, if appropriate. The assessor can look up every food in the table of food composition (Appendix C) and manually determine nutrient intakes, or can use a computer program that does the same thing automatically. Nutrition in Practice 13 more fully describes the use of computers in estimating nutrient intakes.

Once you have determined nutrient intakes, compare them with standards such as the RDA to estimate the adequacy of the diet. Keep in mind that the RDA were not intended to describe the individual's nutrient requirements. They are only guidelines and should be interpreted cautiously.

To estimate the nutrients in foods is informative but time-consuming, even when done with the help of a computer. The information tends to imply an accuracy greater than can actually be obtained from data as uncertain as those that provide the starting information. Because foods vary, the nutrient contents of foods are merely averages. Many history takers use shortcut systems to obtain rough estimates of nutrient intakes, then use the calculation method to pin down any suspected nutrient deficiencies or imbalances. One shortcut method is to compare food intake with the Four Food Groups (see Table 1–2).

Once an estimate of nutrient intake has been obtained by means of a diet history, you can use it along with other sources of information to confirm or eliminate the possibility of suspected nutrition problems. Be alert to the fact that a sufficient intake of a nutrient does not guarantee adequate nutrient status for an individual. The individual's needs may be high; or nutrient absorption, utilization, or excretion may be abnormal. The client may not have a primary nutrient deficiency but may have a secondary one.

Anthropometric Measures

Anthropometrics are physical measurements that reflect growth and development. An individual's measurements are compared with standards specific

FORM 13–4.
Food Diary

Name _____

Date _____

TIME	PLACE	WITH WHOM	EMOTIONAL STATE	HUNGRY OR NOT HUNGRY	FOOD EATEN (AMOUNT)

(etc.)

for sex and age. Those standards, in turn, ideally are derived from measurements taken on large numbers of people of the same race and geographic location as those being measured.

Height and weight are well-recognized anthropometrics. Others include fatfold measurements and various measures of lean tissue. Some are used in specific situations. In infancy, a head circumference measurement may be useful to help assess brain development. In liver disease, a measurement of abdominal girth provides information on abdominal fluid accumulation (see Chapter 22). Anthropometrics are particularly useful when taken at regular intervals.

Appendix B provides a description of procedures used in taking anthropometric measurements and tables of standards used in their interpretation.

Height and Weight

Height and weight are among the most common and most useful measurements. The height measurement may not be critical in itself, but it is used to estimate desirable weight and to interpret other assessment data. Once adult height has been reached, changes in body weight are useful in assessing overnutrition and undernutrition as well as dehydration and overhydration.

Weight measurements can be compared with desirable weight tables (see inside back cover), which are specific for height, sex, and frame size. (The limitations of these tables are discussed in Chapter 9.) The height and weight tables use a weight range rather than pinpointing one weight. This is a good reminder that we cannot determine a "perfect" weight for anyone.

A comparison of a person's actual weight with the ideal weight is used to calculate the *percent ideal body weight* (%IBW), which provides a rough estimation of the degree of overnutrition or undernutrition. A %IBW greater than 115–120 is indicative of obesity; less than 90 is indicative of undernutrition (see Appendix B).

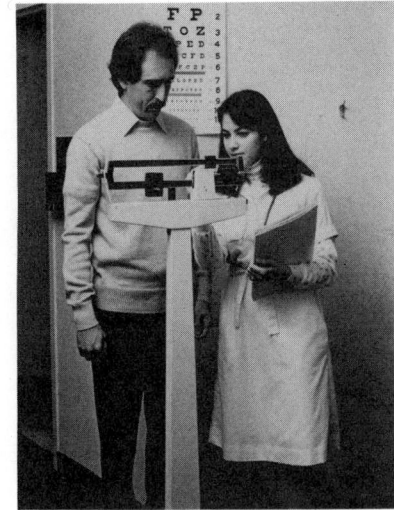

Weigh each client regularly.

B.J. is a 45-year-old male of medium frame with a height of 5′8″. He currently weighs 115 pounds. He has lost 15 pounds in the past month.

$$\%IBW = \frac{\text{actual body weight}}{\text{ideal body weight}^*} \times 100$$

*Use the midpoint of the ideal weight range.

$$\%IBW = \frac{115 \text{ lbs}}{145 \text{ lbs}} \times 100 = 79\%$$

$$\%UBW = \frac{\text{actual weight}}{\text{usual weight}} \times 100$$

$$\%UBW = \frac{115 \text{ lbs}}{130 \text{ lbs}} \times 100 = 89\%$$

Recent weight change—weight loss is significant (almost 4 lb/week).

A more valuable parameter for assessing weight measurements is the *percent usual body weight* (%UBW), which considers what is normal for a particular individual. The client, family, or friends and older medical records are sources of information regarding usual weight. Malnutrition can be more easily detected in an obese subject by using %UBW rather than %IBW (see Appendix B).

Any *recent weight change* can be determined by relating the %UBW to the time period over which a change, if any, has occurred. A five percent weight loss might be significant if it occurred within a month, yet might not be significant if it occurred over five months. Always ask the person about the weight change. Was the change intentional? Why does the client feel his or her weight has changed?

Keep in mind that weight measurements are difficult to evaluate in people who are ill. Diseases or therapy can cause fluid retention and mask significant weight loss. Similarly, a large mass such as a tumor can also mask weight loss.

For children, measurements of height and weight taken at regular intervals provide powerful insight into their overall health, including their nutrition status. Growth charts are presented in Appendix B. Although individual growth measurements may vary, in general, growth should be maintained along the same percentile throughout childhood. In growth-retarded children, it is desirable that height and weight reach a higher percentile. In overweight children, weight should remain relatively stable as height increases, until weight becomes appropriate for height.

Fatfolds and Midarm Muscle Circumference

Significant weight changes in both children and adults can reflect overnutrition and undernutrition with respect to kcalories and protein. To determine the degree to which various body compartments (fat stores or lean body mass) are affected by malnutrition, fatfolds and midarm muscle circumference measurements are used. The triceps fatfold measurement provides an estimate of body fat and together with the midarm circumference (MAC), can be used to mathematically derive the midarm muscle cirumference (MAMC)—an estimate of lean body mass. The methods used to determine these measurements, reference standards for comparing these measurements to norms, and additional information about various anthropometric measurements can be found in Appendix B. Table 13–4 describes the use of anthropometric measurements in nutrition assessment.

Anthropometric measures can be easy to take and require little equipment. Their accuracy and value, however, are limited by the skills of the measurer, the accuracy of the equipment used for measurement, changes in body composition related to different disorders (fluid retention, dehydration), and misinterpetation of measurements. Triceps fatfold measurements can be difficult to determine for people who are obese or for elderly individuals with loose, hanging skin on the upper arm. Mastering the correct techniques for some of the measurements takes time. An assessor must practice for reliable results. Furthermore, significant changes in measurements occur slowly in adults. When changes do occur, they represent prolonged alterations in nutrient intake. Therefore, anthropometrics cannot be used to describe small changes in body composition that occur over short periods of time.[1] Furthermore, fatfold mea-

TABLE 13–4. Anthropometric Measures Used in Nutrition Assessments[a]

Measurement	Reflects
Height-weight	Overnutrition and undernutrition
	Growth in children
%IBW, %UBW, Recent weight change	Overnutrition and undernutrition
Midarm circumference	Muscle mass and subcutaneous fat
Fatfold	Subcutaneous fat and total body fat
Midarm muscle circumference	Muscle mass (i.e., protein status)
Head circumference	Brain growth and development in children

[a]Appendix B provides a more detailed description of anthropometric measures.

surements and the derived MAMC must be interpreted with extreme caution for people in the hospital. We do not know if internal fat stores change at the same rate as triceps fatfold or if changes in total body water markedly influence the triceps fatfold measurement during severe stress.[2] It is conceivable that fatfold measurements could remain constant in spite of the fact that internal fat stores are being depleted. Any error in the fatfold measurement would affect the derived MAMC as well.

Two additional methods for assessing body fat are underwater weighing and bioelectrical impedance techniques. Both of these techniques are popular with athletes and commercial health clubs. Underwater weighing measures body density. The subject is submerged in water, and the amount of water displaced is measured. A mathematical equation translates the body density measurement into a percent body fat measurement. The percent body fat measurement is compared to a standard reference for men and women as appropriate.

Although the underwater weighing technique provides a good estimate of body fat when the test is administered appropriately, the method is not without drawbacks. Errors can result from the mathematical equation used to translate body density measurements into percent fat measurements. The standards used for comparing values to norms were developed on adults. Since the elderly and the young have different body densities (for which standards are not available), interpretation of data in these age groups is difficult.

The use of the bioelectrical impedance technique to determine body composition is gaining popularity because the technique is inexpensive, the equipment is portable, and the procedure is painless.[3] To measure body fat using the bioelectrical impedance technique, a very low intensity electrical current is sent through the body by way of electrodes placed on the wrists and ankles. The amount of water in the body influences the conductivity of the electrical current. Theoretically, the total body water directly reflects lean body mass.

In healthy adults, the bioelectrical impedance technique compares favorably with underwater weighing.[4] However, the subject's state of hydration on any given day as well as individual differences in skin resistance can significantly influence measurement results.[5] In one study of people with cardiac and pulmonary disorders, body fat was underestimated by 23 percent to 35 percent using the bioelectrical impedance technique as compared with underwater

The measurement of body density using the underwater weighing technique is called **hydrodensitometry.**

bioelectrical impedance: a method for estimating body fat using low-intensity electrical current.

weighing.[6] Although the bioelectrical impedance technique may be a promising method for measuring body fat for the future, the proper applications and interpretation of the technique must be established before it can be recommended as a clinical assessment tool.[7]

Up to this point, we have looked at anthropometric measurements that seek to define changes in body composition. More recently, investigators and clinicians have begun to take the nutrition assessment process further. Methods of relating changes in body composition to organ function are receiving emphasis. One method of assessing skeletal muscle function that is gaining popularity is measurement of hand grip strength. An instrument called the dynamometer is used to see how tightly a person can grip. Low grip strength indicates that the person is at risk for poor nutrition status. At least one study has shown that hand grip strength can be used as a simple and inexpensive tool for screening people at risk for poor nutrition status.[8]

Physical Findings

Clues to a person's nutrition status can be identified by examining the person for physical signs of malnutrition (see Table 13–5). However, many of these signs are nonspecific; they can be associated with many nutrient deficiencies or can be unrelated to nutrition at all. So, again, physical findings can be interpreted only in light of other assessment findings.

Physical signs of malnutrition appear most rapidly in parts of the body where cells are being replaced at a high rate, such as in the hair, skin, and GI tract. Chapters 7 and 8 present many symptoms of vitamin and mineral deficiencies and toxicities, indicating the many tissues and organs that would reflect signs of malnutrition. Appendix B lists some easily detected signs of malnutrition and the nutrient deficiencies to which they are related.

TABLE 13–5. Physical Findings Used in Nutrition Assessments[a]

Anatomical Sites	Reflects
Hair	PCM
Face	PCM; vitamin A and iron status
Eyes	Vitamin A, B vitamin, zinc, and iron status
Lips	B vitamin status
Tongue	B vitamin status
Teeth	Mineral status
Gums	Vitamin C status
Glands	PCM and iodine status
Skin	PCM; vitamin A, B vitamin, and vitamin C status
Nails	Iron status
Subcutaneous tissue	PCM and obesity

[a]Findings are listed in their approximate physical order on the body to help the caretaker remember to look for physical signs from "head to toe." Appendix B provides a more detailed description of physical signs of malnutrition.

Laboratory Tests

Biochemical or clinical lab tests help to determine what is happening inside the body. Blood and urine samples are used to directly measure a nutrient or a metabolite (end product or enzyme) that is affected by that nutrient. Biochemical measurements often are sensitive to early signs of malnutrition.

The most common lab tests used to assess nutrition status help uncover protein-kcalorie malnutrition (PCM). They include tests for albumin levels, transferrin levels, total lymphocyte count, urinary creatinine excretion, and urinary urea nitrogen excretion for nitrogen balance studies. All of these laboratory tests, with the exception of urinary creatinine excretion, are measures of the protein status of the blood and internal organs. Measurement of urinary creatinine reflects the protein status of skeletal muscle. Table 13–6 shows how the various laboratory tests are used in nutrition assessments.

Albumin accounts for over 50 percent of the total serum proteins. Because there is so much albumin in the body and because albumin is not broken down quickly, albumin concentrations change slowly with changes in nutrition status. Therefore, low albumin levels indicate prolonged protein depletion. These levels are slow to reach adequate concentrations as nutrition status improves.

Transferrin is a serum protein that transports iron between the intestine and sites of hemoglobin synthesis and degradation. It is considered a more sensitive indicator of protein malnutrition than albumin, because it responds more promptly to changes in protein intake.

More recently, other serum proteins such as prealbumin, retinol-binding protein, fibronectin, fibrinogen, haptoglobin, and C-reactive protein have been studied as indicators of visceral protein status. Although the results of many of these studies have been promising, these indicators are frequently less practical and more expensive to measure and are not in common use.

Various forms of PCM have been associated with depression of the immune system. The lymphocytes (white blood cells that defend against infection) appear to be reduced in number as protein depletion occurs. This is why the total lymphocyte count is a useful index in nutrition assessment. Another measure of immune function is antigen skin testing. Organisms (usually three to four kinds) to which most people are immune are injected just under the skin. After 48 hours, the sites of the injections are inspected for raised, hardened areas. Such areas will be apparent in well-nourished persons. In malnourished

Serum is the watery portion of the blood that remains after the cells and clot-forming material are removed; **plasma** is unclotted blood. In most cases, serum and plasma concentrations are similar. Serum samples usually are preferred, because plasma samples occasionally clog mechanical blood analyzers.

Protein of the blood and internal organs is often called **visceral** (VISS-er-ul) **protein.** The protein of skeletal muscle is called **somatic protein.**

albumin:
the chief blood protein used to assess nutrition status.

transferrin:
an iron-carrying protein in the blood. The concentration of this protein rises if the person's iron stores are depleted; it falls in protein malnutrition.

total lymphocyte count:
a count of the white blood cells; a measure of immune function that may or may not reflect nutrition status.

antigen skin testing:
a test of the immune system's competence in which an antigen is injected just under the skin. A reaction means the immune system is working normally.

The reaction to a skin test—a raised, hardened area of skin—is called **induration.**

TABLE 13–6. Laboratory Tests Used in Standard Nutrition Assessments[a]

Lab Test	Reflects
Urinary creatinine excretion	Skeletal muscle mass (i.e., malnutrition)
Albumin	Protein status
Transferrin	Protein and iron status
Total lymphocyte count	Protein status and immune function
Nitrogen balance	Protein status
Vitamin and mineral tests	Vitamin and mineral status

[a]Appendix B provides a more detailed description of laboratory tests.

persons, however, they will not appear or will be very small, because the body is unable to mount a response to the antigens. Many disorders other than PCM can affect the immune system. Therefore, test results can only be interpreted in light of other diagnostic tests.

creatinine (cree-AT-in-een or cree-AT-in-in) **excretion:**
an indicator of lean body mass. Creatinine is a waste product produced by active muscle.

Urinary creatinine excretion reflects the amount of skeletal muscle mass. By collecting urine over a 24-hour period and determining the total creatinine in the sample, it is possible to estimate muscle mass. Standards for creatinine excretion have been developed based on sex and height (see Appendix B). They are used along with the measured creatinine to derive the creatinine-height index. The validity of the creatinine-height index as a measure of protein status has been questioned.[9] Difficulties arise in collecting complete 24-hour urine samples and in using creatinine standards that fail to consider the age of the subject.[10] A diet high in meat can also contribute to the inaccuracies of the test. The test is invalid if the subject shows signs of kidney disease, since the disease might reduce the body's ability to excrete creatinine.

Nitrogen balance
   nitrogen intake = nitrogen output
Positive nitrogen balance
   nitrogen intake > nitrogen output
Negative nitrogen balance
   nitrogen intake < nitrogen output

Nitrogen balance studies are useful in estimating the degree to which protein is being depleted or repleted in the body. A simple approach is to measure the nitrogen excreted during a 24-hour urine collection. During the same 24-hour period, an accurate record of the subject's nitrogen (protein) intake must be kept to complete the balance study.

Nitrogen intake is calculated by dividing protein intake (in grams) by 6.25 (grams of nitrogen per gram of protein). Nitrogen output per day equals the urine urea nitrogen (UUN) plus a factor of four grams to account for nitrogen lost through the lungs, hair, skin, and nails as well as nonurea nitrogen losses in the urine. As with creatinine excretion, the kidneys must be functioning properly for measurement to be accurate.

Nitrogen balance studies provide a prime example of the need for communication and cooperation between health care providers, departments within the health care facility, and the client. The client must understand the study and cooperate in saving urine specimens and accurately accounting for food intake whenever possible. The nurse must collect the urine specimens. The lab must carefully handle and analyze the urine sample. The dietitian, nurse, or dietetic technician records food intake data, and the dietitian analyzes the data. The physician analyzes the client's medical condition to interpret the validity of the data obtained. You can see that if coordination is not acheived, results would be inaccurate and useless.

Besides helping to assess PCM, laboratory testing can help assess nutrition status with respect to vitamins and minerals. As is true throughout the nutrition assessment procedure, the assessor must use caution in interpreting results of tests like these. Vitamin and mineral levels present in the blood may reflect disease processes, abnormal hormone levels, or other aberrations rather than dietary intakes. Even if these levels reflect dietary intakes, they may be affected by what the person has been eating recently and may not give a true picture of the person's nutrient stores. This sometimes makes it difficult for the assessor to detect a subclinical deficiency. Furthermore, many nutrients interact. The assessor has to keep in mind that an abnormal lab value for one nutrient may reflect abnormal status with respect to other nutrients. Recall, for example, that a zinc deficiency presents symptoms of vitamin A deficiency.

Nutrition Assessment Completed

Once all the available pieces of the puzzle have accumulated from the many types of data, the assessor assembles them into a complete picture. All these pieces are needed to make sense of a person's nutrition status. The ultimate diagnosis is appropriately tentative and is confirmed only after careful remedial steps have been taken and have been shown to successfully alleviate the observed problems.

Research continues in the field of nutrition assessment to identify methods of accurately determining body composition. As you have read through the components of nutrition assessments in this book, you may have noticed that each method has drawbacks and possible inaccuracies. These methods were presented to you because they are the most practical and commonly used methods in general practice—not because they are the best indicators of nutrition status. It is hoped that researchers will discover still more practical and cost-effective assessment techniques that will provide a clearer picture of a person's nutrition status.

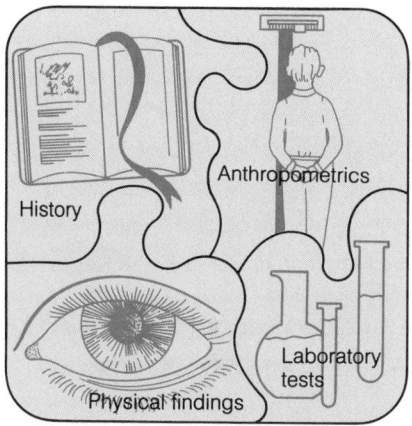

The pieces of nutrition assessment fit together to form a complete picture of the person's nutrition status.

The nutrition assessment procedure just described is a far cry from the kind of experience the person on the street may encounter when she walks into a "nutrition clinic" and is offered a "nutrition assessment" by a "nutritionist." People today are easily led to believe that "computer diet analysis" or "hair analysis" or urine tests will accurately determine their nutrition status. They do not understand all the processes involved in doing such tests. They see, however, that the "experts" seem to know a lot and that the systems being used are complicated, so they think there must be some validity to the "results."

Although computers are invaluable for doing rapid calculations on valid data that have been assembled with care, they turn out utterly meaningless nonsense when used to process data that are meaningless from the start. A computer program using assigned values for nutrients that have not been carefully studied or a program that has been assembled hastily and carelessly cannot accurately compute nutrient intakes.

Similarly, you may have noticed that hair analysis was not mentioned as one of the clinical tests from which nutrition status information is obtained. Hair analyses are still in the experimental stage. They are being studied to determine what their validity and usefulness may be. In several instances, hair contents of minerals have been demonstrated *not* to reflect body contents of minerals in any consistent way.[11] Too many confounding variables interfere: air and water pollution, shampoos and dyes, and water hardness, among others.

We have singled out computer and hair analyses as two nutrition assessment practices that are being used by unscrupulous practitioners to elicit belief and extract money from an unsuspecting public. We could give many other examples, however. The rule for the cautious consumer should be to stay skeptical. The fact that the consumer doesn't understand or hasn't heard of the method a "nutritionist" is using to test nutrition status may not be a reflection of the consumer's limited knowledge. The test may simply be a fraud.

To know what is wrong with a person's nutrition status is not to remedy it. All the effort you have expended in evaluating a person's nutrition problems will be for naught if you do not use the information to formulate a plan of action that will correct the problems.

The Nutrition Care Plan

Objectives of a nutrition care plan:
· To meet the client's nutrient needs.
· To educate the client.

A nutrition care plan translates assessment data into a strategy for meeting the client's nutrient and nutrition education needs. It concentrates on intervention and defines the goals of intervention. Once you have completed a nutrition assessment, you have generated a data base from which you can assemble valuable information. The first step in formulating a nutrition care plan is to analyze nutrition assessment data to generate a nutrition problem list. Determine current and past problems that affect nutrition status. Be sure to consider possible drug-nutrient interactions if the person is taking medication.

Once you have generated a problem list, you should define strategies for tackling each nutrition problem. The plan you identify will be dependent on the reason for the problem. If the nutrition problem is diarrhea, it is important to know the cause before you can work out a strategy for dealing with it. If, for example, the diarrhea is caused by a milk allergy, eliminating milk and milk products from the diet would be an important strategy in solving the problem. Another part of your plan in such a case would be to counsel the client on a diet that eliminates milk and milk products. It would also be important to provide ample fluid and electrolytes to prevent dehydration. You will be learning more about the specific strategies for dealing with a variety of medical disorders in Chapters 16 through 22.

Educating the client is a vital part of the nutrition care plan. Whenever possible, the client and those who care for her should be aware of and understand the importance of the measures being taken to maintain or improve nutrition health. For example, a client in the hospital will be prescribed a liquid diet for a day in preparation for a diagnostic test. Explain to the client why she will be receiving only liquids for that day and caution her not to eat foods other than those on the hospital tray.

Often the nutrition care plan involves more than a short-term simple dietary adjustment. For such situations, nutrition counseling is appropriate. Nutrition counseling has been defined as the "total process of providing individualized guidance so that the client acquires the ability to self-manage his/her own nutrition care, i.e., successfully effect behavior change that results in more healthful behaviors."[12] Nutrition education is but one part of nutrition counseling. Nutrition education involves the provision of information, whereas nutrition counseling helps the client use information to change her eating habits.

An important part of the nutrition care plan is to determine specific goals. If, for example, a person needs a weight reduction diet, you might determine that the client should lose one pound a week for three months and design a diet to meet that goal. You must determine specific objectives of the diet, determine the content of the counseling session, and develop a tentative time frame for accomplishing the objectives. The dietitian most frequently assumes responsibility for nutrition counseling. However, in some hospitals, outpatient clinics, and nursing homes, a dietitian may not be available. The nurse, dietetic technician, or other health care professional may be expected to assume this responsibility.

Implementing and Evaluating the Nutrition Care Plan

Once you have used assessment data to identify the client's nutrition and nutrition education needs, you must take the next step: Implement the nutrition care plan. Use the strategies you have developed to reach your goals for the client's care. Equally important, you must evaluate the effectiveness of your care plan. Are the strategies you have developed meeting the goals for the client? Have other events occurred in the client's life that have changed his nutrition status or altered his nutrient needs? Are the nutrition counseling strategies working, or is the client unable to make the necessary diet changes?

The care process is continuous. The initial nutrition care plan may change frequently as new needs are identified. For example, a person admitted to the hospital for a diagnostic workup may later become a candidate for surgery. As your client's needs change, adjust the care plan to meet them. Be on the alert for changes in medical status so that nutrition needs are not neglected; try a new plan when original approaches fall short.

The involvement of the entire health team in planning, implementing, and evaluating the nutrition care plan will help ensure that the client's needs are met. Strong professional communication networks are beneficial to both the client and the health care team in order to ensure that common goals are understood.

Professional Communication Networks

One way professionals communicate is through the medical record. The medical record is a compilation of the history, the diagnosis and therapy, and the prognosis for each client. It is an important way of sharing information with the health care team. You can continuously assess your client's condition and response to therapy by regularly reading the medical record. You can use this information to determine how to provide the best possible care.

medical record:
a continuous written account of a client's medical care.

diagnosis:
the disease a person has or is thought to have.
dia = through
gnosis = knowing

prognosis:
the predicted course and outcome of a disease.
pro = ahead of time, before

An entry made in a POMR is generally written in the form of a **SOAP note.** SOAP stands for Subjective, Objective, Assessment, and Plan.

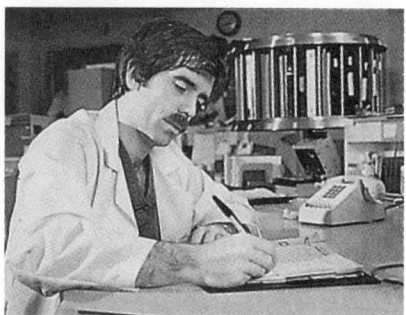

Take time to record important nutrition information in the client's medical record.

Medical records can be organized in many ways. The problem-oriented medical record (POMR) is in common use today. To use this approach, health care team members list each medical problem of the client to generate a problem list. Subsequently, each entry made in the record addresses the actions being taken to deal with the problems. New problems are added to the list as they arise.

Learn how to effectively use the record in the facility where you work. Regardless of the type of medical record used, however, you should always record important nutrition information in the client's medical record. The following are some examples of important information:

- Evaluation of the client's current diet.
- Nutrition assessment data.
- Recommended nutrition therapy.
- The client's acceptance and tolerance of the diet.
- Documentation of diet counseling.
- Any planned followup or referral to another person or agency.
- The client's response to nutrition care.
- The client's response to diet counseling.

Various health care professionals generally keep records of their own in addition to the formal medical record. For example, a nurse keeps a nursing care plan, and a dietitian keeps a nutrition care plan. These records contain some of the information contained in the formal medical record. However, they also include plans and notes that are more detailed and pertinent to the individual health care team member. For example, a nutrition care plan may have more details regarding a client's reaction to a diet, which will later be considered in preparation for diet counseling. Because nurses are involved with direct client care more often than other team members, it is wise to ensure that the nursing care plan contains information regarding special nutrition needs.

Health care team members can share other avenues of communication in addition to medical records. Team members within a health care facility can be phoned or paged when problems are identified or questions arise. In emergencies, team members can be reached in another facility, at the office, at home, or through an answering service.

In an institutional setting, bedside rounds provide an ideal opportunity for professional communication. During rounds, clients are visited and examined as necessary. The health care team members discuss the clients' cases either before or after the visits. Use these discussions to talk over nutrition problems and to exchange information about the clients' concerns and attitudes.

Nurses also report to one another at the end of each shift. This time can be used to pass along information regarding a client's special nutrition needs or requests.

This chapter describes how to assess nutrition status and reviews the procedure through which such data can be translated into a plan for the maintenance or improvement of nutrition health. The next chapter looks more closely at meeting the nutrition needs of people in health care facilities.

Bedside rounds provide an excellent opportunity to discuss your concerns regarding a person's nutrition status.

Nutrition Assessment and Care

Mrs. Evans, a 38-year-old computer scientist, was admitted to the hospital for testing following a car accident. Her injuries included several broken bones and a collapsed left lung. Her lab report revealed a mildly depleted serum albumin and a moderately depleted total lymphocyte count. After reviewing her medical record, the health care team decided that a complete nutrition assessment was necessary. The following significant information resulted:

Anthropometrics
 Height: 5'7".
 Weight: 150 lb.
 Frame size: medium.

Physical Findings
 Hair: dull, easily plucked.
 Others: none noted.

Medical History
 Injuries sustained in the car accident imply increased nutrient requirements.

Laboratory Findings
 Serum albumin: 3 g/dl (mildly depleted).
 Total lymphocyte count: 1,000 mm^3 (moderately depleted).

Diet History
 Usual weight: 175 lb.
 Weight loss intentional.
 Very low-kcalorie, low-carbohydrate diet over the past six weeks.

Drug History
 One standard multivitamin-mineral pill daily.
 No other drugs.

1. Determine Mrs. Evans' ideal body weight and calculate percent ideal body weight.

2. Calculate percent usual body weight.

3. Consider Mrs. Evans' recent weight change. What is a safe rate of weight loss (see p. 000)? How does Mrs. Evans' weight loss compare with the safe rate? Does her recent weight change heighten her risk of poor nutrition status?

4. What do Mrs. Evans' lab values indicate with respect to her protein status (see Appendix B)?

5. Are there any other factors in Mrs. Evans' medical and drug history or physical findings suggestive of malnutrition (see Appendix B)?

6. Describe the steps that would go into the preparation of a nutrition care plan for Mrs. Evans. After you have prepared a plan, what other measures must you take to complete the nutrition care process?

7. Consider opportunities for discussing your concerns about Mrs. Evans' nutrition status with other health professionals.

Notes

1. S. B. Heymsfield and K. Casper, Anthropometric assessment of the adult hospitalized patient, *Journal of Parenteral and Enteral Nutrition* 11 (Supplement 1987): 36S–41S.

2. J. P. Grant, Nutritional assessment in clinical practice, *Nutrition in Clinical Practice* 1 (1986): 3–11.

3. Bioelectrical impedance to measure body fat, *Nutrition and the MD* 13, March 1987, pp. 4–5.

4. Lukaski and coauthors, Assessment of fat-free mass using bioelectrical impedance measurement of the human body, *American Journal of Clinical Nutrition* 41 (1985): 810–817.

5. A. S. Jackson and M. L. Pollock, Practical assessment of body composition, *The Physician and Sportsmedicine* 13, May 1985, pp. 76–90.

6. F. I. Katch and coauthors, Letter to the editor: Validity of bioelectrical impedance to estimate body composition in cardiac and pulmonary patients, *American Journal of Clinical Nutrition* 43 (1986): 972–973.

7. N. W. Solomons, How valid are bioelectrical impedance measurements in body composition studies? *American Journal of Clinical Nutrition* 44 (1986): 306–307.

8. D. R. Hunt, B. J. Rowlands, and D. Johnston, Hand grip strength—A simple prognostic indicator in surgical patients, *Journal of Parenteral and Enteral Nutrition* 9 (1985): 701–704.

9. Grant, 1986.

10. M. Walser, Creatinine excretion as a measure of protein nutrition in adults of varying age, *Journal of Parenteral and Enteral Nutrition* 11 (Supplement 1987): 73S–78S.

11. L. M. Klevay and coauthors, Hair analysis in clinical and experimental medicine, *American Journal of Clinical Nutrition* 46 (1987): 233–236.

12. C. E. Vickery and P. A. Hodges, Counseling strategies for dietary management: Expanded possibilities for effecting behavior change, *Journal of the American Dietetic Association* 86 (1986): 924–928.

13

The Computer in Nutrition Care

Computers are a fixture in our lives today. We use computers at home and in school, for business and for pleasure. Most students today are so accustomed to computers that they may have little appreciation for the way computers have changed our lives. If you are not impressed by the role of computers in our lives, consider the words of Christopher Evans, author of *The Micro Millenium:* "If the automobile industry had developed at the same rate as computers and over the same amount of time, you would be able to buy a Rolls-Royce today for $2.75; it would get 3 million miles to the gallon and would deliver enough power to drive the *Queen Elizabeth II* oceanliner. And, if you were interested in miniaturization, you could put half a dozen of them on a pinhead." This Nutrition in Practice highlights some of the ways that the health care professional can use computers to provide effective nutrition care. The Miniglossary defines some specific terms you may hear about with respect to computers.

I have used a computer in several classes that I have taken, so I know something about how they work. But I really don't know how they are used in health care facilities. Can you give me some information?

In hospitals and other health care settings that use computers, the system generally consists of one computer that is accessed through a network of computer terminals conveniently located at various

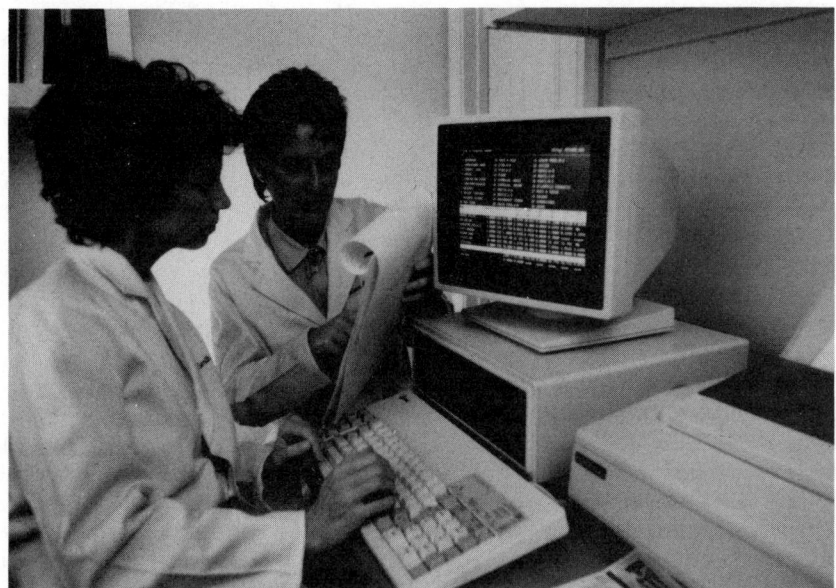

Computers aid health care professionals in providing effective health care.

stations throughout the facility. For example, in the hospital each nursing station has a terminal. Other terminals are found in various departments, such as the dietary department and the pharmacy. The number of terminals and their locations depend on the needs of the facility.

The network of computer terminals in a health care facility can dramatically save time and reduce operating costs. As an example, consider the computer billing systems currently in use in most hospitals. Everything that is ordered for a client while in the hospital is ordered via

computer. Drugs, diet, IV fluids, x-rays, physical therapy treatments, and other supplies and professional services are ordered and billed using the computer. In years past, nurses would have to call in numerous orders for each of many clients to different departments and then ensure that each client was appropriately billed for the supplies or services. You can see how much time this would take, not only for the nurses but also for the departments receiving orders for supplies and services.

From this example you can probably see that computer systems significantly reduce human error. When orders are transmitted verbally, communication errors are more likely to occur. If a nurse is ordering an IV feeding by phone while worried about the client in room 425 and the pharmacist at the other end of the line is in a noisy room, the chances of an error in communication are great. When the communication is printed (as it would be if ordered by computer), the information can be checked and verified.

OK. I can see why computers are useful in a health care facility. But how can they specifically help me in the area of nutrition?
More than 200 computer software programs are available in the field of food science and human nutrition.[1] Computers can help health care professionals with each step of the nutrition care process.[2] First, they can help with nutrition assessment and the interpretation of assessment data. To perform a nutrition assessment, you must collect many pieces of information, compare the anthropometric and biochemical information with standards, analyze nutrient intake, perform some mathematical calculations (%IBW, %UBW, midarm muscle circumference), and determine nutrient needs. After health care professionals collect assessment data, they can use computer programs to analyze anthropometric and biochemical information to identify individuals at risk for poor nutrition status. These programs quickly perform mathematical functions to save valuable time.

Among the most commonly used programs in dietetics are diet analysis programs that estimate the nutrients in a client's diet and enable the dietitian to compare these intakes to dietary standards such as the RDA. To complete this task without the aid of a computer is tedious and time consuming. A sample printout from a diet analysis program is shown in Figure NP13–1.

How can computer programs help develop a nutrition care plan?
Computer programs can be used to formulate an appropriate feeding program. An example is the selection of a tube-feeding formula. As you will see in Chapter 15, a good deal of information must be taken into account when choosing a tube-feeding formula and a method of delivery. The decisions can be overwhelming, especially when the person requiring the formula has several medical conditions that affect nutrient needs. A computer program to help manage these many considerations has been developed.[3] Similarly, computer programs are available to help practitioners plan intravenous therapy as well.[4]

Another way computers can help health care professionals develop nutrition care plans is with programs that assist in the development of diet patterns for people with diabetes (Chapter 19).[5] The diet for a person with diabetes is carefully calculated to include controlled portions of carbohydrate, protein, and fat. Calculating the diet can be very time consuming, as the process requires many mathematical manipulations. Computer programs can simplify the task significantly.

Similar computer programs have been developed to assist dietitians in filling diet prescriptions for clients with phenylketonuria (PKU).[6] PKU is an inherited disorder of metabolism that requires strict adherence to a very restricted diet. To calculate the diet manually is time consuming and difficult.

How can computers help to implement and evaluate nutrition care plans?
To help implement nutrition care plans, computer programs can assist with nutrition education. Computers can help clients understand the concepts of good nutrition. For clients who need special diet advice, software programs are available to teach the rationale and the mechanics of the diets they need. Such programs are available in the areas of weight control, diabetes, and hyperlipidemias, to name a few. Programs to help clients understand the association of sodium with hypertension and how to identify the sodium content of foods are other examples.

Additional programs are available to educate the public. Some of them are intended to educate consumers about general food and nutrition facts. Others give consumers information about shopping and food costs. These programs may cover such topics as reading labels, using coupons, unit pricing, meal planning, and reducing the amount of food wastage.

Once any nutrition care plan has been implemented, computer programs can assist the health care team in monitoring the client's response to therapy. A large volume of data must be considered in determining whether or not an individual is responding adequately to nutrition care. Computer programs

NUTRITION IN PRACTICE 13

FIGURE NP13–1 Sample printout from a diet analysis program.

Nutrition summary

QUANTITY	NAME	WGT (G)	CAL	PROT. (G)	FIBER (G)	CARB. (G)	CHOL (MG)	FAT-UN (G)	FAT (G)	VIT A (IU)	B1 (MG)	B2 (MG)	B6 (MG)	B12 (MCG)	FOL. (MCG)
2 ea	Cooked Egg	100	158	12.1	0	1.2	526	5.9	11.1	520	.074	.286	.114	1.31	49
1 cup	2% lowfat milk	244	121	8.12	0	11.7	22	1.62	4.78	500	.095	.403	.105	.888	12
2 pce	Whole Wheat Bread-soft	56	130	5.2	2.8	27.6	0	.8	1.4	2	.18	.060	.076	0	31.2
2 tsp	Butter	9	67.7	.080		.005	21.4	2.5	7.66	289	.000	.003	.000	.000	.291
	TOTALS:	409	477	25.5	2.8	40.5	569	10.8	25.0	1311	.349	.752	.295	2.20	92.4

Nutrition summary

QUANTITY	NAME	WGT (G)	NIAC. (MG)	PANTO (MG)	VIT C (MG)	VIT E (MG)	CA (MG)	CU (MG)	IRON (MG)	MG (MG)	PHOS. (MG)	POTAS. (MG)	SEL. (MCG)	NA (MG)	ZINC (MG)
2 ea	Cooked Egg	100	.060	1.72	0	.77	56	.096	2.08	12.2	180	130	9.56	138	1.44
1 cup	2% lowfat milk	244	.21	.781	2.32	.146	297	.073	.12	33	232	377	5.66	122	.963
2 pce	Whole Wheat Bread-soft	56	1.6	.238	.002	.868	48	.134	1.79	43.6	142	144	26.4	296	1.06
2 tsp	Butter	9	.004			.149	2.25	.002	.015	.166	2.16	2.41	.062	77.9	.004
	TOTALS:	409	1.87	2.74	2.32	1.93	403	.305	4.00	88.9	556	653	41.6	634	3.47

```
Name: Nutrition summary

Items analyzed:

    2    ea   Cooked Egg
    1    cup  2% lowfat milk
    2    pce  Whole Wheat Bread-soft
    2    tsp  Butter

                    NUTRITIONAL ANALYSIS
                 (Plus % RDA for EXAMPLE)

           Weight:   409   Grams   (14.4 Ounces)

    Calories           477     (22%)**   Carbohydrates   40.5 G   ( 13%)*
    Protein           25.5 G   (54%)     Cholesterol      569 MG  (190%)*
    Dietary Fiber      2.8 G   (13%)*    Fat-unsat.      10.8 G   ( 23%)*
    Vitamin A         1311 IU  (33%)     Fat-total       25.0 G   ( 35%)*
    Thiamin-B1        .349 MG  (32%)     Calcium          403 MG  ( 50%)
    Riboflavin-B2     .752 MG  (58%)     Copper          .305 MG  ( 12%)*
    Pyridoxine-B6     .295 MG  (15%)     Iron            4.00 MG  ( 22%)
    Cobalamin-B12     2.20 MCG (73%)     Magnesium       88.9 MG  ( 30%)
    Folacin           92.4 MCG (23%)     Phosphorus       556 MG  ( 70%)
    Niacin-B3         1.87 MG  (13%)     Potassium        653 MG  ( 17%)*
    Pantothenic acid  2.74 MG  (39%)*    Selenium        41.6 MCG ( 33%)*
    Vitamin C         2.32 MG  ( 4%)     Sodium           634 MG  ( 21%)*
    Vitamin E         1.93 MG  (24%)     Zinc            3.47 MG  ( 23%)

         * No specific RDA; suggested values.
        ** Average value; individual needs may vary.

         Calories from:    Protein         21%
                           Carbohydrates   33%
                           Fats            46%
```

can help integrate this information and save team members' time.

From what you're saying, it sounds as if computers can do everything! If computers can do all these things, what is left for the health care professional?

You can take comfort in knowing that computers can never take the place of the health care professional. Our increasing dependence on computers sometimes makes it difficult to keep in mind that computers are only machines. They can do only what they have been programmed to do by human beings. They are not inherently foolproof. Therefore, we must depend on our own knowledge and common sense to interpret the information generated by computers. Diet analysis programs are a case in point.

Diet analysis programs estimate the amounts of various nutrients consumed in a diet and compare them to a standard such as the RDA. Their accuracy depends not only on the record of foods eaten that is presented to the computer but also on the food composition values that were entered into the data base. Remember that data bases are not perfect; they too are created by human beings. If there are inaccurate values in the data base, the results of the analysis become meaningless. Furthermore, even with complete and accurate values, the program user must know how to interpret the results appropriately. To adequately interpret the computer analysis, a user must have enough nutrition knowledge to know that nutrient values are only estimates, that food composition varies, and that individual requirements for different nutrients also vary.

Another point to keep in mind is that computers can't be programmed to deal with human elements such as feelings and emotions. A computer program that helps a client to learn a special diet cannot see the client's reaction to the instructions. It cannot detect changes in the client's body language that might tell a professional that the client was uncomfortable with a diet. Computer programs can be a valuable tool, but they cannot replace a thinking human being.

So far everything we've talked about is related to direct client care. Are there ways the computer can help me personally with nutrition?

Miniglossary of Computer Terms

bit short for *binary digit:* the smallest unit of computer information.

byte a sequence of bits.

data base the body of information stored by the computer.

diskette a thin, flexible magnetic disk protected in a jacket and used to store or read computer information.

display screen the televisionlike monitor, part of the terminal, that allows computer users to see what they are working on.

floppy disk another name for a diskette.

hard copy a printed copy of the information stored in the computer.

hardware mechanical, magnetic, or electronic equipment used to process data. The hardware limits the type of software that can be used (see also *software*).

input the information that is entered into the computer.

mainframe computer a large computer capable of storing more data than a microcomputer.

Mainframe computers can perform multiple functions very rapidly and are used by many large businesses, research centers, and universities.

microcomputer a smaller computer capable of performing functions similar to mainframe computers. Microcomputers are smaller, less expensive computers frequently found in hospitals and small businesses.

output the information that the computer prints out on paper or displays on the terminal screen.

program the set of step-by-step instructions that tells the computer how to perform a task (see also *software*).

software computer programs that allow the user to perform various functions. Not all software can be used with every computer; hardware and software must be compatible (see also *hardware*).

terminal a keyboard and display screen that allow the user to access and process the information stored in a computer.

Yes, there are many ways. Computers are useful in teaching students about nutrition. Clinical case studies that simulate real-life situations give students practice in dealing with clients and their special needs. The students can work at their own pace, and the instructor has a record of the students' responses. Other programs teach nutrition by giving students information and then asking them to answer questions based on the information given. Students frequently use diet analysis programs to see how their own nutrient intakes compare to the RDA.

You have looked at several of the numerous applications of computers in nutrition. No doubt computers will continue to play a greater and greater role in the way we function as health care professionals as well as in other aspects of our lives. Use the computer to your advantage; be aware of the computer programs available in the facility where you work and of others that you might want your facility to purchase. Computer programs will help you do your job more efficiently and save you valuable time.

Notes

1. R. A. Sager, The software search: A dilemma, *Journal of Dietetic Software* 3 (1986): 8–9.

2. D. A. August and coauthors, Computers and nutritional support, *Nutritional Support Services* 6 (1986): 47–54.

3. J. B. Krasner, A technique for optimization of enteral feeding regimens: Implementation on a microcomputer, *Journal of Parenteral and Enteral Nutrition* 10 (1986): 208–212.

4. F. M. Edwards, Computer assisted planning of parenteral hyperalimentation therapy, *Critical Care Medicine* 10 (1982): 539–543.

5. J. L. Balintfy and L. M. Lancaster, Computing "best fit" calorie-controlled diet patterns by microcomputer, *Journal of the American Dietetic Association* 87 (1987): 73–74.

6. K. Anderson, B. Kennedy, and P. B. Acosta, Computer-implemented nutrition support of phenylketonuria, *Journal of the American Dietetic Association* 12 (1985): 1623–1625.

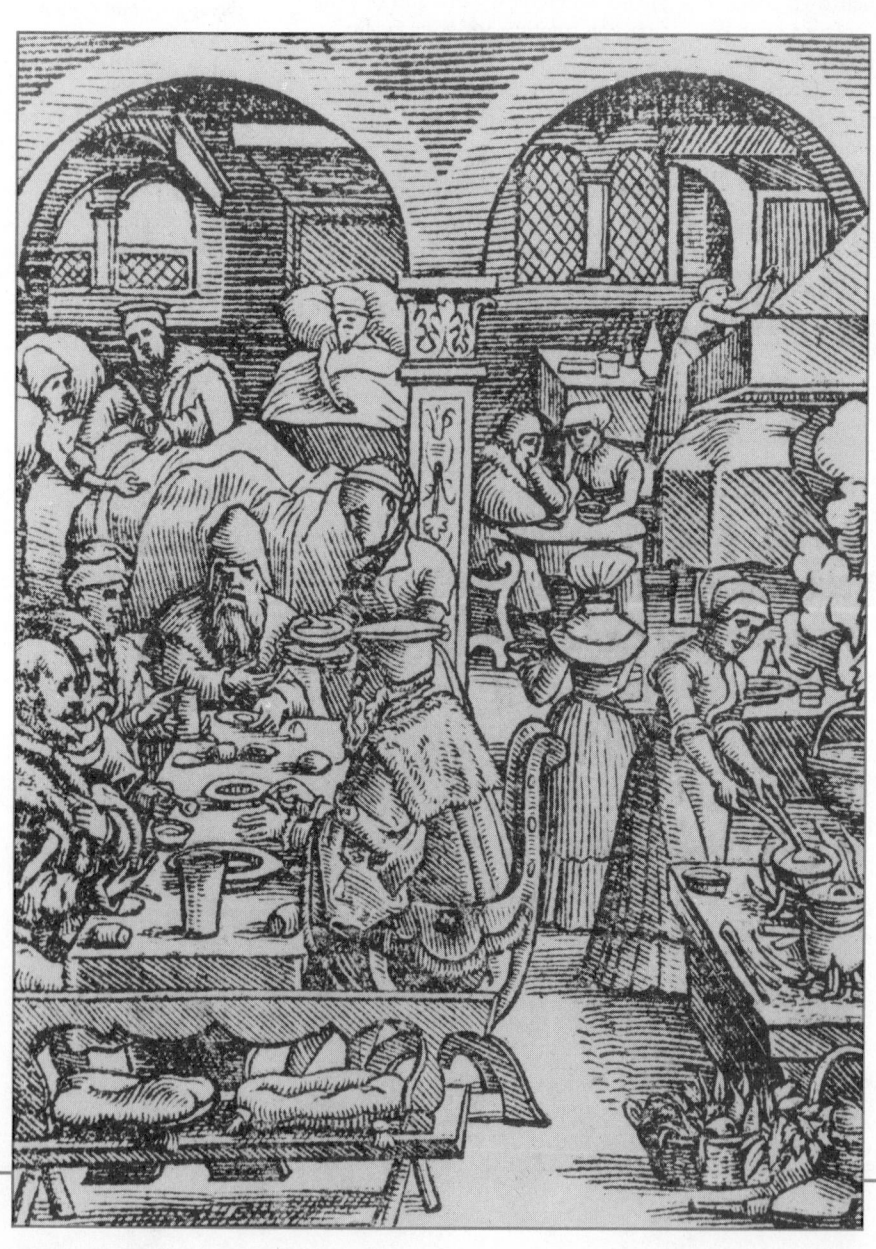

14

Nutrition and Illness

CONTENTS

Hospital Kitchen, Anonymous. Woodcut Courtesy of National Library of Medicine.

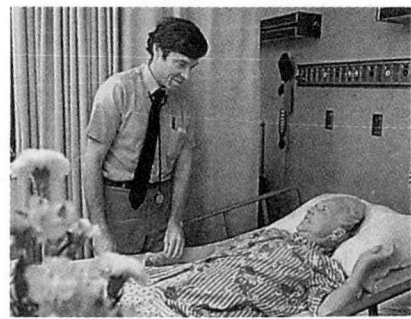

Illness can severely affect nutrition status.

The word **illness** as used in this chapter refers to any medical condition that alters nutrition status. Not all such conditions are diseases. For example, major surgery can have a significant impact on nutrition status (see Chapter 16), although it is not a disease.

It is technically incorrect to speak of body protein stores, because proteins (amino acids) are not stored in the body. All protein is functional; that is, it is being used in some capacity (as part of cell structure, as skeletal muscle, as enzymes or immune factors, or as other body protein components).

Thus far, the focus of our study of nutrition has centered on the basic principles of nutrition, how nutrient needs change throughout life, and how to assess nutrition status. In this and the remaining chapters of this book, we will be looking more specifically at how medical disorders affect nutrition and nutrient needs. This chapter introduces the general concepts of modified diets and diet therapy and identifies some of the unique problems encountered when people are fed in health care facilities.

The Effect of Illness on Nutrition Status

The impact of nutrition on all people, regardless of their state of health, should be obvious at this point. The effect of good nutrition and other health habits on wellness were discussed at length in Chapter 9. Now we turn our attention to illness, specifically, how illness affects nutrition status and how nutrition status can affect the course of an illness.

The effect that an illness has on nutrition status depends on both the severity and the duration of the illness. Disorders that markedly change a person's metabolic rate over long periods greatly enhance the risk of nutrient deficiencies. A person who is unable to eat or retain nutrients (severe vomiting, diarrhea, or malabsorption) is also at risk. Nutrition status may be further compromised by drug therapy used to treat a disorder as well as by the inactivity that frequently accompanies illness. For now, we turn our attention to serious illness and its effect on nutrition status.

Protein-kCalorie Malnutrition and Illness

PCM is of particular concern for the person with serious illness for many reasons including those just discussed. However, to more fully understand the relationship of PCM to serious illness, a basic knowledge is needed of how the body responds to such a stress.

Since the body's requirement for protein and energy increases remarkably during stress, a person's ability to respond to stress depends to a large extent, on available energy reserves and protein status. When energy is not supplied in adequate amounts from the diet, the body uses protein to meet energy needs. When this adaptation occurs, functional protein is lost from skeletal muscle, organs (liver, gut, and lungs), and circulating pools of protein (albumin and immune factors).

For the well-nourished person, loss of *some* protein is not critical, since adequate protein remains to support vital functions. However, during prolonged stress or when malnutrition occurs, the protein loss can be serious. For example, loss of protein in a malnourished person following surgery can result in pneumonia. The loss of a critical number of functioning lung cells combined with a reduced synthesis of immune factors leads to deterioration of lung function and depression of the immune system.

Organs where cells are being replaced rapidly are among the first to be affected by PCM. One such organ system is the GI tract. Once a person develops PCM, the intestinal microvilli gradually shrink and become nonfunctional. Up to 90 percent of them can be lost. The person then has serious difficulty absorbing nutrients which makes the PCM worse.

Within the cell, PCM affects the synthesis of enzymes and other protein molecules necessary for proper metabolism and maintenance of the cell's structure. These protein molecules usually are synthesized and degraded rapidly in the body to help the body adapt promptly to changes in the environment. Losing this ability to adapt is critical.

Protein and fat are used to meet energy requirements once glycogen stores are depleted. Thus, the body's protein and fat compartments are of particular concern in nutrition assessment of the person who is ill (see Chapter 13). Deficiency of vitamins and minerals can also occur simultaneously and further compromise nutrition status. PCM interferes with the body's ability to heal wounds, mount an immune response, and maintain the function of vital organs and skeletal muscle. Furthermore, malnutrition can result in higher morbidity and mortality rates, a greater incidence of postoperative complications, and longer hospital stays, all of which raise health care costs.[1]

In summary, to understand the relationship of protein-kcalorie malnutrition to serious illness, think of energy stores and protein status as money in a savings account. Illness can be compared to a major expense that arises unexpectedly. The person who has saved enough money can cover the expense without too much difficulty. However, if more and more unexpected expenses arise, there may not be enough money to pay them all. The person with little or no savings faces the same problem but is unable to pay even a small expense.

PCM in the Hospital

PCM is a significant problem among people who are hospitalized. A recent study of people in a hospital found that 55 percent were likely to be malnourished.[2] Furthermore, only one in twenty of these people received appropriate nutrition therapy either before developing complications or early in their hospitalization. It may seem inconceivable that something as basic as sound nutrition can be neglected in hospitals where the latest technology abounds. Part of the problem may be a basic failure of health care professionals to recognize the prevalence of PCM and to fully appreciate PCM's consequences to a person who is battling an illness.

Take a moment to imagine you are in a foreign country where you do not understand the language. As you walk down the street, you see signs that describe and direct. But the signs are meaningless to you, for you have yet to learn how to think, speak, or read this new language. Many health care professionals travel through hospitals looking at signs of malnutrition without recognizing them. They look at a person's pale complexion and lack of appetite and see only that the person has a disease; they see a person's poor posture and lethargic attitude and attribute these signs to old age. They have yet to learn to think "nutrition." Malnutrition is easy to miss if you are not looking for it. Caring for people requires that you at least consider the *possibility* that ill health may be due not just to a disease but perhaps to nutrient deficiencies. To overlook nutrition is to provide less than adequate care. The signs of malnutrition are there if you know where to look and how to read them.

People in the hospital may be deprived of food for days at a time while they undergo medical tests and diagnostic procedures. During the very time when their nutrient needs may be high, they are not being given adequate amounts of nutrients; as a result PCM quickly develops. They may also be taking medications that interfere with their appetites.

PCM is preventable. Lack of understanding of the role of nutrition in recovery from disease may explain why weight loss often goes unnoticed, diets often are inadequate, and people in the hospital are allowed to reach an advanced stage of depletion (which may be irreversible). Poor communication among various health care providers is probably a major contributor to PCM. PCM is more likely to occur when a physician orders that a person receive nothing by mouth or orders drugs that interfere with nutrition status or procedures that interfere with nutrient intake. Because PCM results not only from another disease but also from the treatment of that disease, it can be referred to as *physician-induced* or *hospital-induced malnutrition*.

Preventing Protein-kCalorie Malnutrition

The best way to prevent PCM is to assess nutrition status frequently and remedy any problems before they become serious. However, performing complete nutrition assessments takes time. It is often impossible for a dietitian to assess every person being followed in a clinic or treated in a health care facility. For this reason, many health care facilities rely on nutrition screening procedures to identify people at risk for poor nutrition status.

Basically, nutrition screening is a brief nutrition assessment to help identify those who need a more in-depth assessment. All members of the health care team can be a part of the nutrition screening process. Many different procedures have been identified for nutrition screening.[3] Here are some ways that you can help with the nutrition screening process:

- Review the individual's diet, drug, and medical history. Does the person's history reveal risk factors for poor nutrition status?
- Check lab reports on tests that have already been run. Do urinary creatinine excretion, serum albumin, transferrin, or total lymphocyte count suggest malnutrition?
- Weigh each person regularly. (See Appendix B for instructions on how to measure weight.) Is the person's weight for height adequate but not excessive? Has the person been losing or gaining weight? How much? How fast?
- Look at the person. Are there obvious signs of malnutrition? Is the client emaciated? Obese? Extremely pale?
- If the person is being treated in a health care facility, check the person's tray frequently to see if food is being eaten. If the client is to receive nothing by mouth (NPO) and therefore is unable to eat, how long has it been since the client has eaten? Is the client expected to be able to eat soon? Are adequate nutrients being delivered by vein? (See the box "How to Calculate the Nutrient Content of IV Solutions" in Chapter 15.)

Physician-induced malnutrition, technically, is **iatrogenic** (eye-AT-ro-GEN-ic) **malnutrition.** This term includes malnutrition caused by prescription medications.
iatros = physician
genic = arising from

nutrition screening:
the use of preliminary nutrition assessment techniques to identify people who are malnourished or who are at risk for malnutrition.

To identify people at risk for poor nutrition status:

Check the client's history for risk factors for poor nutrition status.

Check lab test results.

Weigh each client regularly.

Look for physical signs of malnutrition.

Observe what and how much the client eats.

Get help if you suspect a problem

NPO:
An order that means that nothing is to be given to the person orally (including food and medications). NPO stands for *nil per os*, which means "nothing by mouth." On the other hand, PO stands for *per os*, which means "by mouth" or "orally."

- Most important, communicate any problems that you discover to someone who can help. The problem may go unnoticed if you do not speak up. A dietitian can perform an in-depth nutrition assessment. Be persistent if you suspect that a problem is being ignored.

Nutrition screening is vital. A recent study showed that nutrition screening at admission in 33 hospitals identified risk of poor nutrition status in over 50 percent of the clients for whom enough information was available to perform the screening.[4] Always check for signs of malnutrition. Remember that a person's nutrition status can deteriorate rapidly during the course of hospitalization.

Because people being treated in the hospital are likely to be seriously ill, the individual who is hospitalized is also more likely than an outpatient to be malnourished. An advantage of inpatient treatment, though, is that the health care team has more control over nutrition care. You may advise an outpatient to drink plenty of fluids to aid recovery from a bladder infection, but you really cannot encourage this intake once the person goes home. However, in a health care facility, team members can bring the person fluids, encourage the person to drink them, and record the amounts of fluid actually consumed. Ways of meeting people's nutrient needs in health care facilities are discussed next.

inpatient:
a person being treated or residing in a health care facility. Hospitals, nursing homes, rehabilitation centers, some eating disorder centers, and some drug and alcohol centers provide inpatient services.

Food Service in Health Care Facilities

To prepare and serve food in a health care setting is a challenge. The overall responsibility for food service rests with either a chief administrative dietitian or a food service manager. These individuals direct all aspects of food service from purchasing to delivery of food to the client.

The clinical dietitian works directly with clients to assess the clients' nutrition status, to plan appropriate diets, and to provide nutrition education. The nurse often reinforces the nutrition education given by the dietitian. In some facilities, dietetic technicians assist the dietitians in both administrative and clinical duties. Among the other employees of the dietary department are clerks, aides, cooks, and porters.

Many health care facilities provide clients with menus from which they can select the foods they will receive while in the facility. This system helps to ensure that clients will receive acceptable foods. It also gives clients a feeling of having some control over their lives in the hospital environment.

In facilities where it is not possible to offer a selective menu, the dietary department serves a balanced diet, altering the basic diet according to diet orders. Such menus are generally very flexible. For example, if the vegetable served at dinner is broccoli, a food the client doesn't like, green beans might be substituted.

You can help your client greatly and save yourself needless aggravation and time by learning something about the food service system in the health care facility where you work. Some of the things you will want to know include:

- The number to call and the procedure to follow if you request a diet the physician has ordered, make diet changes, or report problems with the client's tray.

administrative dietitians:
dietitians primarily concerned with the management of foodservice systems that provide optimal nutrition and quality food, although they sometimes assume some clinical duties as well.

clinical dietitians:
dietitians who are responsible for direct client care—assessing nutrition status, developing and implementing nutrition care plans, and evaluating and reporting the results.

selective menu:
a menu from which clients select the foods they will receive while hospitalized. *House diets* are preselected by the dietary department.

In facilities that utilize a **centralized food service** system, meals are prepared and served from a main kitchen. In a **decentralized food service** system, food is generally prepared in a central kitchen but heated and distributed from smaller satellite kitchens located throughout the institution.

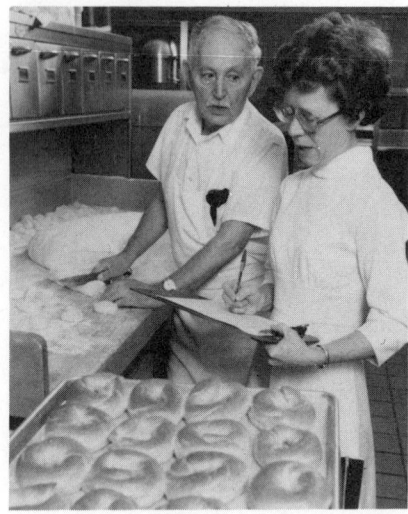

Coordinating food service in a health care facility is a demanding job.

- The number where you can reach the dietitian in case a client needs special nutrition advice.
- The times when meals are plated so that you can call in any requests before those times.
- The location of the diet manual (usually available at each nursing station) and familiarity with its contents.

Once you understand how the dietary department operates, you will know where to turn for help when your client is having problems with food or nutrition.

The hospital is used as the main example of a health care facility in this chapter because it is a setting familiar to most health care providers. Long-term care facilities, such as nursing homes and mental institutions, use similar systems, and most of the information presented in this chapter applies to those settings as well, but some special concerns arise in long-term care facilities. A person in a short-term care facility may not eat well while hospitalized but can make up for nutrient deficits by eating well at home. The resident in a long-term care facility eats in the same place continuously and depends on the foodservice department to provide nutritious and acceptable foods. To provide nutritious foods that a person cannot or will not eat does no good. Therefore, the foodservice personnel must ensure that clients on special diets receive and eat appropriate foods; they cannot rely on deficits being made up later.

Hospital Foods: The Professional Perspective

The primary goal of diet therapy is to achieve or maintain optimal nutrition status. Optimal status is achieved when the cells are provided appropriate amounts of energy, protein, carbohydrate, fat, vitamins, major minerals, trace minerals, and water. These nutrients, in turn, must be provided in a form that is easy for the body to use. For example, if a person's GI tract is not functioning, it will do no good to provide that person with a standard diet.

Each diet prescribed for an individual has its own rationale and purpose. The rationale of a weight reduction diet is to provide less energy from food so that the person will use stored energy and lose weight. The purposes of weight reduction may vary from improving self-image to gaining better control of blood glucose levels.

A person benefits most from diet therapy if his or her nutrition needs have been correctly identified and an appropriate nutrition care plan has been designed. The diet therapy is then selected to meet specific needs and to complement other medical therapy. For example, a diet for an individual with insulin dependent diabetes mellitus (IDDM) must be coordinated so that food is available during the times when the body will have insulin.

Standard and Modified Diets

Regular or *standard diets* are typical diets that provide the recommended daily allowances of nutrients and include all foods. Modifying the regular diet is much like tailoring a suit. A tailored suit is the same suit after alterations—only it fits better. So it is with the modified, or therapeutic, diet. A modified diet is a basic nutritious diet that emphasizes a variety of foods. It is "tailored" by adjusting the consistency; adjusting the level of individual nutrients, energy, or fluid; altering the number of meals; or eliminating certain foods. Table 14–1 gives examples of modified diets used to treat diseases involving different organ systems.

It's helpful to think about modified diets in terms of the symptoms or conditions they relieve rather than in terms of the diseases they are used to treat. People are different, and so are the diets they need. Two people with the same disease may need different diets. Conversely, people in two completely different states of health may benefit from the same diet. Consider two people with cancer and a third who is pregnant. One person with cancer may be nauseated and may need dietary suggestions for controlling nausea. The other person with cancer may be overweight and not experiencing any nausea. The dietary suggestions you make to each cancer client will be different. However, a pregnant woman with nausea may benefit from the same recommendations that you make for the person with cancer who has nausea.

> In the chapters on modified diets that follow, you will be introduced to different diets and the rationales for their uses. You will be given examples of at least one disease or situation for which each diet may be used. As you read, keep in mind the advice you were given previously; diets should be used to treat people rather than diseases. If you know when a diet can help, you can apply your knowledge to help any individual regardless of the actual diagnosis.

The exact foods excluded from or included on a specific modified diet differ among hospitals, generally in minor ways. The variations reflect different schools of thought regarding diet. You can familiarize yourself with a particular institution's diets by reading the institution's diet manual.

In larger hospitals, the diet manual is compiled by the staff of dietitians and approved by the hospital administrator, several physicians, and representatives of the nursing service. A smaller hospital may adopt the diet manual of another hospital or an organization such as the state dietetic association. The diet manual describes what foods are allowed and not allowed on each diet, the rationale and indications for use of the diets, sample menus, and information regarding the nutritional adequacy of the diets. The diets listed in the manual are those available through the dietary department.

The physician prescribes the client's diet and writes the diet order in the medical record. However, the dietitian or other health care team member may consult with the physician about a diet prescription or make recommendations when changes in the diet orders appear warranted. Similarly, the dietitian or nurse may make recommendations to physicians when diet orders are unclear. Keep in mind that many employees in the dietary department do not have formal training in nutrition. Such employees may have difficulty interpreting vague diet orders. Whenever possible, the health care team should jointly recommend the most appropriate diet.

modified or therapeutic diet:
a regular diet that is adjusted to meet special nutrition needs. Such diets can be adjusted in consistency, total food energy, nutrients, amount of fluid, and number of meals or by the elimination of certain foods.

diet order:
a physician's written statement in the medical record of what diet a client should receive.

TABLE 14.1 Summary of Modified Diets by Organ System

Disorders	Possible Diet Modifications	Chapter Reference
Conditions affecting or involving the GI tract, liver, and exocrine pancreas[a]		
Broken jaw	Mechanical soft	16
Celiac disease	Gluten-restricted	22
Cirrhosis	Protein-restricted, sodium-restricted, fluid-restricted	22
Constipation	High-fiber, increased fluids	16
Cystic fibrosis	Low-fat, high-kcalorie, high-protein	20
Dental caries	Mechanical soft	16
Difficulty swallowing (dysphagia)	Mechanical soft, tube feeding, total parenteral nutrition (TPN)	16
Diverticulitis	Low-fiber	16
Diverticulosis	High-fiber	16
Dry mouth	Mechanical soft	16
Dumping syndrome:	Carbohydrate-restricted; no concentrated sugars; small, frequent feedings; fluid and electrolyte replacement	19
Gallbladder disease	kCalorie-restricted, regular	20
Gastritis	Low-fiber, bland	16
Hepatic coma	Protein-restricted, sodium-restricted, fluid-restricted	22
Hepatitis	Regular, high-kcalorie, high-protein	22
Hiatal hernia	Small, frequent feedings; low-fat; bland; weight loss	16
Ill-fitting dentures	Mechanical soft	16
Indigestion (dyspepsia)	Low-fiber; bland; small, frequent feedings	16
Inflammatory bowel disease	Low-fiber, low-fat, high-kcalorie, high-protein, fluid and electrolyte replacement, lactose-restricted, tube feeding, TPN	20
Lactose intolerance	Lactose-restricted	19
Malabsorption	Low-fat, high-kcalorie, high-protein, fluid and electrolyte replacement	20
Missing teeth	Mechanical soft	16
Nausea	Low-fiber; bland; small, frequent feedings	16
Oral surgery	Mechanical soft	16
Pancreatitis	Low-fat; regular; small, frequent feedings; tube feeding; TPN	20
Peptic ulcer	Bland	16
Periodontal disease	Mechanical soft	16
Plastic surgery of head of neck	Mechanical soft, tube feeding, TPN	16
Reflux esophagitis	Small, frequent feedings; low-fat; bland; weight loss	16
Short bowel syndrome	Low-fat, high-kcalorie, high-protein, fluid and electrolyte replacement	20
Ulcers of mouth or gums	Mechanical soft, bland	16
Vomiting	Fluid and electrolyte replacement	16
Conditions of the endocrine pancreas[a]		
Diabetes mellitus	Carbohydrate-controlled, kcalorie-restricted, fat-controlled, high-fiber	19
Hypoglycemia	No concentrated sweets; small, frequent feedings	19

(continued)

TABLE 14–1. Summary of Modified Diets by Organ System (continued)

Disorders	Possible Diet Modifications	Chapter Reference
Conditions affecting the heart and blood vessels		
Atherosclerosis	Fat-controlled, kcalorie-restricted, sodium-restricted, high-fiber	21
Congestive heart failure	Sodium-restricted; kcalorie-restricted; low-fiber; bland; small, frequent feedings; fluid-restricted	21
Coronary heart disease	(see *Atherosclerosis*)	21
Hyperlipidemias	Fat-controlled, kcalorie-restricted, carbohydrate-controlled	21
Hypertension	Low-sodium, kcalorie-restricted, high-potassium; fat-controlled	21
Myocardial infarction	Low-sodium; kcalorie-restricted; low-fiber; bland; small, frequent feedings; moderate-temperature foods; fat-controlled	21
Conditions affecting the kidneys		
Acute renal disease	Protein-restricted, high-kcalorie, fluid-controlled, sodium-controlled, potassium-controlled, fat-controlled, carbohydrate-controlled	22
Chronic renal disease	Protein-restricted, low-sodium, fluid-restricted, potassium-restricted, phosphorus-restricted, fat-controlled, carbohydrate-controlled	22
Kidney stones	Increased fluid intake, calcium-controlled, low-oxalate	22[b]
Nephrotic syndrome	Sodium-restricted, high-kcalorie, high-protein, potassium-restricted	21
Conditions affecting many organ systems		
Acquired immune deficiency syndrome	High-kcalorie, high-protein, increased fluid intake, mechanical soft, tube feeding, TPN	17
Burns	High-kcalorie, high-protein, increased fluid intake	17
Cancer	High-kcalorie, high-protein (see also specific related conditions: dry mouth, indigestion, malabsorption, nausea, plastic surgery of head or neck, ulcers of mouth or gums, vomiting, and so on)	17
Food sensitivities	Elimination of offending substance	11
Galactosemia	Galactose-restricted	19
Obesity, overweight	kCalorie-restricted, high-fiber	18
Phenylketonuria (PKU)	Phenylalanine-restricted	22
Stroke	Mechanical soft, regular, tube feeding	16
Surgery	Regular, high-kcalorie, high-protein, increased fluids	17
Underweight	High-kcalorie, high-protein	17

[a]The pancreas produces both external (exocrine) and internal (endocrine) secretions. The external secretions (enzymes) play an important role in the digestion of food; the internal secretions (insulin and other hormones) play a primary role in the regulation of glucose metabolism.
[b]See Nutrition in Practice 22.

The name given to the diet should be consistent with the name given in the diet manual. To avoid miscommunication, the physician must describe exact modifications when appropriate. For example, a 1,200-kcalorie diet, rather than a low-kcalorie diet, should be specified. A low-sodium diet request should specify the amount of sodium; otherwise, it could be interpreted as containing anything from 500 to 3,000 milligrams of sodium.

When a physician's order for a diet is unclear, ask the physician to clarify the order. In many cases, however, the physician is not available, and the dietitian will determine the exact modification. The dietitian will then record the exact diet being requested in the medical record. If a dietitian is not available and the dietary department receives vague orders from the nursing station, a house diet (usually specified in the diet manual) will be sent.

Because the physician is ultimately responsible for a client's diet order, it is easy for others to follow the order without further consideration. But *all* health care providers are responsible for the client's care.

Ideally, a dietitian or dietetic technician visits all clients and reviews the charts of every person admitted to the hospital. But often the dietitian is assigned to so many people that this is virtually impossible; therefore, most clinical dietitians see only people on modified diets or people they have been asked to see. Some smaller hospitals may not even employ a full-time clinical dietitian.

Mistakes occur daily because of inappropriate diet orders. Consider, for example, the following:

- A grossly overweight individual is described as "well-nourished" and placed on a regular diet. Because the person is not on a modified diet, the dietitian does not see him, and he receives an inappropriate diet and no nutrition advice.

- A physician orders that a person be kept NPO after midnight for a lab test to be run in the morning. Because of a miscommunication, the doctor thinks that the order is changed after the test, but it isn't. The individual is needlessly starved for several more days.

- A person routinely enjoys foods low in sugar and salt. Foods served on the regular diet are too salty for her, so she eats very little food. Furthermore, she feels the hospital has totally neglected its responsibility to provide nutritious foods to its clients.

Why isn't the diet ordered correctly in the first place? In cases where many doctors, interns, and residents are caring for a client, miscommunication can easily occur. The individual may communicate needs more clearly and more often to the nurse or other health care provider than to the physician. Furthermore, the client's doctor may not consider nutrition to be a significant part of the client's care. Whatever the reason, be aware that written diet orders are not always correctly chosen. When they are not, contact the dietitian or alert the physician.

Alternative Feeding Methods

The majority of people in the hospital are given oral diets— either regular or modified—to provide for nutrient needs. If a person cannot eat adequate amounts of ordinary foods to meet these needs, however, other methods of feeding can be used. These methods include supplemental feedings, tube feedings, and intravenous feedings (see Chapter 15).

When a client can't eat enough food from regular meals, the first step is to supplement the diet. Try to give nutritious snacks between meals. Many clients do well with such snacks. For clients who find it easier to drink than to eat, liquid supplements are useful. Psychologically, liquids seem to be less filling, and they are much easier for debilitated, weak, or tired individuals to handle.

Liquid supplements can include common drinks like milk, milkshakes, or instant breakfast drinks. Commercially prepared liquid formulas also are available (some of these formulas are listed in Appendix E). These liquids can be fortified with powdered milk to make them higher in protein. kCalories can be increased by adding a source of carbohydrate such as corn syrup or sugar. Commercial products (also listed in Appendix E) can be used to raise the protein, fat, or carbohydrate content of any liquid supplement.

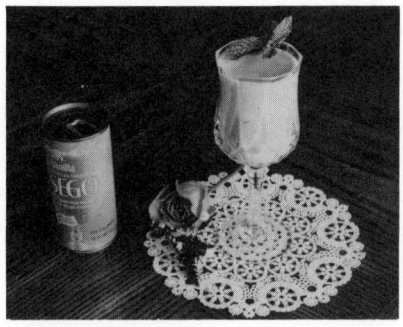

Which would you rather drink?

Even when a person enjoys a liquid supplement, palatability becomes a problem after long-term use. You can help relieve boredom by using more than one type of supplemental feeding. Experiment with flavorings such as chocolate, decaffeinated instant coffee, or strawberry or other fruit flavorings to the supplement. Commercially prepared flavor packets are available in a wide variety of flavors and can be conveniently kept at bedside for use as desired.

Serve liquid feedings attractively. Liquids served from a can are far less appealing than those served in a glass. Remember to serve the formula cold and to provide an ice bath to keep it cold so that it can be sipped as desired.

A liquid formula that supplies all the necessary nutrients is called a complete formula. A complete formula always should be used when the liquid formula is the sole source of nutrients. However, complete formulas can be (and often are) used as supplemental feedings. When used in this way, they augment the nutrient level of the diet even though they may not be given in quantities large enough to meet all nutrient needs.

complete formula:
a liquid formula that, when given in sufficient volume, supplies all the nutrients needed.

Hospital Foods: The Client's Perspective

Hospital food—what do you think of when you see or hear these words? What are your own experiences with hospital food, or the experiences of someone close to you?

People in the hospital often look forward to eating. They enjoy the chance to select foods, because it is one of the few experiences in the hospital in which they have a choice. Clients cannot choose when they will get different tests, how much blood they will have drawn, what nurse will care for them, or what time they will have surgery.

To the client, food is also something familiar in an unfamiliar environment. Unlike many things imposed on the client, food can be eaten or refused. It is the one aspect of the hospital situation the client can control.

Complaints about food are often a way of venting fear, frustration, anger, and physical pain. People who are worried about their health, upset over their progress, disturbed by the way they are being treated, or in pain are likely to complain about food.

Problems with foodservice unrelated to the client's physical or mental state can interfere with appetite. For one, hospital food is not cooked as food is at home—a considerable problem when the client must eat three meals a day for many days in the hospital. Food may be served at times when the client just isn't hungry. A client who has just undergone a painful treatment may be too upset to eat. The client may be on medications that interfere with food intake (see Table 14–2). Unfortunately, the food may also be cold by the time it arrives in the room. The client often must eat alone, in bed, which can make mealtimes more of a chore than a pleasurable experience. Food is so important to most people that a bad experience with it in the hospital can make such people as well as hospital workers agitated and angry.

All this is not to say that every person in the hospital has problems with food. The majority of people will eat adequate amounts of food, even if they complain about it. If their intakes decrease somewhat, the deficit will be easy to correct once they are eating familiar foods in their home environments.

The loss of appetite can have a serious effect on the health or recovery of some people, however. Such individuals lose their appetites at a time when they can least afford a nutrient deficit. Use the steps discussed earlier to identify clients at risk for poor nutrition status. In such cases, it is especially important to improve the appetite and otherwise ensure that adequate nutrients are provided.

Helping the Client Eat

Of all health professionals, nurses and nursing assistants have the closest and most frequent contact with a client. These professionals most often shoulder the responsibility for delivering food to the client's room, preparing the client to eat, observing problems the client may be having with food, and communicating the client's needs to the appropriate person or department.

If a client has a poor appetite or is constantly complaining about food, try to get to the root of the problem. Reassure the client who is frightened, angry, or confused. Simply showing that you care can help improve a client's appetite. Be sure the client understands that nutrition is a part of the recovery process. When it is permissible and possible, a friend or family member can bring favorite foods from outside the hospital if these foods will help the client eat better. This may be especially useful if the client is a child.

Ask yourself and your client these questions to help improve the client's appetite:

- Does the client understand the importance of nutrition to the recovery process?

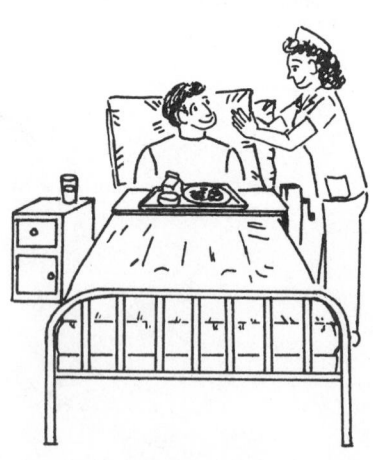

To get clients to eat well, make them feel comfortable and cared for.

TABLE 14–2. Examples of Drugs Affecting Food Intake[a]

Depress appetite

Amphetamines
Antineoplastic drugs
Alcohol (chronic use)
Laxatives (methyl cellulose, guar gum)
Cardiac glycosides
Diuretics

Stimulate appetite

Antihistamines
Tranquilizers
Antidepressants (chlorpromazine, chlordiazepoxide, diazepam)
Hypoglycemic agents (insulin, tolbutamide, chlorpropamide)
Corticosteroids

Induce nausea and/or vomiting

Analgesics
Antibiotics
Anticonvulsants
Antineoplastic drugs
Anti-inflammatory drugs
Chelating agents
Cardiac glycosides
Diuretics
Mineral preparations

Alter taste sensitivity

Antineoplastic agents
Amphetamines
Anesthetics
Penicillamine
Levodopa
Clofibrate

[a]This list is not all-inclusive. Furthermore, not every drug within each major classification causes the effect (e.g., not all antibiotics cause nausea and vomiting).

- If the client is on a modified diet, does he or she understand why? Does the client know which foods are allowed and not allowed on the diet?
- Does the client understand how to mark his or her menu correctly so as to receive the desired foods?

If clients need help in any of these areas, give them the advice they need. Dietitians are the professionals to call if the problem is too big to handle alone. The dietitian or dietetic technician works closely with the client to find acceptable foods.

Health care professionals' attitudes about the hospital's food can affect clients. Try to be positive. Rather than saying, "I couldn't eat this stuff either," say,

"The dietary department really tries to make foods the way you like them. Let me call the dietitian. I'm sure she can help you." When a dietitian or foodservice manager is unavailable, a list of alternative foods available from the dietary department can generally be found at each nursing station.

All clients can benefit from a few steps that help make mealtimes more enjoyable. Encourage clients to wash their faces and hands and to brush their teeth or rinse their mouths before eating. Be sure they are comfortable, either in bed or sitting in a chair. Make sure the extension table is placed at a comfortable height and distance and that the table is clean. Make sure the room is clean and odor-free, too. Take these steps before the tray arrives so that the client can enjoy the meal while foods are still at the right temperature.

When the food cart arrives on the floor, check each tray:

- Verify that the client's name is correct. A client's room number may have been incorrectly recorded, or a new client may have been admitted to a room.
- Check to see that the client is receiving the right diet.
- Look at the tray to see if the client has received the foods that were ordered.
- Scan the tray for overall appearance. The client will eat better if the food is served attractively. Order a new tray if foods are not servable.

Once you have checked the trays, serve them immediately—while warm foods are still warm and cold foods are still cold.

These suggestions may seem a bit overwhelming at first glance. However, when you look at them more closely, you will realize that many of the steps become routine, and they are not as time consuming as they originally appear. Furthermore, your effort can mean a lot to the client whose illness, fears, and frustrations significantly interfere with the desire to eat.

The Sick Child

A sick child often requires special care to ensure that nutrient needs are met. Those who care for children must be sensitive to their feelings and needs. Many of the hints given in Chapter 11 for helping children to eat are useful for working with ill children as well. Additional pointers from people experienced in working with children are:

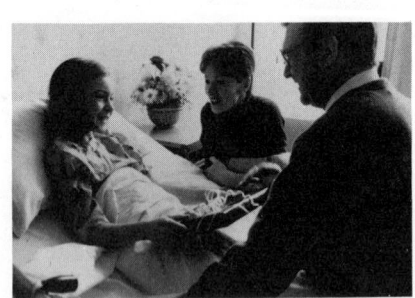

A loved one can ease tensions of the child who is hospitalized.

- Notice the child's posture. Body language will tell you if a child is frightened, hurting, or uncomfortable.
- Touch the child often and lovingly. Your touch communicates more than your words.
- As with adults, let the child choose what to eat as much as possible. Foods brought from outside the hospital can help, if they are allowed.
- Make sure the child eats the food; notice if he or she doesn't. Putting it in front of the child is not enough.
- Stay with the child during the meal, or make sure a loved person is there. The child will eat and assimilate food better if anxiety and loneliness are minimized.

- Encourage the child to eat what he or she needs most first. This will ensure that nutritious foods get eaten before the child gets too full to complete the meal.

- Let the child eat with other children if possible. The child will enjoy mealtimes more, accept more food, and eat for a longer period.

- Avoid painful procedures near mealtimes. The stress of pain or fear shuts down digestion and turns off interest in food.

Nutrition care is an important contribution to a child's recovery, even though its effects may not be immediately obvious.

The Elderly Person in a Long-Term Care Facility

The elderly represent the fastest-growing segment of our population today. As more of our citizens age, the number of people residing in nursing homes will also increase. As discussed in Chapter 12, many factors can influence the nutrition status of the older person. Normal physiologic changes that occur as a result of aging, underlying illness, and prescribed medications taken over long periods of time all compromise nutrition status. Health team members who treat the elderly in long-term care facilities are morally obligated to provide the best care possible.

Nutrition status assessment at regular intervals is of utmost importance in the care of the elderly.[5] Because of the problems listed in the previous paragraph, nutrition status can deteriorate rapidly if it is not assessed regularly.

Pay particular attention to helping the client to eat. Many of the suggestions given earlier for people in the hospital can be useful for the geriatic client as well. Appetite may be affected by medical conditions, pain, depression, boredom, diminished sense of taste or smell, unfamiliar foods, and lack of companionship. The client may have physical or mental disabilities that interfere with the ability to eat. The absence of teeth or improperly fitted dentures can limit the amount and types of foods the client can enjoy.

Some of these problems are correctable, others are not. These measures can help stimulate the appetite:

- Treatment of underlying medical conditions.

- Adminstration of pain medications at the appropriate time before meals to reduce physical discomfort during meals.

- Provision of a varied menu to relieve boredom. The client's likes and dislikes should be considered, and whenever possible, favorite foods should be offered.

- Arrangement of a variety of activities during the day to relieve boredom. Interaction with other residents at mealtime as well as at other times during the day can help provide companionship.

For people who are unable to eat, other measures such as tube feedings or parenteral feedings (see Chapter 15) should be initiated before they reach an advanced state of nutrition depletion.

Clients with physical or mental disabilities often require special assistance with feeding and food. Clients in wheelchairs must be positioned so that they can comfortably reach the table. Occupational therapists can help adapt feeding equipment for people who have trouble grasping feeding utensils or problems coordinating the muscles required to eat. Whenever possible, encourage clients to feed themselves. When a client must be fed, plan ahead. Be sure a staff member will be available to feed the person while the food is still at the right temperature. Be sure the client is ready as well—positioned, clean, comfortable, and ready to eat.

Food and Drug Considerations

Medicine is often given with juice, milk, or food to make the medicine easier to take. Although the nurse is responsible for ensuring that the client in a health care facility is given all prescribed medications, all members of the health care team should be aware of possible interactions that can occur between foods and drugs when given simultaneously. Table 14–3 provides recommendations for administering drugs with respect to food intake.

Food can enhance, delay, or reduce the absorption of a drug. Food in the stomach triggers the secretion of gastric acid, which lowers the pH of the stomach. Therefore, drugs that are negatively affected by an acid environment should be taken on an empty stomach.

For example, Mary is told to take a prescribed antibiotic on an empty stomach (one hour before or two to three hours after meals), because the drug is degraded by high acidity. Sam, on the other hand, has been prescribed a capsule with specific instructions not to drink milk at the same time he takes the capsule. Why? The capsules Sam is taking are specially coated to dissolve in the low acidity of the intestine, and milk alters the acidity of the stomach so that the capsule dissolves there instead. This is undesirable, because the drug can irritate the stomach lining and cause discomfort.

The presence of food in the stomach also stimulates the secretion of bile acids into the intestine, and these acids enhance fat digestion and absorption. Some medications dissolve in and are better absorbed along with fat. Such drugs should be given with food. (The antifungal drug griseofulvin, for example, is well absorbed with fat.)

Food delays the rate at which the stomach empties. Therefore, for a drug to work rapidly, it should be taken on an empty stomach. For example, aspirin taken on an empty stomach works faster than when it is taken on a full stomach. However, aspirin also can be irritating to the GI tract. The presence of food can act as a buffer and reduce irritation. As a guideline, then, if rapid action is not essential, food taken simutaneously with aspirin (or other drugs that irritate the GI tract) can help reduce nausea, lessen irritation, and prevent damage to the lining of the GI tract. A note of caution: The effects of some drugs are actually reduced (not delayed as in the aspirin example) when taken with meals. Drugs in this category include tetracycline, penicillin, levodopa, methyldopa, captopril, and phenobarbital.[6]

Additionally, there are instances in which the desired action of a drug must be timed with food intake. For example, some drugs used to treat ulcers reduce

drug administration terms:
ac: *ante cibes;* before meals.
bid: *bis in die;* twice daily.
c: *cum;* with.
hs: *hora somni;* at bedtime.
pc: *post cibum;* after meals.
qid: *quater in die;* four times daily.
tid: *ter in die;* three times daily.

TABLE 14—3. Drug Administration and Food Intake

Drugs	Give on Empty Stomach*	Give ½ Hour before Meals	Give with Food or Milk	*Don't* Give with Milk or Dairy Products	*Don't* Give with Fruit Juices	Can Give with or without Meals
Acetosulfone sodium			X			
Adrenocorticosteroids		X				
Allopurinol			X			
Ambenonium chloride		X				
Aminophylline			X			
Aminosalicylic acid	X					
Amoxicillin						X
Ampicillin	X				X	
Anisotropine methylbromide	X					
Aspirin			X			
Atropine sulfate		X				
Belladonna		X				
Bethanechol chloride	X					
Bisacodyl				X		
Busulfan			X			
Carbamazepine			X			
Carbenicillin indanyl sodium	X					
Carisoprodol			X			
Cephalexin						X
Cephradine	X					
Chloral hydrate			X			
Chlordiazepoxide		X				
Chlorothiazide			X			
Chlorpromazine			X			
Chlorpropamide			X			
Chlorthalidone			X			
Cimetidine			X			
Cloxacillin sodium	X				X	
Colchicine			X			
Co-trimoxazole	X					
Cyclacillin	X					
Cyclandelate						X
Cyclophosphamide						X
Demeclocycline	X					
Dicloxacillin sodium	X					
Digoxin				X		
Dipyridamole	X					
Doxycycline hyclate				X		X
Erythromycin	X					
Erythromycin, enteric coated						X
Erythromycin estolate or succinate						X
Erythromycin stearate	X					
Estradiol			X			
Estrogen			X			
Ethacrynic acid			X			
Fenoprofen calcium	X					

*(1 hour before or 2 to 3 hours after meals)

(continued)

TABLE 14–3. Drug Administration and Food Intake (continued)

Drugs	Give on Empty Stomach*	Give ½ Hour before Meals	Give with Food or Milk	*Don't* Give with Milk or Dairy Products	*Don't* Give with Fruit Juices	Can Give with or without Meals
Ferrous sulfate, fumarate, lactate, or gluconate				X		
Furosemide			X			
Glycopyrrolate		X				
Griseofulvin			X			
Hydralazine hydrochloride			X			
Hydrochlorothiazide			X			
Hydroflumethiazide			X			
Hydroxyurea			X			
Ibuprofen	X					
Indomethacin			X			
Isoniazide			X			
Isoxsuprine			X			
Levodopa hydrochloride			X			
Lincomycin	X					
Lithium carbonate			X			
Lomustine	X					
Magnesium oxide			X			
Meclofenamate sodium						X
Mefenamic acid			X			
Melphalan	X					
Mepenzolate bromide	X					
Methylthiouracil			X			
Methysergide maleate			X			
Metoprolol tartrate			X			
Metronidazole			X			
Minocycline						X
Mitotane			X			
Nafcillin sodium	X					
Nalidixic acid						X
Naproxen	X					
Nitrofurantoin			X			
Oral contraceptives			X			
Oxacillin sodium	X					
Oxyphenbutazone			X			
Oxytetracycline	X			X		
Penicillin G	X					
Penicillin K						X
Phenformin hydrochloride			X			
Phenmetrazine hydrochloride		X				
Phenobarbital	X					
Phentolamine			X			
Phenylbutazone			X			
Potassium salts			X			
Prednisolone			X			
Prednisone			X			
Procainamide hydrochloride						X

*(1 hour before or 2 to 3 hours after meals)

(continued)

TABLE 14–3. Drug Administration and Food Intake (continued)

Drugs	Give on Empty Stomach*	Give ½ Hour before Meals	Give with Food or Milk	*Don't* Give with Milk or Dairy Products	*Don't* Give with Fruit Juices	Can Give with or without Meals
Promethazine hydrochloride			X			
Propantheline bromide		X				
Propoxyphene hydrochloride			X			
Propranolol hydrochloride			X			
Quinidine sulfate			X			
Rauwolfia serpentina			X			
Reserpine			X			
Rifampin	X					
Salicylamide			X			
Spironolactone			X			
Sulfinpyrazone			X			
Sulfonamide	X					
Tetracycline	X			X		
Theophylline			X			
Thioguanine			X			
Tolbutamide			X			
Triamterene			X			
Trihexyphenidyl hydrochloride			X			
Triameprazine tartrate			X			
Uracil mustard			X			
Valproic acid			X			
Warfarin			X			
Zinc sulfate			X			

*(1 hour before or 2 to 3 hours after meals)

gastric acid secretion and gastric motility. They should be taken just before a meal so that they will be effective while gastric acid secretion is stimulated.

Specific nutrients in food also can have a negative effect on drug absorption. A classic example is the interactions of tetracycline, calcium, and iron. Clients are instructed not to take tetracycline with milk or dairy products. The calcium from dairy products binds to the drug and reduces the amount that is absorbed. Other minerals can also bind tetracycline so that the drug is unavailable for absorption. Antacids that contain calcium carbonate (such as Tums) also can reduce the absorption of tetracycline. In addition, iron supplements should not be taken at the same time as tetracycline; the absorption of each is reduced by the other when taken simultaneously.

This chapter has looked at the unique effects that illness can have on nutrition status and has reviewed some of the considerations of feeding people who are treated in or reside in health care facilities. The next chapter looks at ways of feeding people who are unable to eat by conventional means.

CASE STUDY

Woman with a Poor Appetite

Mrs. Phillips is a 72-year-old woman admitted to the hospital with pneumonia. Her weight has dropped from 135 pounds to 120 pounds over the past month. She is 5 feet, 2 inches tall. She was initially placed on penicillin injections but now is taking 250 mg of pencillin K every six hours. She has a poor appetite and refuses to eat. In talking with her you discover that one of her closest friends has died recently.

1. What factors in Mrs. Phillips's history should alert you to the possibility of poor nutrition status? Determine %IBW and %UBW (see Chapter 13). How would you interpret your findings?

2. List some reasons why Mrs. Phillips's appetite might be poor? Suggest ways to improve her appetite. Consider ways to help Mrs. Phillips maintain her appetite once she goes home. What suggestions can you give her (see Chapter 12)?

3. If Mrs. Phillips were a resident in a nursing home, what additional concerns might you have about her appetite?

4. Describe how Mrs. Phillips's medications should be given with respect to food intake (see Table 14–2). Check Table B–1 in Appendix B for possible drug-nutrient interactions.

Notes

1. Presented at a Congressional Briefing on the Cost Effectiveness of Nutrition Support hosted by the American Dietetic Association, 23 January 1986. Report based on a study conducted by Arthur Anderson and Company and Ross Laboratories.
2. Congressional Briefing, 1986.
3. K. McManus, A malnutrition screening program, *Nutritional Support Services* 8 (1988): 8. M. Garavel and coauthurs, Determining nutritional risk: Assessment, implementation, and evaluation, *Nutritional Support Service* 8 (1988): 18–19.
4. S. K. Kamath and coauthors, Hospital malnutrition: A 33-hospital screening study, *Journal of the American Dietetic Association* 86 (1986): 203–206.
5. D. Sullivan, R. Chernoff, and D. A. Lipschitz, Nutritional support in long-term care facilities, *Nutrition in Clinical Practice* 2 (1987): 6–13.
6. S. M. Garabedian-Ruffalo and R. L. Ruffalo, Drug and nutrient interactions, *American Family Physician* 33 (1986): 165–174.

Food As A Source of Illness

We have seen that nutrition plays a pivotal role in the prevention of disease and the recovery from illness, but foods that provide nutrients can also be a source of illness. Food hazards such as food poisoning and food contaminants compel people to wonder about the safety of the food supply. Nutrition in Practice 14 discusses these concerns.

It seems that I've been hearing many reports about serious cases of food poisoning. What causes food poisoning?
Food poisoning is a real and frequent threat to people who consume food that has been contaminated by toxic microorganisms during processing, packaging, transport, storage, or preparation. Food poisoning can affect large numbers of people whenever batches of contaminated foods escape detection and are distributed and consumed. However, commercial processors are less frequently responsible for incidents of food poisoning than are individuals who prepare food in home kitchens or restaurants, catering firms, and institutions where food is served to large groups.

All foods contain bacteria. Bacteria are widely distributed in nature but are usually harmless. For growth and reproduction, they require warmth, moisture, and a source of food. When the conditions are right, such as in leftover foods improperly stored, bacteria will proliferate. The growth of harmful bacteria causes food poisoning.

What are some types of harmful bacteria?
One type is *Salmonella*. Salmonella infection is estimated to affect more than a million people each year—in the United States alone. *Salmonella* organisms are frequently found on raw meats and poultry and on egg shells. *Staphylococcus aureus* microbes, found on human skin, are the most common cause of food-borne illness in the United States. *Clostridium botulinum* is a toxin-producing bacterial species found in low acid, vacuum-sealed products that are held at room temperature. Botulism is rare but is so deadly that a teaspoonful of the toxin is sufficient to kill five million adults.

Viruses can also cause food-borne illness transmitted from sick people to well ones through seafood. Certain types of seafood, such as oysters and clams, that are grown in water contaminated with human or animal waste products can collect viruses from that waste. For example, waste can contain the virus that causes hepatitis. If the clams or oysters have filtered the virus out of the water and have it in their bodies, there is a good possibility that a consumer of those shellfish will contract hepatitis. However, most seafood that is commercially harvested is safe, because it is harvested from uncontaminated water that is tested.

How do you know if you have food poisoning?
Food poisoning can be very painful. Symptoms of the illness are intestinal distress, fever, vomiting, headache,

and gut pain. Any food-borne illness can be fatal, especially in infants, the elderly, or those already weakened from other illnesses.

What steps can I take to prevent food-borne illness?
We cannot keep all harmful organisms out of the foods we eat. Every day, we ingest small numbers of microbes with no ill effects. Our task is not to eliminate but to kill or control the multiplication of those organisms that are present. Table NP14–1 lists some measures that can be useful in preventing food-borne illness. The person who follows the suggestions provided in the table regarding the selection, storage, and preparation of food will reap many benefits, over a lifetime.

If you suspect that you have a food-borne illness, these steps may be helpful:

1. Call your physician.
2. Wrap and label the remainder of the suspected food, along with its container, so that it can't be mistakenly used; place it in the refrigerator; and hold it for possible inspection by health authorities. Ask your physician whether the food should be saved for examination.
3. Notify the Health Hazard Evaluation Board of the U. S. FDA's Bureau of Foods. The sole purpose of this panel of scientists and health experts is to assess how serious a threat to health the food may be.

TABLE NP14–1 Suggestions for the Prevention of Food-Borne Illness

To prevent illness from *Salmonella*:

- Avoid cross-contamination by using hot, soapy water to wash hands, utensils, cutting boards, or counter tops that have been in contact with raw meats, poultry, or eggs.

- Do not thaw meats or poultry at room temperature. If it is necessary to hasten the thawing of a turkey, use cool running water or a microwave oven.

- Do not stuff poultry until just before cooking, or cook the stuffing separately. Use a meat thermometer to avoid undercooking. The thermometer should be inserted between the thigh and the body of the bird, making sure the tip is not in contact with the bone. Cook to an internal temperature of 190°F. If not using a thermometer, allow about 20 minutes per pound for birds up to 6 pounds, 15 minutes per pound for larger birds. In either case, add five minutes to the pound if the bird is stuffed. Do not stuff poultry that will be microwaved.

- Refrigerate leftovers promptly and heat them thoroughly before serving. (Freshly cooked foods seldom cause illness.)

- Use clean eggs without cracked shells.

- Do not keep susceptible foods at room temperature or at warm holding temperatures.

- Do not use hands to mix foods; keep hands away from mouth, nose, and hair.

- A person with a skin infection or infectious disease should not prepare food. Any healthy person, however, may be a carrier of bacteria and should avoid coughing or sneezing over food.

To prevent poisoning from *Clostridium botulinum*:

- Use only the pressure-canner method of canning vegetables, meats, or poultry. High temperatures required to kill spores cannot be achieved by other home-canning methods. Pickled vegetables and some fruits that are sufficiently acidic to prevent bacterial growth and toxin formation, however, may be canned in a boiling water bath.

- Obtain reliable canning instructions, such as those available from the USDA, and make certain that equipment is functioning properly.

- Throw out foods with off-odors. (An off-odor, however, is not necessarily detectable in a food containing the toxin.)

- Do not even taste food that is suspect. If doubtful about the home-canning procedure used, boil meats, poultry, corn, or spinach for 20 minutes and other vegetables for at least 10 minutes.

- Discard food from cans that leak or bulge. Dispose of the food in a manner that will protect other people and pets from its accidental use.

Additional reminders:

- Do not buy foods stored above the frostline in store freezers.

- Do not buy or use items that appear to have been opened or tampered with.

- Refrigerate perishables promptly. Do not leave groceries in the car while running errands.

- Follow label instructions for storing and preparing packaged and frozen foods.

- When holding foods before serving, keep hot foods at 150°F or higher and cold foods at 45°F or lower. (The refrigerator temperature should be 40°F or lower if foods are kept longer than three or four days.)

- Cooked foods that are not to be served right away should be refrigerated immediately in shallow containers—the foods will cool faster.

- Maintain a clean, dry kitchen that is free of flies and insects. Wash or replace dirty sponges and towels; clean up food spills and crumb-filled crevices. Use hot soapy water for counter tops as well as for dirty dishes. Hot water and soap will immobilize bacteria and wash them away; cold water will not.

Illness from foods can also occur when nonnutrient substances find their way into the food supply. Such contaminants are of concern because they are present in the environment and inevitably may find their way into foods.

What are contaminants?

Contaminants are compounds, such as toxic heavy metals, pesticides, and drugs, that get into foods by accident. The number of contaminants and the amount of information available about them is far beyond the scope of this book. However, a list of chemical contaminants of greatest concern in foods is presented in Table NP14–2.

An example of one contaminant of particular concern today is lead. In 1981, 535,000 U.S. children aged six months to five years were screened for lead poisoning. Twenty-two thousand were found to have symptoms caused by lead toxicity, reflecting a prevalent national health problem. A recent report of the Agency for Toxic Substances and Disease Registry states that every year lead from air, drinking water, and food lowers the IQ of 240,000 children, complicates the pregnancies of 680,000 women, and raises the blood pressure of 130,000 men.[1] One out of every 50 children in rural areas and more than 1 out of every 10 inner city children are affected with lead poisoning reflecting a serious national health problem.[2]

What factors determine whether or not a contaminant will be harmful?

One factor in the potential harmfulness of a contaminant is the extent to which it lingers in the body. If a contaminant enters the system and is rapidly metabolized to some harmless compound or is rapidly

TABLE NP14–2. Chemical Contaminants of Concern in Foods, U.S., 1970 to 1980

Heavy Metals	Halogenated Compounds	Others
Lead	Chlorine	Asbestos
Mercury	Iodine	Dioxins
Cadmium	Vinyl chloride	Acrilonitrile
Selenium	Ethylene dichloride	Lysinoalanine
Arsenic	Trichloroethylene	Diethylstilbestrol
	Polychlorinated biphenyls (PCBs)	Heat-induced mutagens
	Polybrominated biphenyls (PBBs)	Antibiotics (in animal feed)

Source: E. M. Foster, How safe are our foods? *Nutrition Reviews* (supplement), January 1982, pp. 28–34.

excreted, its ingestion may not give cause for concern. If it enters the body, interacts with the body's systems, is not metabolized or excreted, and fools the cells' protein machinery into accepting it as part of the cells' structure, then it is dangerous. All these things are true of lead. Other contaminants may be metabolized to harmful compounds. In either case, additional doses will be piled on top of the first ones, and the dangerous substance will accumulate. This brings us to another factor. It is the *amount* of contamination that makes a difference. If the dose is low enough, it can be tolerated without ill effects.

Other factors can also affect the potential toxicity of a contaminant. One of these factors is nutrition. For instance, total food intake, fat intake, and calcium, iron, and zinc intakes are known to alter animals' (and probably people's) susceptibility to lead toxicity.

Isn't our food supply guaranteed to be safe by the government?

Contaminants are hard to regulate, because they are sometimes difficult to identify. At times we do not even know that they are present. There is no systematic procedure for

monitoring or controlling the presence of contaminants in food, except in individual cases. It will take vigilance and determination to detect these substances and control them appropriately.

The food supply is probably well protected from contaminants, but you need to take stock of the situation and act on your own convictions with regard to specific contaminants. The best protection against the toxicity of food contaminants is an adequate, varied diet and optimal health.

As far as the bacterial contamination of food is concerned, the USDA seal on raw meat or poultry shows that the food has been inspected for quality but does not guarantee that the food is free of potentially harmful bacteria. When buying a product, the consumer assumes the responsibility of handling the product in such a way that the bacteria present won't cause food poisoning.

Notes

1. C. Seabrook, Lead poisoning more widespread, CDC says, *Atlanta Constitution* July 19, 1988, p. 1D.
2. Update: Childhood lead poisoning, *Journal of the American Dietetic Association* 80 (1982): 592, 594.

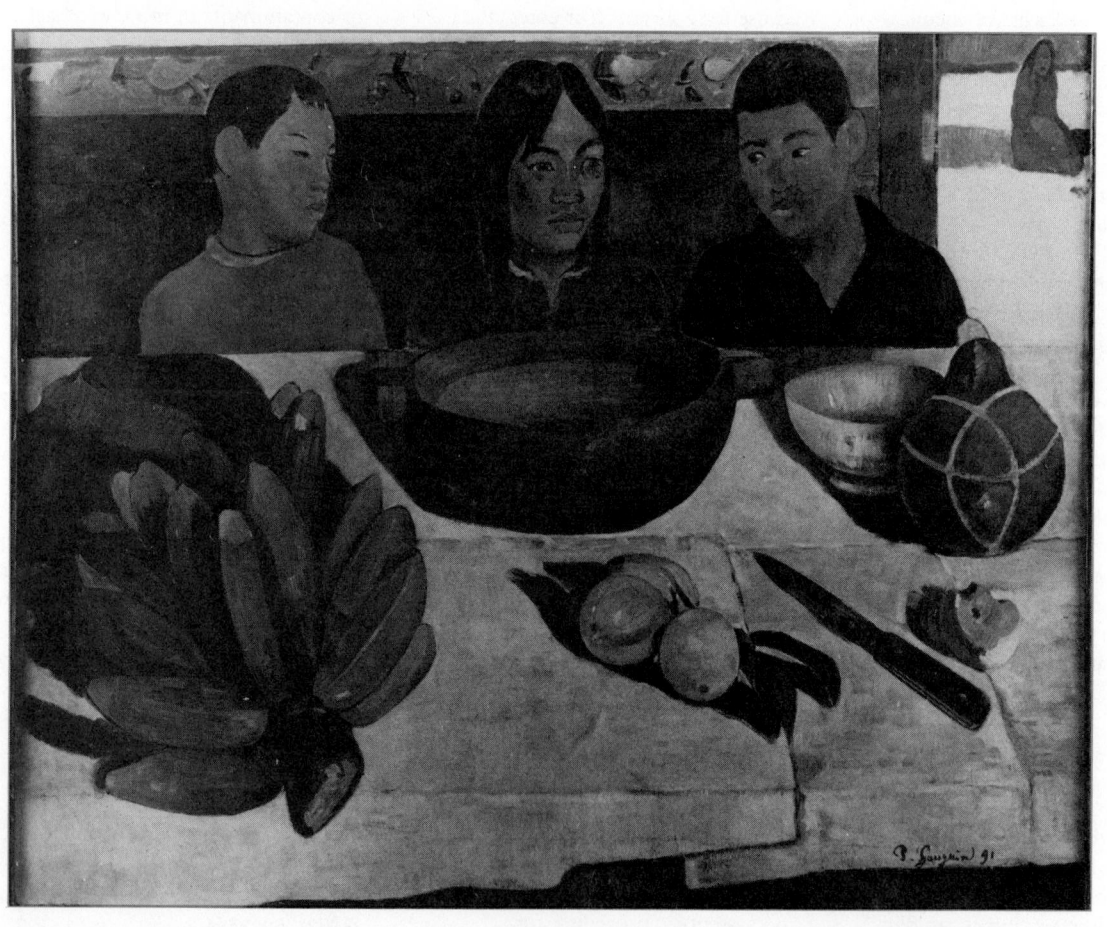

15

Specialized Nutrition Support

CONTENTS

Le Repas des Jeunes Tahitiens by Paul Gauguin. Cliché des
Musées Nationaux, Paris, France.

Chapter 14 described ways that illness can affect nutrient needs. The necessity of providing effective nutrition care to the person who is ill often means attention to many details to ensure adequate intake. This chapter looks at alternative ways of providing nutrients for people who cannot eat by mouth or who are unable to consume enough nutrients from conventional foods.

Tube Feedings

As discussed in Chapter 14, the majority of people in the hospital consume oral diets, either regular or modified, to provide for nutrient needs. These diets can be supplemented with a variety of foods or liquid formulas to help improve nutrient intake. However, in some cases either lack of appetite or other medical conditions can make it impossible for a person to meet nutrient needs. If the problem is expected to be long-term or if the person is in poor nutrition status, aggressive measures to ensure appropriate nutrient intake should be initiated. These measures include tube feedings and total parenteral nutrition. Figure 15–1 demonstrates some factors to consider in the selection of a feeding method.

Tube feeding is the preferred method of feeding the person who is unable to meet nutrient needs orally, providing that the individual has a functional GI tract.[1] The candidate for a tube feeding may have physical problems that

tube feedings:
delivery of nutrients through a tube. *Enteral nutrition* refers to the delivery of nutrients into the intestines; oral diets and tube feedings are types of enteral nutrition.
enteron = intestine

total parenteral nutrition (TPN):
a method of providing all nutrients by vein.

FIGURE 15–1
Selecting the feeding method.

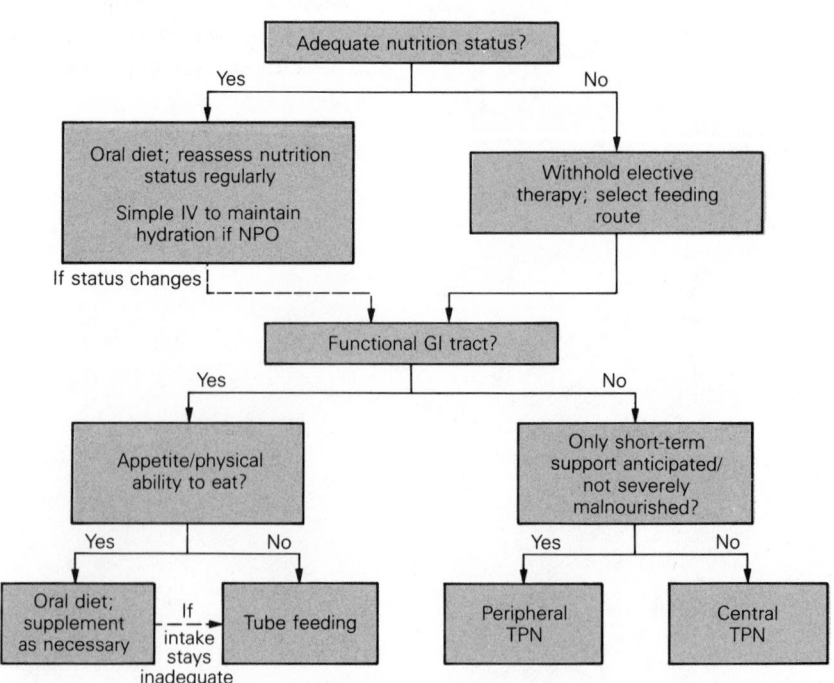

interfere with chewing or swallowing, may not have an appetite, may be in a coma, or may have very high nutrient requirements. Table 15–1 lists indications and contraindications for feeding the person by tube. The Miniglossary of Tube Feeding Terms defines some words you may encounter while working with clients who are fed by tube.

Feeding tubes are most commonly inserted through the nose and passed into the stomach or intestine. They can also be inserted through surgically made openings in the esophagus, stomach, or jejunum. Figure 15–2 illustrates the location of various feeding tube placement sites and Table 15–2 compares features of each.

TABLE 15–1 Indications and Contraindications for the Use of Tube Feedings

Situations in Which Tube Feedings Should Be Recommended

PCM with inadequate oral nutrient intake for 5 or more days
Less than 50% of required nutrient intake orally for 7–10 days
Severe dysphagia (difficulty swallowing)
Major burns
Major bowel resections (see Chapter 20) when used along with TPN
Low output enterocutaneous fistulas (abnormal openings between an internal organ and the skin)

Situations in Which Tube Feedings May Be Useful

Major trauma
Radiation therapy
Mild chemotherapy
Liver failure
Kidney dysfunction

Situations in Which Tube Feedings Are of Limited or Undetermined Value

Intensive chemotherapy
Immediate postoperative or poststress period if adequate oral intake is anticipated in 5–7 days
Enteritis (inflammation of the intestine due to radiation therapy, infection, or inflammatory bowel disease)
Major small bowel resections without the use of TPN

Situations in Which Tube Feedings Are Generally Not Recommended

Intestinal Obstruction
Ileus (paralysis of the intestine)
Hypomotility of the intestine (lack of normal intestinal contractions)
Severe diarrhea
High output enterocutaneous fistulas
Severe acute pancreatitis (inflammation of the pancreas)
Shock
Client or legal guardian does not desire aggressive nutrition support
Prognosis does not warrant aggressive nutrition support

Source: Adapted from A.S.P.E.N. Board of Directors, Guidelines for the use of eternal nutrition in the adult patient, *Journal of Parenteral and Enteral Nutrition* 11 (1987): 435–439.

FIGURE 15–2
Feeding tube placement sites.

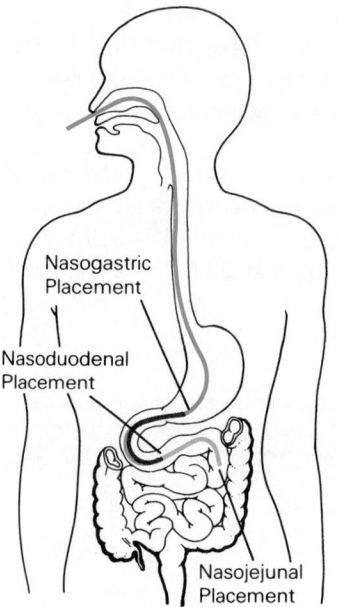

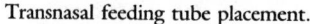

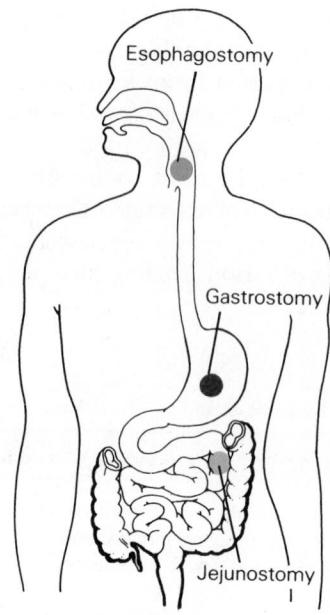

Transnasal feeding tube placement.   Feeding ostomy sites.

Miniglossary of Tube-Feeding Terms

bolus delivery   giving a 4- to 6-hour volume of feeding solution within a few minutes.

continuous drip administration   giving a feeding solution continuously over a 16- to 24-hour period.

feeding ostomy   a surgically made opening through which a feeding tube is passed. An **esophagostomy** is such an opening made in the esophagus. A **gastrostomy** is such an opening in the stomach. A **jejunostomy** is such an opening in the jejenum (small intestine).
ostomy = a surgically formed opening

hypertonic formula   a formula more concentrated than blood serum.
hyper = greater, more

intermittent feeding by slow drip   giving a 4- to 6-hour volume of feeding solution over 20 to 30 minutes.

isotonic formula   a formula with the same concentration as blood serum.
iso = the same
ton = tension

transnasal feeding tube   a feeding tube that is passed through the nose. A **nasogastric (NG) tube** passes from the nose to the stomach. A **nasoenteric tube** passes from the nose to the intestine. Nasoenteric feedings include both **nasoduodenal (ND)** and **nasojejunal (NJ) feedings.**

TABLE 15–2 Features of Various Feeding Tube Placement Sites

Site	Insertion	Potential Irritations	Risk of Regurgitation[a]	Long-term Tolerance	Chance of Removal by Uncooperative Client
Nasogastric	Nonsurgical	Nasal passages, esophagus	High	Fair[b]	Likely
Nasoduodenal	Nonsurgical	Nasal passages, esophagus	Low	Fair[b]	Likely
Nasojejunal	Nonsurgical	Nasal passages, esophagus	Low	Fair[b]	Likely
Esophagostomy	Surgery required	—	High	Good	Unlikely
Gastrostomy	Surgery required	Skin irritation	Moderate	Good	Unlikely
Jejunostomy	Surgery required	Skin irritation	Low	Good	Unlikely

[a]Relative to the other feeding sites. The absolute risk of regurgitation is small.
[b]When the appropriate type and size of tube are used.

Feeding tubes in wide use today are soft, flexible, and small in diameter. These feeding tubes help improve client comfort and are safer to use than older types of feeding tubes. The inner diameter of the tube is an important consideration in selecting the appropriate tube. Generally, the diameter that is selected is the smallest through which the feeding will flow. Because the tubes are small, they can become clogged if the formula does not flow readily through the tube. Unclogging a tube is difficult and frequently unsuccessful.[2] If a new tube must be inserted, the client will be subjected to additional stress and anxiety.

The type of tube is also important. Tubes come in various lengths—shorter tubes for placement in the stomach, longer tubes for placement in the intestines. Some tubes are weighted at one end to facilitate placement and retention in the intestine. However, whether or not weighted tubes actually assist in placing tubes in the intestine and help keep them in place is controversial.[3] Recent studies suggest that unweighted tubes are just as effective as weighted tubes for this purpose.[4]

Although the newer tubes have greatly enhanced client comfort during tube feeding, some complications have been associated with their use.[5] The most common complications result from inadvertent placement of the tube in the lungs and from obstruction of the tube itself. Complications can be serious and sometimes life threatening.

Formula Characteristics

Over 50 products are available to feed people either orally or by tube.[6] (Many of these products are listed in Appendix E). Formulas are designed to meet a variety of medical and nutrition needs and can be modified with respect to individual nutrient components to meet an even wider range of needs.

The formula used as a tube feeding is selected after the client's needs have been identified by a careful nutrition assessment. Many ways of grouping formulas have been reported.[7] For our purposes, it is reasonable to think of

The term **monomeric** (mon-oh-MERR-ic) describes formulas that have hydrolyzed protein or free amino acids as the source of protein. **Polymeric** (POLL-ee-MERR-ic) formulas contain an intact protein source.
monomer = single unit
polymer = chain of units

intact protein formula:
a liquid diet that contains a complete protein that has not been altered.

blenderized diet:
a liquid diet made from a combination of table foods. Blenderized diets usually contain pureed meat, vegetables, fruits, milk, and starches with vitamins and minerals added as necessary. They can be made in a blender or purchased commercially.

protein isolate:
a type of intact protein; a protein with high biological value that has been separated from a source containing a variety of proteins. A *protein isolate formula* contains a protein isolate as the source of protein.

hydrolyzed protein:
an intact protein treated with acids or enzymes to yield a combination of free amino acids and short peptide chains. A *protein hydrolysate formula* contains hydrolyzed protein as a source of protein.

modular formulas:
incomplete formulas that contain specific nutrients and are used as supplements.

osmolality:
the number of molecular and ionic particles (measured in osmoles) per kilogram of water in a solution.

isotonic formula:
a formula with an osmolality similar to that of blood serum (300 mOsm).
iso = the same
ton = tension

hypertonic formula:
a formula with an osmolality higher than that of blood serum.
hyper = greater, more

two major types of formulas. Those that contain protein, carbohydrates, and fats of higher molecular weights are called intact formulas. A person must be able to digest and absorb nutrients without difficulty to use this type of formula. Intact formulas can be blenderized diets or protein isolate formulas. A protein isolate formula contains a purified protein.

The second type of formula is hydrolyzed formula. Such formulas contain breakdown products of protein, fat, and carbohydrate. They are, in a sense, predigested, and require only minimal further digestion in the intestinal tract. People who lack digestive capabilities or who have a smaller than normal area for absorbing nutrients may benefit from them.

Commercially available formulas are available in ready-to-use liquid form, as liquid concentrates, or in powdered form, depending on the formula. Standard formulas provide about one kcalorie per milliliter. Formulas containing 1.5 and 2.0 kcalories per milliliter are also available. Other formulas meet the specific needs of people with diseases who require different amounts or types of protein, amino acids, carbohydrate, and fat. Electrolyte concentrations, vitamins, and fiber content also vary. Special formulas are of particular value to those with liver, kidney, and lung diseases and trauma.

A small number of formulas are termed *modular formulas*. These products contain different forms of individual nutrients (see Appendix E). A module can be added to another formula to alter the composition of that formula (for example, to add protein to a formula) or can be used with other modules to construct totally individualized formulas. Modular formulas can be constructed to more closely meet nutrient requirements than regular commercial formulas and can be less expensive in some cases.[8] However, the person formulating a modular feeding must have an in-depth nutrition knowledge to design a formula that will meet all of a client's nutrient needs.

Osmolality

Osmolality is a measurement of the concentration of molecular and ionic particles in a solution. The greater the number of particles in a solution, the greater the osmolality. The osmolality of normal blood serum is about 300 milliosmoles (mOsm) per liter. The osmolality of formulas ranges from about 250 to over 800 milliosmoles. A formula that approximates the osmolality of the serum is referred to as an isotonic formula. A formula with a higher osmolality than serum is hypertonic.

A hypertonic formula in the intestine can cause water to be drawn from in and around the body cells into the intestine. If the body has had time to adapt to the hypertonic solution, this is usually not a problem. However, if adaptation has not occurred, diarrhea, vomiting, cramps, or nausea can result. Therefore, all else being equal, the most desirable formulas are those as near isotonic as possible.

A hydrolyzed protein formula may contain exactly the same amount of protein as an intact formula, but it contains many more particles. Hydrolyzed formulas are therefore higher in osmolality than most intact protein formulas and are more likely to cause the GI symptoms just mentioned.

Residue and Fiber

Dietary fiber is the portion of food that cannot be digested by the human digestive tract. Residue is a combination of undigested and unabsorbed food in the colon. Intestinal secretions, bacteria, and the turnover of intestinal cells also contribute residue. The residue content of the diet is largely responsible for fecal bulk. As you will see in later chapters, people with certain GI disorders need diets that are low in residue. High-fiber diets may help stimulate normal bowel function in people who do not need low-residue diets. People who may benefit from high-fiber tube feedings include those with diarrhea or constipation and those on tube feedings for long periods of time.[9] Furthermore, recent studies in rats suggest that certain fibers (pectins) may be fermented in the intestine to short-chain fatty acids that may actually provide a fuel source to the lining of the intestine, enabling it to adapt more readily after large portions of the small bowel have been resected (see Chapter 20).[10]

Since hydrolyzed formulas are almost completely absorbed, they leave little residue in the gut. Protein isolate formulas have a low to moderate residue content. Blenderized diets are higher in fiber, as are some commercially prepared formulas to which additional fiber has been added.

Other Characteristics

Formulas can be made from many different ingredients. For example, some contain lactose, while others are lactose free. One formula may derive its protein from a source of higher biological value than another formula. These characteristics are important when a formula is chosen for a client.

Another characteristic of different formulas that varies widely is cost. Costs vary greatly for individual products in different parts of the country and for different hospitals. However, as a general rule, hydrolyzed formulas are more costly than intact formulas, because they require more commercial modification. Nutrition in Practice 18B describes the importance of cost considerations in health care today.

No formula is perfect. In general, the more digestible the formula, the higher its cost and osmolality, and the lower its palatability. As a rule of thumb, because hydrolyzed formulas are more costly and more likely than other formulas to cause complications, they should be used only for people who can't adequately digest and absorb nutrients.

Formula Selection

With so many formulas available, how do you select the best one for your client? The ideal formula for an individual is one that meets nutrient needs with the least risk of complications and at the least cost. A person benefits from a diet only if energy, protein, carbohydrate, fat, vitamin, and mineral needs are met. Attention to formula selection is especially important, since the person on a tube feeding is basically depending on one food source to meet all nutrient needs. Furthermore, people receiving liquid formulas often have altered nutrient needs due to illness. Therefore, a careful and thorough nu-

fiber:
the portion of food that is found in the colon because we don't have the enzymes to digest it.

residue:
the total amount of material in the colon; it includes undigested food, intestinal secretions, bacteria, and the turnover of intestinal cells.

trition assessment is paramount before a formula is selected. If a formula does not meet all nutrient needs, it should be supplemented with the appropriate nutrients.

A formula given orally should taste good. As a general guide, the more hydrolyzed a formula and the lower its fat content, the less tasty it will be. However, remember that people's likes and dislikes vary greatly and what might seem quite unpalatable to you or me might be perfectly acceptable to someone else. Figure 15–3 shows some of the considerations required to select the appropriate formula.

In summary, factors in formula selection include:

• The client's digestive and absorptive function. People who don't have a functioning GI tract are not candidates for oral or tube feedings. However, people with minimal GI function may be able to benefit from hydrolyzed formulas.

FIGURE 15–3
Narrowing the choice of formulas.

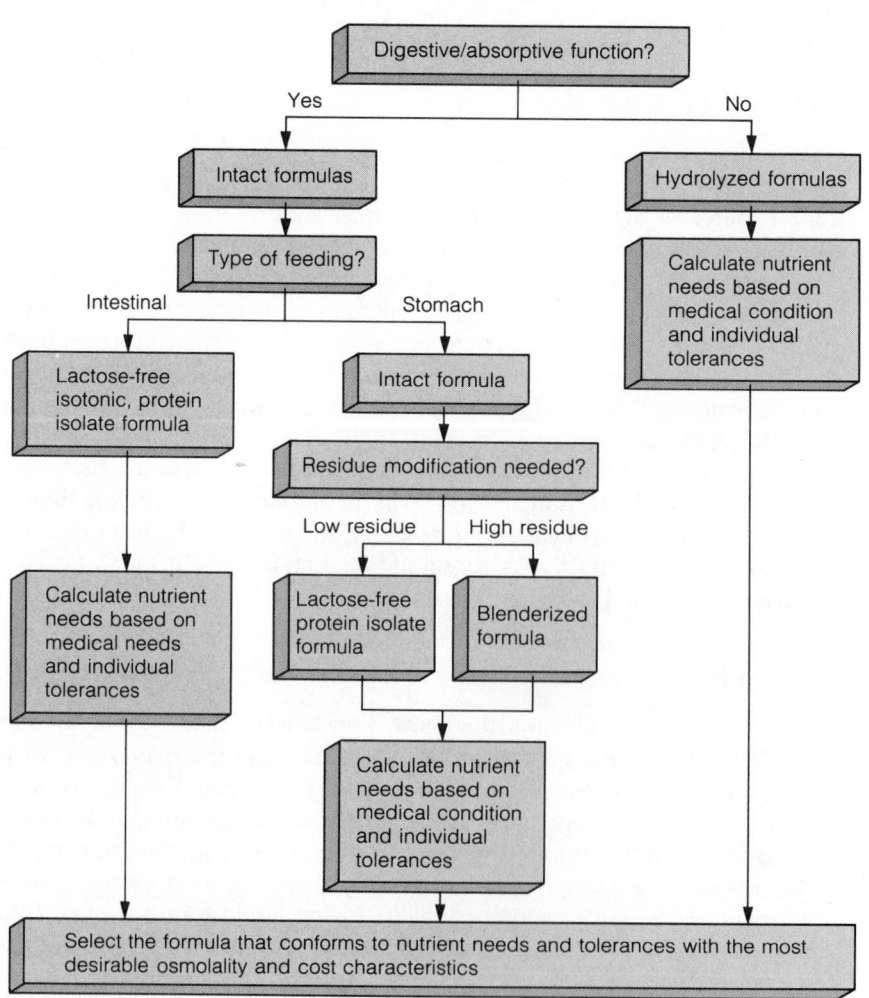

- The placement of the feeding tube (stomach versus intestine). Feedings delivered directly into the intestine must be easily digested, but they do not have to be hydrolyzed if the GI tract is functional. Isotonic formulas are preferred for intestinal feedings, because the intestine is more sensitive than the stomach to hypertonic formulas.
- Nutrient requirements. Nutrient requirements are estimated based on careful nutrition assessment. The client's medical condition, nutrition status, and metabolic rate are all important considerations in estimating nutrient requirements.
- Individual tolerances (food allergies and sensitivities). Lactose-free formulas are frequently selected, because temporary and permanent lactose intolerances are common problems.

In the final analysis, you really can make only an educated or informed guess about the best formula for an individual. Therefore, it becomes critical to monitor each person's nutrition status and tolerance to the formula to ensure that individual needs are being met. Table 15–3 lists the major steps in monitoring people on tube feedings.

Many adults who normally tolerate milk become temporarily lactose intolerant following GI surgery or during radiation therapy or chemotherapy. When such people are given a formula with lactose, they become bloated and develop cramps and diarrhea. The nurse or dietitian who is alert to this possibility can save these people much misery and pain by using a formula that is lactose free.

Administering a Tube Feeding

Attention to formula preparation and administration is critical to appropriate use of tube feedings. Prepare formulas in a clean environment with clean equipment and clean hands. Reduce bacterial contamination by giving only formula made fresh within the last 24 hours. Store unopened cans of formula unrefrigerated. Once a can is opened or a powder is mixed with water, however, refrigerate the formula and label it with the date and time of preparation, the client's name, and the client's room number. Discard opened containers of formula not used within 24 hours. Never add fresh formula to formula still in the feeding container—rinse the feeding container and the tubing attached to it before adding fresh formula. Flush the feeding tube itself with water. The feeding container and tubing (not including the transnasal tube) should be changed every 12 to 24 hours to reduce the risk of bacterial growth. Tube feedings sometimes come prepackaged in containers that can be used to dispense formula directly without being transferred to another feeding container. A recent study suggested that these containers significantly reduce the risk of bacterial contamination.[11]

People placed on tube feedings often have had surgery or have not eaten for several weeks and may not be able to tolerate large volumes or highly concentrated formulas. Therefore, formulas may at first need to be diluted to

TABLE 15−3 Checklist for Monitoring the Tube-fed Individual

Frequency of Monitoring	Procedure
Before starting a new or intermittent feeding:	Complete a nutrition assessment. Check tube placement. Check residual formula in stomach (if 150 ml, consider possible reasons for delayed gastric emptying).
Every half hour:	Check gravity drip rate, when applicable.
Every hour:	Check pump drip rate, when applicable.
Every 2−4 hours of continuous feeding:	Check residual.
Every 4 hours:	Check vital signs, including blood pressure, temperature, pulse, and respiration.
	Check sugar and acetone in urine; monitoring sugar and acetone can be discontinued after 48 hours if test results are consistently negative in a nondiabetic client.
	Refill feeding containing.
Every 8 hours:	Check intake and output.
	Check specific gravity of urine.
	Chart client's acceptance of and tolerance to tube feeding.
Every day:	Weigh client.
	Change feeding bag and tubing.
	Check electrolytes, blood urea nitrogen, and blood glucose daily until stabilized.
Every 7−10 days:	Check all laboratory findings.
	Reassess nutrition status.
As needed:	Observe client for any undesirable responses to tube feeding, for example, nausea, vomiting, or diarrhea.
	Check tube placement (for nasogastric placement only).
	Check nitrogen balance.
	Check laboratory data.
	Clean feeding equipment.
	Chart significant details.

Start the feeding at 50 ml/hour at half strength and progress the feeding as follows:

- After 8 hours
  75 ml/hour at half strength.
- After 16 hours:
  100 ml/hour at half strength.
- After 24 hours:
  125 ml/hour at half strength.
- After 36 hours:
  125 ml/hour at full strength.

one-half or one-third strength (see Figure 15−4). Initially, give the formula slowly, at about 50 milliliters per hour. If the person tolerates the formula, the rate of feeding can be increased by 25 milliliters per hour every 8 to 12 hours. Once the final desired rate has been reached, the strength is increased. If a new rate or strength is not tolerated, you can back up and try increasing it more slowly, giving the person more time to adapt.

In the past, almost all people were placed on diluted formulas when tube feedings were initiated. However, recent studies suggest that in people with normal GI functioning and those with inflammatory bowel diseases (see Chapter 20), diluting formula is unnecessary.[12] Another study suggests that as a rule of thumb, people who have serum albumin levels less than 3.5 grams per 100 milliliters are likely to have problems tolerating concentrated formulas.[13]

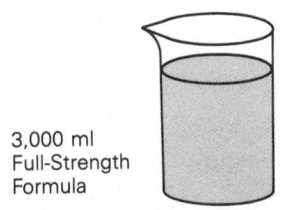

3,000 ml
Full-Strength
Formula

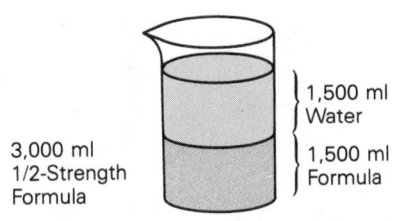

3,000 ml
1/2-Strength
Formula

{ 1,500 ml
Water

{ 1,500 ml
Formula

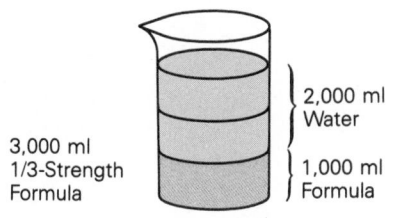

3,000 ml
1/3-Strength
Formula

{ 2,000 ml
Water

{ 1,000 ml
Formula

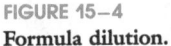

FIGURE 15–4
Formula dilution.

Water is an important consideration for the individual who is fed by tube. As a guideline, adults require from 1,500 to 2,000 milliliters of water daily. A person with a high fever may require an additional 500 to 1,500 or more milliliters. Other conditions such as excessive sweating, severe vomiting, diarrhea, blood loss, and some types of kidney disease increase water requirements. In other types of kidney, liver, and heart diseases, total water may need to be restricted.

Attention to indices of body water balance can help determine individual water requirements. Thirst is a good regulator of water needs in alert adults. A person complaining of thirst generally needs water. Body weight changes can also help determine if fluid needs are being met. An unexplained body weight change of 2.2 pounds (one kilogram) can represent a fluid loss or gain of one liter.[14] Serum electrolytes, hematocrit, and blood pressure should also be monitored regularly. High values for these indices are suggestive of dehydration. Water used to flush the feeding tube before and after a feeding or when the feeding apparatus is being changed not only helps prevent the feeding tube from becoming clogged but also helps keep the client hydrated.

Methods of Delivery

A day's volume of a formula can be given in many ways. For example, a person can be fed four to six times daily. In such a case, the total volume of formula needed for the day is divided by four or six, respectively. Feedings given intermittently allow the client freedom of movement between meals.

If the amount of formula necessary for each feeding is given within a few minutes, it is called a bolus feeding. Feedings given by this method may be poorly tolerated—they lead to more complaints of abdominal discomfort, nausea, fullness, and cramping. Feedings delivered intermittently (four to six times a day) but allowed to infuse over a longer period (20 to 30 minutes) are often better tolerated. This makes sense. After all, you do not gobble down a meal in just a few minutes, especially when you are not feeling well.

Feedings also can be delivered slowly over a 16- to 24-hour period. This feeding method is called continuous drip. Pumps (similar to those used for delivering intravenous solutions) can be used to ensure that the formula is given slowly. Continuous drip administration is useful for people who have poor tolerance to large volumes of formula. Generally, intestinal feedings (particularly jejunal feedings) are delivered by continuous drip.

Formulas themselves contain considerable amounts of water. A standard formula (1.0 kcal/ml) contains about 850 ml of water per liter of formula. Higher-kcalorie formulas contain less water: Formulas, that contain 1.5 kcal/ml and those with 2.0 kcal/ml provide about 775 ml and 600 ml of water per liter of formula, respectively.

If our client, J.K., received her formula intermittently six times a day, at each feeding she would need 500 ml of formula.

3,000 ml ÷ 6 feedings = 500 ml/feeding.

If she received the formula only four times a day, she would need 750 ml of formula at each feeding.

3,000 ml ÷ 4 feedings = 750 ml/feeding.

She would probably tolerate this volume of solution very poorly if it were given to her within a few minutes at each feeding.

bolus delivery:
delivery of a 4- to 6-hour volume of feeding solution within a few minutes.

intermittent feeding by slow drip:
delivery of a 4- to 6-hour volume of feeding solution over 20 to 30 minutes.

continuous drip administration:
delivery of a feeding solution continuously over a 16- to 24-hour period.

If J.K. received continuous drip feedings over 24 hours, she would receive 125 ml/hour.

3,000 ml ÷ 24 hours = 125 ml/hour.

If J.K. received the total volume of solution by continuous drip for 16 hours, she would receive 187.5 ml/hour.

3,000 ml ÷ 16 hours = 187.5 ml/hour.

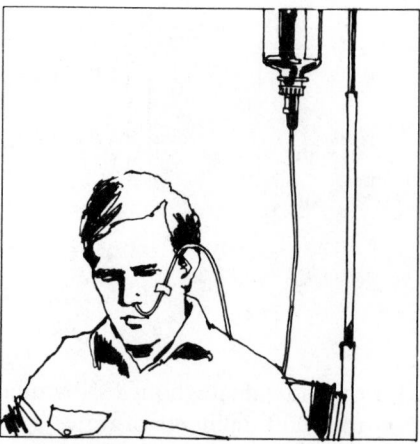

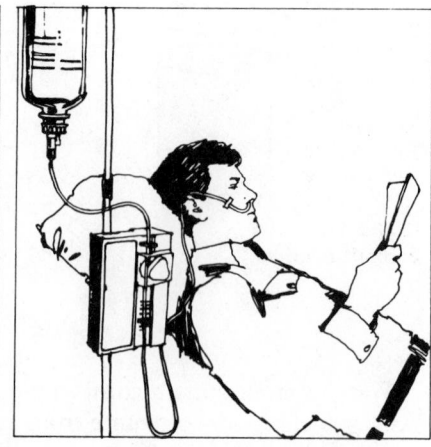

A person being fed by tube. This feeding is being delivered by gravity drip.

Tube feedings can also be delivered by pump. A typical setup is shown here.

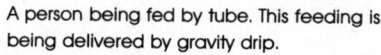

Source: Illustrations courtesy of Ross Laboratories.

Regardless of the method used to deliver a formula, elevate the client's head to at least a 30-degree angle during the feeding and for 30 minutes following an intermittent feeding to minimize the possibility of regurgitation.

Drug Administration Through Feeding Tubes

Advances in our understanding of nutrition as well as the availability of many new products to feed people by tube has resulted in a dramatic growth in the use of this feeding method. Furthermore, a person placed on a tube feeding is generally quite ill and may therefore be receiving numerous medications. Often these medicines are delivered through the feeding tube, and in some cases, undesirable interactions can occur.

Crushing tablets and mixing them with water so that they will flow through the feeding tube is a common practice that should be avoided if possible.[15] If the particles are too large for the lumen of the feeding tube, the tube becomes clogged and may need to be reinserted at considerable discomfort to the client. Also, some types of tablets and capsules are intended to release their contents slowly and should not be crushed, or the person might be exposed to an excessive dose of the drug at one time. Liquid forms of medications should be used whenever available. If tablets are the only available form of the medicine, they should be finely crushed and mixed with water before administering. The feeding tube should be flushed with water before and after any form of medicine is given to help prevent the drug from sticking to the sides of the tube and ensure delivery to the GI tract.

The place where a feeding is delivered is also of considerable importance. A drug that dissolves in the acidic environment of the stomach may not be as readily absorbed if delivered directly to the duodenum or jejunum. Similarly, a drug that is absorbed optimally in the duodenum may be poorly absorbed in the jejunum.

lumen:
the inner open space of a tube.

Some drugs are not compatible with feeding solutions. These drugs are frequently highly acidic, and they result in thickening and clumping of formulas and clogging of the feeding tube. In some cases, drugs added to formulas are incompatible because the drug effects are hindered. One example is phenytoin (a drug used to control seizures). Absorption of phenytoin may be reduced by as much as 70 percent for the person who is on continuous drip tube feedings.[16] Stopping the feeding for two hours before and two hours after giving phenytoin is recommended whenever possible. A similar interaction may occur when tetracycline is administered with tube feedings.[17] Certain electrolytes present in formulas can bind tetracycline and cause it to pass unabsorbed through the intestinal tract.

An important consideration in delivery of a medication through a feeding tube is the medication's osmolality. Hyperosmolar medications that are given rapidly cause the same undesirable side effects associated with hyperosmolar formulas. If the medications are compatible with the tube feeding formula, they can be added directly to the formula and given slowly over a longer period of time.[18] Incompatible drugs should be mixed with water and administered slowly or given by vein to prevent problems.

Drugs delivered through a feeding tube should not be mixed together and given all at once. Give each drug individually and flush the feeding tube with water after each drug is given. This measure reduces the likelihood of drug-drug interactions.

Drugs can trigger GI side effects similar to those associated with tube feedings (see next section). Nausea, vomiting, diarrhea, and electrolyte disturbances are a few of these possible complications. When tube feedings are being given, side effects of drugs should be considered as a possible source of problems. In some cases, a substitute drug with similar pharmaceutical action but without the side effects can be used to reduce GI problems.

Finally, keep in mind that tube feeding formulas can interact with drugs in the same ways that everyday foods can (see Appendix B). Drug therapy should be carefully considered when determining nutrient requirements.

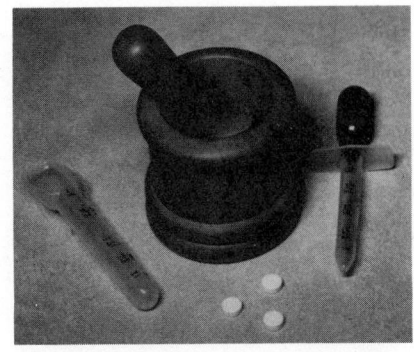

Use liquid medicines for delivery through feeding tubes whenever they are available; if not, finely crush the tablets and mix them with water.

Complications Associated with Tube Feedings

People with carefully placed feeding tubes who receive the proper formula, prepared and administered correctly, seldom have problems with tube feeding. Several types of complications may be associated with tube feedings, however. Some are related to the tube itself, such as inappropriate placement, clogging of the lumen of the feeding tube, displacement of the tube, and skin irritation around a feeding ostomy site.

Problems related to the formula or the way it is administered frequently result in GI complaints. Nausea, vomiting, diarrhea, cramps, constipation, delayed gastric emptying, and abdominal distention are among the more frequent GI complaints.[19] Metabolic problems such as dehydration, electrolyte imbalance, and elevated blood glucose levels can also occur. Many of these complications can be prevented through careful monitoring. Table 15–3 provides a checklist of how to monitor the tube-fed individual. Table 15–4 summarizes some complications associated with tube feedings and identifies steps that can be taken to prevent or correct them.

TABLE 15–4 Causes and Prevention or Correction of Tube-Feeding Complications[a]

Complication	Cause	Preventive/Corrective Measures
Aspiration pneumonia	Regurgitation of formula, which is subsequently inhaled into lungs	Use nasoenteric, gastrostomy, or jejunostomy feedings in high-risk clients; use small-diameter transnasal tube; elevate head of bed during feeding; use continuous drip method of delivery; check gastric residual.
Clogged feeding tube	Formula too thick for tube	Select appropriate tube size; dilute formula with water; flush tubing with water before and after giving formula.
	Medications given through tube inadequately crushed	Use liquid medications whenever possible; Crush tablets finely and mix with water; Flush tubing with water before and after medicines are given; give medicine individually.
Constipation	Low-fiber formula	Provide additional fluids; use high-fiber formula; give laxatives or enemas if necessary.
	Lack of exercise	Encourage walking and other activities, if appropriate.
Dehydration and electrolyte imbalance[b]	Excessive diarrhea	See items under diarrhea.
	Inadequate fluid intake	Provide additional fluid.
	Carbohydrate intolerance	Use continuous drip administration of formula; monitor glucose levels in blood and urine; consider administering insulin; change amount or type of carbohydrate.

[a]Many of the complications presented here can be caused by the client's primary disorder rather than the tube feeding itself. In such a case, the corrective measure would include treatment of the disorder.

[b]This cluster of symptoms is sometimes called the tube feeding syndrome. Imbalances of any electrolytes are possible, and corrective measures would vary.

(table continued on next page)

Psychological Implications of Tube Feedings

Chapter 1 discussed many reasons why people choose the foods they eat. The person fed by tube is denied the right to select food for any purpose, even to obtain nourishment. Feeding becomes mechanical, not an expression of personal preference, social pressure, or cultural tradition. To compound the problem, the person may experience physical and emotional discomforts from the tube, tube feeding, the illness itself, or hospitalization.

Help allay the client's fears as much as possible. Explain the procedure for inserting the tube and administering the formula. Answer all questions and try to gain the client's cooperation. Be sure the client and the client's family understand the objective of the tube feeding and how it will aid in recovery.

The person may also feel self-conscious about how the tube looks and may feel tied down by the feeding equipment. Show the client how to manipulate the equipment so that he can get out of bed. Encourage him to walk about and socialize whenever possible. Walking around will help the client realize that movement is not impossible and that exercise feels good. Socializing may help the individual to forget about the tube.

TABLE 15—4 Causes and Prevention or Correction of Tube-Feeding Complications[a] (continued)

Complication	Cause	Preventive/Corrective Measures
Diarrhea, cramps, and distention	Excessive protein intake	Monitor blood electrolyte levels; reduce protein intake.
	Bacterial contamination	Use fresh formula every 24 hours; store opened or mixed formula in a refrigerator; rinse feeding bag and tube before adding fresh formula; change feeding bag every 24 hours; prepare formula with clean hands using clean equipment in a clean environment.
	Lactose intolerance	Use lactose-free formula in lactose-intolerant and high-risk clients.
	Hypertonic formula	Dilute formula and increase concentration gradually; use isotonic formula.
	Rapid formula administration	Use continuous drip administration of formula.
	Malnutrition/low serum albumin	Dilute formula and increase concentration gradually.
	Drug therapy	Use antidiarrheal agents; change drug therapy if possible.
	Low-fiber formula	Provide high-fiber formula.
Hyperglycemia	Diabetes, hypermetabolism, drug therapy	Check glucose in blood and urine; slow administration rate; provide adequate fluids; limit type or amount of carbohydrate; consider hypoglycemic drug therapy.
Nausea and vomiting	Obstruction	Discontinue tube feeding.
	Delayed gastric emptying	Check gastric residual; use continuous drip method of administration.
	Intolerance to concentration or volume of formula	Dilute formula, increasing strength gradually; use continuous drip method of administration.
	Drug therapy	Change drug therapy if possible; Use antinausea and antiemetic drugs.
	Psychological reaction to tube feeding	Address clients' concerns.
Skin irritation around feeding ostomy site	Leakage of GI secretions and friction caused by the tube	Keep site clean; inspect area for redness, tenderness, and drainage.

You can take other steps to make the tube-feeding experience tolerable. The person who is allowed to eat or drink other foods should be given the foods she prefers. Sometimes a person can "drink" a favorite beverage or food (blenderized) through a tube for psychological satisfaction.

The more complex the procedure that a health care provider is responsible for, the more likely she is to focus on the procedure and forget the client's feelings. Remember, no matter how many technicalities you have to keep in mind, you must never forget the person who is the object of your care.

What to Chart

We have previously discussed the medical record and its importance as a communication tool. Use the medical record to prevent tube feeding complications and to ensure that the client is reaching the nutritional goals that have been set for her. The following information about tube feeding should be documented:

- Type of feeding tube.
- Tube placement.
- Client's response to tube insertion.
- Administration schedule (concentration and rate).
- Method of delivery (intermittent or continuous).
- Client's tolerance to tube feeding (note any complications and any corrective actions taken).
- Client's response to tube feeding.
- Drugs delivered through the feeding tube.
- Education about feeding received by client.

When changing the feeding bag or adding fresh formula to a bag, check the amount of formula left from a previous feeding. Is the client receiving the amount of formula that has been ordered? If not, why not? Has the formula been labeled to be sure the client is getting the right formula? Has the formula been stored properly? Be sure to correct any problems early. Appropriate charting helps all members of the health care team to maintain an optimal level of care.

In many situations, tube feedings can provide a practical solution to feeding the person who is unable to consume adequate nutrients by mouth. However, a person without a functional GI tract cannot benefit from a tube feeding. In such a case, intravenous nutrition can be a life-saving treatment option.

Intravenous Nutrition

intravenous (IV) or parenteral:
through a vein. *Parenteral nutrition* refers to the delivery of nutrients through a vein, bypassing the intestines.
intra = within
vena = vein
para = opposite
enteron = intestine

dextrose:
a form of glucose that is very soluble in water and is therefore used in IV solutions. Dextrose contains a little water; therefore, while glucose provides 4 kcal/g, dextrose provides only 3.4 kcal/g.

A variety of nutrient solutions can be administered by vein to people unable to eat or drink. These intravenous (IV), or parenteral, solutions may consist of all or a combination of the essential nutrients: Water, dextrose, electrolytes, amino acids, fat, vitamins, and trace elements.

The routine use of simple parenteral solutions given by peripheral vein is widespread in the hospital. Simple IV solutions provide water and combinations of dextrose, electrolytes, and occasionally other nutrients. These solutions help maintain fluid and electrolyte as well as acid-base balances. For the well-nourished person who is expected to eat within 7 to 10 days following surgery, simple IV solutions are very useful.[20]

Generally, adults in good nutrition status with normally functioning kidneys can benefit from a simple IV solution that provides from 2½ to 3½ liters of a five percent dextrose solution following trauma or surgery. Electrolytes are replaced as needed. Three liters of a five percent dextrose solution contribute about 150 grams of glucose, or about 510 kcalories per day (see the box, "How to Calculate the Nutrient Content of IV Solutions"). Simple IV solutions are far from complete nutritionally. Given for short periods of time, however, they are not harmful. People who can't eat for long periods of time, those who are malnourished, and those who have high nutrient requirements need more complete solutions.

How to Calculate the Nutrient Content of IV Solutions

You will have more confidence in IV solutions if you know what's in them. The basic thing to remember is that the percentage of a substance in a solution tells you how many grams of that substance are present in 100 milliliters. For example, in a five percent dextrose solution, there are five grams of dextrose per 100 milliliters. A 3.5 percent amino acid solution contains 3.5 grams of amino acids (protein equivalents) per 100 milliliters. A 0.9 percent normal saline solution contains 0.9 gram of sodium chloride per 100 milliliters.

A person receiving 1,500 milliliters of 50 percent dextrose and 1,500 milliliters of 7 percent amino acid solution would get:

$$\frac{50 \text{ g dextrose}}{100 \text{ ml}} \text{ as } \frac{X \text{ g dextrose}}{1,500 \text{ ml}}$$
$$(50 \text{ g} \times 1,500 \text{ ml}) \div 100 \text{ ml} = 750 \text{ g dextrose}$$

$$\frac{7 \text{ g amino acids}}{100 \text{ ml}} \text{ as } \frac{X \text{ g amino acids}}{1,500 \text{ ml}}$$
$$(7 \text{ g} \times 1,500 \text{ ml}) \div 100 \text{ ml} = 105 \text{ g amino acids}$$

To calculate the total kcalories in the mixture, simply multiply by kcalories per gram:

$$750 \text{ g dextrose} \times 3.4 \text{ kcal/g} = 2,550 \text{ kcal}$$
$$105 \text{ g protein} \times 4.0 \text{ kcal/g} = \underline{420 \text{ kcal}}$$
$$2,970 \text{ kcal}$$

Several abbreviations are used to name IV solutions:

D: dextrose

W: water

NS: normal saline (0.9% sodium chloride solution)

These abbreviations are combined to specify IV solutions as follows:

D_5W

Read as: 5% dextrose in water (the subscript following the *D* tells you the percentage of dextrose required).

$D_{10}W$

Read as: 10% dextrose in water.

$D_5\frac{1}{2}$ normal saline

Read as: 5% dextrose in a ½ normal saline solution (0.45% sodium chloride).

How would you read $D_{50}W$?

IV Fat Emulsions and Peripheral Total Parenteral Nutrition

Simple glucose solutions or those solutions containing amino acids only present a major drawback—they fall far short of meeting total nutrient needs. The problem is that the small-diameter peripheral veins become irritated and eventually collapse when highly concentrated nutrient solutions are infused. If less concentrated solutions were used, it would take 12 to 15 liters of solution a day to deliver all the needed nutrients. This volume is more than the body can safely handle in a day.

IV fat emulsions make it possible to deliver needed nutrients by peripheral vein for two reasons. First, they provide a concentrated source of kcalories. Ten percent fat emulsions provide 1.1 kcalories per milliliter, and 20 percent

peripheral vein:
the small-diameter veins that bring blood to the extremities (arms and legs).

peripheral total parenteral nutrition (PTPN):
the provision of nutrient solution that meets nutrient needs by peripheral vein.

A typical PTPN solution contains
750 ml of 2.5% amino acid solution
750 ml of 6.25% dextrose solution
1,500 ml of 10% fat emulsion

bilirubin:
a pigment in the bile whose concentration in the blood may become elevated as a result of some disorders.

hyperlipidemias:
elevated levels of fats in the blood. See Chapter 21.

palpitations:
rapid fluttering or throbbing of the heart.

cyanosis:
a bluish or grayish color of the skin.

total parenteral nutrition (TPN):
a method of meeting all nutrient needs by using large-diameter central veins.

central veins:
the larger-diameter veins located close to the heart (see Figure 15–5).

fat emulsions provide 2.0 kcalories per milliliter. Second, IV fat is isotonic to blood and does not irritate the veins the way hypertonic glucose and amino acid solutions do.

IV fat is also important because it provides essential fatty acids, thus preventing deficiencies. IV fat can safely provide from 50 to 60 percent of the total daily energy requirement for the unstressed client.[21] Some studies suggest that in the stressed client fat may be less effective than glucose in promoting nitrogen balance.[22] However, other studies have failed to confirm these findings.[23] Animal studies suggest that burns may alter lipid metabolism and it may be desirable to limit fat to less than 15 percent of the total kcalorie requirements.[24] Again, however, further studies are needed in animals and humans to determine optimal fat intake for the person who is severely burned.

The use of IV fat, amino acids, and dextrose given by peripheral vein to meet all energy needs is called *peripheral total parenteral nutrition (PTPN)*. IV vitamins, minerals, and trace elements can also be given to provide for other nutrient needs.

People who need only short-term nutrition support (about 7 to 14 days), people with normal renal function who do not have excessive energy requirements, people in whom inserting an IV catheter into a central vein might be difficult, and people on oral or tube feedings may benefit from PTPN. IV fat emulsions are contraindicated in newborns with markedly elevated bilirubin levels and in people with some types of hyperlipidemias, severe liver disease, and those with severe egg allergies. Cautious use of IV fats is recommended for people with atherosclerosis, moderate liver disease, blood coagulation disorders, pancreatitis, and some types of lung problems.

Although infrequent, adverse reactions to IV fat emulsions occur in some people, particularly when IV fats are given in excessive doses or administered too rapidly. Immediate reactions can include fever, warmth, chills, backache, chest pain, allergic reactions, palpitations, rapid breathing, wheezing, cyanosis, nausea, and an unpleasant taste in the mouth. Irritation and inflammation of the vein are also possible. After long-term administration, the most commonly observed adverse effect is the deposition of a brown pigment in certain liver cells. These pigments disappear after parenteral therapy is stopped, and their effect on liver function is unknown. Other effects of long-term administration can include enlarged liver and spleen and a reduced number of blood platelets and white blood cells.

TPN by Central Vein

Another method used to meet all nutrient needs by vein is called *central total parenteral nutrition (TPN)*. When the term *TPN* is used alone, it refers to total parenteral nutrition by central vein. In central TPN, the IV catheter is surgically placed in a large-diameter central vein (see Figure 15–5). Almost a gallon of blood rushes through one such vein—the superior vena cava—each minute. Here, highly concentrated solutions can be quickly diluted. By the time these solutions reach the peripheral veins, they are not irritating. Therefore, central TPN can deliver concentrated nutrient solutions even without the use of IV fat.

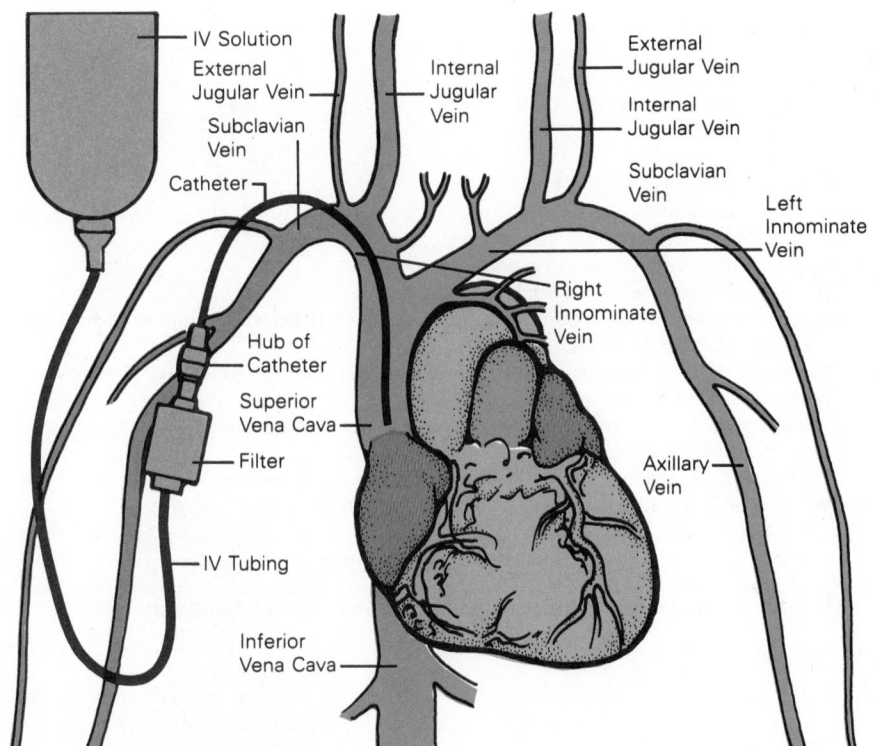

IV Solution
External Jugular Vein
Subclavian Vein
Catheter
Internal Jugular Vein
External Jugular Vein
Internal Jugular Vein
Subclavian Vein
Left Innominate Vein
Right Innominate Vein
Hub of Catheter
Superior Vena Cava
Filter
IV Tubing
Axillary Vein
Inferior Vena Cava

FIGURE 15–5

The central veins used for TPN. The superior vena cava is one of the largest-diameter central veins and is usually used for giving TPN solutions. When it cannot be used, the internal jugular vein is the next choice, followed by the external jugular vein. Can you see why?

Enteral nutrition is always preferred to parenteral nutrition (by central or peripheral vein) for many reasons. First of all, enteral nutrition helps maintain normal gut function. When the GI tract is not used for long periods of time, the cells of the intestine (the villi) shrink and enzyme activity in the gut is reduced. Enteral nutrition is associated with fewer complications, even when tube feeding is necessary. A transnasal feeding tube can be inserted at bedside without an anesthetic. Insertion of an IV catheter for central TPN is a minor surgical procedure that requires local anesthesia. Care of the catheter site is more demanding than care of the feeding tube. Finally, enteral nutrition is far less costly than TPN. Cost containment (see Nutrition and Practice 15B) is an important consideration in client care. One study suggested potential cost savings of over $70,000 for 14 clients who received nutrition support for 280 days had enteral nutrition been given rather than parenteral nutrition.[25]

People who cannot or should not be fed through the GI tract are candidates for TPN, which is indicated whenever long-term parenteral nutrition will be required, when nutrient requirements are high, or when people are severely malnourished. Some specific conditions that may necessitate its use are listed in Table 15–5. The actual need for TPN must be determined by the individual's medical and nutrition needs. Ideally, the person should not reach a severely depleted state before TPN is initiated. It is much easier to maintain nutrition status than to try to replenish lost nutrient stores with TPN.

IV catheter:
the thin tube inserted into a vein through which nutrient solutions or medications can be given directly.

TABLE 15–5 Possible Indications for TPN by Central Vein.

Major small bowel resections.
Radiation enteritis (inflammation of intestine caused by radiation).
Severe diarrhea.
Intractable vomiting.
Intensive chemotherapy.
Bone marrow transplants.
Inflammatory bowel disease (see Chapter 20).
Moderate to severe acute pancreatitis.
Severe malnutrition when GI tract is nonfunctional.
Hypermetabolic disorders, or major surgery, when it is anticipated that the GI tract will be unusable for 5–7 days.
Moderate stress if adequate nutrient intake cannot be achieved for over 7–10 days.
Enterocutaneous fistulas.
Hyperemesis gravidarum (severe nausea and vomiting associated with pregnancy) when it lasts for over 5–7 days.
Moderate malnutrition if surgical or intensive medical intervention is necessary.
When adequate enteral nutrition cannot be established within 7–10 days of hospitalization.

Source: Adapted from A.S.P.E.N. Board of Directors, Guidelines for the use of total parenteral nutrition in the hospitalized adult patient, *Journal by Parenteral and Enteral Nutrition* 10 (1986): 441–445.

The TPN Solution

The actual concentrations of amino acids and dextrose that compose the final TPN solution are determined by each person's unique nutrient needs. People who are extremely malnourished or highly stressed (by burns or infection) require more protein and kcalories than moderately malnourished or mildly stressed individuals.

Traditionally, TPN solutions provide energy primarily from dextrose. IV fat is given periodically (two 500-milliliter bottles per week) to meet essential fatty acid requirements. Currently, however, the trend is to use IV fat emulsions more frequently as an energy source.[26] This is particularly true for people in respiratory failure, because oxidation of glucose in the body produces more carbon dioxide per kcalorie than does fat and can lead to respiratory acidosis.

Electrolytes, vitamins, and trace elements are added to the TPN solution in addition to dextrose, amino acids, and fat. The normal ranges of requirements for these nutrients are listed in Tables 15–6 and 15–7. Essential fatty acid requirements are met by giving IV fat. Other possible additions to the TPN solution include:

- Albumin, to raise serum albumin concentration.
- Heparin, to prevent clots, which might obstruct the flow of the TPN solution from forming on the IV catheter.
- Insulin, to help regulate blood sugar levels.

Adding albumin, heparin, and insulin directly to the TPN solution is a controversial practice. Not all institutions consider these substances TPN additives. Where they are used, only those additives needed by each individual are given.

One liter of a typical TPN solution contains 25% dextrose and 3.5% amino acids. Often, 3 L of the solution are given daily and provide 3,000 kcal and 105 g protein.

respiratory acidosis:
a condition of too much acid in the blood caused by failure of the lungs to ventilate properly. Excess acids are normally released from the lungs during exhalation; diseased lungs, however, are unable to perform this function adequately.

TABLE 15–6 Normal Range of Daily Vitamin and Mineral Requirements During TPN

Vitamin[a]	Recommended Amount
Vitamin A (IU)	3,300
Vitamin D (IU)	200
Vitamin E (IU)	10
Vitamin C (mg)	5
Folacin (μg)	400
Niacin (mg)	40
Riboflavin (mg)	3.6
Thiamin (mg)	3.0
Vitamin B_6 (mg)	4.0
Vitamin B_{12} (μg)	5.0
Pantothenic acid (mg)	15
Biotin (μg)	60

Mineral[b]	Normal Range
Sodium (mEq)	60 to 150
Potassium (mEq)	70 to 150
Chloride (mEq)	Equal to sodium
Calcium (mEq)	0.2 to 0.3/kg
Magnesium (mEq)	0.35 to 0.45/kg
Phosphorus (mmole)	7 to 10 per 1,000 kcal

[a]Data from American Medical Association, Department of Foods and Nutrition, Multivitamin preparations for parenteral use: A statement by the Nutrition Advisory Group, *Journal of Parenteral and Enteral Nutrition* 3 (1979): 258–262.

[b]Data from J. P. Grant, *Handbook of Total Parenteral Nutrition* (Philadelphia: Saunders, 1980), p. 98.

Like a tube feeding, a TPN feeding is started slowly to give the client time to adapt to the high nutrient concentrations of the TPN solution. Health team members monitor the client regularly to ensure that the nutrient solution is appropriate for the person's needs and that the person is tolerating the solution. Guidelines for monitoring the person on TPN are given in Table 15–8.

TABLE 15–7 Guidelines for Trace Element Use in Parenteral Nutrition

Trace Element	Suggested IV Intake	Comments
Zinc	2.5 to 4.0 mg	Add 2.0 mg for adult in acute catabolic state; add 12.2 mg/l of small bowel fluid lost; add 17.1 mg/kg of stool or ileostomy output.
Copper	0.5 to 1.5 mg	
Chromium	10 to 15 μg	Add 20 μg for stable adult with interstinal losses.
Manganese	0.15 to 0.80 mg	

Source: Adapted from American Medical Association, Department of Foods and Nutrition, Guidelines for essential trace element preparations for parenteral use, a statement by an expert panel, *Journal of the American Medical Association* 241 (1979): 2051–2054.

TABLE 15–8 Guidelines for Monitoring People on TPN

Frequency of Monitoring	Clinical or Biochemical Parameter
Every 4–6 hours:	Urinary glucose Vital signs (respiration, pulse, temperature)
Daily:	Weight Strict intake and output Urine specific gravity
Daily until stable; then 2–3 times weekly:	Serum glucose Serum electrolytes Blood urea nitrogen
Weekly:	Nutrition assessment Serum protein Serum calcium Serum phosphorus Serum ammonia Complete blood count

Transitional/Combination Feedings

Once the need for tube feedings or intravenous nutrition has ended, the client is gradually weaned onto an oral diet while the volume of the special feedings is tapered off. Care must be taken to ensure that the individual's nutrient needs will continue to be met. For example, a person on a tube feeding should be eating adequate amounts of food by mouth before the tube feeding is discontinued. The person can eat "around the tube" as the volume of the tube feeding is gradually tapered off. In many cases, the person can drink the same formula as is delivered by tube.

The transition from intravenous feeding to an oral diet can be accomplished in several ways. One way is to place the client on a tube feeding. The volume of the IV nutrition solution is reduced as a greater volume of tube feeding is tolerated. If the tube feeding is not tolerated, the person can still rely on TPN to meet nutrient needs. The person can also be weaned from the TPN solution while oral intake is resumed, avoiding the use of a tube.

The transition to enteral nutrition after a person has been on intravenous feedings for long periods of time is especially important. Following long periods of disuse, the intestinal villi shrink and lose some of their function. The return to enteral nutrition must be gradual to avoid problems of malabsorption and other GI discomforts. The gradual introduction of nutrients to the GI tract stimulates the progressive return of the villi to normal structure and function.

The return to oral intake for the person who has been fed either intravenously or by tube can have a variety of effects. Some people may be eager to eat again, and food can be an important morale booster. Others may be apprehensive about eating, particulary if they had extensive GI problems. Appetite may be slow to return for others. In such circumstances, all members of the health care team can play a pivotal role in the successful reintroduction of food.

Recognize the person's concerns and reassure the person that you will be there to help him through the process.

Specialized Nutrition Support at Home

Occasionally a client must continue to receive specialized nutrition support (tube feedings or parenteral nutrition) after the primary medical condition has stabilized. In such a case, hospitalization remains necessary largely so that the client can continue to receive specialized nutrition support. An alternative to continued hospital care is continuance of nutrition support at home.

The main objective of home parenteral and enteral nutrition (HPEN), as with TPN and tube feedings in the hospital, is to maintain or achieve adequate nutrition status. However, HPEN has an added dimension: it permits a person to get the needed nutrition care at home, in familiar surroundings. If you have ever been in the hospital yourself, or even taken a long trip for that matter, you probably remember what comfort and relaxation you experience when you return to your own bed, can get things when you need them, and know where things are. The familiarity of home is comforting. In some cases, people who require HPEN can resume many activities, such as going to work, driving, and playing sports. In general, HPEN allows people the opportunity to lead more normal lives than in the hospital.

An additional benefit of HPEN is cost savings. It is less expensive to maintain a person on parenteral or tube feedings when that person or the family assumes responsibilities formerly performed by hospital staff. On the average, home parenteral nutrition (HPN) costs about half what the care would cost in the hospital, whereas for home enteral nutrition (HEN), costs are reduced by 75 percent.[27]

Since the first report of a person sent home successfully on HPN in 1969,[28] the use of HPEN has expanded rapidly. The number of people benefiting from HPEN programs continues to grow, and health care professionals who work with HPEN are gaining valuable experience to improve the quality of specialized nutrition support at home. Although the exact number of people on HPEN programs is unknown, it is estimated that from 2,000 to 5,000 people are on HPN and from 15,000 to 20,000 are on HEN.[29] Many medical supply companies provide the equipment, formulations, and service necessary to support the person on HPEN.

While one person may require HPEN for a relatively short time (for example, a few months), another may require HPEN permanently. In addition to medical considerations, the candidate for HPEN and those who care for that person must have rational, stable personalities so that problems can be successfully handled as they arise. The person or those who care for him must be capable of learning the techniques of HPEN and of dealing with complications. Additionally, the person must have financial resources to support the program as well as access to the equipment, supplies, and professional support that are integral components of a successful HPEN program. The members of the nutrition support team most frequently decide if a client is a candidate for HPEN.

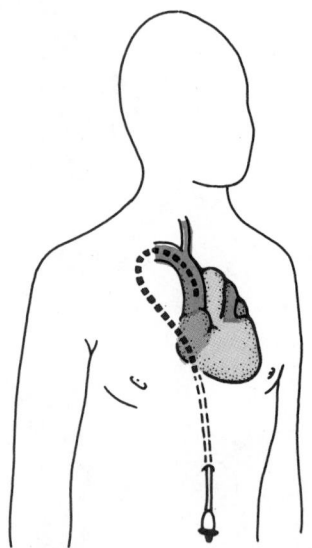

FIGURE 15–6
Placement of an HPN catheter. In this
case, the catheter is tunneled under the skin
before going into the subclavian vein; in
other cases, the catheter may enter the
subclavian directly. The catheter has a
Dacron cuff; connective tissue from the
person's skin grows into this cuff and helps
hold it in place.

Home Parenteral Nutrition

Different types of HPN programs are in current use. Ideally, clients are given as much responsibility for their own care as they can handle. For example, a client who is capable of mixing the solutions and changing the catheter dressings is trained to do so. Typically, family members also learn the techniques so that they can assist in the procedures whenever necessary.

A special type of catheter often is inserted for HPN; it enters near the middle of the chest, is tunneled under the skin, and eventually enters the subclavien vein (see Figure 15–6). The use of this technique makes it possible for the client to see the catheter site and to inspect it for changes as well as to perform dressing changes.

Another method for infusing HPN solutions that is quickly gaining popularity is the subcutaneous port. Unlike a typical catheter that has an outside portion exposed, the port is totally implanted under the skin. Totally implanted devices appear to be associated with a lower infection rate, and they do not require a dressing except when the nutrient infusion is being delivered.[30] The port is cosmetically superior (an advantage for the adolescent), and it results in less restriction of activity (an advantage for young children and other active people). However, disadvantages are also associated with the subcutaneous port. Obese clients and those who are noncompliant or misuse the port may have a more difficult time with this method.[31]

The most common method of nutrient administration is for the client to use an infusion pump set at a rate that delivers the total volume of solution needed for the day within 8 to 12 hours. Most people can tolerate solutions delivered this way. The total volume of solution can be placed in large-capacity IV bags so that the client can infuse the solution while sleeping or at any other convenient time. This method of delivery allows freedom of movement during much of the day.

The client starts the solution slowly to avoid hyperglycemia and tapers it off at the end of the feeding to avoid hypoglycemia. Each time the client disconnects the IV tubing, heparin is injected into the catheter to prevent clotting.

For people who cannot tolerate an 8- to 12-hour infusion rate, nutrients are infused over 24 hours. Those who are ambulatory can benefit from a lightweight vest that holds a small pump and IV bags. This system allows the client to move around freely with little inconvenience.

Some people prepare their own HPN solutions from bottles of IV dextrose and amino acids. Others receive their bottles premixed. Premixed solutions are more convenient and are essential when the client's (or family member's) ability to correctly mix the solution is questionable. The costs of premixed versus self-mixed solutions vary widely. In some cases, self-mixed solutions are actually more expensive. A significant and shocking variablity in the costs of home TPN solutions has been reported. In a survey of home care costs, 12 home care vendors were asked to provide price quotes for a given home TPN formula.[32] The price for self-mixed formulas varied from $63,430 to $133,431 annually; as you can see, the difference between the least expensive and most expensive vendor was about $70,000 annually! Similarly, the difference between the least expensive and most expensive vendor for premixed formulas was over $60,000 annually. Although the authors note that the services provided by the different vendors are not accounted for in this survey, it is obvious that health care team members need to look closely at the vendors in their area who provide home care services.

Home Enteral Nutrition

HEN programs are similar to HPN programs in many ways. HEN is the choice of feeding method for the person who must continue special nutrition support at home. Enteral nutrition preserves normal bowel function, it is simpler to prepare and deliver, it is less expensive, and it has fewer complications than parenteral nutrition.

Feeding ostomies often are placed for long-term tube feedings. Some people learn to use a transnasal tube, which they insert at each feeding. When possible, an intermittent feeding schedule is arranged so that the person is free to move around between meals. Generally, infusion pumps are used only if necessary; they are expensive to purchase or rent. People who must receive a continuous drip feeding are trained to use the pump. Small pumps, easily concealed in clothing, are available to allow more freedom of movement for clients on continuous drip feedings. The person on HEN either makes a tube feeding from blenderized table food or purchases a commercially prepared, premixed formula. Most clients prefer to purchase formula. A premixed formula should be used whenever the person's ability to mix the formula is questionable.

Generally, a nurse visits the person on HEN at home, and the client sees a physician at regular intervals. In some programs, dietitians make home visits also. A qualified nurse, dietitian, or physician must be available to answer questions as they arise.

How Do People on HPEN Cope?

Several social and psychological problems accompany the use of HPEN.[33] Such problems must be recognized and dealt with to successfully implement an HPEN program. Clients worry about the substantial costs associated with HPEN, and common problems include body image problems, depression, drug dependency, delirium, grief, and anxiety. People on HPEN must learn to cope with their inability to eat or drink normally and their dependency on a machine for survival.

However, many people in successful HPEN programs have a reasonable quality of life.[34] HPEN allows people to resume many activities, including employment, sexual activity, recreation, swimming, social activity, and travel. Women on HPN successfully carry and deliver babies. Students return to college. One person on HPN was quoted as saying, "Do I miss the taste of real food? Sure. But you get used to it. Look at the alternative. Ten years ago I would have been dead of starvation."[35]

The tremendous growth of HPEN programs offers new hope for many people who otherwise could have survived only in the hospital. As more and more people begin HPEN programs, health professionals continue to find better methods of helping people help themselves. In the future, more will be learned about the technical, psychological, and social implications of HPEN, and the quality of care will continue to improve.

CASE STUDY

A Client Requiring Total Parenteral Nutrition

Mr. Small has been admitted to the hospital for a diagnostic workup. He has been steadily losing weight. He appears emaciated and states that he can't swallow and has lost his appetite. He was afraid to come to the hospital and has waited a long time before checking in. After a thorough examination, Mr. Small has been found to have an obstruction in his esophagus. The nutrition assessment reveals severe PCM. Surgery will be required as soon as possible. Mr. Small is placed on central TPN before surgery. He progresses well, gains weight, and undergoes surgery about two weeks after admission. During surgery, a feeding jejunostomy is made.

1. What factors in Mr. Small's history indicate the need for central TPN?

2. How would you explain the need for TPN to Mr. Small?

3. Is the placement of a feeding jejunostomy during surgery a good idea? Why or why not?

About two days after surgery, Mr. Small begins to receive feedings through the jejunostomy. His digestive and absorptive capacity are intact.

4. Specifically, what type of formula would you recommend for Mr. Small's tube feedings?

5. How does the feeding route influence your selection of formula?

6. How would you begin the tube feeding? How would you progress it? How would you deliver it? How would you monitor its effectiveness?

7. When should Mr. Small be taken off central TPN? How should this be accomplished?

8. After several weeks, Mr. Small is ready to take some food by mouth. How does this affect his tube feeding?

9. If Mr. Small's medical condition stabilized but he was unable to consume enough food by mouth to go off tube feedings, he might be a candidate for HEN. Discuss some considerations in selecting a candidate for HEN. What are some of the advantages of such a program?

Notes

1. A.S.P.E.N. Board of Directors, Guidelines for the use of enteral nutrition in the adult patient, *Journal of Parenteral and Enteral Nutrition* 11 (1987): 435–439.

2. L. J. Nicholson, Declogging small-bore feeding tubes, *Journal of Parenteral and Enteral Nutrition* 11 (1987): 594–597.

3. K. E. Fagerman and L. K. Lysen, Enteral feeding tubes: A comparison and history, *Nutritional Support Services* 7, September 1987, pp. 10–14.

4. D. B. Silk and coauthors, Clinical efficacy and design changes of "fine bore" nasogastric feeding tubes: A seven year experience involving 809 intubations in 403 patients. *Journal of Parenteral and Enteral Nutrition* 11 (1987): 378–383; R. Levenson and coauthors, Do weighted nasoenteric feeding tubes facilitate duodenal intubations? *Journal of Parenteral and Enteral Nutrition* 12 (1988): 135–137.

5. B. K. Bohnker, L. E. Artman, and W. J. Hoskin, Narrow bore nasogastric feeding tube complications, *Nutrition in Clinical Practice* 2 (1987): 203–209.

6. S. Bell and coauthors, Modular enteral diets: Cost and nutritional value comparisons, *Journal of the American Dietetic Association* 87 (1987): 1526–1530.

7. A. Bloch, Enteral formulas, *Nutritional Support Services* 1, March 1987, pp. 23–24.

8. Bell and coauthors, 1987.

9. D. H. Raigman and C. Braunschweig, Fiber in enteral feedings, *Nutritional Support Services* 6, June 1986, pp. 29–33.

10. M. J. Koruda and coauthors, The effect of a pectin-supplemented elemental diet on intestinal adaptation to massive small bowel resection, *Journal of Parenteral and Enteral Nutrition* 10 (1986): 343–350.

11. L. Vaughan, M. Manore, and D. Wilson, Bacterial safety of a closed-administration system for enteral nutrition solutions, *Journal of the American Dietetic Association* 88 (1988): 35–37.

12. P. P. Keohane and coauthors, Relation between osmolality of diet and gastrointestinal side effects in enteral nutrition, *British Medical Journal* 288 (1984): 678–680.

13. J. L. Rombeau, Advances in enteral feeding, an address presented at the Georgia Dietetic Association Annual Meeting, 17 July 1986.

14. C. Austin, Water: Guidelines for nutritional support, *Nutritional Support Services* 6, September 1986, pp. 27–29.

15. B. Wright and L. Robinson, Enteral feeding tubes as drug delivery systems, *Nutritional Support Services* 6, February 1986, pp. 33–37, 47.

16. J. Saklad, R. Graves, and W. P. Sharp, Interaction of oral phenytoin with enteral feedings, *Journal of Parenteral and Enteral Nutrition* 10 (1986): 322–323.

17. K. Fagerman, D. McGuigan, and B. Pixley, Potential interaction between enteral feeding solutions and oral tetracycline, *Nutrition and Clinical Practice* 1 (1986): 257–258.

18. P. Egging, Enteral nutrition from a pharmacist's perspective, *Nutritional Support Services* 7, April 1987, pp. 17–18, 34.

19. C. L. Breach and L. G. Saldanka, Tube feeding complications, Part I: Gastrointestinal, *Nutritional Support Services* 8, March 1988, pp. 15–17.

20. A.S.P.E.N. Board of Directors, Guidelines for use of total parenteral nutrition in the hospitalized adult patient, *Journal of Parenteral and Enteral Nutrition* 10 (1986): 441–445.

21. M. Roesner and J. P. Grant, Intravenous lipid emulsions, *Nutrition in Clinical Practice* 2 (1987): 96–107.

22. H. Shizgal and R. Forse, Protein and calorie requirements with total parenteral nutrition, *Annals of Surgery* 192 (1980): 562–569; J. Long and coauthors, Effect of carbohydrate and fat intake on nitrogen excretion during total intravenous feeding, *Annals of Surgery* 185 (1987): 417–421.

23. J. Nordenstrom, J. Askanazi, and D. Elwyn, Nitrogen balance during total parenteral nutrition: Glucose vs fat, *Annals of Surgery* 197 (1983): 27–33; J. Macfie and coauthors, Glucose or fat as a nonprotein energy source? *Gastroenterology* 80 (1981): 103–107.

24. M. M. Gottschlich and J. W. Alexander, Fat kinetics and recommended dietary intake in burns, *Journal of Parenteral and Enteral Nutrition* 11 (1987): 80–85.

25. D. D. O'Brien and coauthors, Recommendations of nutrition support team promote cost containment, *Journal of Parenteral and Enteral Nutrition* 10 (1986): 300–302.

26. H. Gilder, Parenteral nourishment of patients undergoing surgical or traumatic stress, *Journal of Parenteral and Enteral Nutrition* 10 (1986): 88–99.

27. Howard and coauthors, A review of the current national status of home parenteral and enteral nutrition from the provider and consumer perspective, *Journal of Parenteral and Enteral Nutrition* 10 (1986): 416–424.

28. M. E. Shils and coauthors, Long term parenteral nutrition through an external arteriovenous shunt, *New England Journal of Medicine* 283 (1970): 341–344.

29. Howard and coauthors, 1986.

30. S. L. Beck, N. R. Rose, and A. J. Zagoren, Home total parenteral nutrition utilizing implantable infusion ports, *Nutrition in Clinical Practice* 2 (1987): 26–29.

31. J. H. Bodzin, Homecare open forum, *Nutritional Support Services* 6, July 1986, pp. 23, 25.

32. R. J. Baptista and coauthors, The cost of home total parenteral nutrition, *Nutrition in Clinical Practice* 2 (1987): 14–22.

33. A. D. Gulledge and coauthors, Psychosocial issues of home parenteral and enteral nutrition, *Nutrition in Clinical Practice* 2 (1987): 183–194.

34. C. Marein and coauthors, Home parenteral nutrition, *Nutrition in Clinical Practice* 1 (1986): 179–192; J. R. Wesley, Home parenteral nutrition: Indications, principles, and cost-effectiveness, *Comprehensive Therapy* 4 (1983): 29–36; K. Ladefoged, Quality of life in patients on permanent home parenteral nutrition, *Journal of Parenteral and Enteral Nutrition* 5 (1980): 132–137.

35. D. Ingber, People who never need to eat, *Science Digest,* January 1982, pp. 34–35.

NUTRITION IN PRACTICE
15A
Ethical Issues in Clinical Nutrition

Chapter 15 described in some detail the techniques of parenteral and enteral nutrition. Only in recent years have we had at our disposal the capability of providing nutrients for people unable to eat by conventional means. The technical advances made in the areas of enteral and parenteral nutrition have been lifesaving for many. However, as is true with many new technologies, the availability of special nutrition support forces health care professionals to deal with ethical dilemmas—specifically, when it is morally and legally appropriate to use special nutrition support techniques and when these techniques should be discontinued.

The purpose of this Nutrition in Practice is to discuss some of the ethical questions that have been raised regarding the use of enteral and parenteral nutrition. The intent of this section is not to draw conclusions or solve the problem. Rather, we seek to present the issues for your consideration.

What ethical problems face health care professionals with respect to nutrition support?
To put the problem into perspective, consider for a moment the techniques of specialized nutrition support. Under most circumstances, the decision to feed a person by tube feeding or TPN is clear-cut. The person who has a reasonable chance to recover from a disease and sustain an

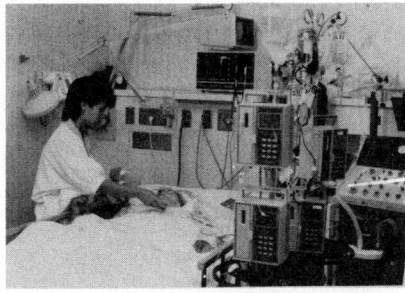

When is it morally and legally appropriate to use special nutrition support techniques?

acceptable quality of life is given whatever form of nutrition support is necessary. Clearly, nutrition support cannot rightfully be withheld because of poor judgment or negligence. If a person were to die because nourishment was withheld, the caretakers would be held responsible. In all likelihood, a malpractice lawsuit would result. In one case, an out-of-court settlement of $400,000 was negotiated by a hospital charged with failure to provide needed care, including nutrition support, to a person with Crohn's disease.[1]

However, what about the person who is not expected to recover from a disease or the person who is expected to have a very poor quality of life even if recovery is possible? How aggressively do we support the person who is terminally ill or permanently comatose? How do we respond to elderly or physically disabled people who refuse special nutrition support

because they feel the quality of their lives is so poor that they do not wish to be sustained? Do we (as a society) allow such a choice? Are health care professionals morally and legally obligated to comply with or to deny such requests? Furthermore, when people are incompetent and unable to speak for themselves, who, if anyone, should be allowed to make such life-and-death decisions? These questions are but a few of the unanswered concerns that have evolved along with the technology of special feeding techniques.

That's quite a bit to think about. What can legally be done in the situations you described?
Although each specific case is different, in many cases the client's wishes receive primary consideration. Individuals have a legal right to refuse medical treatment even if that treatment is considered necessary to sustain life. From a legal standpoint, refusal of treatment is not considered suicide as long as the person's eventual death results from the underlying disease and not from the person's own doing.

However, the situation changes when the person is comatose, incompetent, or otherwise unable to refuse or accept medical treatment. How can his wishes regarding treatment be made known? To address this concern, many states have enacted laws that authorize the use of living wills.[2]

What is a living will?

A living will is the written statement of a competent person that specifies that no extraordinary treatments should be administered in the event that the person is diagnosed as terminally ill and is unable to make the necessary decisions at that time. Alternatively, a living will may declare a person's wish to have every effort made to keep him alive in the event of terminal illness or irreversible loss of consciousness. People should make their wishes known in writing, even if their state does not have a living will provision. Each individual's preference should be known to her physicians and family and should be a part of the medical record.

An advantage of planning ahead for future care in the case of a terminal illness or irreversible state of unconsciousness is that others are freed from the guilt and anxiety of having to make that decision. Imagine, for example, the anxiety a spouse would have to go through in directing the health care team to stop nutrition support, knowing that it would hasten death. That decision would be far easier if the spouse knew that was what the individual would want or, better yet, if a legal document took the decision out of the spouse's hands altogether.

Living wills are not authorized in some states. In other states, living wills may state that *medical* measures to sustain life should be discontinued but that *nutrition* and *hydration* should proceed. In fact, they may specifically exclude withholding nourishment and hydration as an option. People who prefer that these techniques not be used in the event of imminent death

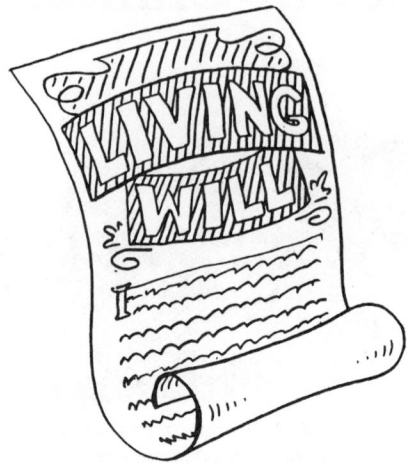

A living will gives competent adults a chance to make known their wishes that no heroic efforts be made to revive them in the event that they become terminally ill or comatose and they are unable to authorize or refuse medical treatments.

or vegetative state may need to take further legal actions to ensure that their wishes be carried out.

What other legal actions can be taken?

The durable power of attorney may be an appropriate alternative.[3] A durable power of attorney allows one competent adult to designate another competent adult as an agent to make decisions in the event of incapacition. The durable power of attorney has yet to be tested in court, but it may be a feasible alternative for ensuring that the individual's requests be carried out in states that do not authorize living wills or in states that do not allow nourishment and hydration to be withheld.

How do parenteral and enteral nutrition fit into the picture of living wills?

As technology has improved to the extent that a person can be fed totally by parenteral and enteral nutrition, questions regarding the use of these feedings to sustain an individual who is terminally ill or in an irreversible coma have surfaced. On the one hand, it is argued that nourishment and hydration do not constitute "extraordinary treatment." Indeed, nourishment is so basic to life that feeding a person, even through mechanical means, should not be considered extraordinary. Furthermore, feeding a person has traditionally not been considered to be painful or obtrusive. Those who argue this side of the case find it totally unacceptable that food or water would be withheld or withdrawn from a living being for any reason.

On the other hand, it is argued that using parenteral and enteral nutrition to replace the normal process of eating is not different from using a respirator to replace the process of breathing. These individuals feel that the placement of a feeding tube or TPN catheter *is* obtrusive and uncomfortable. They feel that withholding and withdrawing nutrition support is morally and legally justified for individuals who request that no heroic measures be made to sustain their lives in the event of terminal illness or irreversible coma.

Often, it is unclear which of these positions the individual with the terminal illness supports. Even those who have signed living wills may not have considered whether nutrition support is an extraordinary treatment. Basically, living wills state that only measures that will preserve the person's comfort and dignity should be taken. It is unclear whether the individual who signs the living will intends to include or exclude the use of parenteral or enteral nutrition as such a measure. As discussed earlier, several states with living will legislation specifically *exclude* the right to withhold or withdraw nourishment or hydration.[4]

To date, the number of court cases that specifically involve withholding or withdrawing nutrition support is relatively small. This suggests that many cases are being resolved among the people involved in the individual's care—the person, her family, and the health care team.

How can health care professionals help deal with these problems?

That is a good question. In some hospitals, ethics committees are formed to deal with problems of this type. Health care professionals should ensure that their disciplines are represented on such committees. Recently, the American Dietetic Association published a position paper on feeding terminally ill adults.[5] The paper provides an excellent review of the subject of ethics in nutrition care, and interested readers would be advised to read it.

The many ethical and legal problems that have evolved with the improved technology for delivering nutrients present tough challenges for individuals, their loved ones, the health care team, and the legal system. It is likely that new questions will

Miniglossary

artificial feeding parenteral and enteral nutrition. Feeding by a route other than the normal ingestion of food.

brain dead having an irreversible loss of the brain function necessary to sustain life.

cerebral palsy a loss of sensation and ability to control movement that results from defects in the brain or trauma at birth.

comatose in a state of deep unconsciousness from which the person cannot be aroused.

gangrene death of tissue.

homicide murder.

living will a document signed by a competent adult that specifically states that the person does not wish any heroic measures to be taken in the event of terminal illness or irreversible coma from which the person is not expected to recover.

organic brain syndrome a group of mental disorders associated with brain damage or impaired brain function.

arise in the future. One thing is clear: The solutions to these problems are as complex as the problems themselves.

Health care professionals, particularly physicians, can find themselves in awkward and difficult positions regarding aggressive

nutrition support. On the one hand, they are obligated to provide optimal care. Negligence could result in a malpractice suit. On the other hand, health care professionals are client advocates. In this role, they must respect the wishes of the people in their care. Again, there is no easy answer to this dilemma. Each case must be carefully decided on its individual circumstances and actions taken as appropriate.

Notes

1. A. Barrocas, J. Farquharson, and M. Fernandez, Legal considerations in nutritional support: 1986 update, *Nutritional Support Services* 6, May 1986: 33.
2. All states except Alaska, Hawaii, Kentucky, Massachusetts, Michigan, Minnesota, Nebraska, New Jersey, New York, North Dakota, Ohio, Pennsylvania, Rhode Island, South Carolina, and South Dakota have authorized the use of living wills. B. Mishkin, Withholding and withdrawing nutritional support: Advance planning for hard choices, *Nutrition in Clinical Practice* 1 (1986): 50–52.
3. Mishkin, 1986.
4. These states include Arizona, Colorado, Connecticut, Florida, Georgia, Illinois, Iowa, Maine, Maryland, Missouri, New Hampshire, and Oklahoma. Indiana requires only that appropriate nutrition and hydration be provided, a vague statement that could be interpreted in many ways. Mishkin, 1986.
5. American Dietetic Association, Position of the American Dietetic Association: Issues in feeding the terminally ill adult, *Journal of the American Dietetic Association* 87 (1987): 78–85.

Cost Containment and Specialized Nutrition Support

Skyrocketing health care costs are of crucial significance to health care facilities, their employees, and their clients as well as government agencies and taxpayers. The cost of hospitalization has risen higher than costs of any other service industry. Efforts to put a cap on these spiraling costs are necessary to ensure that the majority of people will have access to and the ability to pay for health care. It is beyond the scope of this section to discuss the reasons why health care costs continue to rise or all that these rising costs imply. Rather, we will look at some changes in health care delivery prompted by these spiraling costs and how they affect nutrition care, particularly specialized nutrition support.

I was shocked at the cost of my physical exam to get into college, and I'm concerned about what to expect in the future. What steps are being taken to contain health care costs?

One of the primary steps taken by the government to contain health care costs is the introduction of the prospective payment system for paying the medical bills of people on Medicare. Before the prospective payment system was enacted in September 1983, hospitals were reimbursed by Medicare for a portion of the costs that were incurred while an eligible client was hospitalized. Using this system, hospitals had little incentive to reduce costs, because they

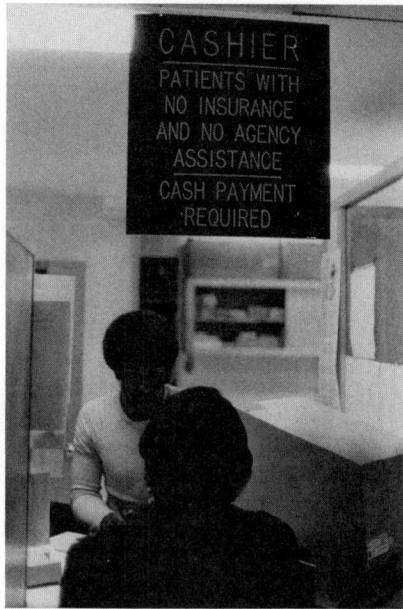

Cost containment is a significant issue in health care today.

were reimbursed for the expenses incurred.

Prospective payment is quite different. Under this system hospitals are paid a fixed price for the care of a client depending on the client's diagnosis. Diagnosis-related groups (DRG) determine how much money will be reimbursed to the hospital for the client once the client is discharged. The payment for hospital costs is independent of actual cost. If, for example, the hospital can care for the

client in fewer days with fewer tests than provided for under the DRG system, the hospital makes money. If the client must be hospitalized longer or if unnecessary tests are performed, the hospital may lose money. Thus, the DRG system encourages hospitals to reduce costs.

That sounds good in a way, but it scares me, too. How can you be sure that the client will not be shortchanged in an effort to reduce costs?

Your concern is shared by others. However, it is important to keep in mind that hospitals and their staffs exist to treat disease and to relieve suffering and pain. In addition, competition between hospitals to attract clients as well as the potential for malpractice suits helps keep the situation in balance. The Prospective Payment Assessment Commission, created by Congress to oversee the DRG system, has found no evidence of reduced quality of care created by the system.[1]

The hospital can receive additional reimbursement for a person who must be hospitalized for much longer than normal or who incurs much higher hospital costs for a particular DRG. However, in such cases, reimbursement is less than actual costs. This is of concern for people who need special nutrition support, because such people are frequently more ill and have longer hospital stays.[2]

I'm confused. In Chapter 13 we learned that attention to good nutrition would result in lower mortality rates, fewer complications, and reduced length of hospital stay. Now it sounds as if the opposite is true. Please explain.

First of all, it's important to note that studies *suggest* that appropriate nutrition support lowers mortality rates, results in fewer complications, and reduces length of hospital stay. Common sense dictates that no disease process benefits from starvation.[3] However, this assertion is difficult to prove for several reasons. One is that people who are malnourished and who need specialized nutrition support are often quite ill. A disease itself may lead to complications or death regardless of the person's nutrition status. Furthermore, the extent of the disease and the degree of malnutrition are not the same in any two people. Therefore, you cannot really look at two different individuals and say positively that any one factor (like nutrition) was responsible for differences you observed during the study.

Although studies have shown that aggressive nutrition support can improve nutrition status, documentation that nutrition support improves outcome from a disease process is limited. The studies that have been done have not shown dramatic effects.[4] All of these factors make it difficult to justify the use of specialized nutrition support services in an atmosphere of cost containment.

How much do TPN and enteral nutrition really cost? How much do they affect the hospital's revenues?

Providing nutrition support, particularly total parenteral nutrition,

Miniglossary

cost effective promoting quality care at the least cost.

cost containment using measures that reduce costs.

diagnosis-related groups (DRG) classification of disorders that provides a basis for reimbursement under Medicare's prospective payment system.

medicare health insurance for eligible recipients that is administered from the Social Security Administration.

prospective payment system a system for reimbursing medical costs for eligible recipients that is based on the person's diagnosis rather than actual costs.

is expensive. Based on a survey completed in 1984, the average cost of parenteral nutrition is about $300 dollars per day.[5] Since the average person placed on parenteral nutrition needs the therapy for about 21 days, the cost of parenteral nutrition alone during an average hospitalization is over $6,000. The cost of providing parenteral nutrition solutions in hospitals in 1984 was estimated to have been three billion dollars.[6]

Enteral nutrition is a far less expensive therapy. The average cost of enteral nutrition is about $25 per day, and the average time required for enteral nutrition is about 18 days.[7] Therefore, the average cost of enteral nutrition during a typical hospitalization is about $450.

The cost of parenteral nutrition combined with the fact that people who require TPN also have longer hospital stays can put serious financial burdens on hospitals. Financial pressures may force hospitals to discontinue the use of specialized nutrition support or to discourage its use.[8] Either of these measures could have a serious impact on the optimal nutrition support of clients.

What can be done to ease the problem?

While some practitioners are pessimistic about the future of specialized nutrition support under the DRG system, others are more optimistic. It is hoped that as more experience with DRG is gained, additional money will be provided under the DRG system to cover the costs of specialized nutrition support. It appears that the DRG system is here to stay—at least for now. It is time to look at how to work within the system to justify the costs of specialized nutrition support.

A nutrition support team can have a significant impact on reducing the costs of specialized nutrition support.[9] The team can reduce costs by:

- Recommending the most cost efficient method of feeding (enteral versus parenteral) as well as the most suitable feeding solution.

- Evaluating and purchasing supplies necessary for nutrition support that will provide the needed service at the least cost.

- Monitoring people on parenteral and enteral nutrition support to avoid or correct metabolic, mechanical, and other problems that can lead to costly complications.

- Identifying people with malnutrition so that malnutrition can be documented as a diagnosis and, in some cases, hospital reimbursement can be increased for the malnourished individual.[10]

- Documenting the positive effects of specialized nutrition support techniques to show that costs would be higher if nutrition support were not provided.

- Continuously evaluating new methods of delivering nutrition support that could save money.

In one study, the potential cost savings of nutrition support recommended by a nutrition support team versus nutrition support initiated by an attending physician was evaluated.[11] In most of the cases where the recommendations of the nutrition support team were not followed, the team had recommended enteral nutrition whereas the physician initiated parenteral nutrition. For the 14 cases that were noncompliant with the team's advice, the potential savings to the client was estimated at over $5,000 per client or over $70,000 for the 14 cases!

Teams help limit the cost of nutrition support by following procedures that reduce the likelihood of complications. One group of authors report an estimated cost savings of $400,000 a year to their hospital due to the low rate of TPN catheter sepsis in their hospital.[12] The authors credit their nutrition support nurse with the much-lowered sepsis rate (1 percent per client catheter) compared to the rate observed in hospitals without a nutrition support nurse (33 percent per client catheter).

To ensure that specialized nutriton support will be safely and readily available for the people who need it, it is imperative that health care professionals understand the problems associated with reimbursement under the prospective payment system. It is only through this understanding that one can begin to take the necessary steps to ensure that clients will have access to optimal nutrition support.

Notes

1. American Society for Parenteral and Enteral Nutrition, *PENline* (newsletter discussing the DRG system), February 1987.

2. G. Robinson, M. Goldstein, and G. M. Levine, Impact of nutritional status on DRG length of stay, *Journal of Parenteral and Enteral Nutrition* 11 (1987): 49–51.

3. A.S.P.E.N. Board of Directors, Guidelines for the use of total parenteral nutrition in the hospitalized adult patient, *Journal of Parenteral and Enteral Nutrition* 10 (1986): 441–445.

4. J. A. Sargent, Assessing the utility and improving the effectiveness of nutritional support, *Nutrition in Clinical Practice* 1 (1986): 29–39.

5. G. F. Anderson and E. P. Steinberg, Prospective payment and nutritional support: The need for reform, *Journal of Parenteral and Enteral Nutrition* 10 (1986): 3–8.

6. Anderson and Steinberg, 1986.

7. Anderson and Steinberg, 1986.

8. Anderson and Steinberg, 1986.

9. J. M. Mirtallo and coauthors, Cost-effective nutrition support, *Nutrition in Clinical Practice* 2 (1987): 142–151.

10. K. S. Christensen, Hospitalwide screening increases revenue under prospective payment system, *Journal of the American Dietetic Association* 86 (1986): 1234–1235.

11. D. D. O'Brien and coauthors, Recommendations of nutrition support team promote cost containment, *Journal of Parenteral and Enteral Nutrition* 10 (1986): 300–302.

12. M. V. Kaminski and coauthors, Confusion of cost containment and cost effectiveness in nutritional support therapy, *Nutritional Support Services* 8, April 1988, pp. 27–28.

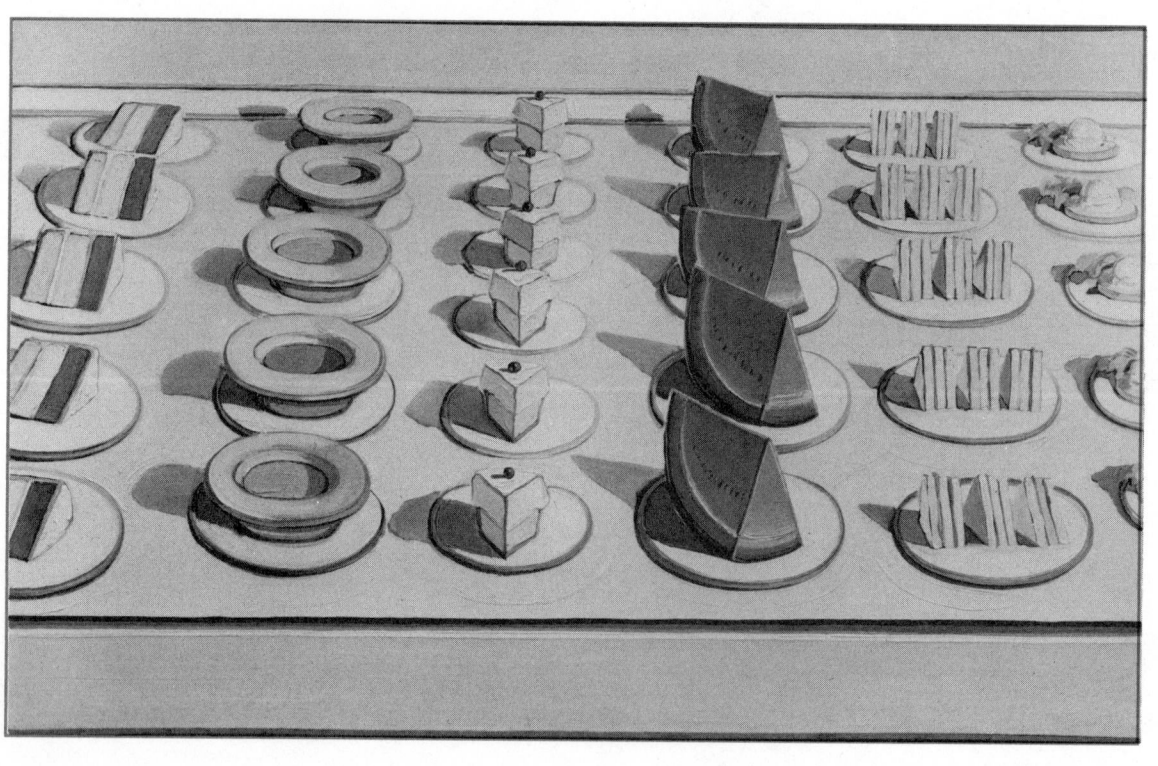

16

Diets Modified in Consistency, Texture, and Number of Meals

DIETS DISCUSSED
Liquid Diets
Low-Fiber Diets
Mechanical Soft Diets
Bland Diets
High-Fiber Diets
Small, Frequent Feedings

Case Study: Businesswoman with a Peptic Ulcer
Nutrition in Practice 16A: Fiber: Facts and Fads
Nutrition in Practice 16B:
A Perspective on Diet Therapy

CONDITIONS DISCUSSED
Dysphagia
Surgery
Indigestion and Nausea
Ileostomies and Colostomies
Strokes
Gastritis
Peptic Ulcers
Constipation
Irritable Bowel Syndrome
Diverticular Disease
Reflux Esophagitis and Hiatal Hernia

Lunch Table by Wayne Thiebaud. Stanford University Museum of
Art 64. 119. Gift of the Committee for Art at Stanford.

$\mathbf{M}$ odified diets complement other medical therapies in the prevention or treatment of many disorders. In some instances, diet therapy is crucial. In others, modified diets are only a small part of the total treatment plan. Sometimes the only diet required is a well-balanced one. Table 16–1 summarizes the diets modified in consistency, texture, and number of meals and shows the conditions for which they are indicated.

This chapter and the next several chapters look closely at modified diets and the reasons for their use in different disorders. This chapter describes diets that differ from the regular diet in consistency, texture, and frequency of

TABLE 16–1. Indications for the Use of Diets Modified in Consistency, Texture, and Number of Meals

Clear Liquids
Postsurgical diet
Bowel preparation for surgery or diagnostic test
Diarrhea
Early refeeding after complete bowel rest
Early feeding in protein-kcalorie malnutrition

Full Liquids
Postsurgical diets
Dysphagia
(see also *Mechanical soft diet*)

Low-Fiber or Soft Diet
Postsurgical diet
Indigestion
Nausea
Esophageal varices (cirrhosis)
Gastritis
Diarrhea
Diverticulitis
Inflammatory bowel disease
Myocardial infarction (heart attack)
Congestive heart failure

Mechanical Soft Diet
Severe dental caries
Missing or no teeth
Ill-fitting dentures
Dry mouth
Periodontal disease
Ulceration of mouth or gums
Oral surgery
Broken jaw
Plastic surgery of the head or neck
Difficulty chewing or swallowing
Stroke
Acquired immune deficiency syndrome (AIDS)

feedings. Such diets often aid in the treatment of GI disorders or conditions that affect the GI tract (surgery, for example). If you think about it, this makes a lot of sense. The consistency or texture of a food makes a difference only in the GI tract. Once digested and absorbed, only the basic units of foods are used by the cells. It makes no difference which foods these units came from.

Liquid Diets

There are two major types of liquid diets—clear liquids and full liquids. Table 16–2 and the sample menus show foods included in these diets. A clear liquid diet consists of foods that are clear and liquid or that liquefy at body temperature. The purpose of a clear liquid diet is to provide fluids and electrolytes to prevent dehydration. Clear liquids are easily digested and absorbed and contribute little or no residue in the GI tract. Clear liquid nutrition supplements are also available.

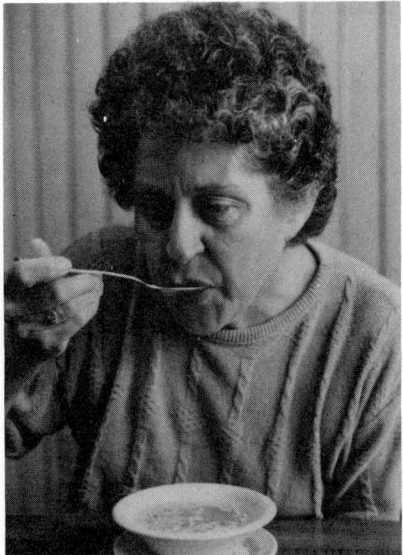
Liquid diets help to prevent dehydration.

residue:
bulk in the colon that includes undigested food, intestinal secretions, bacteria, and intestinal cells that are being shed.

TABLE 16–1. (Continued)

Bland Diet

Ulcers of the mouth or gums
Nausea
Reflux esophagitis
Hiatal hernia
Gastritis
Peptic ulcers
Myocardial infarction
Congestive heart failure

High-Fiber Diet

Constipation
Irritable bowel syndrome
Diverticulosis
Weight loss
Obesity
Diabetes mellitus
Heart disease

Small, Frequent Meals

Indigestion
Nausea
Reflux esophagitis
Hiatal hernia
Dumping syndrome
Hypoglycemia
Pancreatitis
Myocardial infarction

TABLE 16–2. Foods Included on Liquid Diets

Clear Liquid Diets	Full Liquid Diets
Bouillon	All clear liquids
Broth, clear	Butter
Carbonated beverages	Cheese, cottage[a]
Coffee, regular and decaffeinated	Commercially prepared liquid formulas (all)
Commercially prepared clear liquid formulas	Cooked cereals, strained
Fruit drinks	Cream
Fruit ices	Custard
Fruit juices, strained	Egg, soft cooked or scrambled[a]
Gelatin	Flavorings
Hard candy	Ice cream, plain
Honey	Instant breakfast drinks
Lemonade	Margarine
Popsicles	Milk, all types
Salt	Potatoes, mashed and diluted in cream soups
Salt substitutes	Pudding
Sugar	Sherbet
Sugar substitutes	Soups, strained vegetable, meat, or cream
Tea	Sour cream
	Vegetable juices, strained
	Vegetable purees, diluted in cream soups
	Yogurt

[a]As tolerated.

The clear liquid diet may be used to prepare the intestine for surgery or diagnostic tests or as a first diet after surgery. It may also be used to treat diarrhea or as a first feeding in a malnourished person or in a person who has

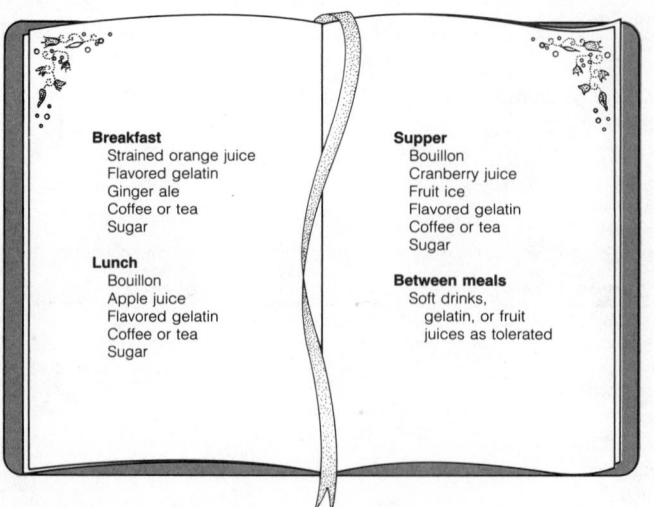

Breakfast
Strained orange juice
Flavored gelatin
Ginger ale
Coffee or tea
Sugar

Lunch
Bouillon
Apple juice
Flavored gelatin
Coffee or tea
Sugar

Supper
Bouillon
Cranberry juice
Fruit ice
Flavored gelatin
Coffee or tea
Sugar

Between meals
Soft drinks,
gelatin, or fruit
juices as tolerated

Sample clear liquid diet menu.

not had any oral intake for some time. The diet is usually temporary; as the client can tolerate other foods, they are added to the diet.

The full liquid diet includes both clear and opaque liquid foods and those that liquefy at body temperature. It may be used as a second diet (after clear liquids) following surgery or for a person who is unable to chew or swallow (see mechanical soft diet later in the chapter). A sample full liquid diet menu is shown in the text. Any liquid nutrition formula can be included on a full liquid diet to provide nutrients.

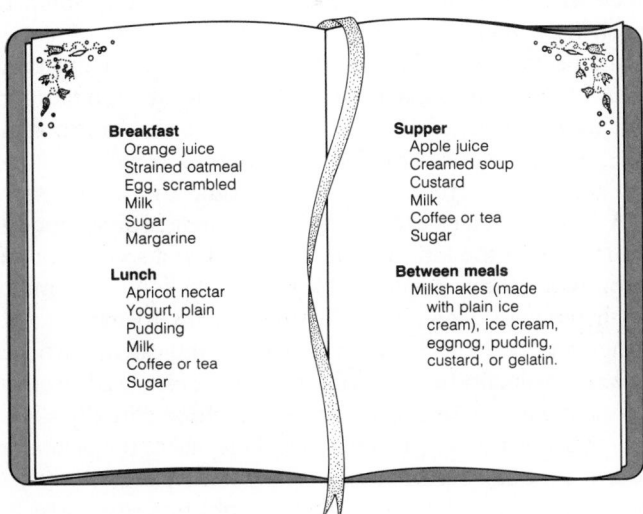

Breakfast
Orange juice
Strained oatmeal
Egg, scrambled
Milk
Sugar
Margarine

Lunch
Apricot nectar
Yogurt, plain
Pudding
Milk
Coffee or tea
Sugar

Supper
Apple juice
Creamed soup
Custard
Milk
Coffee or tea
Sugar

Between meals
Milkshakes (made with plain ice cream), ice cream, eggnog, pudding, custard, or gelatin.

Sample full liquid diet menu

Take a close look at the foods allowed on a standard liquid diet. You can imagine why someone who is sick would find these foods unappetizing. Even more disturbing, consider the nutritional quality of the diet. If not supplemented, it is deficient in kcalories and most nutrients for the normal person. A stressed person has even greater requirements. Therefore, care must be taken to ensure that no one is kept on an unsupplemented liquid diet for more than a few days. After that, nutrition formulas that meet the client's nutrient needs should be given either orally or, if necessary, by tube. Both clear and full liquid formulas are available.

Liquid diets can be adapted to meet other dietary requirements. For example, a person may need a low-sodium liquid diet or a low-residue liquid diet. In such cases, only liquids that meet the diet requirements would be allowed. On a low-sodium clear liquid diet, low-sodium broth would be substituted for regular broth.

Dysphagia

The esophagus transports food from the mouth to the stomach and is important in swallowing. Disorders of the esophagus can therefore affect the ability to swallow and cause dysphagia. Dysphagia can be the result of psy-

dysphagia (dis-FAY-gee-ah): difficulty in swallowing.
dys = bad
phagein = to eat

achalasia (ack-ah-LAY-zee-ah): dysfunction of the esophagus. Achalasia is sometimes called *esophageal dyssynergia* (ee-SOF-ah-GEE-al dis-sin-ER-gee-ah) or *cardiospasm*.

a = not

chalasis = relaxation

dys = bad

synergia = cooperation

The **cardiac sphincter** is often called the **lower esophageal sphincter (LES)** or the **gastroesophageal sphincter.** (The passage of food through the GI tract is described on pp. 00).

The fear of eating is called **sitophobia** (SIGH-toe-FOE-bee-ah).

sitos = food

phobos = fear

When an organ, such as the esophagus, becomes enlarged beyond normal dimensions, it is said to be **dilated.** To make an organ or vessel larger is called **dilation** or **dilatation.**

reflux esophagitis (ee-sof-ah-JIE-tis): the backflow or regurgitation of gastric contents from the stomach into the esophagus, causing inflammation of the esophagus. Dietary therapy for reflux esophagitis is discussed later in this chapter.

re = back

fluxus = flow

chological problems as well as physiological ones; we will discuss only those causes of dysphagia that can be helped by diet.

One such cause of dysphagia is achalasia, the cause of which is unknown. In achalasia, nerves that control the motility of the esophagus do not function properly, and the muscles of the esophagus are unable to propel the food bolus downward toward the stomach. Additionally, the cardiac sphincter does not relax and open during swallowing to allow the food to pass from the esophagus into the stomach. Foods and fluids accumulate in the esophagus of a person with achalasia, which explains the sensation of food sticking in the throat. Gradually, either the pressure of the food causes the cardiac sphincter to open or the person regurgitates the food.

At first, the person with achalasia may experience only temporary and mild dysphagia. As the condition worsens, the symptoms become more painful. The esophagus widens as achalasia progresses. The person becomes fearful of eating and gradually reduces food intake. Marked weight loss and nutrient deficiencies are likely to be present by the time the person seeks medical attention. A further danger exists—the person may aspirate food stagnating in the esophagus into the lung which could lead to a serious lung infection.

The person with achalasia will be able to tolerate liquid or semiliquid foods only in small servings. Suggest liquid supplements to meet nutrient needs. Tube feedings and parenteral nutrition may be indicated, particularly if the person is severely malnourished or unable to orally consume adequate nutrients.

The treatment for achalasia is to either stretch or partially slit the cardiac sphincter so that it is no longer functional. This makes the person more comfortable, but it does not restore motility to the esophageal muscles. Because the cardiac sphincter remains open, reflux esophagitis (discussed later in this chapter) is a common complication.

Nutrition and Surgery

Whenever possible, a person's nutrition status should be optimal before surgery. Optimal nutrution status may be difficult to achieve, however, since the illness that necessitates the surgery or the psychological stress associated with it may interfere with food intake or nutrient utilization. To prepare for many diagnostic and laboratory tests that frequently are performed before surgery, the person must fast or follow a clear liquid diet, which further taxes nutrition status.

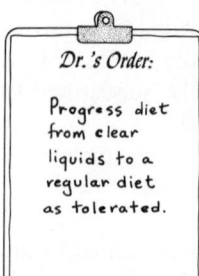

Dr.'s Order:

Progress diet from clear liquids to a regular diet as tolerated.

Before surgery a regular diet is generally adequate for well-nourished people who are expected to have no complications afterward. Regular hospital diets provide ample kcalories and generally exceed the RDA for protein. For people who are malnourished, diets high in kcalories and protein are recommended (see Chapter 17). In most hospitals, these clients receive high-kcalorie, high-protein supplements and snacks between meals. For people with functioning GI tracts who cannot orally consume an adequate intake, tube feedings are indicated. TPN may be initiated before surgery if use of the GI tract is contraindicated.

All foods and fluids are generally withheld for at least eight hours before surgery to prevent regurgitation and aspiration, which can occur during anesthia or recovery. For people undergoing GI surgery, liquids or foods low in residue are given for two or three days before surgery to minimize the amount of fecal material in the gut and help prevent distention after surgery. Low-residue and residue-free supplements are available to meet all the nutrient needs of people on liquid diets.

The immediate nutrition-related concern following surgery is the maintenance of fluid and electrolyte balance. The loss of blood, fluid, and electrolytes from the body during surgery can lead to dehydration and shock. Additional fluids may be lost thereafter from fever, draining wounds, vomiting, and diarrhea. Fluids and electrolytes are replaced by IV infusion after surgery, because peristalsis in the GI tract stops in the immediate postoperative period. Until peristalsis returns, food and fluids cannot be given orally.

Nutrition plays an important role in a person's ability to recover from surgery. If you consider what you know about the roles nutrients play, you'll be keenly aware of this. Consider protein alone: It is the material of antibodies needed to fight infection, of collagen to form scars, of all cells to rebuild damaged tissue, of plasma proteins that maintain fluid balance, of the matrix on which bones are rebuilt after fractures, and of many more crucial tissue constituents. The person who is protein deficient is handicapped by being inadequately supplied with all these factors and more.

Table 16–3 shows the nutrition consequences of various types of surgery. A person who develops complications following surgery is even more likely to become malnourished because of the additional stress placed on the body.

The objective of postsurgical nutrition support is to prevent weight loss and depletion of nutrients. Generally, the diets of people who are not receiving specialized nutrition support progress from clear liquids or full liquids to a low-fiber diet (discussed next), then to a regular diet as tolerated.

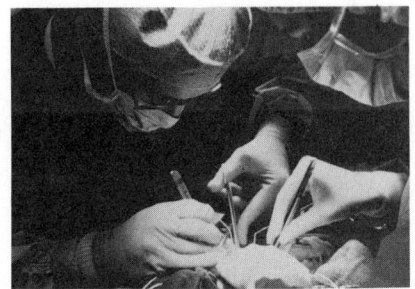

A person's nutrition status affects that person's ability to respond to the stress of surgery.

progressive diet:
the general progression of diets after surgery from clear liquids to full liquids to a low-fiber diet to a regular diet.

Often the postsurgical diet order simply says "diet as tolerated." Nursing personnel consult with the client and use their discretion in advancing the diet from liquids to a regular diet. Many times someone forgets to advance the diet. Other times a person truly cannot tolerate foods except for clear liquids; in such cases, further steps must be taken. Occasionally, tube feedings or total or supplemental intravenous nutrition may be necessary.

If you work with people after surgery, remember to check their diets. If they must stay on liquid diets for several days, alert the dietitian or suggest to the physician that a supplemental formula be considered.

A standard hospital diet adequate in all nutrients is the diet of choice after uncomplicated surgery for the well-nourished person who can tolerate solid foods. People with depleted nutrient stores and people with postsurgical complications need high-kcalorie, high-protein diets. If they cannot consume adequate nutrients by mouth, tube feedings or TPN should be considered. People placed on tube feedings or parenteral nutrition before surgery will likely stay on specialized nutrition support until they are able to meet most of their nutrient needs with an oral diet.

TABLE 16–3. Possible Effects of Surgery on Nutrition Status

Head and neck resection	
Difficulty in chewing/swallowing	Inability to chew/swallow
Esophageal resection	
Reduced gastric motility	Steatorrhea (Fat malabsorption)
Reduced gastric acid production	Fistula formation (Chapter 20)
Diarrhea	Stenosis (constriction)
Stomach resection	
Dumping syndrome	Vitamin B_{12} malabsorption
Hypoglycemia	General malabsorption
Lack of gastric acid	
Intestinal resection	
General malabsorption	Hyperoxaluria (Chapter 20)
Steatorrhea	Fluid and electrolyte imbalance
Diarrhea	Blind loop syndrome (Chapter 20)
Pancreatic resection	
General malabsorption	Diabetes mellitus

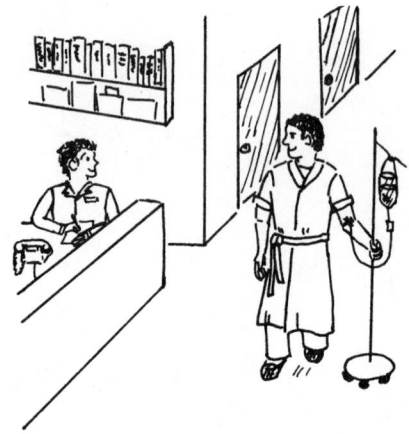

Exercise helps improve a client's appetite.

anorexia:
loss of appetite.

A low-fiber diet and a low-residue diet are very similiar. However, milk is restricted on a low-residue diet.

Depending on the type of surgery and the quality of the diet, supplements of some nutrients may be necessary. The need for many of the B vitamins increases when energy and protein intakes are high. Pay special attention to vitamin C; it helps form collagen, which plays an important role in wound healing. Zinc also plays a role in the healing of wounds. Vitamin K is important after surgery because it functions in blood clotting.

Malnutrition after surgery may be further complicated by anorexia and immobilization. Chapter 14 suggests ways to improve a person's appetite in the hospital. Individualizing the diet is very important. Exercise is important, too: Encourage your clients to get out of bed and to begin minimal exercise, such as walking, as soon as medically safe.

Low-Fiber Diets

The purpose of a low-fiber diet is to provide foods that are least likely to form an obstruction when the intestinal tract is narrowed by inflammation or scarring or when GI motility is slowed. The low-fiber diet is often used as an intermediate diet after intestinal or rectal surgery as a person progresses from a liquid to a regular diet. People with inflammatory bowel diseases (Chapter 20), ileostomies, colostomies, or those with a partial obstruction of the intestine may benefit from a low-fiber diet. Table 16–4 lists foods included in and eliminated from a low-fiber diet. A sample menu is illustrated in the text.

TABLE 16–4. Low-Fiber/Low Residue[a] Diet

Foods Allowed	Foods to be Avoided
Meat and meat alternates	
Baked, broiled, or roasted beef, fish, lamb, liver, poultry, veal, crisp bacon; hard- or soft-cooked eggs	Fried poultry or meats, cold cuts, sardines, fried eggs, peanut butter
Milk and milk products	
Whole, nonfat, or low-fat milk; yogurt; mild cheeses	Milk drinks or yogurt containing whole fruits or berries, seeds, or skins; strongly flavored cheeses
Fruits and vegetables	
Cooked or canned fruits without seeds and skins; ripe bananas, orange sections, grapefruit sections; all fruit juices; cooked asparagus tips, beets, broccoli, carrots, green beans, tomato juice, wax beans, winter squash; strained peas, spinach, summer squash, or potatoes	Berries; avocado; prune juice; raw fruits except those listed; legumes and raw vegetables and all other vegetables except those listed; sweet potatoes
Grains	
Refined, enriched white bread; plain muffins or rolls; white flour crackers (saltines, melba toast, zwieback); refined, ready-to-eat, or cooked cereals; noodles; macaroni; spaghetti; strained oatmeal	Whole-grain breads and cereals or those containing nuts, coconut, bran, or seeds; fried breads such as doughtnuts
Miscellaneous	
Tea, coffee, fruit drinks, carbonated beverages, butter, cream, margarine, mayonnaise	Any dishes made with foods to be avoided; coconut

[a]For a low-residue diet, milk and milk products are limited to two cups per day.

Two terms, *fiber* and *residue,* are used to describe diets that affect the contents of the colon. People often use these terms interchangeably, although it is incorrect to do so. *Fiber* describes the portion of food that is found in the colon because we don't have the enzymes to digest it. *Residue* refers to the total amount of material in the colon. (See margin, p. 311). High-fiber foods are also high-residue foods, but not all high-residue foods are high-fiber foods. Milk is a fiber-free food that leaves a residue of curds in the gut following digestion.

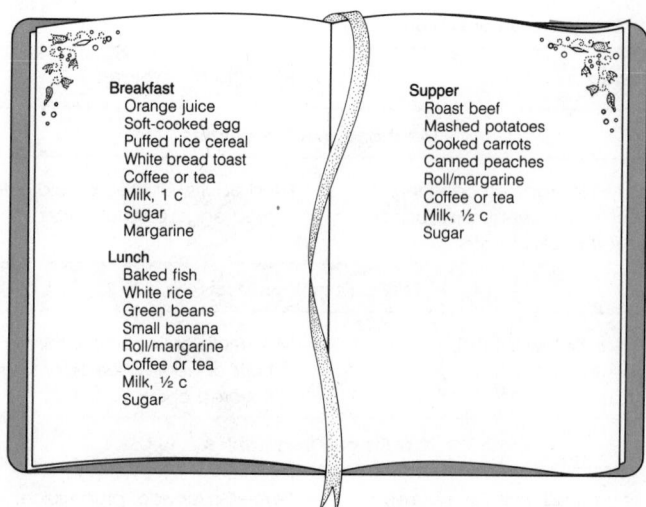

Sample low-fiber/low-residue diet menu.

Soft diets are similar in composition to low-fiber diets. However, in addition to providing low-fiber foods, the soft diet is soft in texture and is moderately seasoned. The soft diet may be used as a transitional diet after surgery or for some minor GI complaints, such as indigestion and nausea.

Indigestion and Nausea

Indigestion and nausea are common GI complaints. They are not diseases, they are symptoms and can be associated with many disorders.

dyspepsia:
vague abdominal discomfort. Dyspepsia is a symptom, not a disease.

Dr.'s Order:

Low-fiber diet, no alcohol, no caffeine.

Indigestion or dyspepsia is a vague term used to describe any discomfort in the GI tract. Indigestion can be caused by emotional tension, underlying medical conditions, eating too much, eating too rapidly, or chewing poorly.

Generally, no diet modifications are necessary for a temporary bout of indigestion. When indigestion occurs frequently, the cause should be identified. You can give some dietary advice that may help: Eat slowly, at regular times, and in a relaxed atmosphere; follow a low-fiber or soft diet (temporarily); and avoid excessive amounts of alcohol and caffeine-containing beverages. Of course, people should avoid any food that they know gives them indigestion. Antacids may provide relief.

All drugs, even over-the-counter drugs such as antacids, should be used cautiously. A serious problem can be masked by covering up symptoms. For example, a person who repeatedly takes antacids for stomach discomfort may be ignoring the signs of an ulcer.

Antacids also contain ingredients that may be undesirable. Some antacid contribute significant amounts of sodium or calcium. Although these ingredients may not be a problem for healthy individuals, they can aggravate some medical conditions. Aluminum-containing antacids can lead to phosphorus depletion and bone disease.[1] Therefore, we repeat: All drugs—prescription and nonprescription alike—should be taken with caution.

A person with persistent indigestion may habitually eat too little and become malnourished. Chronic indigestion may be a symptom of two disorders discussed later in the chapter: Gastritis and peptic ulcers.

Nausea is also a vague term describing a feeling that one is about to vomit. Nausea can be a symptom of many conditions from pregnancy to cancer. Certain smells or disturbing sights can trigger nausea. Generally, a nauseated person does not want to eat, which is fine when nausea is temporary. When nausea is persistent, as it may be in people with cancer or during pregnancy, the individual must eat or malnutrition will result.

Dr.'s Order:

Low-fiber diet with small meals and liquids between meals.

You can make several suggestions that may help: Follow a low-fiber or soft diet, eat smaller meals, save liquids for between meals, avoid foods with odors that cause nausea, slowly sip clear liquids, or suck popsicles or ice cubes made from a favorite liquid. Loosening the clothing, and getting fresh air can help relieve nausea.

The rationale for recommending a low-fiber or soft diet to treat nausea and indigestion is weak, but it may work if a person believes it will work. The client may think that low-fiber foods are easier to digest—although this is not true—and less likely to form gas. Although high-fiber foods are more likely to cause gas and possibly discomfort, certain low-fiber foods can also cause gas in some people.

If nausea leads to vomiting, other concerns may arise. Simple vomiting is certainly unpleasant and wearying for the nauseated person but is no cause for alarm. It is merely one of the body's adaptive mechanisms to rid itself of something irritating.

Prolonged vomiting can be serious and dangerous enough to require a doctor's care, because fluid is lost from the body's cells. Leaving the cells with the fluid are electrolytes—particularly sodium, potassium, chloride, and bicarbonate—that are absolutely essential to the life of the cells. Dehydration and electrolyte imbalances can occur. Fluids and electrolytes may be difficult to replace if vomiting continues. If possible, fluids and electrolytes are replaced orally. Soft drinks, fruit drinks, or other clear liquids are often used. Otherwise, IV feedings of saline and glucose with electrolytes added are frequently necessary while the doctor diagnoses the cause of the vomiting and institutes corrective therapy.

Ileostomies and Colostomies

stoma (STOH-ma):
a surgically formed opening; after an ileostomy or colostomy, a stoma is formed from the cut off end of the intestine through which excretion of wastes occurs.

In some people who have suffered from certain intestinal obstructions or lesions, a portion or all of the large intestine may need to be removed. An ileostomy involves the removal of the entire colon and rectum; a stoma, or opening, is made from the ileum and brought out through the abdomen to allow for defecation (see Figure 16–1A). In a colostomy, only the rectum and anus are removed and the stoma is formed from the remaining part of the colon (see Figure 16–1B). A watery stool will result from an ileostomy, while a more formed stool is produced by a colostomy.

Dr.'s Order:

Progress from a low-fiber, bland diet to a regular diet as tolerated.

After oral intake is initiated following surgery, the client is generally placed on a low-fiber, bland diet to help promote healing of the stoma and prevent irritation. However, encourage the client to resume a normal diet as soon as possible. Foods should be added individually and in small amounts so that their effects can be assessed. If a new food causes problems, it can be tried again a few months later.

ostomate (OSS-toe-mate):
a person who has a surgically-formed opening from the bowel to the outside of the body, bypassing the anus. An *ileostomate* (ILL-ee-OSS-toe-mate) has had an *ileostomy;* a *colostomate* (ko-LOSS-toe-mate) has had a *colostomy.*
stoma = window

Ostomates are often concerned about gas, odor, and loose and watery stools. Foods that cause excessively watery stools must be determined individually for each person. Certain raw fruits and vegetables and highly spiced foods cause problems for some ileostomates. Beer and other alcoholic beverages may cause diarrhea and gas. Gas and odor can be caused by such foods as beans, onions, green peppers, cabbage, turnips, and beets.

FIGURE 16–1
Ileostomy and colostomy .

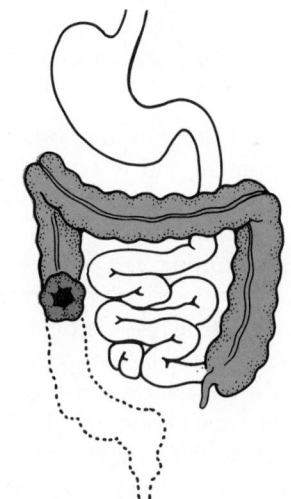

A. Ileostomy. The entire colon and rectum are removed, and the stoma is formed from the ileum.

B. Colostomy. The rectum and anus are removed, and the stoma is formed from the remaining colon.

Stress to the ostomate the importance of drinking plenty of fluids and reassure the individual that excess fluid, taken above and beyond the amount lost through the ostomy, will be absorbed and excreted by the kidneys and will not make the diarrhea worse.

New ostomates have many adjustments to make after surgery. They may feel they have lost control over a basic and private function. The retraining required to care for the ostomy and maintain bowel function may be difficult. Ostomates may also be worried that loved ones, particularly spouses, may find them unattractive. The health care team must work closely with each client and family to help them make the necessary adjustments for the ostomate to resume normal activities.

A health care professional specially trained to assist ostomates in learning the proper methods of caring for ostomy sites and adjusting to the ostomy is the **enterostomal** (en-ter-oh-STOME-al) **therapist (E.T.).**

Mechanical Soft Diets

The diet used to ease the task of chewing and swallowing is a highly individualized modification of a regular diet called a mechanical soft diet. This diet merely eliminates those foods the person cannot easily chew or swallow. The permitted foods may be liquid, chopped, pureed, or regular foods with a soft consistency. Unlike the soft diet described earlier, spices and fibrous foods are not restricted in a mechanical soft diet unless the person cannot chew or swallow such foods.

A variety of dental, medical, and surgical conditions can lead to temporary or permanent problems with chewing or swallowing. Table 16–5 lists some of these conditions. In these cases, the diet must be adjusted, or the person will eat too little, lose weight, and suffer the consequences of a deteriorating nutrition status.

People's tolerances of food consistency vary greatly. Health care professionals should work closely with individuals to identify those tolerances and to make needed adjustments. Provide foods that are as similar as possible to those of a regular diet. These foods will offer the most variety, enhancing the client's acceptance of them and lessening the likelihood of nutrient deficiencies. For example, although a person with a newly broken jaw may be able only to handle liquids, a person without teeth may be able to eat baked chicken or fish, ground beef, casseroles, canned fruits, and many soft-cooked vegetables.

mechanical soft diet:
a diet that excludes foods difficult for an individual to chew or swallow; also called a *dental soft diet.*

TABLE 16–5 Conditions That Interfere with Chewing or Swallowing

Acquired immune deficiency syndrome (AIDS)	Oral surgery
	Periodontal disease
Broken jaw	Radiation therapy of the head and neck
Dental caries	Sensitivity to hot or cold
Dryness of the mouth	Stroke (sometimes)
Ill-fitting dentures	Surgery of the head and neck
Missing teeth	Ulceration of mouth or gums
No teeth	

As stated earlier, any person who cannot eat enough soft foods or drink enough liquids to meet nutrient needs should be fed by tube.

All seasonings and types of foods are allowed on a mechanical soft diet. However, you should be aware that highly seasoned or acidic foods (citrus fruits, tomatoes) can cause pain to someone with mouth ulcers. Also, suggest that a person with mouth ulcers avoid foods containing nuts or seeds (such as breads with sesame or poppy seeds) that can easily get trapped in the ulcer and cause discomfort.

Take a moment to think about a pureed diet. A typical dinner of baked chicken, boiled potatoes, and green beans is now white mush, more white mush, and one green blob added for color. In many hospitals baby foods routinely replace pureed foods. Baby foods are nutritious, but they often taste bland, since they are prepared without salt or spices. Whether food is pureed or baby food, the consistency of the food creates a psychological block to eating. Malnutrition can result.

Can you improve the situation? The answer is yes. First, be sure your client needs pureed rather than chopped foods. Second, help your client select colorful meals. For example, substitute mashed sweet potatoes for mashed white potatoes. Such a change adds appetizing color to the meal. Serve the food attractively and at the right temperature. Lastly, unless the physician has ordered otherwise, suggest spices that will improve the taste of the food. Many people think that because they are on a special diet they are not allowed to have additional seasonings.

Talk to the administrative dietitian or food service manager, if pureed diets are consistently a problem. Whenever possible, regular foods that have been pureed should be served instead of baby foods. Pureed foods should be smooth and thick—not watery or thin.

FIGURE 16-2

Special feeding devices.

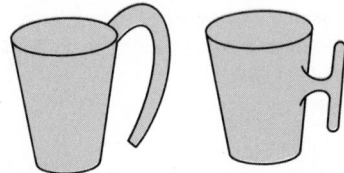

These cups can be used by people who cannot grasp well.

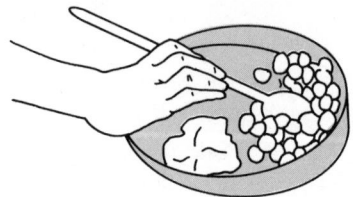

Using a plate with a built-up side allows food to be pushed onto a spoon or fork with one hand.

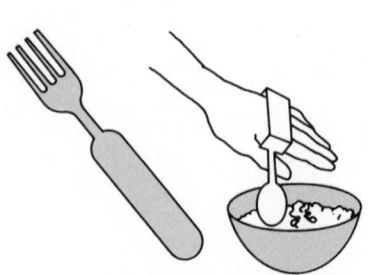

Utensils with built-up handles or cuffs are also helpful for people who cannot grasp well.

The Stroke Victim

When blood flow to the brain is insufficient or when blood vessels burst and blood flows into the brain, a stroke or cerebrovascular accident (CVA) results. Recovery for some stroke victims is unremarkable. The optimal diet in such a case is based on the stroke victim's underlying medical condition (hyperlipidemia, hypertension, obesity).

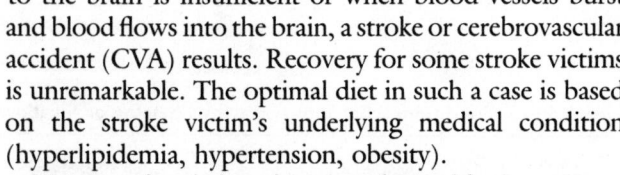

Dr.'s Order:

Mechanical soft diet.

Many stroke victims, however, have either temporary or permanent problems with chewing, swallowing, and the physical process of eating. Tube feedings often are indicated initially. Later, a mechanical soft diet may be useful. Some people also have problems with the physical aspects of eating. They can be helped a great deal through the use of special feeding devices, several of which are shown in Figure 16–2.

Bland Diets

Bland diets eliminate foods that stimulate gastric acid secretion or those that are irritating to the gastric mucosa. It is important to individualize the diet based on each person's tolerances. Most practitioners recommend that alcohol and both regular and decaffeinated coffee be avoided. There is less agreement about pepper and beverages other than coffee that contain caffeine.[2] More recent studies suggest that the essential fatty acids linoleic acid and arachidonic acid may be useful in preventing injury to the gastric mucosa.[3] However, far more research will be necessary before the value of fatty acids in preventing gastric injury can be determined.

Bland diets are frequently prescribed for gastritis, ulcers, and reflux esophagitis (discussed later in this chapter). People who suffer heart attacks or people with congestive heart failure (see Chapter 20) may benefit from a temporary bland diet. Bland foods are thought to be less gas forming. Gas can distend the stomach, causing the diaphragm to be pushed upward toward the heart, adding to the heart's workload.

The bland diet has changed dramatically over the years from the bland diet of the past. Table 16–6 illustrates the differences between the traditional bland diet and the liberal bland diet currently in use. You can see that the client was expected to avoid many foods, and milk was a part of each meal and snack. Three meals were replaced by six, small feedings (see peptic ulcers for more information about this diet). These restrictive diets are high in cholesterol and saturated fat, which may be related to the development of atherosclerosis (see Nutrition in Practice 21A). As it became evident that the rationale for many of the restrictions was not supported by scientific evidence, the more liberal diet approach was adopted by most dietitians and physicians. However, some practitioners still continue to use traditional bland diets even though they offer no proven benefit.

Gastritis

Gastritis is a common disorder characterized by inflammation of the mucosal lining of the stomach. The person with gastritis may complain of anorexia, nausea, vomiting, belching, a feeling of fullness, and stomach pain.

gastritis
inflammation of the lining of the stomach.

TABLE 16–6 Comparison of the Traditional and Liberal Bland Diets

Diet modification	Traditional bland	Liberal bland
Frequency of feedings	Six small feedings	Three feedings
Milk	Use liberally	Not encouraged
Caffeine and caffeine-containing beverages	Restricted	Restricted
Decaffeinated coffee	Not restricted	Restricted
Alcohol	Restricted	Restricted
Pepper and spicy foods	Restricted	As tolerated
High-fiber foods	Restricted	Not restricted

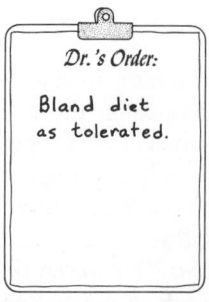

Acute gastritis is most often caused by ingesting aspirin or other drugs that irritate the gastric mucosa. Alcohol abuse, food irritants, food allergies, food poisoning, radiation, stress, and infections can cause gastritis. Keep these two principles in mind for the dietary management of acute gastritis:

- Eliminate irritating foods.
- Reduce gastric acidity.

If the person with gastritis cannot eat because of nausea or vomiting, food is generally withheld for one or two days. The diet is then progressed from liquids to bland as tolerated. Antacids may also be given.

Chronic gastritis has the same symptoms as acute gastritis but persists for longer periods of time. Chronic gastritis has no known cause, and finding the appropriate diet may be a matter of trial and error. A bland diet may help relieve gastrointestinal symptoms in some cases.

Peptic Ulcers

Ulcers can occur in many places inside and outside the body. Used alone, however, the term *ulcer* generally refers to an ulcer in the stomach or duodenum. The term *peptic ulcer* includes both of these. An ulcer is an erosion of the top layer of cells from the wall of the stomach or intestine, leaving the second and succeeding underlying layers of cells exposed to gastric juices. The erosion may proceed until the acid reaches the capillaries that feed the area and the nerves, leading to bleeding and pain. If the erosion penetrates all the way through the stomach or duodenum, a major infection known as peritonitis can rapidly develop and can be fatal.

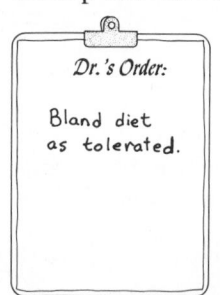

A person with an ulcer may experience a gnawing, burning pain that lasts up to several weeks. Although symptoms generally disappear for periods of time, they usually recur. People with gastric ulcers almost always have chronic gastritis.

Currently there is no cure for ulcers. Instead, treatment is aimed at relieving pain, healing the ulcer, and minimizing the likelihood of recurrence. The treatment for both gastric and duodenal ulcers is the same.

The objectives of peptic ulcer therapy are to neutralize gastric acidity and to reduce gastric acid secretion. These measures help protect the stomach and duodenum wall from the eroding effect of gastric acid. In the past, diet was a major part of the treatment of peptic ulcer disease. As more has been learned about the effects of various foods on the gastric mucosa, drug therapy has become the primary therapy for ulcers, with diet playing a smaller role. The client with ulcers may be instructed to:

- Follow prescribed drug therapy, which may include cimetidine, ranitidine, sucralfate, or anticholinergics.
- Use antacids, taken one hour after meals when gastric acid secretion is high.

peptic ulcer:
an eroded lesion of the stomach (gastric ulcer) or duodenum (duodenal ulcer).

cimetidine:
a drug that reduces gastric acid secretion by interfering with histamine. Histamine stimulates gastric acid secretion.

ranitidine:
a drug that inhibits gastric acid secretion and effectively reduces the pain of an ulcer almost immediately.

sucralfate:
an ulcer medication that works by sticking to the stomach's lining, forming a protective coating that allows the ulcer to heal.

anticholinergics:
drugs that reduce gastric acid secretion and gastric motility.

- Eliminate drugs that irritate the stomach (aspirin).
- Reduce stress, which stimulates gastric acid secretion.
- Reduce or eliminate cigarette smoking, which also stimulates gastric acid secretion.
- Eliminate any food that routinely causes indigestion or pain.

People with ulcers can eat any spicy foods they can tolerate. Individuals who do not routinely eat highly spiced foods may have discomfort if they do eat such foods. However, individuals who routinely consume highly spiced foods are probably not at higher risk of developing ulcers or having ulcers reoccur.[4] Generally, the person with an ulcer is advised to avoid caffeine and alcohol.

At one time, the person with an ulcer was advised to eat small, frequent meals. Milk was given with each meal and between meals. However, since food stimulates gastric acid secretion, three regular meals a day are indicated for people with healed ulcers. Milk may actually have a negative effect for people with duodenal ulcers. In one study of people with ulcers who were taking cimetidine, the ulcers healed in 78 percent of the people who ate a normal diet but in only 53 percent of those whose main food was milk.[5]

High-Fiber Diets

One of the most frequently recommended diets in use today is the high-fiber diet. You may recall that the *Dietary Guidelines* recommend increasing the consumption of whole-grain breads and cereals, fruits and vegetables, dried beans and peas, and nuts to increase fiber intake. The role of fiber in preventing various disorders is discussed in Nutrition in Practice 16A. The addition of high-fiber foods is often recommended for weight loss (Chapter 18) and for people with diabetes mellitus (Chapter 19) or heart disease (Chapter 21). However, the most clearly defined and least controversial use of high-fiber diets is in the treatment of constipation and diverticular disease.

The amounts of fiber in foods are difficult to estimate. Chemists can analyze food for fiber content in the laboratory by digesting it with acids and bases. Whatever remains is called crude fiber. If you eat the same food the chemists analyzed, subjecting it to the action of your own enzymes, the undigested residue will be greater, because the body's enzymes are less harsh than the laboratory treatment. The amount of fiber that remains in the intestine after the normal human digestive process is dietary fiber. As a rule of thumb, for every gram of crude fiber in a food, there are probably about two or three grams of dietary fiber.

Many types of fiber can be found in foods; the effects that fiber has in the body depend on the type of fiber. Table 16–7 lists some conditions that may be affected by fiber and which type of fiber exerts an effect.

The major impact of dietary fiber is on the colon. The high-fiber diet acts by adding volume and weight to the stool, speeding the transit of undigested materials through the intestine, and minimizing pressure within the colon. Table 16–8 lists foods useful for adding fiber to the diet. A sample menu is

crude fiber: see p. 26.

dietary fiber: see p. 27.

Some of the different types of fibers in foods are **cellulose, hemicellulose, gums, pectins,** and **lignins.** Table 16–7 lists some foods that contain each type of fiber.

TABLE 16–7. Effects of Different Kinds of Fiber

Conditions and Effects of Fiber	Fiber Type		
	Cellulose, hemicellulose (from fruits; vegetables; legumes; wheat bran, oat bran, and other cereal brans; nuts and seeds; whole-grain flours)	Gums, pectins (from fruits, vegetables, seeds, legumes, oats, barley)	Lignins (from whole grains, seeds, woody parts of vegetables)
Obesity—displaces kcalories (gel forming)?	Yes	Yes	No
Constipation/ hemorrhoids— effect on stool bulk, ease of passage	Reduces pressure, softens stools[a]	None	Make stools move faster
Cancer—increases bile acid excretion?	No[b]	Yes	Yes
Diabetes and other disorders of blood glucose regulation— improves glucose tolerance?	Yes[c]	Yes—some help control blood sugar in diabetes	—
Cardiovascular disease—lowers blood cholesterol?	No—except oat bran lowers it	Yes	Yes
kCarlorie intake— how completely digested?	60 to 95% digested	Mostly digested	Not digested
Blocks mineral absorption?	Yes	No	Yes

[a]Wheat bran improves both constipation and diarrhea. M. S. Mathur, H. Ram, and V. S. Chadda, Effect of bran on intestinal transit time in normal Indians and in intestinal amoebiasis, *American Journal of Proctology Gastroenterology and Colon and Rectal Surgery*, November/December 1978, pp. 30–32, 34.
[b]Wheat bran binds bile acids in vitro but does *not* affect bile acid excretion in man. M. A. Eastwood and R. M. Kay, An hypothesis for the action of dietary fiber along the gastrointestinal tract, *American Journal of Clinical Nutrition* 32 (1979): 364–367.
[c]Wheat bran improves glucose tolerance; pectins do not. J. W. Anderson and W.-J. L. Chen, Plant fiber: Carbohydrate and lipid metabolism, *American Journal of Clinical Nutrition* 32 (1979): 346–363.

given in the text. High-fiber diets provide about 20 to 25 grams of dietary fiber daily. Bran can be used to significantly increase the fiber content of the diet. Bran can be sprinkled on cereal, salads, applesauce, and many other food items or it can be added to beverages. Many breakfast cereals contain a considerable amount of crude fiber.

TABLE 16–8. Foods to Provide 25 Grams of Fiber per Day

Fruit group: About 2 g fiber per serving; use four or more per day.

Apple, 1 small	Orange, 1 small
Banana, 1 small	Peach, 1 medium
Strawberries, ½ c	Pear, ½ small
Cherries, 10 large	Plums, 2 small

Bread and cereal group: About 2 g fiber per serving; use four or more per day.

Whole-wheat bread, 1 slice	All Bran, 1 tbsp
Rye bread, 1 slice	Corn flakes, ⅔ c
Cracked wheat bread, 1 slice	Oatmeal, dry, 3 tbsp
Shredded wheat, ½ biscuit	Wheat bran, 1 tsp
Grape Nuts, 3 tbsp	Puffed Wheat, 1½ c

Vegetable group: About 2 g fiber per serving; use four or more per day.

Broccoli, ½ stalk	Lettuce, raw, 2 c
Brussels sprouts, 4	Green beans, ½ c
Carrots, ⅓ c	Potato, 2 inch diameter
Celery, 1 c	Tomato, raw, 1 medium
Corn on the cob, 2-inch piece	Baked beans, canned, 2 tbsp

Miscellaneous group: About 1 g fiber per serving.

Peanut butter, 2½ tsp	Pickle, 1 large
Peanuts, 10	Strawberry jam, 5 tbsp

Source: Adapted from Recommendation for a high-fiber diet, *Nutrition and the MD,* July 1981; in turn adapted from D.A.T. Southgate and coauthors, A guide to calculating intakes of dietary fiber, *Journal of Human Nutrition* 30 (1976): 303–313.

Help a client adjust to a high-fiber intake by advising that fiber gradually be added to the diet. During the first few weeks on the diet, the person may feel bloated, pass gas frequently, or experience heartburn. Forewarn the person

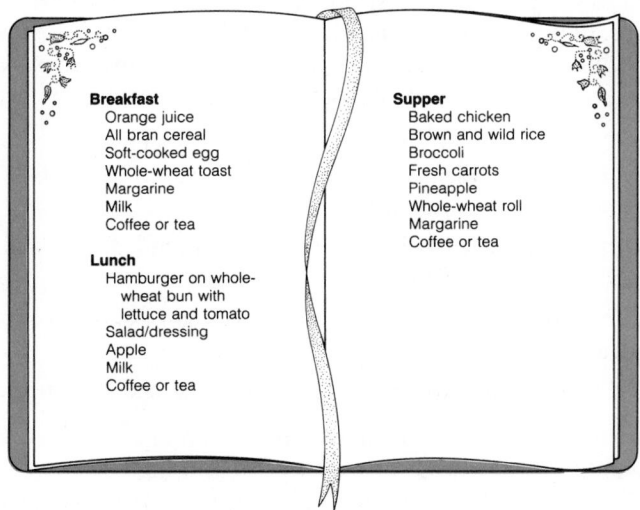

Breakfast
Orange juice
All bran cereal
Soft-cooked egg
Whole-wheat toast
Margarine
Milk
Coffee or tea

Lunch
Hamburger on whole-wheat bun with lettuce and tomato
Salad/dressing
Apple
Milk
Coffee or tea

Supper
Baked chicken
Brown and wild rice
Broccoli
Fresh carrots
Pineapple
Whole-wheat roll
Margarine
Coffee or tea

Sample high-fiber diet menu.

phytobezoar (FIGH-toh-BEE-zor): a collection of plant fibers that forms a ball in the stomach or intestine.

Some types of gastric surgery and a condition of reduced gastric motility that sometimes affects people with diabetes mellitus (Chapter 19) are associated with an increased risk of phytobezoar formation.

about these symptoms to dispel unnecessary fears and to foster compliance. It won't be a problem for long.

The cautious use of some high-fiber foods is recommended for people with disorders that affect gastric emptying and people with reduced gastric acidity.[6] Such individuals are prone to form phytobezoars, which can interfere with normal GI tract function or lead to ulcers or abdominal infections. Foods to avoid include oranges, persimmons, coconut, berries, green beans, figs, apples, sauerkraut, brussels sprouts, and potato peels.

Constipation

You may joke about or be irritated by laxative commercials on TV, but most people believe the message they are sending. For example, Mrs. X must have a daily bowel movement or else she will be headachy and irritable. The screen then shows Mrs. X the next day feeling her old jovial self because her pharmacist persuaded her to take a laxative.

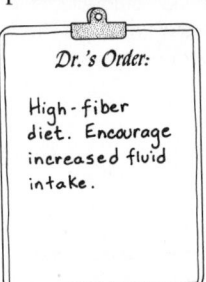

Dr.'s Order:

High-fiber diet. Encourage increased fluid intake.

constipation: difficult or painful bowel movements; elapsed time between movements is irrelevant.

Each person's GI tract responds to food in its own way, with its own rhythm, so that the fecal matter arrives at the rectal area in a fairly constant number of hours. If several days pass between movements but these movements take place without discomfort, the person is not constipated. The person who experiences bowel movements that are hard and passed with difficulty, discomfort, or pain is constipated. The amount of time that has elapsed since the previous bowel movement is irrelevant.

Constipation occurs when the muscles of the colon are loose and fail to push the intestinal contents along. Hospitalized or institutionalized individuals often suffer from constipation. Stress from disease, nervous tension, inactivity, and failure to respond to signals to defecate can all be contributing factors. Constipation can also occur as a result of irregular and excessive contractions of the colon. This disorder—the irritable bowel syndrome—is discussed in the following section.

In some cases, constipation is a symptom of organic diseases such as intestinal obstructions, tumors, or diverticular disease (discussed later). More often constipation is functional rather than organic, and corrective measures can be taken to alleviate the problem. Recommend these measures to help relieve constipation:

- Follow a high-fiber diet. Several types of fiber (see Table 16–8) can aid in the treatment of constipation.
- Drink more fluids. It has been suggested that added fluid adds bulk in the upper intestine, which promotes peristalsis.
- Eat prunes and drink prune juice; prunes contain a substance that acts as a laxative.
- Exercise regularly and follow a consistent eating and sleeping schedule.

Adding fat to the diet can help relieve constipation in some cases. Fat in the intestine stimulates the release of bile which has a high salt content. Water from the intestinal wall is mobilized to equalize the high osmolality in the intestine which in turn stimulates peristalsis and softens the fecal matter.

If diet and lifestyle changes do not correct the constipation, a physician should be consulted. Laxatives may be indicated. Chronic constipation is associated with other problems. The constant pressure of straining to defecate may result in hemorrhoids or the formation of diverticula (discussed later).

Irritable Bowel Syndrome

Irritable bowel syndrome is a very common disorder of the GI tract. The person experiencing this disorder frequently complains of a variety of symptoms, including indigestion, nausea, abdominal pain, flatulence, diarrhea, constipation, or both diarrhea and constipation in alternating sequence. The disorder is characterized by a disturbance in GI tract motility.

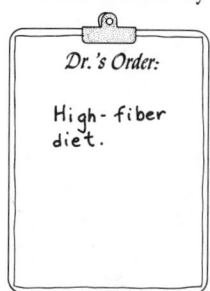

Dr.'s Order:

High-fiber diet.

For the person whose primary symptom is alternating diarrhea and constipation, adding fruits and vegetables to the diet may be helpful.[7] The addition of bran or hydrophyllic colloids generally returns bowel function to normal.

People with irritable bowel syndrome that complain of gas and abdominal pain might benefit from avoiding foods that contain certain complex carbohydrates. These particular carbohydrates cannot be digested and absorbed. However, when they reach the colon, bacteria metabolize them and produce gas in the process. Foods that contain these gas-forming carbohydrates are shown in Table 16–9. People who complain of both gas and problems with diarrhea and constipation can use hydrophillic colloids but should not use bran.

Diverticular Disease

Sometimes pouches, or diverticula, form along the intestine in areas where the intestinal muscles are weak, often at points where blood vessels enter the muscles. Evidence suggests that the pouches result from high pressures in the intestinal lumen. Diverticulosis is the condition in which diverticula have formed in the intestine.

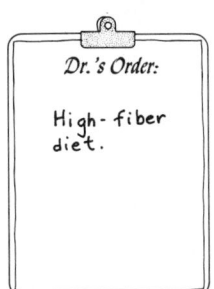

Dr.'s Order:

High-fiber diet.

The person with diverticulosis is symptom free and may not know she has the disorder. But in some people, fecal material gets trapped in the diverticula, causing inflammation and infection. This condition is called diverticulitis and it can be dangerous because the diverticula may burst. People with diverticulitis may complain of cramps, alternating periods of diarrhea and constipation, dyspepsia, gas, and abdominal distention.

For many years, people with diverticulosis were advised to adopt low-fiber diets. It was believed that fiber could become trapped in the diverticula and cause irritation. This advice has changed dramatically in recent years, however; and it is now widely believed that a high-fiber diet may reduce the incidence of diverticulosis. Many people with established diverticular disease remain symptom free while following a high-fiber diet. However, foods with seeds, such as okra and strawberries, may need to be avoided; they may get trapped in the diverticula and cause irritation.

TABLE 16–9. Foods that Can Cause Gas

Artichokes, Chinese
Barley
Beans
Brussels sprouts
Cabbage
Celery
Coconut
Eggplant
Figs
Honey
Kohlrabi
Melons
Milk
Molasses
Mulberries
Nuts
Onions
Radishes
Rye seeds
Soybeans
Wheat
Yeast

The complex carbohydrates associated with gas formation are **raffinose** and **stacchyose.**

hydrophillic colloids:
a type of laxative that attracts water in the intestine to form a bulky stool, which then stimulates peristalsis.

diverticulosis (DYE-ver-tic-you-LOH-sis):
the condition of having outpocketings of weakened areas of the intestinal wall (like air bubbles in a tire). The danger of diverticulosis is that it can give rise to *diverticulitis* (-EYE-tis), in which the pockets become infected or inflamed and may rupture. About one in every six people in Western countries develops diverticulosis in middle or later life.
divertir = to turn aside
osis = disease
itis = inflammation or infection

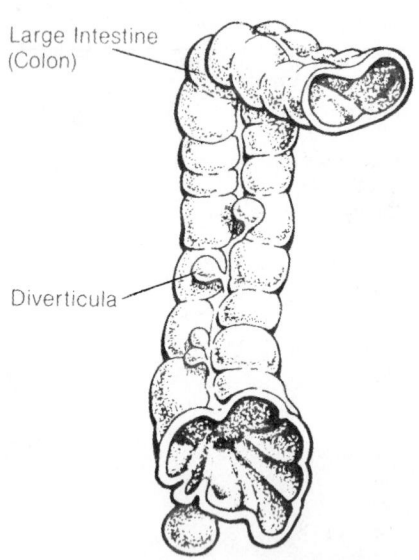

Large Intestine
(Colon)

Diverticula

The outpocketings of the intestinal wall that balloon through the weakened muscles of the intestinal wall are known as **diverticula**.

Often people with diverticulosis, particularly older people, have been following a low-fiber diet for many years. They may be apprehensive about switching to a high-fiber diet. After all, they had been told that the low-fiber diet would prevent symptoms, and they may be fearful of trying once forbidden foods. They may be skeptical about any diet after having received such contradictory advice. What can you do to relieve their anxiety? In addition to following the advice given earlier for gradually introducing a high-fiber diet, you can acknowledge their concerns and try to stress the value of the diet. Also, try gaining their involvement and cooperation during the teaching process.

Small, Frequent Feedings

Any regular or modified diet can be given in small, frequent feedings. Small feedings are useful whenever distention of the stomach causes pain or discomfort. Thus, as we have already discussed, people suffering from indigestion or nausea may benefit from small, frequent feedings—for example, six a day, each half the size of a regular meal. People who lack the energy to eat regular meals or who have problems with chewing or swallowing may also benefit from this modification. Small, frequent feedings also aid in the treatment of reflux esophagitis and hiatal hernia.

Reflux Esophagitis and Hiatal Hernia

hiatal hernia (high-AY-tal HER-knee-uh):
a protrusion of a portion of the stomach up through the opening of the diaphragm where the esophagus comes through. There are several types: sliding (see Figure 16–3B), rolling, and short esophagus.

In reflux esophagitis, the lower esophagus is irritated. The cardiac sphincter does not close tightly enough, and highly acidic gastric contents splash backward into the esophagus, irritating the esophageal mucosa. Table 16–10 lists some foods and substances that affect cardiac sphincter pressure. People with hiatal hernias often develop reflux esophagitis, and the goal for the nutrition care for the person with either condition is the same. Figure 16–3 shows the relationship of the upper GI tract to the diaphragm and the changes that occur in the presence of a hernia.

TABLE 16–10 Substances That Affect Cardiac Sphincter Pressure

Elevates Pressure	Lowers Pressure
Bethanechol	Alcohol
Metoclopropamide	Anticholinergic agents
Protein	Atropine
	Caffeine-containing beverages
	Chocolate
	Cigarette smoking
	Fat
	Peppermint and spearmint oils

FIGURE 16–3
Relation of upper GI tract to diaphragm.

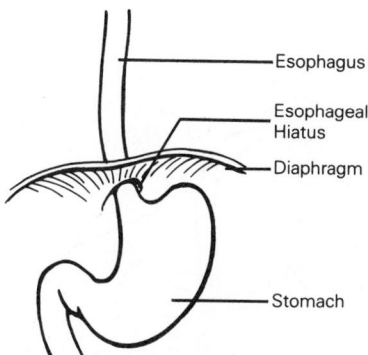

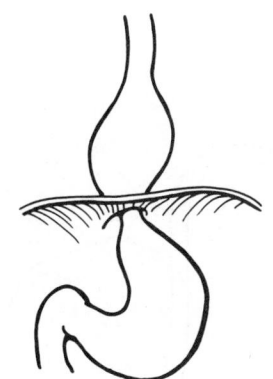

A. Normally, the stomach lies below the diaphragm, and the esophagus passes through the esophageal hiatus (opening in the esophagus).

B. A *sliding hiatal hernia* is the most common type of hiatal hernia.

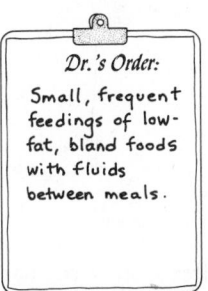

Dr.'s Order:
Small, frequent feedings of low-fat, bland foods with fluids between meals.

A burning pain (heartburn) occurs when the gastric juices splash back into the esophagus. The pain is severe enough to awaken a sleeping person. Heartburn usually hurts behind the sternum (see Figure 16–4), often spreading into the neck and back of the throat in waves. Heartburn is especially likely when pressure in the stomach exceeds pressure in the esophagus, so it occurs most frequently when a person lies down or bends over.

The best treatment of reflux esophagitis is prevention. Instruct clients to avoid substances that lower cardiac sphincter pressure and activity that raises pressure in the stomach. Dietary advice is an important part of the treatment of reflux esophagitis. Instruct the client to:

- Eat small, frequent meals and drink liquids one hour before or after meals to avoid distending the stomach.
- Refrain from lying down or bending over and from wearing tight-fitting garments, particularly after eating, to avoid elevating pressure in the stomach.
- Lose weight, if necessary.
- Limit fat, alcohol, caffeine, and peppermint and spearmint oil intake to avoid lowering cardiac sphincter pressure.
- Limit caffeine-containing foods and beverages, decaffeinated coffee, and red pepper to avoid stimulation of gastric acid secretion.
- Avoid acidic juices such as orange, grapefruit, and tomato juice when experiencing symptoms of reflux esophagitis to minimize irritation to the esophagus.

Other measures can also be helpful. Advise clients not to smoke cigarettes, since cigarette smoking can reduce cardiac sphincter pressure. In addition, antacids or other drugs may be prescribed to neutralize gastric acidity. Suggest that to prevent reflux the person sleep with the head of the bed elevated, so that the chest is higher than the stomach. Generally, these measures can control esophagitis. However, in some cases, surgery may be indicated if medical management fails.

FIGURE 16–4
Effect of gastric pressure on reflux.
Whenever the pressure in the stomach is greater than the pressure in the esophagus, the chance of reflux increases. Overeating and overdrinking can cause the stomach to be overdistended, increasing the pressure in the stomach.

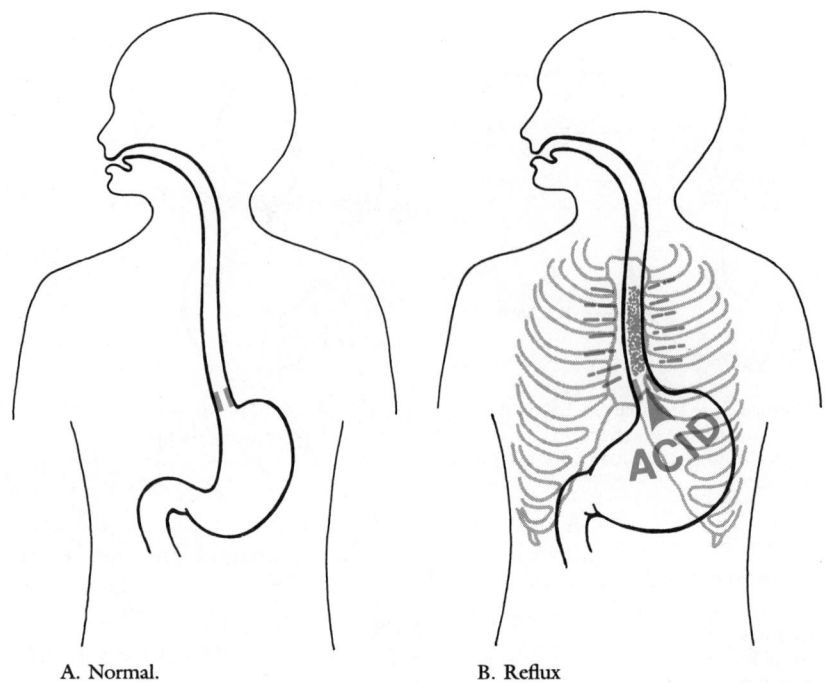

A. Normal.   B. Reflux

This chapter has presented an overview of diets that differ from a regular diet in consistency, texture, and number of meals. In addition, you have seen how each diet is used in at least one condition or disorder. The following chapters look at different types of modified diets—those modified in nutrients.

CASE STUDY

Businesswoman with a Peptic Ulcer

Ms Kelly is a busy executive in a high-pressure job. She entertains many clients, so she eats many meals out and drinks alcoholic beverages regularly. She smokes and gets little sleep. Ms Kelly visited her physician after she began experiencing severe, gnawing stomach pain. A diagnosis of peptic ulcer was made.

1. What changes in lifestyle will help Ms Kelly with treatment of her ulcer? Assess Ms Kelly's medical situation and make suggestions for correcting her problems.

2. What diet should Ms Kelly follow? From the limited information that you have been given about her eating habits, what suggestions can you give Ms Kelly about her diet? What questions could you ask Ms Kelly to help her design a diet she could live with? How could you help her identify foods that irritate her ulcer?

Notes

1. A. Lione, Aluminum intake from non-prescription drugs and sucralfate, *General Pharmacology* 16 (1985): 223–228.

2. D. Hollander, Diet therapy in peptic ulcer disease, *Nutrition and the MD,* February 1988, pp. 1–2; Effect of pepper on the gastrointestinal mucosa, *Nutrition and the MD,* February 1988, p. 3.

3. D. Hollander and A. Tarnawski, Dietary essential fatty acids and the decline of peptic ulcer disease—a hypothesis, *Gut* 27 (1986): 239.

4. K. Holt and D. Hollander, Gastric mucosal injury, *Annual Review of Medicine* 37 (1986): 107.

5. N. Kumar and coauthors, Effect of milk on patients with duodenal ulcers, *British Medical Journal* 293 (1986): 666.

6. A. P. Emerson, Foods high in fiber and phytobezoar formation, *Journal of the American Dietetic Association* 87 (1987): 1675–1677.

7. A. D. Schwabe, Dietary management of the irritable bowel syndrome, *Nutrition and the MD,* July 1987, pp. 1–2.

Fiber: Facts and Fads

For several years, fiber has received increasing attention as an important component of the diet. The "fiber hypothesis" suggests that consumption of unrefined, high-fiber carbohydrate foods protects against many Western diseases. The purposes of this Nutrition in Practice are to discuss what is known about fiber today and to dispel some myths about it.

I have been hearing a lot about fiber lately. Exactly what disorders have been associated with low-fiber diets?

Constipation, hemorrhoids, diverticular disease, appendicitis, colon cancer, heart disease, diabetes, and obesity are some disorders associated with low-fiber intakes. Rural Africans naturally consume a diet very high in fiber and show a lower incidence of these chronic conditions. However, it is important to note that the Western diet is not only lower in fiber but also higher in salt, sugar, and fat, especially saturated fat, so it's hard to single out fiber as the causative factor.

That's quite an impressive list of diseases. How could fiber possibly help to prevent so many different disorders?

Remember that the fiber hypothesis is not proven. However, some of the ways in which food fibers are thought to prevent disease states are:

- It attracts water into the digestive tract, thus softening the stools and preventing constipation.

- It softens the stools. Because the person doesn't have to strain to

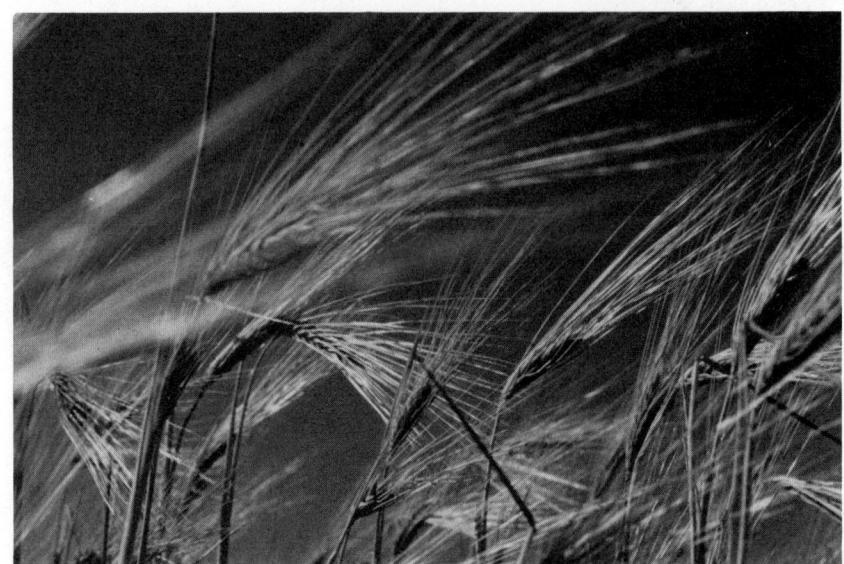

Many health-related organizations advise us to increase our intakes of complex carbohydrates and fiber.

defecate, abdominal pressure is reduced, and rectal veins are less likely to swell and enlarge into hemorrhoids.

- It exercises the muscles of the digestive tract so that they retain their health and tone; thus, the muscles can resist bulging out into the pouches characteristic of diverticulosis.

- It prevents the formation of hard fecal matter that can become lodged in the appendix and permit bacteria to flourish there, resulting in appendicitis.

- It may speed the passage of food through the digestive tract, thus shortening the "transit time" and helping to prevent exposure of the tissue to cancer-causing agents in food.

- It binds lipids, such as cholesterol and bile, and carries them out of the body with the feces so that the blood lipid concentrations are lowered. Possibly the risk of heart and artery disease are lowered as a consequence.

- Complex carbohydrates, in the presence of fiber, may moderate the rise in blood glucose that occurs following ingestion of other carbohydrates, preventing blood glucose levels from getting too high.

- Fiber may promote weight loss by contributing bulk to the diet, thus enhancing satiety and displacing the kcalories of concentrated sweets and fats. Foods high in fiber tend to be low in fat and simple sugars. High-fiber breads have fewer kcalories per pound than refined breads. High-fiber foods add bulk, thanks to their water-holding capacity.

Not all fibers have similar effects, however. For example, wheat bran, which is composed mostly of cellulose, has no cholesterol-lowering effect, whereas oat bran and the fiber of apples (pectin) do lower blood cholesterol. On the other hand, wheat bran seems to be one of the most effective stool-softening fibers, especially if a certain particle size is used. Fibers that form gels in water (pectin, guar) prolong the transit time of materials through the intestine, whereas insoluble fibers (cellulose) tend to shorten it. Table 16−7 shows the effects of different types of fiber.

A compound not classed as a fiber but often found along with fiber in foods is phytic acid. Most of the phytic acid in the diet comes from seeds, such as the cereal grains. (The role of phytate in the plant seed may be to hold these ions in storage during germination.)

You say all the evidence is not in, but fiber sounds pretty impressive to me. How much fiber should I be getting every day?

There is no recommended daily allowance (RDA) for fiber. An average of six grams of dietary fiber a day is perhaps sufficient for minimum body needs, but to receive all the benefits of fiber claimed by high-fiber diet advocates, you would have to eat about three to four times this amount, as do the populations of people studied in Africa. At the present time, the question remains unanswered.

If foods are used as the fiber sources, then 25 grams of dietary fiber is probably a safe intake (see Table 16−8). Don't go overboard in adding purified fiber (for example, bran) to foods, because it can cause dehydration and carry off needed minerals with the lost water. Use a variety of whole grains, nuts, fruits, and vegetables to obtain a mixture of dietary fibers and improve the diet's overall nutritive value.

The consistency of your stools will help tell you if you are getting enough fiber. If your stools are hard and compact, you may not be. If they are easy to pass and occur regularly, you probably are getting enough fiber.

Is it possible to get too much fiber?
Most clinical reports are concerned with the influence of the lack of fiber in the diet on health and disease. The ideal range of fiber intakes and the harm caused by excess intakes remain to be defined.

When foods are too bulky, it can be hard to eat enough to remain adequately nourished, or even to get enough kcalories. Vegetarian children are especially vulnerable to this possibility because their stomachs are small and they can't eat much at a

time. People who have marginal or inadequate intakes of the vitamins and trace minerals—including elderly people, people on low-kcalorie diets, and children—may also be likely to develop nutrient deficiencies on high-fiber diets.

Maximum absorption of iron occurs early during digestion. If high-fiber foods move fast through the intestine, there may be less chance that iron and other nutrients will be absorbed. Also, a high-fiber diet is likely to be high in phytic acid, which binds many minerals. On a diet high in phytic acid, minerals may be lost.

Clearly, fiber is like the nutrients in that "more" is only "better" up to a point. Too much is not better for you than too little. Purified fiber is not as beneficial as the fiber of foods; the purified version is empty of nutrients, while the food version is loaded with them.

I see that I'll want to aim at getting enough, but not too much, fiber. Can you give me an idea of what my diet might be like with 25 grams of fiber a day?
Yes. Chapter 16 illustrates a sample high-fiber diet menu. From Table 16−8 you can plan a high-fiber diet: Four slices of whole-grain bread, three servings of fruit, one serving of whole-grain cereal, and two to three cups of cooked vegetables will provide this much fiber. However, as you may have noticed, eating such a diet involves the consumption of large quantities of whole grains, fruits, and vegetables. There is little room in the diet for fats, meats, and dairy products—a way of eating to which some people could find it hard to adjust.

NUTRITION IN PRACTICE
16B

A Perspective on Diet Therapy

In Nutrition in Practice 1, we tried to stimulate your interest in nutrition by pointing out that what you learn about nutrition is relevant to you in both a personal and professional way. Since then you have explored concepts of normal nutrition and have begun to explore how diets are adapted to accommodate various levels of health. Before you continue your study of diets in the treatment of different disorders, it is important to understand how the things you have learned about clinical nutrition apply to real situations. Our intention is to help you see that a therapeutic diet is only one part of a client's treatment plan; the diet must be considered in relation to the whole person before it can be useful. A prescribed diet may be critical at times. In other situations, it may be only slightly beneficial, or even contraindicated.

Are you saying therapeutic diets are not always important?
As you read the chapters on diet therapy, you are learning about different diets and how they are used in the treatment of different disorders. You may recall that there are proven benefits to using some diets and less evidence for using others. You are reading about some disorders, such as indigestion, where diet "might" help and others, such as renal disease, where diet is "critical."

What determines when a diet is critical?
To put a diet in perspective, consider the following:

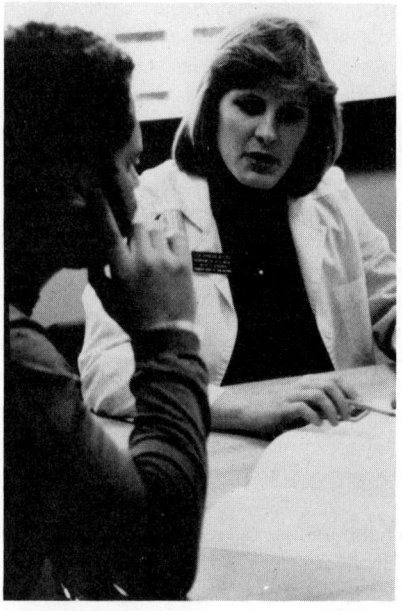

Successful dietary intervention is planned to consider the client's lifestyle and habits.

• What are the proven benefits of the diet?

• What are the negative effects of the diet?

• What are the proven risks of *not* following the diet?

After you have reflected on these questions, consider other factors—the intangibles of actual life situations. Consider the effect of the diet on the whole person rather than on the disease, and exercise clinical judgment in deciding how important a diet is to a client's health. From your

evaluation, you can learn when a client's dietary indiscretions are a real concern that require further intervention and when it may be best to leave well enough alone.

Can you give me an example?
Yes. Let's take a look at Ted, a busy executive who is constantly on the go. Last year, Ted found out that he had a peptic ulcer. His doctor prescribed a traditional bland diet with six small meals a day and told Ted to drink plenty of milk and to take antacids between meals.

Ted is very upset about the diet. You have gotten to know him pretty well during his hospital stay and can appreciate his problems. He barely has time to eat three meals a day, let alone six. He hates milk. The only thing he likes about the diet is that he can still have his usual bedtime snack. Ted confided in you that he has no intention of sticking to the diet. He was outraged when the nurses refused to bring him his morning coffee.

What should you say to Ted? First of all, consult the facts. The traditional bland diet is of little proven value. Eating frequent meals and drinking milk actually stimulates gastric acid secretion (see Chapter 16). Couple these facts with your knowledge about Ted's not wanting to follow the diet anyway and you have identified several major factors weighing against Ted's proposed dietary regimen.

And what about coffee? True, coffee, even decaffeinated, increases gastric acid secretion. But will Ted's stomach secrete even more acid if he gets worked up about not having coffee? You can't know the answer to this question, but you do know Ted, so you must draw a conclusion from what you know. All in all, it seems to you that the minuses outweigh the pluses in this case.

You decide to discuss your concerns with the dietitian. She contacts Ted's physician and suggests an alternative approach, which the doctor approves. The dietitian instructs Ted to follow a liberal bland diet with three meals a day. As for coffee, you reinforce what the dietitian has told him: It's not recommended, and you explain why. But you add that if he does drink coffee, he should limit it to his one favorite cup in the morning and not drink it on an empty stomach.

Can you give me an example of when the diet might be more important?
Well, let's say that Ted doesn't have an ulcer but rather has a hiatal hernia. This time the doctor prescribes a liberal bland diet with five small meals and no eating before bedtime. Ted still doesn't see how he can squeeze in two extra meals, and he doesn't want to give up his bedtime snack; but now the ratio of benefits to disadvantages has changed. You decide to tell Ted why.

This time the diet is more justifiable. Smaller feedings will help prevent stomach distention, which can aggravate the hiatal hernia. Furthermore, heartburn can result if the diet is not followed and it can be quite painful. Lying down after eating increases the risk of reflux esophagitis and heartburn, so a bedtime snack is unwise. Coffee lowers the cardiac

sphincter pressure, which also aggravates the problem.

The major drawback of the diet is that Ted will have to change his lifestyle somewhat. He will have to find time to squeeze in extra feedings and to live without a bedtime snack.

This time the benefits of the diet outweigh the disadvantages. If Ted wishes to avoid the pain of heartburn and the possible complications of hiatal hernia, he will have to find a way to make the necessary adjustments. Ask the dietitian to talk with Ted. He or she can suggest foods that are convenient for Ted to eat. You can reinforce the dietitian's suggestions.

OK. I think I understand what you mean. Can you give me an example of when a diet is critical?
Yes, that's a good idea. Let's look at Jennifer, a healthy young woman of 25 who was born with phenylketonuria (PKU). PKU is discussed in more detail in Chapter 22. For now it is enough to know that the diet is very difficult to follow, but without the diet, a healthy baby gradually develops mental retardation. Strict adherence to the diet is critical. Jennifer's PKU was diagnosed within three days' time; therefore, her parents instituted the PKU diet immediately to promote Jennifer's normal development. The diet was discontinued when Jennifer was six years old, and she has led quite a normal life since then. Now she is pregnant, and her doctor has told her that she must go back on the PKU diet. She is expressing resentment at the necessity of following the diet's myriad rules and of buying its expensive special products. She

remembers that the diet cramped her lifestyle and prevented her from participating fully in many social activities even when she was only five.

What should you say to Jennifer? First, consult the facts. To evade the doctor's orders would in this case pose considerable risks, not to Jennifer herself but to her unborn infant. The diet does not provide a perfect guarantee that Jennifer's baby will be mentally and physically normal, but severe disability is inevitable if she does *not* follow the diet. It is your responsibility to present her with the facts, and to make sure that she receives meticulous instructions about all the intricacies of the diet. Jennifer will make her own decision, but you can't in good conscience support her in a choice not to comply with the doctor's orders. Inform the doctor and dietitian about Jennifer's feelings so that all of you can work together to help Jennifer through a difficult time.

Other diets that are of critical importance are those that bring about life-sustaining changes in metabolism. Among these diets are those for liver failure, renal failure, and insulin-dependent diabetes. All your efforts should be directed toward ensuring compliance with these diets. A client's complaint that such a diet is restrictive is not a cue for you to tell the person, "Never mind, it's all right not to follow the diet."

But clients hate those diets sometimes. Is there anything I can do to help them follow restrictive diets?
Yes, and many practical suggestions are given in the diet therapy chapters. Remember, no diet is so rigid that it cannot be planned to some extent around the individual's lifestyle and

preferences. There are no foods that can't occasionally and with careful planning be worked into most diets. The key is that "forbidden" foods should be used only now and then, in limited amounts, and only when their inclusion in the diet is planned. An occasional lapse from the diet rules will not be fatal, but the better the compliance with a metabolism-normalizing diet, the better the person's recovery and health are supported.

What can I do to help a person who has several different disorders that all require diet modifications?

That's a good question. It's a situation that occurs often, particularly in the elderly. As an example, let's look at Martha, a sweet, elderly (70 years old) lady with several problems:

- Obesity.
- Noninsulin-dependent diabetes.
- Hiatal hernia.
- Type IV hyperlipoproteinemia.
- Chronic constipation.

For the first time, her doctor is recommending a diet for her. Considering her multiple problems, the diet that might be appropriate for Martha would be:

- Low in kcalories.
- Low in total fat, saturated fat, and cholesterol (see Chapter 21).
- Low in concentrated sweets (see Chapter 19).
- Restricted in foods that stimulate gastric acid secretion.
- High in fiber.

These changes entail several problems, however. For one thing, they are quite a few to inflict on someone who has already lived seventy years. For another, Martha would get very confused trying to obey all those rules at once. Let's analyze the pros and cons and establish priorities before deciding what kind of diet would be useful to her.

To make the diet low in kcalories would help with four of Martha's five problems, because a low-kcalorie diet would bring about weight loss, normalize blood glucose, bring down her high triglycerides, and reduce abdominal pressure, which would pacify her hernia. Three of these four advantages would also be gained by making the diet low in concentrated sweets: weight loss, blood glucose control, and lower triglyceride levels. It would seem advisable, then, to help Martha at least work out a low-kcalorie, low-concentrated-sweets diet. This would be a fairly simple process and would not be overwhelming to Martha.

To make Martha's diet high in fiber as well would help with her constipation problem, would facilitate weight loss by displacing kcalorie-rich foods, and might improve her blood glucose control, three of the five goals chosen for her. Martha could probably understand this diet and, with help, might incorporate these changes into her eating habits, especially if you gave her reason to hope that she would notice an improvement in her health.

What about all the proposed changes in the kinds and amounts of fats in Martha's diet? A review of the facts on similar cases suggests that a

fat-controlled diet for a woman Martha's age might not significantly reduce the risk of atherosclerosis. In this case, asking her to change menus she has used for years might not be worth the trouble. As for the elimination of irritating foods to help with the hiatal hernia, perhaps you should discuss this with her. What you and Martha might work out together might be a low-kcalorie diet in which high-fiber foods are emphasized and concentrated sweets are discouraged. You might make Martha aware of the foods likely to irritate her hiatal hernia, then leave the use of those foods to her discretion.

Doing all that seems like a tall order.
Yes, it is. But if you care enough to provide the best nutrition therapy for your clients, you will work hard to develop skill in giving diet advice. You won't simply give everyone who has the same "label" the same diet advice. Furthermore, because research in diet therapy is an active and fast-moving area, you will keep your eyes and ears open for new information on the benefits and risks of alternatives in diet. You will develop your clinical judgment, as all good judges do, by allowing each new fact and each new case to find its proper place in the making of your decisions. As you read the chapters to come, try to keep in mind that you encounter a variety of unique circumstances with each individual you encounter. Although this uniqueness makes your job more difficult at times, it is also challenges such as these that make your job more rewarding.

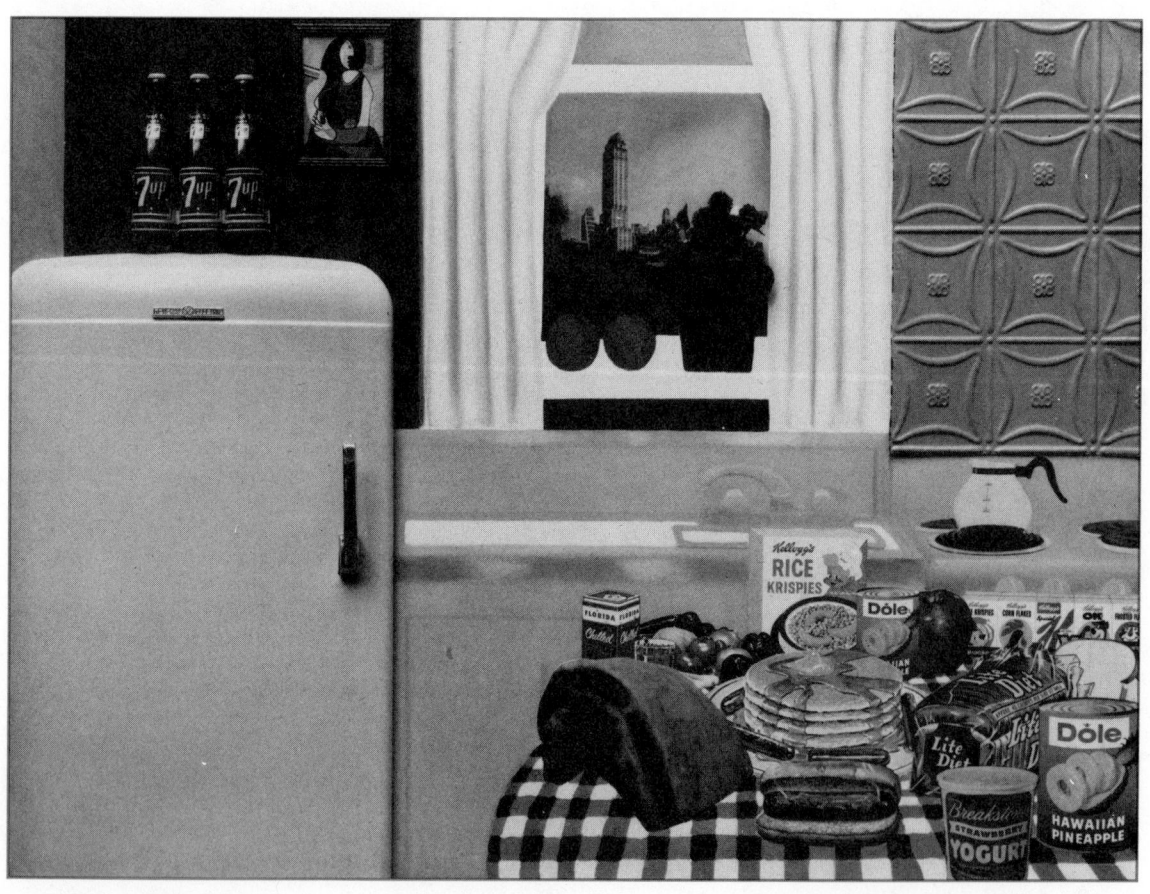

CHAPTER

17

Diets Modified in kCalories, I: High-kCalorie Diets

DIETS DISCUSSED

High-kCalorie Diets

Case Study: Woman with Burns

Nutrition in Practice: Nutrition and Cancer Prevention

CONDITIONS DISCUSSED

Underweight

Severe Stress and Burns

Cancer Cachexia

Chronic Obstructive Pulmonary Disease

Acquired Immune Deficiency Syndrome

Still Life #30 by Tom Wesselman, 1963. Oil, enamel, and synthetic polymer paint on composition board with collage of printed advertisements, plastic artificial flowers, etc., 48½ × 66 × 4″. Collection, The Museum of Modern Art, New York. Gift of Philip Johnson.

High-kcalorie diets are often used to rehabilitate people who are malnourished or underweight and to prevent malnutrition and weight loss in conditions that greatly increase food energy needs. Such conditions include cancer cachexia, chronic obstructive pulmonary disease (COPD), acquired immune deficiency syndrome (AIDS), and severe stress and trauma.

High-kCalorie Diets

High-kcalorie diets are also high-protein diets. A typical high-kcalorie diet provides an extra 1,000 kcalories above those the person normally needs to maintain weight and about 1.5 grams of protein per kilogram of body weight as opposed to the 0.8 gram per kilogram normally considered adequate. A sample menu is shown in the text. Table 17–1 lists indications for the use of high-kcalorie, high-protein diets.

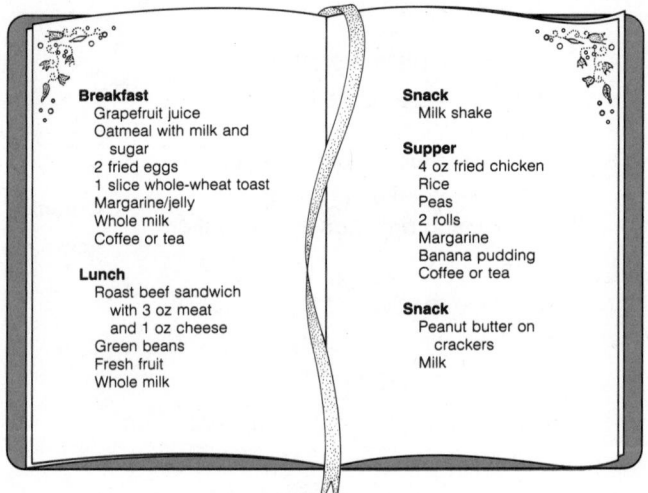

Sample high-kcalorie, high-protein diet menu.

To design a high-kcalorie diet, the planner aims at improving energy intake, using foods that provide as many kcalories in as small a volume as possible so as not to make the client uncomfortably full. Recommended are nutritious, high-kcalorie milk shakes; liberal servings of meat, bread, and starchy vegetables; and desserts. The person on a high-kcalorie diet is urged to select the highest kcalorie items from each food group (see Table 1–2). Encourage the person on a high-kcalorie diet to eat fast and to eat the higher kcalorie items in the meal first. Some practical pointers for adding kcalories and protein are given in Table 17–2.

An effective strategy for gaining weight is to snack systematically between meals. A 400-kcalorie milk shake at midmorning and a 700-kcalorie sandwich

TABLE 17–2. Strategies for Adding kCalories and Protein to the Diet

- Add 2 tablespoons of milk powder to the milk that you drink, use in recipes, or add to soups, puddings, and cereals.
- Add ground meats, chicken, fish, or grated cheese to sauces, soups, casseroles, or vegetables.
- Use extra butter, margarine, or cream cheese on bread.
- Eat peanut butter on fruit, celery, or crackers.
- Use butter or margarine whenever possible (on bread, potatoes, vegetables, pasta, and rice).
- Use yogurt, sour cream, or a sour cream dip with vegetables.
- Use mayonnaise as a salad dressing and on sandwiches.
- Add whipping cream to desserts and hot chocolate or use it to lighten coffee.
- Have snacks available at all times.
- Add nuts and dried fruits such as raisins to desserts or cereals.
- Use cream instead of milk with cereal.
- Try commercially available liquid supplements or instant breakfast mixes for meals or between-meal snacks.

plus shake between lunch and dinner can help to promote a weight-gain rate of 1½ to 2 pounds a week.

Although the advice given to help someone gain weight might sound like a dream come true for the person who is overweight, eating all this extra food could be a nightmare for the person who needs the diet—especially for the person with PCM or for a person suffering from complications after surgery.

Imagine feeling almost too sick to move or too tired to sit up. To someone in this state, the effort of eating even normal amounts of food three times a day seems monumental. It is even harder to eat extra foods.

You can help in several ways. As with other diets, be sure the person knows why the extra food is important. Work closely with the individual to find the high-kcalorie foods she enjoys most and is most likely to eat. Encourage the person to select foods that require little effort to eat. For example, eating a roast beef sandwich requires less effort than cooking, cutting, and eating a steak. Drinking a high-kcalorie creamed soup is easier than eating with a spoon. Finally, let the person know that you understand the difficulty involved.

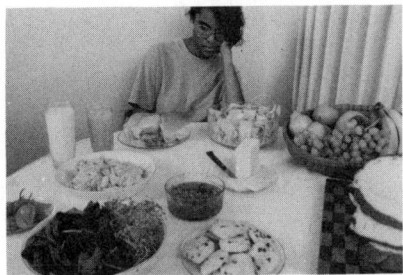

The person needing a high-kcalorie diet may be overwhelmed by the thought of eating large quantities of food.

Underweight

No serious health hazards are associated with mild degrees of underweight. However, the mildly underweight individual may become more seriously underweight if a condition develops that greatly increases nutrient needs. Furthermore, an individual may wish to add some weight for personal reasons such as to improve his self-image.

atrophy (ATT-ro-fee):
to waste away.
a = without
trophy = growth

homeostasis (HOME-ee-oh-STAY-sis):
the maintenance of relatively constant
internal conditions in the body.
homeo = same
stasis = staying

Metabolically, fasting and starvation have the
same consequences in the body. In fasting,
food intake is voluntarily discontinued,
whereas in starvation, lack of food intake is
involuntary.

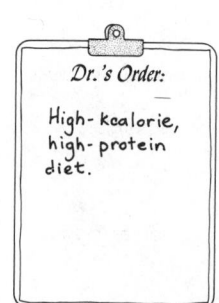

Dr.'s Order:
High-kcalorie,
high-protein
diet.

Whenever a person becomes extremely underweight, PCM develops. The problems associated with PCM are discussed in Chapters 4 and 13. Refeeding a person with PCM should be gradual. Recall from Chapter 14 that disuse of the GI tract results in atrophy of the intestinal villi. Digestive enzyme concentrations may be markedly reduced. To prevent malabsorption, nutrients must be reintroduced gradually to allow time for the intestinal villi and enzyme activity to return to normal. A person who has not been eating an oral diet for some time should first be given clear liquids, then full liquids, then a regular diet, and finally a high-kcalorie, high-protein diet as tolerated.

A condition that results in PCM is anorexia nervosa, the self-starvation eating disorder. This and the related disorder, bulimia, are discussed in Chapter 12. PCM can develop from any type of stress (infection, trauma, or burns) that causes energy needs to increase significantly as well as in people with cancer, COPD, and AIDS.

Severe Stress and Burns

Under normal circumstances, the body is a finely tuned instrument that operates efficiently to maintain an internal balance. Even small changes in the internal environment set in motion a series of metabolic events to restore balance. More drastic changes in the internal environment, such as surgery, a broken bone, infection, or a burn, require more complex mechanisms to restore balance. These complex changes are collectively called the stress response.

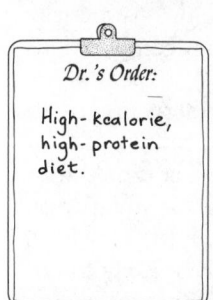

Dr.'s Order:
High-kcalorie,
high-protein
diet.

The response to each type of stress is unique—mending bones requires a different response than healing a wound or fighting an infection—but the general metabolic responses to stress are similar. To understand what happens inside the body in response to stress, it is helpful to review what happens during fasting, which is also a stress to the body. Chapter 6 provides this information (see pp. 86 to 87). The metabolic changes that occur during fasting present a fairly uncomplicated picture of the stress response. If you can visualize this picture, you can use it to understand the more complex changes that occur when more severe stresses are imposed on the body. Initially, the body's metabolic rate accelerates (hypermetabolism) and the breakdown of the body's energy reserves occurs rapidly. During recovery, the metabolic rate returns to normal and the body resumes its normal balance. Figure 17–1 summarizes the metabolic stress response.

The amount of time it takes for the body to regain normal balance depends on the type of stress and its severity. A well-nourished person undergoing minor elective surgery is only mildly stressed, whereas a person with extensive burns suffers the most severe type of stress. In severe stress or malnutrition, a person may not have enough protein available to meet the metabolic demands of severe injury without sacrificing vital proteins. As you may recall from

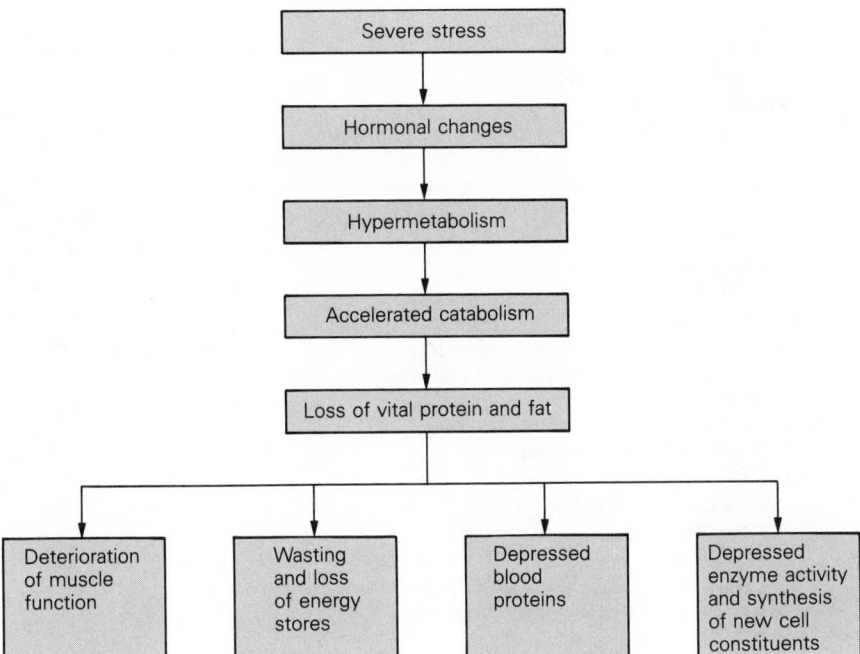

FIGURE 17–1
Metabolic response to stress. The degree to which the body is affected by stress depends on the severity and duration of the insult.

Chapter 13, this person is more likely to develop complications, such as infection or organ failure, that can be fatal.

As discussed in Chapter 16, the well-nourished person who has undergone uncomplicated surgery can do well on a regular diet. The malnourished person or the person with complications is given a high-kcalorie, high-protein diet. Table 17–3 provides guidelines for determining energy needs during stress. The need for many B vitamins increases when kcalorie and protein intakes increase. Vitamins and minerals are important cofactors in the metabolic reactions that are occurring, and their levels are also being drained. However, diets higher in kcalories and protein normally will contain higher amounts of vitamins as well. A person who is accepting a variety of foods often needs no supplements.

The person with extensive burns rapidly uses up the energy reserves and vital protein necessary for survival; therefore, the nutrient needs of the burned individual are very high. Moreover, people with burns often experience anorexia, which compromises their ability to meet nutrient demands. The burn injury itself can make eating difficult because of the pain associated with it or because of its physical location, such as the hands. Burn therapy, immobilization, and lack of exercise further aggravate the situation.

Immediately after a person is burned, dramatic changes take place in the circulatory system. Blood proteins, mainly albumin, and electrolytes leak through the capillaries into the spaces between the blood vessels and the cells and into the burned area causing considerable edema. Blood volume can be reduced by half or even more in people with burns over 40 percent of their bodies.

TABLE 17–3. Stress and Energy Needs

Basal Energy Expenditure (BEE)[a]
  Women
    BEE = 655 + [9.6 × wt in kg[b]] + [1.7 × ht in cm[b]] + [4.7 × age in years]
  Men
    BEE = 66 + [13.7 × wt in kg] + [5 × ht in cm] + [6.8 × age in years]
Add to BEE for activity
    20% Sedentary
    35% Moderately active
    50% Advice
Add to BEE for stress
    10–15% Uncomplicated elective surgery
    20–40% Complicated surgery or fractures
    50% Major burn
Add to BEE for fever (if present)
    13% per degree centigrade[b]
Add to BEE for growth (if necessary)
    5% Moderate weight loss
    10–15% Severe weight loss

---

[a]This is the Harris-Benedict equation frequently used to estimate energy needs.
[b]See inside back cover for equations to convert kg, cm, and °C.

During this time, then, the primary consideration of therapy is to provide enough fluid, electrolytes, and albumin to maintain blood volume and prevent shock. Isotonic fluids are given intravenously, because severely burned people experience a temporary absence of peristalsis and cannot take fluids by mouth. On an average, 3 to 5 liters are needed to replace fluid losses daily. In some cases, as many as 10 or more liters of fluid may be required.

Bowel activity usually resumes in the period following fluid replacement, and attention to adequate nutrition then becomes paramount. Hypermetabolism reaches a peak at about the end of the first postburn week and gradually becomes normal over a period of several weeks. During this time, a high-kcalorie, high-protein diet can be crucial to survival. The typical person will need about 4,000 kcalories (two times the basal energy expenditure) and 200 grams of protein (2.5 grams per kilogram body weight) daily. If the client cannot or will not eat adequate amounts of food by mouth, tube feeding or intravenous nutrition is in order. Animal studies suggest that enteral nutrition is preferred to parenteral nutrition in the immediate postburn period.[1] Enteral nutrition helps maintain the normal function of the intestinal cells and may inhibit the secretion of hormones that stimulate catabolism.

The proportion of nutrients supplying energy for the person who is burned may also be important. Although further research is necessary to define optimal nutrition care, studies suggest that carbohydrate may be a more effective source of nonprotein kcalories than fat for the person who is burned.[2] Restricting fat to 10 to 15 percent of the nonprotein kcalories is suggested. Furthermore, the type of fat may be important. Use of fish oil to supply 50 percent of the fat kcalories has proven beneficial in a preliminary study of children with burns.[3]

Specific vitamin and mineral requirements for people with burns have not been established. However, in consideration of the high-energy and high-protein needs and of the nutrients needed for tissue repair and replacement of blood and skin losses, additional vitamins are generally given. These nutrient needs are so high that they are not met by eating a high-kcalorie, high-protein diet. Adults might be given two standard multivitamins per day with an additional one to two grams of vitamin C. Children might be given one to two doses of a pediatric multivitamin preparation in addition to 500 to 700 milligrams of vitamin C. Since many liquid vitamin preparations commonly used for children do not contain vitamin K and folacin, these vitamins may require additional supplementation. Generally, mineral requirements are met with a diet adequate in protein and kcalories, although some studies suggest that supplemental zinc may help burn wounds heal more quickly. If iron-deficiency anemia is present, iron supplementation should be given.

Your support in helping the client to eat is important. Remember to keep the total person in mind. Understandably, food may seem uninviting to the person who faces a lengthy hospital stay, a great deal of pain, and fear of permanent disfigurement. Burn therapy, which generally includes whirlpool baths and the cutting away of dead skin and tissue, is extremely painful. If possible, these treatments should be scheduled so as not to interfere with mealtimes. Pain medication can be timed so that the person is feeling less pain at mealtime.

Some individuals may feel awkward about eating when the location of a burn interferes with self-feeding. Sometimes this problem can be worked out with the aid of an occupational therapist, who might be able to adapt feeding utensils for the client. The client also should be encouraged to walk around and begin physical therapy as soon as possible. This measure helps to prevent further tissue breakdown associated with injury, improves morale, and may also help to stimulate the appetite.

Cancer Cachexia

At least 50 percent of all people with cancer develop cancer cachexia, a syndrome characterized by loss of appetite (anorexia), wasting of lean body mass, and metabolic abnormalities.[4] A downward spiral develops. The appetite loss and metabolic changes lead to muscle wasting and poor health, which further contribute to the inadequate intake of nutrients. Malnutrition interferes with quality of life and contributes to the morbidity and mortality associated with the disease process. Some of the known causes of cachexia and the cancer syndrome are summarized in Figure 17–2.

Reduced food intake in the person with cancer can be due to:

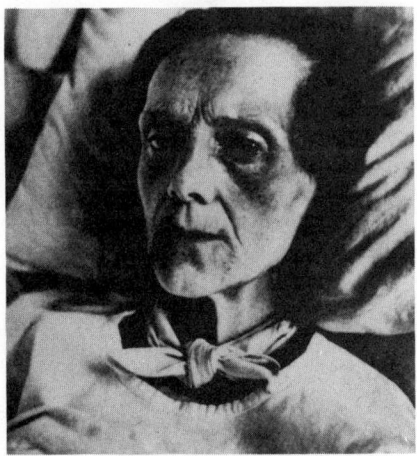

Cancer cachexia can be induced by many cancers. The major symptoms are anorexia with inadequate food intake, speeded-up metabolism and wasting, and general ill health associated with cancer.
kakos = bad, poor
hexis = condition

- Psychological stress.
- Cancer itself. Often anorexia and weight loss are the complaints that bring the person to visit the doctor in the first place.
- Premature feeling of fullness.
- Lack of energy to prepare and eat food.
- Obstruction in the upper GI tract, which interferes with the ability to chew or swallow.

FIGURE 17–2
Causes of the cancer cachexia syndrome. Anorexia and cachexia contribute to each other. Cancer itself and the available treatments for it make both problems worse.

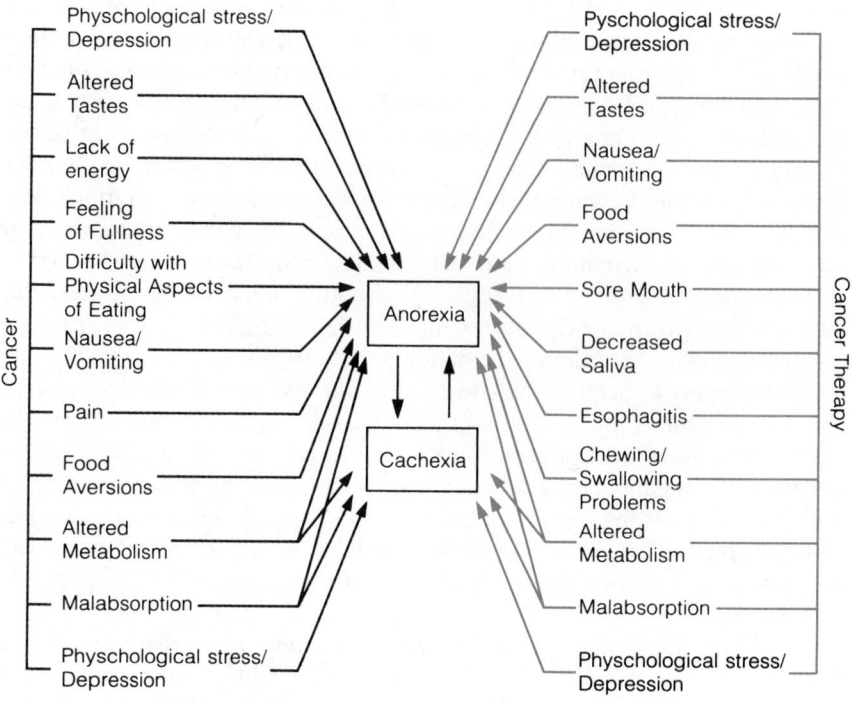

chemotherapy:
the use of drugs to arrest or destroy cancer cells. Chemotherapeutic drugs are sometimes called *antineoplastic agents.* *chemo* = chemical

radiation therapy:
the use of radiation to arrest or destroy cancer cells.

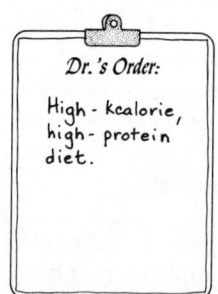

Dr.'s Order:

High-kcalorie, high-protein diet.

• Cancer therapy. The major treatments for cancer are surgery, chemotherapy, and radiation therapy. A summary of the effects of various types of surgery on the individual's nutrition status is presented in Table 16–2. Table 17–4 describes the effects of cancer therapy that can lead to limited nutrient intake.

Although the exact mechanisms of cancer cachexia are unknown, it appears that changes in the metabolism of carbohydrate, protein, and fat, along with reduced food intake, play a role. Metabolic changes may occur that raise energy needs or cause nutrients to be used ineffectively (see Table 17–4). Some studies suggest that people with certain types of cancer are not hypermetabolic.[5] Other studies show conflicting results. It may be that metabolic changes vary with different types of tumors or vary depending on lean body mass, weight loss, or body size.

For many years, the deteriorating nutrition status that accompanies cancer was largely ignored. Many practitioners believed that emaciation and physical debilitation were an inevitable result of cancer. Others believed that if you fed the host, you also fed the tumor and should therefore starve the person with cancer. Another problem was the state of the art of feeding people who could

TABLE 17–4. Effects of Radiation and Chemotherapy on Nutrition Status

Radiation	Chemotherapy
Reduced nutrient intake	
Anorexia	Abnominal pain
Damage to teeth and bones	Anorexia
Esophagitis	Intestinal ulcers
Nausea	Nausea
Reduced salivary secretions	Taste alterations
Taste alterations	Vomiting
Thick salivary secretions	
Vomiting	
Accelerated nutrient losses	
Chronic blood loss from intestine and bladder	Diarrhea
Diarrhea	Malabsorption
Fistula formation	
Intestinal obstructions	
Malabsorption	
Altered metabolism	
(Secondary to malnutrition)	Fluid and electrolyte imbalance
	Hyperglycemia
	Interference with vitamins or other metabolites
	Negative nitrogen and calcium balance

not eat. The widespread use of tube feedings and total parenteral nutrition (TPN) is a recent advance.

Today, attitudes regarding the benefits of nutrition for the person with cancer have changed dramatically. Attention to the diet can prevent or reverse poor nutrition status, and we now recognize the advantages of maintaining optimal nutrition status. Concern for nutrition status should be given before the person becomes seriously depleted. It is much harder to build up a person's nutrient reserves than to prevent them from being depleted.

People with cancer, particularly those who feel they cannot be helped by therapy, are easy targets for peddlers of cancer "cures." Such people may take massive doses of vitamins and/or minerals, some of which may be toxic. Generally, people will not volunteer information about their use of vitamin supplements. Health care professionals should try to find out what and how many supplements their clients may be taking.

People with cancer often benefit from a high-kcalorie, high-protein diet. A diet that daily supplies from 40 to 45 kcalories with 1½ to 2 grams of protein per kilogram of body weight is frequently recommended.[6] The following suggestions can be valuable to help improve a person's appetite:

- Eat the most during the times when you feel the best.
- Use foods that are easy to prepare and easy to eat.
- Eat small, frequent meals.
- Use high-kcalorie, high-protein liquids often.

Suggestions for controlling nausea and vomiting are given in Chapter 16 (see pp. 350–351). These as well as other suggestions are summarized in Table 17–5. If chewing and swallowing are a problem, a mechanical soft diet (see p. 353) can help.

TABLE 17–5. Suggestions for Controlling Some Symptoms of Cancer Through Diet

To improve the appetite

- Explain why eating is important.
- Encourage clients to eat the most when they feel the best.
- Suggest foods that are easy to prepare and eat.
- Recommend smaller meals.
- Advise the client not to drink liquids with meals.
- Recommend the use of time-saving food preparation appliances.

To combat bitter or metallic tastes

- Encourage the use of eggs, fish, poultry, and dairy products instead of meats.
- Recommend adding sauces and seasonings to meats.
- Suggest that meats be served cold or at room temperature.
- Advise the client to brush teeth or use a mouthwash before eating.

To control nausea and vomiting

- Recommend small meals.
- Advise the person to avoid high-fat foods and smells that cause nausea.
- Encourage the individual to sip clear liquids or to suck Popsicles to prevent dehydration.
- Suggest that the client get fresh air, loosen clothing, or lie down after meals.
- Advise clients to avoid eating their favorite foods during the times of the day when they frequently experience nausea or vomiting.

To alleviate problems with chewing and swallowing

- Work with the client to find the consistency of food that will be easiest to handle.
- Recommend that the person experiment with tilting his/her head forward and backward to see if swallowing can be made easier with the head positioned differently.
- Suggest a straw for drinking.
- Advise the client with mouth ulcers to avoid foods that are spicy, acidic, or coarse or that contain seeds that can be trapped in the ulcer.
- Encourage the client who suffers from a reduced flow of saliva to rinse the mouth frequently and to avoid concentrated sweets. Artificial saliva from the pharmacy can also help.

People with cancer frequently complain of a bitter or metallic taste in their mouth. Because of this taste alteration, they may dislike red meat and may prefer fish, poultry, eggs, or dairy products. Meat casseroles or soups and meats served in sauces may be more appealing than meats served alone, and meats served at room temperature or cold meats may taste better than hot meats. Suggest marinating poultry and meats in sweet wines, Italian dressing, or sweet-sour sauces. Recommend that they try strong seasonings such as oregano, basil, mint, or tarragon. Using a mouthwash or brushing the teeth before eating is recommended to start the meal with a fresher, more pleasant taste in the mouth.

When anorexia persists, particularly during and immediately after treatment, tube feedings or parenteral nutrition may be indicated. Animal studies suggest that defined formula diets (containing only free amino acids as the source of protein) may be contraindicated when methotrexate (a chemotherapeutic drug) is being administered.[7] In the study, all the animals given only free amino acids died from severe inflammation of the intestine, whereas survival improved as protein in the form of polypeptides or a regular diet was provided.[8] Further studies will need to be conducted to determine if the results of these studies are applicable to human beings.

Although enteral and parenteral nutrition may be beneficial for many people, the use of aggressive nutrition support for the person with terminal cancer may be contraindicated (see Nutrition in Practice 15A). Studies of people with cancer who receive TPN have not been promising in terms of improved survival or tolerance to therapy.[9] While TPN can improve body weight, weight gain appears to be mostly water and fat rather than lean body tissue. The inability of TPN to replete lean body mass most likely results from metabolic abnormalities that accompany cancer cachexia. A promising study in rats with cancer cachexia suggests that insulin may be useful for preserving weight without promoting tumor growth.[10] It is hoped that further study will demonstrate effectiveness of insulin for people with cancer.

Any discussion of nutrition and cancer pales in relation to actual experience in working with the person with cancer. There are so many variables that only experience can teach you. Every type of cancer as well as every person with cancer changes the way nutrition care is delivered. To provide one brief illustration of how many effects and variables there can be, we would like to share with you an example from a personal experience. Kathy was a 36-year-old, vibrant, intelligent woman who developed a malignant brain tumor that progressively affected her speech center and the right side of her body. Because this type of tumor grows rapidly, the prognosis was poor, with an expected length of survival of six months.

As Kathy's ability to communicate declined, it became progressively more difficult for her to express her desires and needs regarding foods she would like to eat. Simultaneously, she was less able to prepare and physically eat foods herself because of loss of function on the right side of her body. Kathy was right-handed, and learning to use her left hand, particularly to handle feeding utensils, was a difficult task. One solution to this problem was to serve foods that could be finger fed. The type of food was important in preserving Kathy's dignity—she was an intelligent adult who did not want to be treated like a child. Breads, cheeses, fruits, and luncheon meats were easy to handle. Depression and frustration that resulted from the inability to communicate and the poor prognosis made it even more difficult for Kathy to eat.

Another problem occurred when foods were too small. Kathy lost the ability to move her tongue back and forth, and when small foods lodged in the right side of her mouth, she could not feel them and could choke.

Kathy was taking a steroid medication to reduce swelling in the brain as well as narcotics to deal with the severe headaches associated with the tumor. Both the steroids and the tumor caused nausea, although in Kathy's case, she ate more rather than less because of the nausea. Kathy stated that she felt much more nauseated when she had an empty stomach. The tumor itself and the narcotics made her sleepy, which compounded the difficulty she had with physical aspects of eating.

As you can see, many factors affect nutrition status in the person with cancer. Consider also that nutrition is only one part of many treatments in the care of the person with cancer. In Kathy's case, prognosis was poor, so the need to maintain long-term nutritional health was not as critical as helping Kathy preserve feelings of self-esteem, dignity, comfort, and independence. Such considerations are certainly important, particularly for the person whose disease is terminal. When time is short, you want the person to enjoy, rather than be burdened by, the routine experiences of everyday life.

Chronic Obstructive Pulmonary Disease

Chronic obstructive pulmonary disease (COPD) is a persistent obstruction of airflow through the lungs. The two major types of COPD are emphysema and chronic bronchitis. The primary risk factor for COPD is smoking. Other risk factors that may play a role include exposure to environmental pollution (including exposure of nonsmokers to cigarette smoke); alcohol consumption; family history of respiratory disorders; and, possibly, repeated respiratory tract infections in young children.

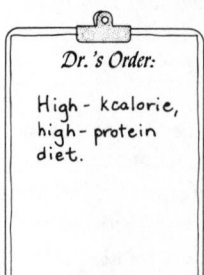

Dr.'s Order:

High-kcalorie, high-protein diet.

In emphysema, the small passages and air sacs (alveoli) within the lungs lose their elasticity. The victim has trouble exhaling to remove air taken in during inspiration. Stale air containing an excess of carbon dioxide becomes trapped in pockets in the lung, and the lung enlarges to accommodate the increased air volume. As the air pockets in the lungs expand, their walls thin out; they then tend to collapse during exhalation. Emphysema is believed to be caused by the destruction of elastin, the major structural protein in the normal lung.

chronic obstructive pulmonary disease (COPD):
a disease that causes blockage of the lung's air passages and thus interferes with the exchange of gases between the air and the body.

emphysema (EM-fe-SEE-ma):
a type of COPD in which the lungs lose their elasticity and the victim becomes breathless.

alveoli (al-VEE-oh-lie):
air sacs in the lungs (one sac is an *alveolus*).

elastin:
a structural protein in the lung.

The individual with chronic bronchitis suffers from a different problem. In chronic bronchitis, excessive mucus is produced and clogs the air passages (bronchioles). These passages also become inflamed, and this contributes to the obstruction.

Regardless of the type of COPD, it becomes more and more difficult for the oxygen necessary for metabolism to reach the tissues and for carbon dioxide (a waste product of metabolism) to be removed. No cure for COPD is available; treatment is aimed at relieving the symptoms.

People with COPD frequently experience weight loss, emaciation, and infection. PCM is widespread in people with COPD. One study noted that hospitalized people with cancer and pulmonary diseases have the highest overall prevalence of malnutrition.[11] Measurements of nutrition status and pulmonary function in these people suggest that nutrition status may be related to the severity of the disease.[12]

As COPD advances, weight loss progresses. The lungs are muscles that lose mass and strength as body weight decreases. This in turn negatively affects lung function. Furthermore, infections are likely to occur in a client with poor nutrition status and pulmonary disease. Infections place further demands on nutrient stores (see Severe Stress and Burns earlier in this chapter).

The following are some possible explanations as to why many individuals with COPD are at risk for poor nutrition status:

- Anorexia and poor food intake.
- Increased energy expenditure associated with labored breathing.
- Drug therapy.
- Increased energy needs during periods when mechanical ventilators are used to sustain adequate respiration.
- Repeated infections.

Weight loss in COPD has commonly been attributed to loss of appetite, impaired absorption, and altered metabolism. A recent report suggests that weight loss in COPD is caused predominantly by increased resting energy expenditure.[13] Clients with stable COPD who weighed less than 75 percent of standard body weight reported higher kcalorie and protein intakes than COPD clients with body weights closer to standard.[14] The authors of the study concluded that kcalorie needs increase as the disease progresses. It is increased nutrient needs, not poor intake of nutrients, that explains weight loss in people with stable COPD. Still, anorexia and poor food intake may be a problem for the person with advanced COPD. The person may be unable to verbalize feelings of hunger and may not be able to take adequate nourishment.[15] When on a mechanical ventilator, the person may feel weak, uncomfortable, and overwhelmed.

Steroids used in the treatment of COPD can also raise nutrient requirements and contribute to poor nutrition status in people with COPD. People who require mechanical ventilation are in a hypermetabolic state, which also increases the risk of poor nutrition status.

The frequent respiratory infections seen in COPD also contribute to malnutrition. Infection raises nutrient needs, and nutrient deficiencies, in turn,

bronchitis (bron-KYE-tis):
inflammation of the lung's air passages.
bronchos = wind pipe
itis = inflammation

bronchioles (BRON-key-ohls):
the small air passages from the trachea to the lungs.

mechanical ventilator:
a machine that "breathes" for the person who can't.

can increase the likelihood of infection. The severe weight loss that can occur in COPD may create a vicious cycle of malnutrition and infection.

Respiratory failure can occur as a result of many disorders including advanced COPD. Respiratory failure occurs when the lungs are no longer able to perform their function in exchanging gases. People with respiratory failure spend more energy, especially during attempts to wean them from mechanical ventilation. The type of nutrients used to provide this energy appears to be important. Such people are often candidates for TPN or tube feedings, and standard formulas are high in glucose. However, glucose generates more carbon dioxide when metabolized than does fat. High-glucose formulas may put additional stress on the lungs to rid the body of excess carbon dioxide. For this reason, many authorities currently recommend that the TPN solution derive half its nonprotein kcalories from fat and half from glucose.[16]

Acquired Immune Deficiency Syndrome

Acquired immune deficiency syndrome (AIDS) is a devastating disorder rapidly approaching epidemic proportions. As the incidence of AIDS increases, prevention and treatment are of ever greater concern to health care professionals. AIDS is a disorder of the immune system that leaves its victims defenseless against infections and disorders from which most people are protected. The person with AIDS frequently develops infections of the lungs, central nervous system, GI tract, and skin. Pneumonia, a special type of cancer, and severe diarrhea are frequent and often fatal complications. Currently, AIDS has no cure. Treatment is aimed at controlling the complications and improving the person's comfort and quality of life.

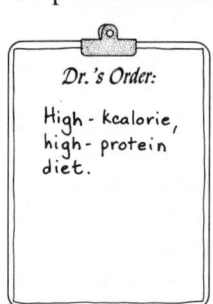

As discussed earlier in the chapter, malnutrition increases the likelihood of infection, and infection can further tax nutrition status. AIDS itself as well as the various treatments for AIDS can interfere with nutrition status. Therefore, it seems logical that attention to nutrition status may play a role in the treatment of AIDS. Currently, there is no direct evidence that aggressive nutrition support can correct any of the complications associated with AIDS. However, clinical observations have demonstrated that nutrition can affect the person's ability to care for himself or herself and that it may affect the course of the disease.[17]

In addition to infection, some of the complications of AIDS with nutrition consequences include anorexia, nausea, vomiting, severe diarrhea, fever, lesions of the mouth and esophagus, malabsorption, and disorientation. Table 17–6 shows some of the causes of these complications. Presently, virtually no controlled studies have documented specific nutrient needs of the person with AIDS. However, practitioners have begun to make recommendations for care based on clinical experiences.[18]

Although dietary intervention is not always successful, it can be very helpful in some cases. A high-kcalorie diet of nutrient-dense foods may be useful. For people with anorexia or nausea, mechanical soft diets (see Chapter 16) or liquid formulas can help improve intake. For the person with lesions of the mouth and esophagus, eating can be very painful. Even liquids can become

respiratory failure:
failure of the lungs to perform.

acquired immune deficiency syndrome (AIDS):
an immune system disorder that leaves its victims vulnerable to numerous infections. AIDS can be transmitted sexually or intravenously or from mother to infant during pregnancy.

Infections from microorganisms that normally do not cause disease in the general population but can infect people whose immune systems are impaired (as with AIDS) are called **opportunistic infections**.

A type of cancer rare in the general population but common in people with AIDS is called **Kaposi's sarcoma.**

TABLE 17–6. Possible Causes of Nutrition Complications in AIDS

Anorexia

Drug therapy
Lack of energy to eat
Pain associated with eating
Fever/infection
Nausea and vomiting
Psychological factors such as fear and depression

Diarrhea and malabsorption

Various bacteria and parasites
Drug therapy
Low serum albumin levels

Nausea and vomiting

Drug therapy
Oral lesions
Inflammation of the stomach (gastritis) or esophagus (esophagitis)

Oral lesions

Bacterial and viral infections
Kaposi's sarcoma

Source: Adapted from information in M. E. Garcia, C. L. Collins, and P. W. A. Mansel, The acquired immune deficiency syndrome: Nutritional complications and assessment of body weight, *Nutrition in Clinical Practice* 2(1987): 108–111 and M. Bentler and M. Stanish, Nutrition support of the pediatric patient with AIDS, *Journal of the American Dietetic Association* 87(1987): 488–491.

difficult for the person to handle. In such cases, tube feedings should be considered if the GI tract is functional. Otherwise, parenteral nutrition may be necessary. The person with nausea and vomiting may benefit from the use of antiemetics.

Nutrition therapy for the person with AIDS is frequently complicated by malabsorption and severe diarrhea. The underlying causes of these complications are not fully understood. In some cases, infectious agents have been identified, but in about half the cases, the cause is unknown.[19] When diarrhea is not severe, the person may benefit from a low-fiber, lactose-free diet as well as antidiarrheal agents. However, in many cases, diarrhea is severe—the person may lose from 10 to 15 liters of diarrheal fluids daily—and is often difficult to treat. In such a case, replacement of fluids and electrolytes is the most critical consideration. Dietary intervention is not effective. For the person with fat malabsorption, a low-fat diet can be useful in controlling steatorrhea.

Obviously, much work in the area of AIDS and nutrition will have to be completed before anyone will know if there are true benefits from maintaining good nutrition status in people with AIDS. One recent report outlined the medical course of a person with AIDS who was able to maintain his weight and protein status on a home TPN program and an unrestricted oral diet.[20]

antiemetics:
drugs used to control nausea and vomiting.

Lactose-free diets are discussed in more detail in Chapter 19.

antidiarrheal agents:
drugs used to control diarrhea.

steatorrhea (stee-ah-toe-REE-ah):
fatty diarrhea associated with fat malabsorption. Chapter 20 gives more information about steatorrhea.

Common sense seems to indicate that careful attention to nutrition status should be attempted for the person with AIDS.

This chapter has discussed high-kcalorie diets and disorders for which such diets are used to help prevent severe consequences for nutrition status. Chapter 18 looks at low-kcalorie diets and the risks that excess weight can have on the body.

CASE STUDY

Woman with Burns

Ms Sampson, a 36-year-old computer scientist, has been admitted to the hospital following a car accident. She has burns on her arms and legs and a fractured leg. She is 5 feet 5 inches tall and weighs 125 pounds.

1. Identify Ms Sampson's immediate post-injury nutrient needs. Should she be fed orally at this time? If not, how will the physician know when she can eat food by mouth?

2. Discuss the appropriate diet for Ms Sampson. What nutrients are of particular concern? What hints can you give her to help her meet her nutrient needs? Explain how a burn causes nutrient needs to increase.

3. What physical factors might interfere with Ms Sampson's ability to eat? What emotional factors?

Notes

1. H. Saito and coauthors, The effect of route of nutrient administration on the nutritional state, catabolic hormone secretion, and gut mucosal integrity after burn injury, *Journal of Parenteral and Enteral Nutrition* 11 (1987): 1–7.
2. M. M. Gottschlich and J. W. Alexander, Fat kinetics and recommended dietary intake in burns, *Journal of Parenteral and Enteral Nutrition* 11 (1987): 80–85.
3. Gottschlich and Alexander, 1987.
4. K. A. Kern and J. A. Norton, Cancer cachexia, *Journal of Parenteral and Enteral Nutrition* 12 (1988): 286–298.
5. H. W. Murrick and coauthors, Energy requirements for cancer patients and the effect of total parenteral nutrition. *Journal of Parenteral and Enteral Nutrition* 12 (1988): 8–14.
6. R. M. Faulk, Nutritional therapy in cancer, *Postgraduate Medicine* 78, no.1 (1985): 83–87.
7. L. P. Harvey and coauthors, Reversibility of elemental liquid diet-enhanced methotrexate toxicity by refeeding with chow, *Journal of Parenteral and Enteral Nutrition* 11 (1987): 119–123.
8. O. J. McAnena and coauthors, Alteration of methotrexate toxicity in rats by manipulation of dietary components, *Gastroenterology* 92 (1987): 354–360.
9. Kern and Norton, 1988.
10. J. L. Peacock and J. A. Norton, Impact of insulin on survival of cachectic tumor-bearing rats, *Journal of Parenteral and Enteral Nutrition* 12 (1988): 260–264.
11. L. Bushman and R. Russell, Malnutrition among patients in an acute-care veterans facility, *Journal of the American Dietetic Association* 77 (1980): 462–465.
12. N. L. Keim and coauthors, Dietary evaluation of outpatients with chronic obstructive pulmonary disease, *Journal of the American Dietetic Association* 86 (1986): 902–906.
13. Keim and coauthors, 1986.

14. S. Goldstein and coauthors, Energy expenditure in patients with chronic obstructive pulmonary disease, *Chest* 91 (1987): 222–224.

15. C. N. Noller and S. Mobarhan, Enteral feeding in patients with advanced chronic obstructive pulmonary disease, *Nutritional Support Services* 6, February 1986, pp. 37–39.

16. Noller and Mobarhan, 1986.

17. D. P. Kotler, Why study nutrition in AIDS? *Nutrition in Clinical Practice* 2 (1987): 94–95.

18. M. E. Garcia, C. L. Collins, and P. W. A. Mansell, The acquired immune deficiency syndrome: Nutritional complications and assessment of body weight status, *Nutrition in Clinical Practice* 2 (1987): 108–111. M. Bentler and M. Stanish, Nutrition support of the pediatric patient with AIDS, *Journal of the American Dietetic Association* 87 (1987): 488–491.

19. Kotler, 1987.

20. T. L. Donaldo and L. S. Natividad, Nutritional management of a patient with AIDS and cryptosporidium infection, *Nutritional Support Services* 6, April 1986, pp. 30–31.

NUTRITION IN PRACTICE
17

Nutrition and Cancer Prevention

Chapter 17 shows how nutrition therapy can support the person who is being treated for cancer. Cancer is a concern for all of us; one out of every four people now alive will eventually contract cancer. Current research has been revealing that the way people eat may make them more or less susceptible to certain kinds of cancer. Consitituents in foods may be cancer causing, cancer promoting, or protective against cancer. This Nutrition in Practice looks at the role of diet in preventing cancer. The Miniglossary defines terms related to this discussion.

I've heard that nutrition was related to cancer causation, but I always think of other environmental factors, like air and water pollution, as being important causes.
They are, but nutrition is one part of the environment. Comparison of high-risk and low-risk areas suggests that 80 to 90 percent of human cancers may be caused by environmental factors.[1] We can't control many aspects of the environment, but we *can* control our food choices. Researchers have thus taken the study of nutrition and cancer as a challenge and are attempting to discover what dietary differences exist between people who do and don't get cancer.

That sounds like a promising approach. What differences have they found?
Seventh-Day Adventists are one group of people with a remarkably lower

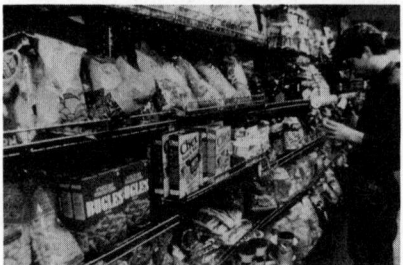

If I don't buy any of the foods I've read about that cause cancer, I won't be able to buy any groceries!

death rate from cancers of all kinds. This religious group has rules against smoking and using alcohol, discourages the use of hot condiments and spices, and encourages a lacto-ovo vegetarian diet. After cancers linked to smoking and alcohol are discounted, Seventh-Day Adventists still have a cancer mortality rate about one-half to two-thirds that of the rest of the population. This may be due to a low consumption of *meat* (and therefore *fat*) and to a high consumption of *vegetables* and *cereal grains*.

In a study involving 37 countries, investigators documented the daily food available per person as well as other indicators of lifestyle. They found many correlations, but one of the most striking showed both breast and colon cancer to be strongly associated "with indicators of affluence, such as a *high-fat* diet rich in *animal protein.*"[2]

In one study, 179 Hawaiian-Japanese people with colon cancer

were carefully matched with 357 Hawaiian-Japanese people without cancer. The people with cancer were found to have a strikingly higher consumption of *meat,* especially beef. An Israeli study showed *fiber* consumption to be lower in colon cancer victims than in comparable people who did not have cancer. A study of U.S. blacks with colon cancer showed them to be eating less *fiber* and more *saturated fat* than others without cancer. These studies have led reviewers to the view that a diet "high in total fat, low in fiber, and high in beef [is] associated with a higher incidence of large-bowel cancer in man."[3]

I see. Have these connections between nutrition and cancer been explained?
No, and attempts to link dietary components with disease should be approached with caution. An increase in one component of the diet causes increases or decreases in others.[4] If a close correlation is shown between a disease and, say, the consumption of animal protein, how can you be sure that the critical factor is the animal protein? It may be increased fat consumption, because fat goes with animal protein in foods. Along with the higher fat consumption, total kcalorie consumption may increase, and this may be a factor. Or the disease may occur because of what is crowded out: Vitamins, minerals, or fiber contained in the missing fruits, vegetables, and cereals.

That's a good point. I know that wherever the diet is high in fat-rich foods, it tends to be low in vegetable fiber. Do you know if the absence of fiber promotes cancer independently of the presence of fat?

These two possibilities are difficult to distinguish, but the association of fat with cancer is stronger than the lack of fiber with cancer. Still, fiber might help protect against some cancer, by promoting the excretion of bile from the body, for example, or by speeding up the transit time of all materials through the colon so that the colon walls are not exposed for long to cancer-causing substances.

Evidence from Finland supports fiber's independent protective effect. The Finns eat a high-fat diet, but unlike other such diets, theirs is very high in fiber as well. Their colon cancer rate is low, suggesting that fiber has a protective effect even in the presence of a high-fat diet.[5]

If fat and meats are implicated in causation of certain cancers, and if fiber and vegetables are associated with prevention, vegetarians should have a lower incidence of those cancers.

They do. The Seventh-Day Adventists have already been mentioned. Vegetarian women also have less breast cancer than do meat eaters. A number of studies examined the relationship between cancer and vegetable consumption. Studies done in Minnesota and in Norway showed that people with colon cancer use vegetables less frequently; a New York study revealed that colon cancer victims specifically use less cabbage, broccoli, and brussels sprouts. Similarly, careful comparisons of stomach cancer victims' diets with diets of case controls showed less use of vegetables in the cancer group—in

Miniglossary

carcinogen (car-SIN-oh-jen) a cancer-causing substance. A carcinogen is one kind of initiator; another is radiation.
carcin = cancer
gen = gives rise to

cruciferous vegetables a group of vegetables named for their cross-shaped blossoms. They have been shown to protect against cancer in laboratory animals. Examples are cauliflower, cabbage, brussels sprouts, broccoli, turnips, and rutabagas.

initiating event an event caused by radiation or chemical reaction that can give rise to cancer.

promoter a substance that does not initiate cancer, but that favors its development once the initiating event has taken place.

one case, *vegetables* in general; in another, *fresh vegetables;* in others, lettuce and other *fresh greens* or vegetables containing vitamin C.[6] One of the suspects for the causation of stomach cancer is nitrosamines, produced in the stomach from nitrites. The vegetables may help in prevention by contributing vitamin C, which inhibits the conversion of nitrites to nitrosamines.

So meat, vegetables, fat, fiber, and vitamins all are involved one way or another. What about alcohol: is there any connection with cancer?

Yes. When environmental causes of head and neck cancer were studied,

the major factor appeared to be the combination of alcohol and tobacco consumption. Again, however, dietary factors have turned up, pointing to a low intake of *fruits* and *raw vegetables,* specifically of the fruits and vegetables that contribute carotene (the vitamin A precursor) and riboflavin. Carotene and its relatives, the retinoids, are also important in preventing cancers of epithelial origin, including skin cancer.[7]

As a matter of fact, I'd heard vitamin A might be related to cancer some way. How do you suppose it works?

Among the known actions of vitamin A are the important roles it plays in supporting immune function. A strong immune system may be able to prevent cancers from gaining control, even after they have gotten started in the body.

In Norway, a five-year prospective study showed lung cancer incidence to be 60 to 80 percent lower in men with a high vitamin A intake than in those with a low intake. In Japan, a study of 280,000 persons showed lung cancer rates to be 20 to 30 percent lower in smokers who ate *yellow* or *green vegetables* daily than in those who did not. In ex-smokers with lung cancer who ingested yellow or green vegetables daily, the reduction was much greater, indicating that the *repair* of damage done by smoking might be enhanced by something in the vegetables.[8]

That "something" in the vegetables would be vitamin A, of course.
Don't be too sure. *Green vegetables* appear to have a protective effect beyond those already discussed for vitamin A, vitamin C, and fiber. These

vegetables also contain folacin, which is involved in DNA replication and may prove to play an important role in cancer prevention. The effects of the members of the cabbage family, for example, may be due to these vegetables' containing substances known as indoles, which may act by inducing an enzyme in the host that destroys carcinogens.[9] Green vegetables also contain significant amounts of riboflavin and calcium, and both of these nutrients have been linked to cancer prevention as well.[10]

Is there any way of testing these possibilities?
Yes. Research on animals is contributing to our knowledge of diet and cancer. Laboratory studies using animals confirm suspicions that fat intake correlates with cancer. One study showed an increase in the number of mammary tumors in rats when dietary fat was raised.[11] The fat was not initiating the cancers, however. To get the tumors started, the animals were exposed to a known carcinogen. After that exposure, the high-fat diet made more cancers develop and made the cancers develop earlier than did low-fat diets. Thus, fat appeared to be a cancer *promoter* rather than an *initiator*.

Do all these findings have any implications for the way I should eat right now, today?
Although we clearly still have much to learn, many researchers believe that we know enough to take the first preventive steps. The Food and Nutrition Board of the National Academy of Sciences published provisional guidelines in 1982.[12] These guidelines include:

1. Reduce the consumption of both saturated and unsaturated fats.
2. Include fruits (especially citrus fruits), vegetables (particularly carotene-rich and cruciferous vegetables), and whole-grain products in the daily diet.
3. Minimize consumption of foods preserved by salt curing, salt packing, or smoking.
4. Minimize contamination of foods with carcinogens from any source and continue to evaluate food additives for carcinogenic activity.
5. Reduce the concentration of mutagens in foods when feasible to do so.
6. Consume only moderate amounts of alcohol, if any.

A summary of the evidence that backed these guidelines included these points:

- Attention should also be paid to nitrates and their relatives in foods.
- Toxic substances in drinking water are also of concern.

The concerns about diet that the guidelines addressed included the following:

- *Total energy intake.* Studies on animals show that reduced food intakes reduce cancer incidence at any age, but the evidence is less clear for human beings.
- *Lipid.* Both animal studies and epidemiological studies support the view that high fat intakes increase the incidence of cancers of the breast and colon. Evidence on cholesterol is unclear.
- *Protein.* High protein intakes may be associated with increased risks of

certain kinds of cancer, but the evidence is not yet firm enough to permit a definitive statement.
- *Carbohydrate.* High simple carbohydrate intakes may contribute to kcaloric excess (with possible risks already discussed); certain fibers may protect against colorectal cancer.
- *Vitamin A.* Inadequate intakes of vitamin A and/or its relatives (carotenoids) seem to correlate with high incidence of cancers of the lung, bladder, and larynx; by inference, adequate intakes must help protect against these cancers.
- *Vitamin C.* Vitamin C may help prevent formation of carcinogens and thereby protect against cancers of the esophagus and stomach.
- *Other vitamins and minerals.* There are suggestive bits of evidence linking other nutrients to cancer, but no firm conclusions can yet be made.
- *Carotene-rich and cruciferous vegetables.* Consumption of carotene-rich and cruciferous vegetables is associated with a reduced incidence of cancer at several sites.

Other links may exist: Between alcohol excess and liver cancer, between alcohol plus cigarette smoking and cancer of the esophagus, between excessive beer drinking and rectal cancer, between certain food contaminants and cancer, and between natural substances in foods and cancer. Additives legally permitted in foods are not implicated in cancer causation.[13]

Obviously, much remains to be learned about the connections between nutrition and cancer. Still, many people working in cancer research believe that we already know enough to take the tentative preventive steps recommended in the "*Interim Dietary Guidelines.*" One pair of reviewers says, "The public is looking for answers regarding this diet-cancer link and will look to anyone willing to provide answers, regardless of his/her qualifications. . . . The recommendations offered here constitute no risk and may help lower the incidence of . . . cancers." The advice agrees with most recommendations made to the public for helping prevent heart disease, diabetes, and many other ills in addition to cancer. To the recommendations made in these guidelines, we would add only one other: Vary your choices. Don't let your diet become monotonous.

Why do you add that suggestion?
This last suggestion is based on an important concept that is specific to the prevention of cancer initiation—dilution. Whenever you switch from food to food, you are diluting whatever is in one food with what is in the others. It is safe to eat *some* processed meats, but don't eat them all the time. Eat many green, yellow, and orange vegetables; they are all needed in the diet for many good reasons.

That makes sense. Would you mind giving me some suggestions on how to go about varying my diet?
Not at all. The variety principle has traditionally meant to eat foods from each of the four food groups. This principle needs to be applied *within* each of the food groups as well. Don't alternate just between corn and

potatoes. Select different vegetables each time you go to the store—broccoli, peas, green beans, squash, or any of some 40 others.

Place emphasis on whole foods, too. Try to select the foods within each group that are the most unaltered from their original farm-grown state; that have the least salt, sugar, and fat added; and that are most likely to be nutrient dense. It is fine to eat *some* processed meats, refined breads, and canned vegetables, but don't eat them all the time.

I don't like vegetables much. Couldn't I just take supplements?
No. Research has shown many food components—including fiber, vitamin A, vitamin C, carotene, riboflavin, indoles, and others—to have preventive effects on cancer development. It's obvious that we don't have *the* answer—just many partial answers. It is also doubtful that there is just one answer, which is why nutrient supplements are not beneficial. By the time you read the results of a spinach study and purchase your vitamin A supplements, folacin will be declared the hero. It's best to rely on foods. Fruits and vegetables will add a healthy array of vitamins, minerals, and fiber to your diet—and color and flavor as well.

Although there are many cancer-causing factors that you cannot control, you can decide which food habits you will keep and which ones you will change. By using the guidelines described here in making your choices, you will have every reason to feel confident that you are providing your body with the best nutrition at the lowest possible risk.

Notes
1. B. S. Reddy and coauthors, Nutrition and its relationship to cancer, *Advances in Cancer Research* 32 (1980): 238–345.
2. B. S. Drasar and D. Irving, Environmental factors and cancer of the colon and breast, *British Journal of Cancer* 27 (1973): 167–172.
3. Reddy and coauthors, 1980.
4. K. K. Carroll, Experimental evidence of dietary factors and hormone-dependent cancers, *Cancer Research* 35, no. 2 (1975): 3374–3383. B. Modan, Role of diet in cancer etiology, *Cancer* 40 (1977): 1887–1891.
5. E. L. Wynder, Dietary habits and cancer epidemiology, *Cancer* 43 (1979): 1955–1961, as cited by S. H. Brammer and R. L. DeFelice, Dietary advice in regard to risk for colon and breast cancer, *Preventive Medicine* 9 (1980): 544–549.
6. Reddy and coauthors, 1980.
7. J. L. Werther, Food and cancer, *New York State Journal of Medicine,* August 1980, pp. 1401–1408.
8. Werther, 1980.
9. L. W. Wattenberg and coauthors, Dietary constituents altering the responses to chemical carcinogens, *Federation Proceedings* 35 (1976): 1327–1331. L. W. Wattenberg and W. D. Loub, Inhibition of polycyclic aromatic hydrocarbon-induced neoplasia by naturally occurring indoles, *Cancer Research* 38 (1978): 1410–1413.
10. Riboflavin and cancer, in An overview of riboflavin, *Dairy Council Digest* 56, November-December 1985, p. 35; M. Lipkin and H. Newmark, Effect of added dietary calcium on colonic epithelial-cell proliferation in subjects at high risk for familial colonic cancer, *New England Journal of Medicine* 313 (1985): 1381–1384.
11. Carroll, 1975.
12. Committee on Diet, Nutrition, and Cancer, National Research Council, *Executive Summary: Diet, Nutrition, and Cancer* (Washington, D.C.: National Academy Press, 1982).
13. Committee on Diet, Nutrition, and Cancer, 1982.

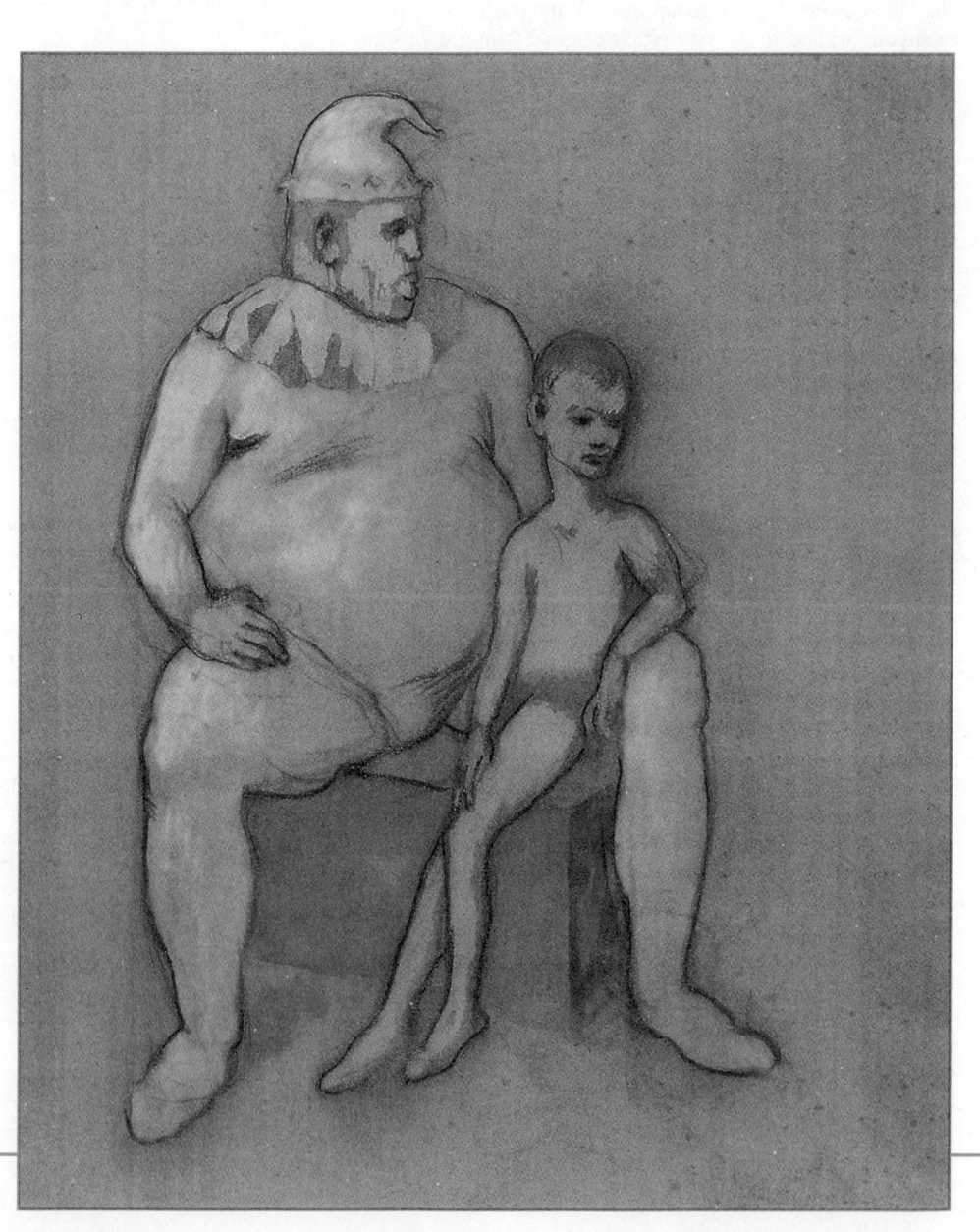

18

Diets Modified in kCalories, II: Maintenance and Low-kCalorie Diets

Seated Saltimbanque with Boy by Pablo Picasso, 1905. The Baltimore Museum of Art: The Cone Collection, formed by Dr. Claribel Cone and Miss Etta Cone of Baltimore, Maryland. BMA 1950.270.

Obesity occurs to an alarming extent and is on the rise in developed countries. For example, in the United States some 10 to 25 percent of all teenagers and some 25 to 50 percent of all adults are obese. This chapter looks at the problems of overweight and obesity and introduces the exchange system for diet planning. The exchange system is useful in the treatment of many conditions and disorders. The most widely used of exchange systems is that employed to plan diets for weight control, diabetes, and other conditions requiring control of kcalories and energy nutrients.

Diet Planning Using Exchange Lists

Unlike a food group system that sorts foods by protein, vitamin, and mineral content only, the exchange system pays special attention to kcalories; proportions of carbohydrate, fat, and protein; and portion sizes. All the food portions on a list have approximately the same number of kcalories and the same amounts of energy nutrients (protein, fat, and carbohydrate). The U.S. exchange system described here is an example of such a system, which consists of six lists of foods. Each list has a typical member—with portion size specified—that you can remember the list by. The six lists and their typical representatives are

1. Milk—1 cup nonfat milk (90 kcalories)

2. Vegetable—½ cup green beans (25 kcalories)

3. Fruit—½ small banana (60 kcalories)

4. Bread/starch—1 slice bread (80 kcalories)

5. Meat/meat alternates—1 ounce lean meat or low-fat cheese (55 kcalories)

6. Fat—1 teaspoon butter (45 kcalories).

Table 18–1 shows the protein, fat, and carbohydrate values that pertain to each list, and Table 18–2 shows the foods on each list with their portion sizes.

The user of the exchange system is encouraged to think of nonfat milk as milk and of whole milk as milk with added fat. A glass of whole milk is described, in fact, as "one milk plus two fats," and a glass of low-fat milk as "one milk plus one fat." The vegetable list includes only low-kcalorie vegetables, so that a half-cup of any of vegetable will provide about 25 kcalories. The fruit list specifies "no added sugar or sugar syrup." Portion sizes are adjusted so that fruit portions are equal in kcalories. One small banana counts as "two fruits." A piece of cherry pie, however, is *not* "a fruit." It *includes* a fruit if it contains 12 large cherries, but it also includes bread and fat exchanges and added sugar. Thus, a piece of cherry pie might be counted as "one fruit, two breads, and three fats with three teaspoons of sugar." The bread list also specifies portion sizes and makes clear which grain products contain added fat. Corn, lima beans, and other starchy vegetables are listed with the breads, not the vegetables, because they are similar to breads in kcalorie and carbohydrate content.

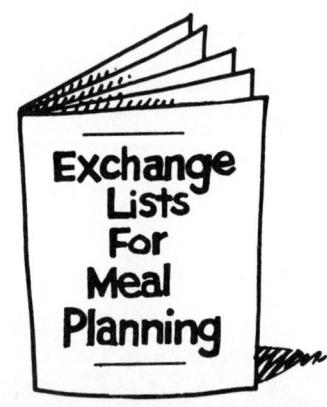

The exchange lists were originally developed for people with diabetes. They proved so useful, however, that they are now in general use for diet planning. Weight-Watchers, a well-known organization that helps people control their weight while eating a nutritious diet, bases its eating plans on the exchange system. (Other kinds of exchange systems also exist—for example, those based on the sodium content of foods.)

TABLE 18–1. The Six Exchange Lists[a]

List	Portion Size	Carbohydrate (g)	Protein (g)	Fat (g)	Energy (kcal)
Starch/Bread[b]	1 slice	15	3	trace	80
Meat[c]	1 oz				
Lean		—	7	3	55
Medium-fat		—	7	5	75
High-fat		—	7	8	100
Vegetable[d]	½ c	5	2	—	25
Fruit	1 portion	15	—	—	60
Milk	1 c				
Nonfat		12	8	trace	90
Low-fat		12	8	5	120
Whole		12	8	8	150
Fat	1 tsp	—	—	5	45

[a]This is the U.S. exchange system. The complete details are shown in Table 18–2.

[b]This list includes starchy vegetables, such as lima beans and corn, as well as cereal, bread, pasta, and other grain products.

[c]This list includes cheese and peanut butter as well as meat.

[d]This list includes low-kcalorie vegetables only.

Meats and cheeses are separated into three categories—lean, medium fat, and high fat. By including such items as bacon and olives, the fat list alerts the user to foods that are unexpectedly high in fat kcalories.

The task of planning an exchange list diet for the client is most often the responsibility of the dietitian. However, those interested in intelligently managing their own diets find the exchange system a useful and versatile tool for many purposes. The system works equally well for planning a weight-loss diet, an ordinary nutritious diet, a prudent diet, or any other diet, including a diabetic diet. The next section is addressed to "you," even if it is not your responsibility to plan diets, because the information may be useful to you as an individual.

The first few times you use exchange lists to plan a diet, it may take an hour or two. With only a little practice, however, you can learn to work out the whole plan in a matter of minutes. The following steps go into planning the diet:

1. *Weigh the client and estimate ideal body weight (IBW)*. We'll illustrate using a woman who is 5 foot 4 inches tall and weighs 140 pounds. To estimate ideal body weight:

Males: Allow 106 pounds for the first 5 foot, then add 6 pounds for each inch over 5 foot.

Females: Allow 100 pounds for the first 5 foot, then add 5 pounds for each inch over 5 foot.

Adjustment: Add 10% for large-framed individuals; subtract 10% for small-framed indivduals.

Children: IBW varies with height for age; refer to growth chart (Appendix B).

TABLE 18–2. The U.S. Exchange System

Starch/Bread List (15 g carbohydrate, 3 g protein, 80 kcal)

Amount	Food
Cereals/Grains/Pasta	
⅓ c	Bran cereals, concentrated[a]
½ c	Bran cereals, flaked[a]
½ c	Bulgur (cooked)
½ c	Cooked cereals
2½ tbsp	Cornmeal (dry)
3 tbsp	Grapenuts
½ c	Grits (cooked)
¾ c	Other ready-to-eat unsweetened cereals
½ c	Pasta (cooked)
1½ c	Puffed cereal
⅓ c	Rice, white or brown (cooked)
½ c	Shredded wheat
3 tbsp	Wheat germ[a]
Dried Beans/Peas/Lentils	
⅓ c	Beans and peas (cooked) (such as kidney, white, split, blackeye)[a]
⅓ c	Lentils (cooked)[a]
¼ c	Baked beans[a]
Starchy Vegetables	
½ c	Corn[a]
1 cob	Corn on cob, 6 in. long[a]
½ c	Lima beans[a]
½ c	Peas, green (canned or frozen)[a]
½ c	Plantain[a]
1 small (3 oz)	Potato, baked
½ c	Potato, mashed
¾ c	Squash, winter (acorn, butternut)
⅓ c	Yam, sweet potato, plain
Bread	
½ (1 oz)	Bagel
2 (⅔ oz)	Bread sticks, crisp, 4 in. long × ½ in.
1 c	Croutons, low fat
½ muffin	English muffin
½ (1 oz)	Frankfurter or hamburger bun
½ loaf	Pita, 6 in. across
1 (1 oz)	Plain roll, small
1 slice (1 oz)	Raisin, unfrosted
1 slice (1 oz)	Rye, pumpernickel[a]
1 tortilla	Tortilla, 6 in. across
1 slice (1 oz)	White (including French, Italian)
1 slice (1 oz)	Whole wheat

[a]3 grams or more of dietary fiber per serving. Average fiber contents of whole-grain products is 2 grams per serving. For starchy foods not on this list, the general rule is that ½ cup of cereal grain, or pasta is one serving; 1 ounce of a bread product is one serving.
[b]400 mg or more of sodium per exchange. Meats contribute no fiber to the diet. Most vegetable servings contain 2 to 3 g of dietary fiber.

TABLE 18–2. The U.S. Exchange System (continued)

Amount	Food

Crackers/Snacks
8 crackers	Animal crackers
3 crackers	Graham crackers, 2½ in. square
¾ oz	Matzoth
5 slices	Melba toast
24 crackers	Oyster crackers
3 c	Popcorn (popped, no fat added)
¾ oz	Pretzels
4 crackers	Rye crisp, 2 in. × 3½ in.
6 crackers	Saltine-type crackers
2–4 slices (¾ oz)	Whole wheat crackers, no fat added (crisp breads)

Starchy Foods Prepared with Fat
(Count as 1 starch/bread serving, plus 1 fat serving.)
1 biscuit	Biscuit, 2½ in. across
½ c	Chow mein noodles
1 (2 oz)	Corn bread, 2 in. cube
6 crackers	Cracker, round butter type
10 (1½ oz)	French fried potatoes, 2 in. to 3½ in. long
1 muffin	Muffin, plain, small
2 pancakes	Pancake, 4 in. across
¼ c	Stuffing, bread (prepared)
2 tacos	Taco shell, 6 in. across
1 waffle	Waffle, 4½ in. square
4–6 crackers (1 oz)	Whole wheat crackers, fat added

Meat/Meat Alternate Lists (Lean meat = 7 g protein, 3 g fat, 55 kcal. Medium-fat meat = 7 g protein, 5 g fat, 75 kcal. High-fat meat = 7 g protein, 8 g fat, 100 kcal).

Lean Meat and Alternates
Beef:	1 oz	USDA Good or Choice grades of lean beef, such as round, sirloin, and flank steak; tenderloin; and chipped beef[b].
Pork:	1 oz	Lean pork, such as fresh ham; canned, cured, or boiled ham[b]; Canadian bacon[b], tenderloin.
Veal:	1 oz	All cuts are lean except for veal cutlets (ground or cubed). Examples of lean veal are chops and roasts.
Poultry:	1 oz	Chicken, turkey, Cornish hen (without skin)
Fish:	1 oz	All fresh and frozen fish
	2 oz	Crab, lobster, scallops, shrimp, clams (fresh or canned in water[b])
	6 medium	Oysters
	¼ c	Tuna[b] (canned in water)
	1 oz	Herring (uncreamed or smoked)
	2 medium	Sardines (canned)
Wild Game:	1 oz	Venison, rabbit, squirrel
	1 oz	Pheasant, duck, goose (without skin)
Cheese:	¼ c	Any cottage cheese
	2 tbsp	Grated parmesan
	1 oz	Diet cheeses[b] (with less than 55 kcalories per ounce)
Other:	1 oz	95% fat-free luncheon meat
	3 whites	Egg whites
	¼ c	Egg substitutes with less than 55 kcalories per ¼ cup

TABLE 18–2. The U.S. Exchange System (continued)

Medium-Fat Meat and Alternates

Beef:	1 oz	Most beef products fall into this category. Examples are: all ground beef, roast (rib, chuck, rump), steak (cubed, Porterhouse, T-bone), and meatloaf.
Pork:	1 oz	Most pork products fall into this category. Examples are: chops, loin roast, Boston butt, cutlets
Lamb:	1 oz	Most lamb products fall into this category. Examples are: chops, leg, and roast.
Veal:	1 oz	Cutlet (ground or cubed, unbreaded)
Poultry:	1 oz	Chicken (with skin), domestic duck or goose (well-drained of fat), ground turkey
Fish:	¼ c	Tuna[b] (canned in oil and drained)
	¼ c	Salmon[b] (canned)
Cheese:		Skim or part-skim milk cheeses, such as:
	¼ c	Ricotta
	1 oz	Mozzarella
	1 oz	Diet cheeses[b] (with 56–80 kcalories per ounce)
Other:	1 oz	86% fat-free luncheon meat[b]
	1	Egg (high in cholesterol, limit to 3 per week)
	¼ c	Egg substitutes with 56–80 kcalories per ¼ cup
	4 oz	Tofu (2 ½ in. × 2 ¾ in. × 1 in.)
	1 oz	Liver, heart, kidney, sweetbreads (high in cholesterol)

High-Fat Meat and Alternates

Beef:	1 oz	Most USDA Prime cuts of beef, such as ribs, corned beef[b]
Pork:	1 oz	Spareribs, ground pork, pork sausage[b] (patty or link)
Lamb:	1 oz	Patties (ground lamb)
Fish:	1 oz	Any fried fish product
Cheese:	1 oz	All regular cheeses[b], such as American, Blue, Cheddar, Monterey, Swiss
Other:	1 oz	Luncheon meat[b], such as bologna, salami, pimento loaf
	1 oz	Sausage[b], such as Polish, Italian
	1 oz	Knockwurst, smoked
	1 oz	Bratwurst[b]
	1 frank (10/lb)	Frankfurter[b] (turkey or chicken)
	1 tbsp	Peanut butter (contains unsaturated fat)

Count as one high-fat meat plus one fat exchange:

1 frank	(10/lb)	Frankfurter[b] (beef, pork, or combination)

Vegetable List (5 g carbohydrate, 2 g protein, 25 kcal) All portion sizes, except as otherwise noted, are ½ c of any cooked vegetable or vegetable juice, 1 c of any raw vegetable.

Artichoke (½ medium)	Mushrooms, cooked
Asparagus	Okra
Beans (green, wax, Italian)	Onions
Bean sprouts	Pea pods
Beets	Peppers (green)
Broccoli	Rutabaga
Brussels sprouts	Sauerkraut[b]
Cabbage, cooked	Spinach, cooked
Carrots	Summer squash (crookneck)
Cauliflower	Tomato (one large)

TABLE 18–2. The U.S. Exchange System (continued)

Vegetable List (continued)

Eggplant	Tomato/vegetable juice[b]
Greens (collard, mustard, turnip)	Turnips
Kohlrabi	Water chestnuts
Leeks	Zucchini, cooked

Starchy vegetables such as corn, peas, and potatoes are found on the Starch/Bread List. For free vegetables, see Free Food List.

Fruit List (15 g carbohydrate, 60 kcal)
All portion sizes, unless otherwise noted, are: ½ c of fresh fruit or fruit juice, ¼ c of dried fruit.

Amount	Food

Fresh, Frozen and Unsweetened Canned Fruit

Amount	Food
1 apple	Apple (raw, 2 in. across)
½ c	Applesauce (unsweetened)
4 apricots	Apricots (medium, raw) or
½ c, or 4 halves	Apricots (canned)
½ banana	Banana (9 in. long)
¾ c	Blackberries (raw)[c]
¾ c	Blueberries (raw)[c]
⅓ melon	Cantaloupe (5 in. across)
1 c	(cubes)
12 cherries	Cherries (large, raw)
½ c	Cherries (canned)
2 figs	Figs (raw, 2 in. across)
½ c	Fruit cocktail (canned)
½ grapefruit	Grapefruit (medium)
¾ c	Grapefruit (segments)
15 grapes	Grapes (small)
⅛ melon	Honeydew melon (medium)
1 cup	(cubes)
1 kiwi	Kiwi (large)
¾ c	Mandarin oranges
½ mango	Mango (small)
1 nectarine	Nectarine (1½ in. across)[c]
1 orange	Orange (2½ in. across)
1 c	Papaya
1 peach, or ¾ c	Peach (2¾ in. across)
½ c, or 2 halves	Peaches (canned)
½ large, or 1 small	Pear
½ c or 2 halves	Pears (canned)
2 persimmons	Persimmon (medium, native)
¾ c	Pineapple (raw)
⅓ c	Pineapple (canned)
2 plums	Plum (raw, 2 in. across)
½ pomegranate	Pomegranate[c]
1 c	Raspberries (raw)[c]
1¼ c	Strawberries (raw, whole)[c]
2 tangerines	Tangerine (2½ in. across)
1¼ c	Watermelon (cubes)

[c]3 or more grams of dietary fiber per serving. Average fiber contents of fresh, frozen, and dry fruits: 2 g per serving.

TABLE 18–2. The U.S. Exchange System (continued)

Dried Fruit
4 rings	Apples[c]
7 halves	Apricots[c]
2½ medium	Dates
1½ figs	Figs[c]
3 medium	Prunes[c]
2 tbsp	Raisins

Fruit Juice
½ c	Apple juice/cider
⅓ c	Cranberry juice cocktail
½ c	Grapefruit juice
⅓ c	Grape juice
½ c	Orange juice
½ c	Pineapple juice
⅓ c	Prune juice

Milk List (Nonfat and very lowfat milk = 12 g carbohydrate, 8 g protein, trace fat, 90 kcal. Lowfat milk = 12 g carbohydrate, 8 g protein, 5 g fat, 120 kcal. Whole milk = 12 g carbohydrate, 8 g protein, 8 g fat, 150 kcal.)

Amount	Food
1 c	Nonfat milk
1 c	½% milk
1 c	1% milk
1 c	Lowfat buttermilk
½ c	Evaporated nonfat milk
⅓ c	Dry nonfat milk
8 oz	Plain nonfat yogurt

Lowfat Milk
1 c fluid	2% milk
8 oz	Plain lowfat yogurt (with added nonfat milk solids)

Whole Milk
1 c	Whole milk
½ c	Evaporated whole milk
8 oz	Whole plain yogurt

Fat List (5 g fat, 45 kcal)

Amount	Food
⅛ medium	Avocado
1 tsp	Margarine
1 tbsp	Margarine, diet[d]
1 tsp	Mayonnaise
1 tbsp	Mayonnaise, reduced-kcalorie[d]

Unsaturated Fats

Nuts and Seeds:
6 whole	Almonds, dry roasted
1 tbsp	Cashews, dry roasted
2 whole	Pecans

[d]If more than one or two servings are eaten, these foods have 400 mg or more of sodium.

TABLE 18–2. The U.S. Exchange System (continued)

Unsaturated Fats (continued)

20 small or 10 large	Peanuts
2 whole	Walnuts
1 tbsp	Other nuts
1 tbsp	Seeds, pine nuts, sunflower (without shells)
2 tsp	Pumpkin seeds
1 tsp	Oil (corn, cottonseed, safflower, soybean, sunflower, olive, peanut)
10 small or 5 large	Olives[d]
2 tsp	Salad dressing, mayonnaise-type
1 tbsp	Salad dressing, mayonnaise-type, reduced-kcalorie
1 tbsp	Salad dressing (all varieties)[d]
2 tbsp	Salad dressing, reduced-kcalorie[d]

Saturated Fats

1 tsp	Butter
1 slice	Bacon[e]
½ oz	Chitterlings
2 tbsp	Coconut, shredded
2 tbsp	Coffee whitener, liquid
4 tsp	Coffee whitener, powder
2 tbsp	Cream (light, coffee, table)
2 tbsp	Cream, sour
1 tbsp	Cream (heavy, whipping)
1 tbsp	Cream cheese
¼ oz	Salt pork[e]

Free Foods (A free food is any food or drink that contains less than 20 kcalories per serving. People with diabetes are advised to eat as much as they want of those items that have no serving size specified. They may eat two or three servings per day of those items that have a specific serving size. It is suggested that they spread them out through the day.)

Drinks:

	Bouillon[e] or broth without fat
	Bouillon, low-sodium
	Carbonated drinks, sugar-free
	Carbonated water
	Club soda
1 tbsp	Cocoa powder, unsweetened
	Coffee/Tea
	Drink mixes, sugar-free
	Tonic water, sugar-free

Nonstick pan spray

Fruit:

½ c	Cranberries, unsweetened
½ c	Rhubarb, unsweetened

Note: Two tablespoons of low-kcalorie salad dressing is a free food.

[e]400 mg or more of sodium per serving.

TABLE 18–2. The U.S. Exchange System (continued)

Vegetables:		
(raw, 1 c)		
	Cabbage	
	Celery	
	Chinese cabbageᶠ	
	Cucumber	
	Green onion	
	Hot peppers	
	Mushrooms	
	Radishes	
	Zucchiniᶠ	
Salad greens:		
	Endive	
	Escarole	
	Lettuce	
	Romaine	
	Spinach	
Sweet substitutes:		
	Candy, hard, sugar-free	
	Gelatin, sugar-free	
	Gum, sugar-free	
2 tsp	Jam/Jelly, sugar-free	
1–2 tbsp	Pancake syrup, sugar-free	
	Sugar substitutes (saccharin, aspartame)	
2 tbsp	Whipped topping	
Condiments:		
1 tbsp	Catsup	
	Horseradish	
	Mustard	
	Picklesᵉ, dill, unsweetened	
2 tbsp	Salad dressing, low-kcalorie	
1 tbsp	Taco sauce	
	Vinegar	
Seasonings:		
	Basil (fresh)	
	Celery seeds	
	Cinnamon	
	Chili powder	
	Chives	
	Curry	
	Dill	
	Flavoring extracts (vanilla, almond, walnut, peppermint, butter, lemon, etc.)	
	Garlic	
	Garlic powder	
	Herbs	
	Hot pepper sauce	
	Lemon	
	Lemon juice	
	Lemon pepper	
	Lime	
	Lime juice	
	Mint	
	Onion powder	

ᶠ3 or more grams of fiber per serving.

TABLE 18–2. The U.S. Exchange System (continued)

Seasonings (continued)

	Onion powder
	Oregano
	Paprika
	Pepper
	Pimento
	Spices
	Soy sauce[e]
	Soy sauce, low sodium ("lite")
¼ c	Wine, used in cooking
	Worcestershire sauce

Combination Foods (Much of the food we eat is mixed together in various combinations. These combination foods do not fit into only one exchange list. It can be quite hard to tell what is in a certain casserole dish or baked food item. This is a list of average values for some typical combination foods. This list will help you fit these foods into your meal plan. Ask your dietitian for information about any other foods you'd like to eat. The *American Diabetes Association/American Dietetic Association Family Cookbooks* and the *American Diabetes Association Holiday Cookbook* have many recipes and further information about many foods, including combination foods. Check your library or local bookstore.)

Food	Amount	Exchanges
Casseroles	1 c (8 oz)	2 starch, 2 medium-fat meat, 1 fat
Cheese pizza[e], thin crust	¼ of 15 oz, or ¼ of 10″	2 starch, 1 medium-fat meat, 1 fat
Chili with beans[ef] (commercial)	1 c (8 oz)	2 starch, 2 medium fat-meat, 2 fat
Chow mein[ef] (without noodles or rice)	2 c (16 oz)	1 starch, 2 vegetable, 2 lean meat
Macaroni and cheese[e]	1 c (8 oz)	2 starch, 1 medium-fat meat, 2 fat
Soup:		
Bean[ef]	1 c (8 oz)	1 starch, 1 vegetable, 1 lean meat
Chunky, all varieties[e];	10 ¾ oz can	1 starch, 1 vegetable, 1 medium-fat meat
Cream[e] (made with water)	1 c (8 oz)	1 starch, 1 fat
Vegetable[e] or broth[e]	1 c (8 oz)	1 starch
Spaghetti and meatballs[e] (canned)	1 c (8 oz)	2 starch, 1 medium-fat meat, 1 fat
Sugar-free pudding (made with nonfat milk)	½ c	1 starch
If beans are used as a meat substitute:		
Dried beans[f], peas[f], lentils[f]	1 c (cooked)	2 starch, 1 lean meat

TABLE 18–2. The U.S. Exchange System (continued)

Foods for Occasional Use Food	Amount	Exchanges
Angel food cake	1/12 cake	2 starch
Cake, no icing	1/12 cake, or a 3″ square	2 starch, 2 fat
Cookies	2 small (1 ¾″) across)	1 starch, 1 fat
Frozen fruit yogurt	⅓ c	1 starch
Gingersnaps	3 cookies	1 starch
Granola	¼ c	1 starch, 1 fat
Granola bars	1 small	1 starch, 1 fat
Ice cream, any flavor	½ c	1 starch, 2 fat
Ice milk, any flavor	½ c	1 starch, 1 fat
Sherbet, any flavor	¼ c	1 starch
Snack chips⁹, all varieties	1 oz	1 starch, 2 fat
Vanilla wafers	6 small	1 starch, 1 fat

⁹If more than one serving is eaten, these foods have 400 mg or more of sodium.

Source: The Exchange Lists are the basis of a meal planning system designed by a committee of the American Diabetes Association and the American Dietetic Association. While designed primarily for people with diabetes and others who must follow special diets, the Exchange Lists are based on principles of good nutrition that apply to everyone. © 1986 American Diabetes Association, Inc., American Dietetic Association.

By comparing the person's actual weight to her ideal weight you can determine whether or not she needs a weight-loss or a weight-maintenance diet. For the person in our example (IBW 120 pounds), a weight loss diet is in order.

2. *Estimate energy needs.* For a weight-loss diet, multiply the current body weight by 10 kcalories per pound to determine the total kcalories for the day.[1] The person in our example would be allowed 1,400 kcalories per day.

$$140 \text{ lbs} \times 10 \text{ kcal/lb} = 1,400 \text{ kcal}$$

You can estimate energy needs for maintaining IBW by multiplying the IBW by 10 to get the basal energy requirement. Add kcalories for activity: For sedentary people, add 30 percent; for moderately active people, add 50 percent; for people who engage in strenuous activity, add 100 percent. Children under 12 require about 1,000 kcal plus 100 kcal per year of age.

3. *Determine the grams of protein, carbohydrate, and fat to be included in the meal plan.*
A good balance for your diet would be:

- 12–20 percent of kcalories from protein.
- 50–60 percent of kcalories from carbohydrate.
- 30 percent of kcalories from fat.

TABLE 18–3. A Balanced 1,400 kCalorie Diet[a]

Exchange Item	Number of Exchanges	Carbohydrate (g)	Protein (g)	Fat (g)	kCalories
Starch/bread	5	75	15	—	400
Meat (lean)	5	—	35	15	275
Vegetable	3	15	6	—	75
Fruit	4	60	—	—	240
Milk (nonfat)	2	24	16	—	180
Fat	5	—	—	25	225
		174	72	40	1,395

[a]This diet supplies about 50% of the kcalories as carbohydrate, 21% of the kcalories as protein, and 26% of the kcalories as fat. The percentages do not add up to 100%, because the kcalorie values used in the exchange system are approximations.

In gram amounts, this balance works out to:

- 42–70 grams protein.
- 175–210 grams carbohydrate.
- 47 grams fat.

Protein should not fall short of the RDA, and you should leave enough fat in the diet to provide satiety. Carbohydrate-containing foods consisting of complex carbohydrates also help you feel fuller at a lower kcalorie cost.

4. *Translate the diet prescription into a meal pattern.* Start by allotting milk, vegetable, fruit, and bread portions, because these four types of foods have to deliver all the carbohydrate you have planned.

5. *Once you have arrived at about the number of grams of carbohydrate you want from these four lists, subtotal the protein they contain to see how much more protein you'll need.* The meat list is the only remaining list that offers protein, so enter a number of meat exchanges that will supply this much protein.

6. *Now subtotal the fat you have so far and enter a number of fat exchanges to round off the diet's total fat to the amount you want.* As a double check, add up the kcalories these exchanges contain; the total should approximate the number you wanted to plan. Table 18–3 shows a pattern you might arrive at for a 1,400 kcalorie weight-loss diet. Table 18–4 shows diet patterns for different kcalorie levels.

Weight: How Much Is Too Much?

It isn't always possible to tell from the bathroom scale if a person is overweight, because body weight says nothing about body fat. An Olympic weight lifter may weigh far more than his "ideal weight" although his body may contain an

ideal weight:
a misnomer; not the desirable but the average weight given in insurance tables for persons of a given sex and height—not necessarily ideal for a given individual.

TABLE 18–4. Diet Patterns for Different kCalorie Levels[a]

Exchange Item	Energy Level (kcal)					
	1,000	1,200	1,500	1,800	2,000	2,200
Starch/Bread	3	4	6	8	10	11
Meat	4	5	5	5	6	6
Vegetable	2	3	4	4	4	6
Fruit	3	3	4	5	5	5
Milk	2	2	2	2	2	2
Fat	3	4	5	7	7	8

[a]These patterns of exchanges supply about 30% of the kcalories as fat in accordance with the view that a moderate fat intake is desirable.

average or less than average amount of fat. A more complete discussion of body weight, including shortcut tips for assessing body fat appears in Chapter 9. Chapter 13 and Appendix B describe clinical methods for assessing body fat.

Even so, scales with the weight tables are the most common tools used to assess body fatness. Here's how they work. After weighing yourself, you turn to the tables published by the insurance companies (see inside back cover). You then discover that for a person of your height and sex, three weight ranges are suggested: One for a small frame, one for medium frame, and one for large frame (see inside back cover). Don't forget your shoes: You are assumed to be wearing one-inch heels. Thus, a person who stands 5 feet 10 inches tall in bare feet would look up the range for a person 5 feet 11 inches. Finally, if you weigh yourself nude, you must adjust for clothing, because the tables assume five pounds of clothes for men, three pounds for women. A person who is more than 10 percent above the weight on the table is considered overweight; if 20 percent or more, a person is considered obese. (Some authorities say that a body weight 15 percent above the table weight constitutes obesity; some say 25 percent.) Similarly, a person who is more than 10 percent below the table weight is considered underweight.

Obviously, many problems exist with defining ideal weight. Rather than consider weight loss successful when one attains an ideal weight, one author suggests that successful weight loss be defined as a loss of 10 to 15 percent of body weight over a 6 to 18 month period.[2] By using this approach, weight loss goals can be reevaluated regularly, and the person and the health care team can better determine when an appropriate weight is attained.

The Need for Weight Reduction

Obesity is a major malnutrition problem in developed countries. Insurance companies report that fat people die younger from a host of causes, including heart attacks, strokes, and complications of diabetes. In fact, gaining weight often appears to precipitate the major type of diabetes. Obese people more often suffer high levels of blood fat, hypertension, coronary heart disease,

frame size:
the size of a person's bones and musculature. A person with a large frame should weigh more than a person the same height with a small frame.

overweight:
body weight more than 10 percent above the average (insurance company table) weight.

obesity:
excessive body fatness; often loosely defined as a condition of being overweight by 20 percent or more.

underweight:
body weight more than 10 percent below normal or average weight.

postsurgical complications, gynecological irregularities, and pregnancy-induced hypertension. For men, the risk of cancers of the colon, rectum, and prostate gland rises with obesity; for women, the risk of cancers of the breast, uterus, ovaries, gallbladder, and bile ducts is greater. The burden of extra fat strains the skeletal system, aggravating arthritis especially in the knees, hips, and lower spine. The muscles that support the belly may give way, resulting in abdominal hernias. When leg muscles are abnormally fatty, they fail to contract efficiently to help blood return from the leg veins to the heart; blood collects in the leg veins, which swell, harden, and become varicose. Extra fat in and around the chest interferes with breathing, sometimes causing severe respiratory problems. Gout is more common, and even the accident rate is greater for the severely obese.

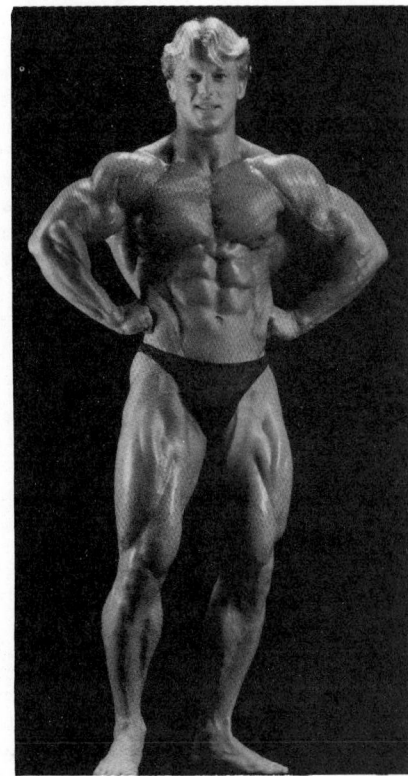

It is not how much one weighs but the proportion of the weight contributed by lean body mass that makes a difference.

Dr.'s Order:

Weight reduction diet.

Social and economic disadvantages also plague the fat person. Obese people are less often sought after for marriage, pay higher insurance premiums, meet discrimination when applying for college admissions and jobs, can't find attractive clothes easily, and are limited in their choice of sports.

It is important to realize that diet is only one part of a successful weight reduction program. To lose weight is a difficult and demanding task. It seems that the only realistic and sensible way for the obese person to achieve and maintain ideal weight is to cut kcalories, to increase activity, and to maintain this changed lifestyle to the end of his life. This is a tall order. Fewer than a third of the people who lose weight manage to keep it off in the long run. To succeed means modifying all the attitudes and behaviors that have contributed to the problem in the first place, sometimes against internal and external pressures that can't be changed. Still, it can be and has been done successfully, as many former fat people can attest. Such people usually attribute their success to a three-pronged approach: Diet, exercise, and behavior modification.

The diet plan most frequently used by dietitians to translate a low-kcalorie diet order into actual foods is the exchange list system. However, many other weight reduction diets are in use. Some are adequate, others are not. Table 18–5 compares various diets and suggests ways for you to evaluate diets. Inappropriate ways of treating obesity are listed in the Miniglossary of Poor Treatment Choices for Obesity.

Dieters are frequently tempted by diet products and diets that promise rapid weight loss. Repeated fad dieting and regaining weight makes each pound of weight loss harder to achieve. Weight—including lean tissue—is lost, and fat is gained, which slows metabolism. Then weight is lost with greater difficulty, again including lean tissue, and fat is again gained, further slowing metabolism. At the end of each round of dieting, kcalorie needs are less, weight zooms higher, and fat is harder to lose the next time—the so-called ratchet or yoyo effect. The only way to lose weight successfully and keep it off is to adopt a balanced low-kcalorie diet, such as the exchange diet demonstrated here, lose weight gradually, and exercise to retain or build lean tissue and support normal metabolism. Chapter 9 provides additional information about the ratchet effect.

yoyo effect:
another term for the ratchet effect. See Chapter 9.

TABLE 18–5. Weight-Loss Diets Compared

With a balanced perspective on foods and a sense of what's important in diet planning and what's not, you can evaluate the many different diets people consume. Here's a summary of the questions you might ask. Start with 100 points, and subtract if any of these criteria are not met:

1. Does the diet provide a reasonable number of kcalories (enough to maintain weight; not too many; and if a reduction diet, not fewer than 1,200 kcal for the average-sized person)? If not, give it a **minus 10**.
2. Does it provide enough, but not too much, protein (at least the recommended intake or RDA, but not more than twice that much)? If not, **minus 10**.
3. Does it provide enough fat for satiety, but not so much fat as to go against current recommendations (say, between 20 and 35% of the kcalories from fat)? If not, **minus 10**.
4. Does it provide enough carbohydrate to spare protein and prevent ketosis (100 g of carbohydrate for the average-sized person)? Is it mostly complex carbohydrate (not more than 20% of the kcalories as concentrated sugar)? If no to either, **minus 5**; if no to both, **minus 10**.

Diet Description	Question 1: kCalories	Question 2: Protein
A low-carbohydrate/high-protein diet that allows unlimited protein and fat, but severely limits carbohydrate. In addition to the hazards of a low-carbohydrate diet, explained in Chapter 6, the diet is high in total fat, saturated fat, and cholesterol. The omission of breads and cereals and the large reduction of fruits, vegetables, and milk characterize the diet.	Yes	No, excessive protein MINUS 10
A diet of six bananas and three glasses of nonfat milk daily, plus vitamin and mineral supplements.	No, provides less than 1,000 kcal MINUS 10	No, low protein MINUS 10
A diet that allows, for the first ten days, no food other than specific fruits. Timing and combining of foods are claimed to cause weight loss, with no scientific basis for the claims. Sometimes causes diarrhea and excess gas in the digestive tract because of the laxative nature of fruit. Physicians warn that shock, low blood pressure, and perhaps death may result.	No, low in kcalories MINUS 10	No, low protein MINUS 10
The plan is a two-weeks-on, two-weeks-off low-carbohydrate, ample-protein diet of about 1100 kcal/day, touted as a no-hunger, no-pills way to lose 20 lb in two weeks. It includes plenty of meat, vegetables, fruits, and some starches, but no milk.	Yes	No, provides approximately 216% of the protein needs MINUS 10
A powdered formula sold directly to the public for use three times daily. One day's worth of the formula provides 33 g protein, 40 g carbohydrate, and 3 g fat, fortified with vitamins and minerals.	No MINUS 10	No, low protein MINUS 10
A fast in which only water is allowed.	No MINUS 10	No MINUS 10
A diet that requires the addition of 2 tsp of bran to be taken with water at each mealtime. The foods provided by the menus are low-fat, low-kcalorie items, with few milk products.	Yes	Yes
A strict diet built around the Four Food Group Plan, which alternates periods of 700 kcal/day and 1500 kcal/day.	The average intake is 1100 kcal/day, but periods of severe restriction are included MINUS 5	Yes

5. Does it offer a balanced assortment of vitamins and minerals from whole food sources in all four food groups (see Chapter 1)? If a food group is omitted (for example, meats), is a suitable substitute provided? The four food groups are milk/milk products; meat/fish/poultry/eggs/legumes; fruits/vegetables; and grains. For *each* food group omitted and not adequately substituted for, **minus 10**.
6. Does it offer variety, in the sense that different foods can be selected each day? If you'd class it as "monotonous," give it a **minus 10**.
7. Does it consist of ordinary foods that are available locally (for example, in the main grocery stores) at the prices people normally pay? Or does the dieter have to buy special, expensive, or unusual foods to adhere to the diet? If you'd class it as "bizarre" or "requiring unusual foods," **minus 10**.

Question 3: Fat	Question 4: Carbohydrate	Question 5: Food Groups	Question 6: Variety	Question 7: Ordinary Foods	Total Score
No, excessive fat MINUS 10	No, inadequate carbohydrate MINUS 10	No, three food groups omitted MINUS 30	No, monotonous MINUS 10	Yes	30 points
No, low fat MINUS 10	Yes	No, three food groups omitted MINUS 30	No, monotonous MINUS 10	Yes	30 points
No, low fat MINUS 10	No, no starch MINUS 10	No, four food groups omitted MINUS 40	No, monotonous; omits most food groups other than fruits MINUS 10	No, requires tropical fruits in large quantities and later suggests lobster and steak MINUS 10	0 points
No, meat has a high fat percentage MINUS 10	No, carbohydrate level is 30% of need MINUS 5	No, milk group omitted MINUS 10	Yes	Yes	65 points
No, low fat MINUS 10	No, low carbohydrate MINUS 10	No food allowed on a regular basis MINUS 40	No, monotonous MINUS 10	No ordinary food; expensive formula required MINUS 10	0 points
No MINUS 10	No MINUS 10	No MINUS 40	No MINUS 10	No MINUS 10	0 points
Yes	Yes	Half the milk allowance MINUS 5	Yes	Requires bran MINUS 5	90 points
Yes	Yes	Yes	Yes	Yes	95 points

TABLE 18–5. Weight-Loss Diets Compared (continued)

Diet Description	Question 1: kCalories	Question 2: Protein
A diet that involves eating only rice and fruit. Vitamin and mineral supplements are recommended.	Yes	No, low protein MINUS 10
A very low carbohydrate, high-fat, high-meat, very-low-kcalorie diet with no milk. One-half grapefruit is required before each meal.	No MINUS 10	No, too high MINUS 10
A diet that severely restricts fat, limits protein to below the recommended levels, and limits dairy products severely. Several levels of kcalories are available from 700 to 1200 per day.	Choosing any plan except 1,200 kcal will not provide the recommended level MINUS 5	No, too low MINUS 10
A diet that uses the exchange system to ensure adequate nutrient intake, while emphasizing complex carbohydrate foods.	Yes	Yes
A diet that alternates 600, 900, and 1200 kcal/day intakes (higher for men) in the first three weeks, then allows moderate intakes for a week, and starts over. It also includes unlimited quantities of selected fruits and vegetables.	Two weeks of severe kcalorie restriction is ill advised MINUS 5	Not likely to have sufficient protein, especially in view of carbohydrate restriction MINUS 5
A high-carbohydrate, low-protein diet that allows no meats or milk products.		No, too low MINUS 10
A diet of powdered herbs or other powders to replace food for one meal a day.	Likely to be inadequate MINUS 10	Depends on how much consumed from food in other meals

Causes of Obesity

Energy is not stored in fat until the body's energy needs have been met. Excess body fat can accumulate only when kcalories are eaten beyond those needed for the day's metabolic, muscular, and digestive activities. Obesity, then, results from eating more than the body needs for its daily activities.

Question 3: Fat	Question 4: Carbohydrate	Question 5: Food Groups	Question 6: Variety	Question 7: Ordinary Foods	Total Score
No, low fat MINUS 10	Yes	No meat, milk, or vegetables allowed MINUS 30	No, monotonous MINUS 10	Yes	40 points
Yes, but so low in kcalories that total fat is low MINUS 10	No, too low MINUS 10	No milk or grains allowed MINUS 20	No, monotonous MINUS 10	Yes	30 points
No, too low MINUS 10	Yes	No, meat and milk groups restricted MINUS 5 MINUS 5	Yes	No, dieters are urged to use special products MINUS 10	55 points
Yes	Yes	Yes	Yes	Yes	100 points
No, too little fat, half the time MINUS 5	No, too little carbohydrate, half the time MINUS 5	No, insufficient milk likely, half the time MINUS 5	Yes	Yes	75 points
No MINUS 10	Yes	No, meat and milk omitted MINUS 20	No, monotonous MINUS 10	Yes	50 points
Likely to be inadequate MINUS 10	Likely to be inadequate MINUS 10	One or more likely to be omitted MINUS 10	No, monotonous MINUS 10	No, dangerous; herbs can be toxic and cause adverse reactions MINUS 10	40 points or less; if meals are omitted and only the powder is taken, score the diet 0 points

But why do people overeat? Is it a hunger problem? An appetite problem? A satiety problem? Is it genetic? Metabolic? Environmental? Is it a matter of habits learned in early childhood? Is it psychological? Might all these factors play a role? To tell the truth, we do not know the cause.

In general, two schools of thought address this problem. One attributes it to inside-the-body causes, the other to environmental factors. One currently

Miniglossary of Poor Treatment Choices for Obesity

diet pills   pills that depress the appetite temporarily; often, physician-prescribed amphetamines (speed). It is generally agreed that these drugs are of little value for weight loss and that their use can cause a dangerous dependency.

fad diets   diets designed to bring about quick weight loss that are usually unbalanced nutritionally and are sometimes dangerous.

gastric stapling   a type of surgery that involves stapling the stomach to make it smaller. Its effectiveness is limited; many obese peole manage to eat enough high-kcalorie foods with small bulk to stay fat, and the procedure can have serious side effects.

glucomannan (glue-co-MAN-an)   a preparation derived from a vegetable (konjac tuber) used in Japanese cooking. In a controlled experiment reported in 1982, glucomannan was ineffective in controlling weight.[3]

HCG or human chorionic gonadotropin (core-ee-ON-ic go-nad-o-TROPE-in):   a hormone excreted in the urine of pregnant women believed to enhance weight loss and reduce hunger. It does neither.

intestinal bypass surgery: surgery that involves removing or disconnecting a portion of the small intestine to reduce absorption of energy nutrients. It has severe side effects, including liver failure and deranged fluid and electrolyte balance. Gastric stapling is preferred, but both are recommended only as a last resort for otherwise healthy people under 30 who weigh more than 300 pounds and who have tried everything else.

starch blockers   products derived from kidney beans that are incorrectly credited with blocking starch digestion in humans. They were banned by the FDA when they were found to cause nausea, diarrhea, and stomach pains, and not to block starch digestion.

water pills   diuretics that promote the excretion of water from the body. The water loss results in some weight loss, but this loss can be dangerous, because the overfat subject has a smaller percentage of body water than a person of normal weight. Dehydration can result from the use of water pills.

Several terms related to eating include hunger, appetite, and satiety. The distinctions among these terms are as follows:

hunger:
the physiological need to eat; a negative, unpleasant sensation.

appetite:
the desire to eat, which normally accompanies hunger; by itself a pleasant sensation.

satiety (sat-EYE-uh-tee):
the feeling of fullness or satisfaction at the end of a meal that prompts a person to stop eating.

popular inside-the-body theory is the so-called set-point theory. Noting that many people who lose weight on reducing diets subsequently return to their original weight, some researchers have suggested that the body "wants" to maintain a certain amount of fat and regulates eating behaviors and hormonal actions to defend its "set point" (see Chapter 9).

The other point of view is that obesity is environmentally determined. Proponents of this view hold that we overeat because we are pushed to do so by factors in our surroundings—foremost among them, the availability of a multitude of delectable foods. The two views are not mutually exclusive, and research with animals suggests that both are possible. Some obesity may arise from one cause and some from the other, and there is no reason why they should not both be operating in the same person.

One way to approach the question of what causes obesity is to ask whether it is hereditary. One way to study this question in human beings is to study twins who have been raised by different families. If genes determine fatness, both twins will be equally fat or thin. But if the environment is responsible, each twin will resemble the family he or she grows up in. Another approach is to study adopted children to see whether they resemble their natural or adoptive parents. Studies of both approaches suggest that the tendency to obesity is inherited but that the environment is influential in the sense that it can prevent or permit the development of obesity when the potential is there.

Do fat babies become fat adults? Ten years ago, most nutrition experts might have answered yes (probably). Today, however, the results of several studies in which people have been followed from infancy to adulthood have suggested the answer to be *not necessarily;* some do, some don't. There is a greater chance, however, that the child will remain obese in families where the parents and grandparents are obese.[4]

Many researchers have the impression that early food habits exert a powerful influence on lifelong tendencies to overeat. Food-centered families encourage such behaviors as overeating at mealtimes, rapid eating, excessive snacking, and eating to meet needs other than hunger.

The possible causes of obesity mentioned so far all relate to the input side of the energy equation. What about output? A person may be obese because he eats too much, but another possibility is that he spends too little energy. It is probable that the most important single contributor to the obesity problem in our country is underactivity.

No two people are alike either physically or psychologically, and the causes of obesity may be as varied as the people who are obese. Many causes may contribute to the problem in just one person. Given this complexity, it is obvious that there is no panacea. The top priority should be prevention, but where prevention has failed, the treatment of obesity must involve a simultaneous attack on many fronts.

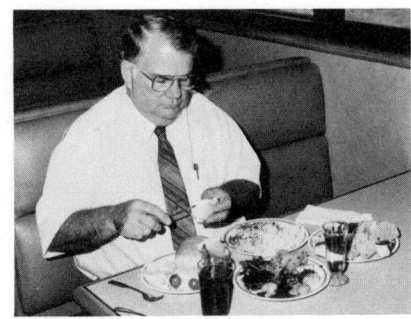

Successful dieting requires modifying the diet, attitudes, and behaviors that contributed to the overweight.

Strategies for Weight Loss

To heighten the sense of individuality, we wrote the following sections in terms of advice to "you." We intend to give you the illusion of listening in on a conversation in which an obese person is being competently counseled by someone familiar with the techniques known to be effective. Notes in the margin highlight the principles involved.

No particular diet is magical, and no particular food must be either included or avoided. Since you are the one who will have to live with the diet, you will need to be involved in its planning. Don't think of it as a diet you are going *on* because then you might be tempted to go *off* the diet once you have lost some weight. The diet can be called successful only if the pounds do not return. Think of it as an eating plan that you will adopt for life. It must consist of foods that you like, that are available to you, and that are within your means.

Choose a kcalorie level you can live with. There is not much point in hurrying, because you will never go *off* this eating plan, and nutritional adequacy can't be achieved on fewer than about 1,400 kcalories—1,200 at the very least. Remember as a rule of thumb to multiply your weight by 10 to find a desirable kcalorie level while losing weight.

Diet Counseling Principles
Diet with the intention of maintaining lost weight.

Be an active participant in the planning process.

Adopt a realistic plan.

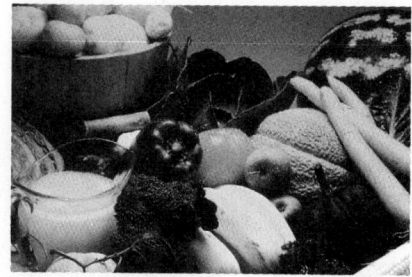

Emphasize nutrient-dense foods.

Plan a nutritionally adequate diet.

Eat at least three regular meals a day.

Save favorite foods for times when you are hungry.

Keep food records.

Weigh weekly or once every two weeks.

Anticipate a plateau.

This recommendation probably doesn't apply to people who are morbidly obese (twice their ideal body weights). Such individuals may need to lose weight more quickly, because they are at high risk for serious medical problems or may already have serious medical problems.

Because you will be eating less food, it is important to select foods of high nutrient density. Put diet adequacy on the list of your priorities. Choose unrefined, complex carbohydrates in place of simple sugars. Use fats cautiously—a slip of the butterknife can add many extra kcalories over the day's allotment. Finally, give up alcohol until you reach your goal weight. If you include alcohol in your diet plan, limit it strictly to no more than 150 kcalories/day. Table 18–6 shows the kcalories in different alcoholic beverages.

Some other tips can help you stay with your plan:

• Eat regularly, and if possible, eat before you are very hungry.

• Save favorite foods or beverages for the end of the day, in case you become hungry once again.

• Keep a record of what you eat each day for at least a week or two until your habits become automatic.

• Weigh yourself only once every week or two and always on the same scale, so that you can clearly see the progress you are making.

• Remember that many dieters reach a temporary plateau after about three weeks of dieting, even if they are strictly following their diets. This is water weight that is gained temporarily while the body is still losing fat. The fat you are hoping to lose must be combined with oxygen (oxidized) to make carbon dioxide and water if it is to leave the body. The oxygen you breathe in combines with the carbons of the fat to make carbon dioxide and with the hydrogens to make water. The carbon dioxide will be breathed out quickly, but the water stays in the body for a longer time. It must work its way into the bloodstream before it can be excreted. While water is making its way into the blood, you have a weight gain, because the water weighs more than the fat that was oxidized. If you faithfully follow your diet plan, one day the plateau will break. You can tell from your frequent urination.

TABLE 18–6. kCalorie Values of Alcoholic Beverages and Mixers

Beverage	Amount (oz)	Energy (kcal)
Beer	12	150
Gin, rum, vodka, whiskey (86 proof)	1½	105
Dessert wine	3½	140
Table wine	3½	85
Tonic, ginger ale, other sweetened carbonated waters	8	80
Cola, root beer	8	100
Fruit-flavored soda, Tom Collins mix	8	115
Club soda, diet drinks	8	1

Note: 100 proof means 50% alcohol; 86 proof means 43%. One oz is 28 g.
One g alcohol = 7 kcal.

- Avoid situations that prompt you to eat. For example, don't do your grocery shopping when you are hungry.

- After losing 20 to 30 pounds, expect to reach a stable plateau. Take this as a good sign. It means you have lost so much weight that you now require fewer kcalories to maintain your weight. Take a deep breath. You knew this was coming and you are courageous; therefore, institute a change. Increase your activity, cut your kcalories further, or both.

- If you slip, don't punish yourself. Go back to your plan and begin again right away.

- If you stop losing weight or gain unexpectedly, get tough on yourself. Check portion sizes. Write down everything you are eating and look at your record closely. Very seldom does an unpredicted weight plateau of any duration have no explanation in the dieter's own choices.

Control external cues.

Use positive reinforcement. Never blame, never punish.

Identify problems and correct them. Check portion sizes.

Finally, if you stop losing weight or begin to gain, be aware that you may be choosing to do so. Your weight is under your control, and you are entirely free to gain if you wish. You may find you are choosing to take a break, to go into a holding pattern, and to get adjusted before going on. Rather than letting yourself suffer from guilt feelings and feelings of failure, hold your head high and take the attitude, "This is me, and this is the way I am choosing to be right now."

Take personal responsibility for your diet.

Exercise

The importance of exercise in a weight loss program was thoroughly discussed in Chapter 9. The health advantages of regular exercise are well documented. Exercise can help speed weight loss and can help you look, feel, and be healthier.

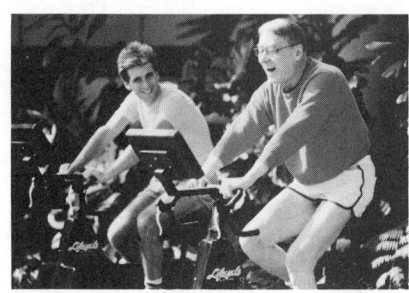

Enjoy exercise as a part of your weight loss strategy.

A conversation overheard in the cafeteria went like this:

Ms A: I'm jogging half an hour every day to lose weight.

Ms B: That's an awfully hard way to lose weight. Half an hour of jogging for someone your size would spend only 150 kcalories. I'd rather leave off a glass of milk every day, myself.

Ms B is right about the kcalories, but she doesn't know the *other* advantages of jogging, and her choice would be wrong. If Ms A keeps up her routine, her body will gradually change. She'll develop more lean tissue so that even her basal metabolic rate *at rest* will be faster. That means she'll burn more kcalories all day and night, not just during exercise. She'll have a higher kcalorie need, so she'll be able to drink that glass of milk (and more besides), obtaining all the nutrients it offers. Also, her muscles will become conditioned, so that she'll be able to jog longer or faster and spend *more* energy. Meanwhile, Ms B will be losing lean body mass as she sits around getting into poorer and poorer shape. Ms B will also be losing out on the nutrients she needs from foods she can't afford to eat. Let's hope Ms A knows enough to defend her choice to Ms B and perhaps even to persuade Ms B to join her on her daily run.

Behavior Modification

People who overeat often need to change their eating behavior—a part of their lives that most are only faintly aware of. How often do they put down their forks (if at all)? How often do they interrupt their eating to converse with a friend? How fast do they chew their food? Do they always clean their plates?

Books and pamphlets on behavior modification techniques abound, but it is beyond the scope of this book to list the techniques in detail. Examples of some suggestions you can make are described briefly:

- Learn to eat slowly. Give your body a chance to recognize that it's full. The satiety signal indicating that you have had enough to eat is sent after a 20-minute lag.

- Join a group, such as TOPS (Take Off Pounds Sensibly), Weight Watchers, or Overeaters Anonymous (OA). The support of people who understand is invaluable.

- Record for a while the circumstances surrounding your eating—the time, the place, the person you are with, the emotions you have at the time, the physical sensations, and other things. An example of such a record is shown in Form 13–4. Looking back, you can see what stimulates you to eat, and you can learn to control these stimuli. You may find that you are indeed eating for the "wrong" reasons—for example, boredom. You can begin to make rules for yourself, such as "Never eat when you're bored."

- If you are especially sensitive to pressure from your family or friends or hosts (you can't say no), get some assertiveness training. Learning not to clean your plate might be one of your first objectives.

From all the behavior changes available to you, you can choose the ones to begin with. Don't try to master them all at once. No one who attempts too many changes at one time is successful. Set your own priorities. Pick one trouble area that you think you can handle. Start with that and practice your strategy until it is habitual and automatic. Then you can select another trouble area to work on.

Enjoy your new, emerging self. Inside of every fat person is a thin person struggling to be freed. Get in touch with—reach out your hand to—your thin self, and help that self feel welcome in the light of day.

Weight Maintenance

As mentioned earlier, it is harder to maintain weight than it is to lose weight. People who lose weight often regain all that they have lost—and more. Paradoxically, those who lose the most, more than 40 pounds, have the greatest tendency to zoom up to levels above their starting points. On arriving at the goal weight after months of self-discipline and new habit formation, the victorious weight loser must at all costs avoid "celebrating" by resuming old eating habits. Buy a new outfit instead. The pounds are gone forever—remember? Membership in an ongoing weight-control organization, such as

OA or Weight Watchers, and continued participation in regular sports or other physical activity can provide indispensable support for the formerly fat person who wants to remain trim.

Obese Young Woman

Allison is a 24-year-old individual of medium frame who weighs 185 pounds and is 5 feet 4 inches tall. She has been obese since her early teen years and has tried dieting unsuccessfully many times. Allison works as a telephone operator. She enjoys needlework and is an avid moviegoer. Although Allison has a few friends, she is frequently lonely. She wants to get out and socialize more often, but she feels awkward about her weight. Allison states that she has tried "every diet in the book." Now she has come to you for help.

1. Using the tables on the inside back cover, estimate Allison's appropriate body weight. What percent is her ideal body weight?

2. Plan a diet for Allison at her current weight. (In real life, you would be helping her plan this diet.) How many kcalories and how much carbohydrate, protein, and fat will you recommend? What tips can you give Allison to help her with her diet?

3. What important concept must Allison understand if she is to maintain her weight?

Notes

1. American Dietetic Association, As cited in M. Hudnall, Dieting goal: 10 calories per pound of weight, *Environmental Nutrition* 10, July 1987, p. 2.
2. G. L. Blackburn, As cited in The primary goal in weight loss change, *Nutrition and the M.D.* 14, April 1988, p. 7.
3. L. Sanders, But do they work? *Health,* September 1982, pp. 29, 52, 62.
4. S. M. Garn and M. LaVelle, Two-decade follow-up of fatness in early childhood, *American Journal of Diseases of Children* 139 (1985): 620–624.

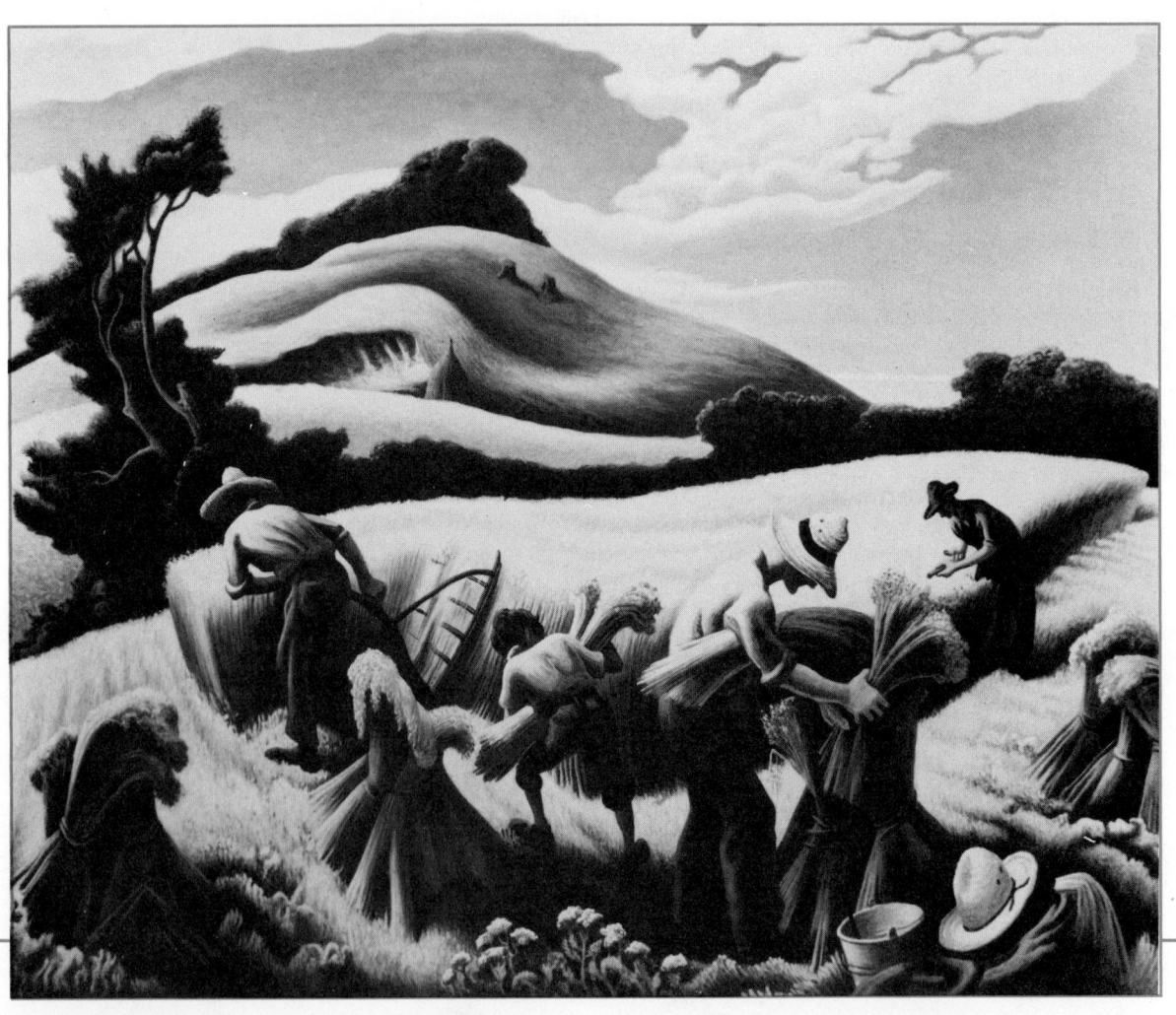

19

Diets Modified in Carbohydrates

DIETS DISCUSSED
Carbohydrate-Controlled Diets
Diets Restricted in Simple Carbohydrate
Lactose-Restricted Diets
Galactose-Restricted Diets

Case Study: Child with Type I Diabetes
Nutrition in Practice: Sugar Substitutes

CONDITIONS DISCUSSED
Diabetes Mellitus
Hypoglyemia
Dumping Syndrome
Lactose Intolerance
Galactosemia

Cradling Wheat by Thomas Hart Benton, 1938. American, 1889–
1975. The Saint Louis Art Museum, museum purchase.

U nlike diets modified in consistency and texture, which have their primary effect in the GI tract, carbohydrate-modified diets affect metabolism. They are used, therefore, in the treatment of some metabolic disorders, including diabetes mellitus, hypoglycemia, lactose intolerance, and galactosemia. Table 19–1 shows other indications for carbohydrate-modified diets.

Carbohydrate-Controlled Diets

A carbohydrate-controlled diet is a carefully planned diet in which the total amount and the type (starch versus sugar) of carbohydrate is controlled. Actually, the other energy nutrients are controlled as well, because when you control one energy nutrient, the others must be adjusted to ensure that daily energy needs are met. A better name for the carbohydrate-controlled diet, then, is a kcalorie-, carbohydrate-, fat-, and protein-controlled diet. For our purposes, we will use the shorter name.

The carbohydrate-controlled diet is useful in the treatment of diabetes mellitus and hypoglycemia. Its purpose is to maintain blood glucose levels in the normal range in order to prevent complications associated with high or low blood glucose levels.

The carbohydrate-controlled diet is most frequently planned using the exchange list system described in Chapter 18. Foods from the bread, milk, vegetable, and fruit lists contain carbohydrate and are used to meet the carbohydrate allowance. For people with diabetes, hypoglycemia, or dumping syndrome, it is currently widely recommended that concentrated sweets be avoided because of the effect they may have on blood glucose levels. It is also suggested that

TABLE 19–1. Indications for the Use of Carbohydrate-Modified Diets

Carbohydrate-controlled diets

Diabetes mellitus
Dumping syndrome
Hypoglycemia
Obesity, overweight

Lactose-free or lactose-restricted diets[a]

Acquired immune deficiency syndrome (AIDS)
Inflammatory bowel diseases
Lactose intolerance
Malabsorption syndromes

Galactose-free diet

Galactosemia

[a]Many conditions can result in temporary or permanent lactose intolerance. Some of them include surgery to the GI tract, cancer of the GI tract, radiation therapy of the GI tract, dumping syndrome, and protein-kcalorie malnutrition.

concentrated sweets be restricted in low-kcalorie diets, but not for metabolic reasons. People on low-kcalorie diets have no room for empty-kcalorie foods. When concentrated sweets are used in low-kcalorie diets, pay careful attention to the kcalories they contribute (see p. 26).

What are the effects of different types of carbohydrates on blood glucose levels? To address this question, researchers study the glycemic effects of foods—how different types of carbohydrates affect blood glucose levels. For years it was widely believed that simple sugars (glucose, sucrose) caused a sharp rise in blood glucose levels, whereas starches caused a slower rise in blood glucose. Now we know that the case is not so simple. Rather, the effects of different foods on blood glucose apparently depend on many factors:

- The digestibility of the starch in the food.
- Interactions of the starch with the protein in the food.
- The amounts and kinds of fat, sugar, and fiber in the food.
- The presence of other constituents, such as molecules that bind starch.
- The form of the food (dry, paste, or liquid; coarsely or finely ground; how thoroughly cooked; and so forth).

All these factors work together to produce a food's glycemic effect. Of all the foods that have been studied, the ones associated with the lowest rise in blood glucose levels appear to be legumes, especially lentils. A source of carbohydrate eaten by itself has a different effect when it is one component of a meal containing different foods. Currently, not enough information is available on the glycemic effect of foods to change advice given to people with diabetes and hypoglycemia.[1]

Diabetes Mellitus

The problem in people with diabetes is that their blood glucose is too high. In diabetes, energy metabolism is altered by either an absolute or relative deficiency of insulin.

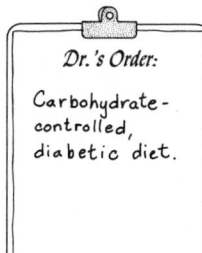

Dr.'s Order: Carbohydrate-controlled, diabetic diet.

Diabetes is not a single disease. Rather, it is a group of disorders with different causes, clinical features, and outcomes. The two major types of diabetes are insulin-dependent diabetes mellitus (IDDM or type I diabetes) and noninsulin-dependent diabetes mellitus (NIDDM or type II diabetes). Some features of the major types of diabetes are summarized in Table 19–2.

Genetic factors are important in both types of diabetes. Fewer than 15 percent of people with diabetes have IDDM, which frequently occurs in childhood and often follows a viral infection. The cells of the pancreas that produce insulin are destroyed, therefore insulin must be provided.

Noninsulin-dependent diabetes mellitus usually develops later in life and is often associated with obesity. Insulin secretion is not the major problem in NIDDM. Rather, the cells of the peripheral tissues—muscle and fat—become

diabetes mellitus (dye-uh-BEE-teez MELL-ih-tus or mell-EYE-tus): a disorder of energy metabolism caused by an absolute or a relative deficiency of insulin. When the word *diabetes* is used alone, it refers to diabetes mellitus.
mellitus = honey sweet (from sugar in the urine)

Another type of diabetes, caused by inadequate secretion of antidiuretic hormone, is called **diabetes insipidus** (in-SIP-id-us). It is treated by giving the hormone.
insipid = without taste (no sugar in the urine)

A type of NIDDM that develops during the teen years has been termed **maturity-onset diabetes in the young (MODY).**

TABLE 19–2. Features of IDDM and NIDDM

	IDDM	NIDDM
Other names	Type I diabetes	Type II diabetes
	Juvenile-onset diabetes	Adult-onset diabetes
	Ketosis-prone diabetes	Ketosis-resistant diabetes
	Brittle diabetes	Lipoplethoric diabetes
		Stable diabetes
Age of onset	Under 40 (mean age, 12)	Over 40
Associated conditions	Viral infection	Obesity
Insulin required?	Yes	Sometimes
Insulin receptors	Normal	Low or normal

The symptoms of diabetes:
  Hyperglycemia
  Glycosuria (GLIGH-cose-YOUR-ee-uh)
  Dehydration
  Polyuria (POLL-ee-YOUR-ee-uh)
  Polydipsia (POLL-ee-DIP-see-uh)
  Weight loss
  Polyphagia (POLL-ee-FAY-gee-uh)
  Acetone breath
  Ketosis
  Ketonuria
  Diabetic coma
  Hyperglycemic nonketotic coma

insensitive to insulin. Obesity makes the insulin resistance worse. Even though the body might make enough insulin, it can't use the insulin adequately. About 85 percent of people with diabetes have type II diabetes, which is usually milder at first and progresses more slowly than type I diabetes. Due to its insidious progression, however, complications may develop before the disease is diagnosed. Type II diabetes is especially health threatening for this reason.

In diabetes, glucose is unable to get into cells. Instead, glucose levels build up in the blood, resulting in hyperglycemia. As the blood glucose concentration rises, water moves from the cells into the blood. Remember that water moves from a less concentrated to a more concentrated solution. The kidneys begin excreting the excess glucose, and water is excreted along with the glucose. Thus, both the intracellular fluid and the extracellular fluid become depleted. The person produces excessive urine (polyuria) and, being dehydrated, may also become excessively thirsty (polydipsia). Polyuria and polydipsia are often early symptoms of diabetes. Figure 19–1 summarizes these events.

Normally, insulin signals the body that it has been fed and directs cellular activities that favor the uptake of amino acids, carbohydrate, and fat. The net effect is to reduce blood glucose levels. When one is fasting, the continued presence of some insulin prevents the body's energy stores from being mobilized excessively.

When not enough insulin is produced or when the cells cannot respond to insulin, the cells are deprived of the substrates they need for energy. Amino acids and glucose may abound in the cells' fluid environment, but the cells have limited access to them and therefore must mobilize their own protein and fats as energy sources. Because of the large amounts of fat being broken down, the liver begins making ketone bodies that also accumulate in the blood. The losses of both glucose and ketone bodies (both energy substrates) in the urine and the breakdown of protein lead to weight loss. This is why the insulin-dependent person with diabetes is likely to be thin. It is also why the person may eat excessively (polyphagia).

People with type II diabetes, as mentioned earlier, tend to be obese rather than thin. They overeat because their cells, lacking energy fuels, are hungry. Then, the insulin they do have slowly takes effect and the body ends up storing fat from the excess energy they have consumed.

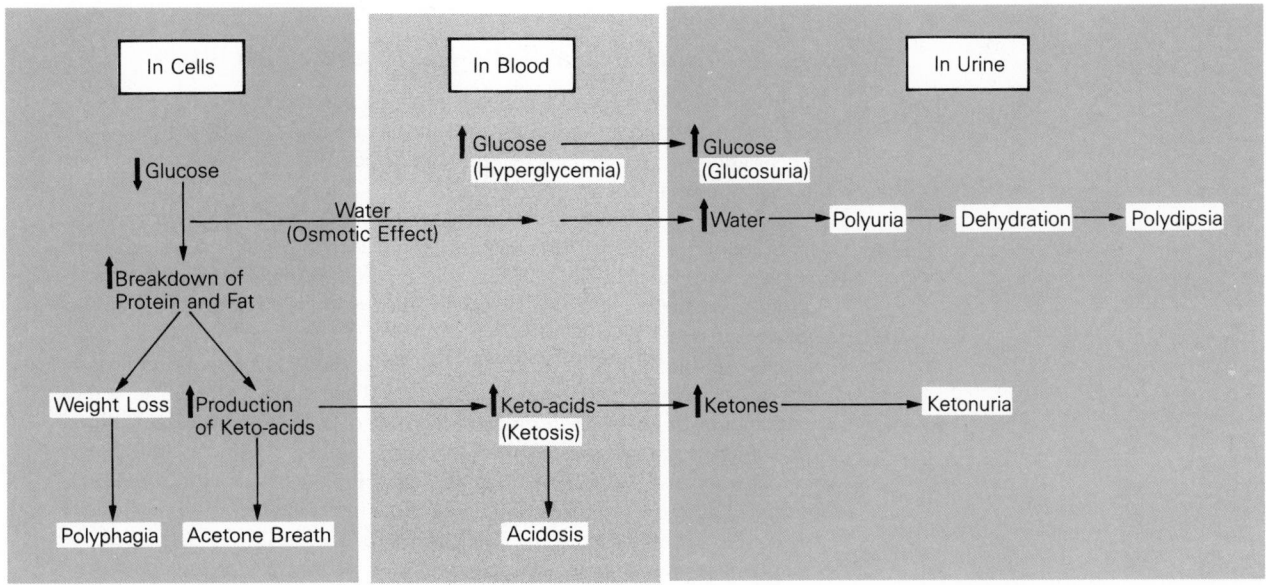

FIGURE 19–1
Overview of diabetes.

If type I diabetes goes uncontrolled, excessive levels of ketones persist in the blood (ketosis). The presence of one type of ketone (acetone) can be detected by a fruity odor on the breath. The ketones are acidic and lower the blood pH (acidosis). Ketones begin to appear in the urine (ketonuria); sodium and potassium are excreted along with them by a mechanism that worsens the acidosis. When acidosis becomes severe enough, the person can lapse into a fatal coma.

People with type II diabetes generally are not prone to ketosis, because they have enough insulin to prevent the excessive buildup of ketones. They can develop another kind of coma, however, caused by extremely high blood glucose levels without acidosis. Logically, this kind of coma is termed hyperglycemic nonketotic coma.

Over the long term, the person with diabetes suffers not only from the acute complications of diabetes just described but also from chronic effects of the disorder:

- Infections, especially of the urinary tract.
- Vascular diseases, including atherosclerosis, gangrene, and microangiopathies. Atherosclerosis is the major cause of death in NIDDM.
- Nerve damage (neuropathy). Neuropathy is often first detected as a loss of sensation in the extremities.

No one knows if maintaining blood glucose levels within a fairly normal range can prevent the chronic complications of diabetes. However, evidence is accumulating that control of blood glucose levels does produce this benefit, and it surely does no harm. Methods of monitoring blood glucose control as well as testing for the presence of diabetes are described in the box entitled "Biochemical Tests for Diabetes Mellitus."

gangrene:
death of tissue that usually occurs when the blood supply is cut off.

microangiopathies (MY-crow-ANN-gee-OP-ah-thees):
disorders of the capillaries, often seen in diabetes. *Retinopathy* (RET-in-OP-ah-thee) is a type of microangiopathy affecting the capillaries of the eye; *nephropathy* (nee-FROP-ah-thee) affects the capillaries of the kidney.
micro = tiny
angio = blood vessel
pathy = disease
retino = of the retina
nephro = of the kidney

Biochemical Tests for Diabetes Mellitus

The diagnosis of diabetes mellitus can be made based on clinical symptoms and the plasma glucose level following an overnight fast. A plasma glucose concentration of greater than 140 milligrams per 100 milliliters on more than one occasion establishes a positive diagnosis.

Another method of diagnosing diabetes is the glucose tolerance test. The person follows a high-carbohydrate diet for at least three days before the test and must not take medication, smoke cigarettes, or exercise during the test. Furthermore, the test may not be valid if the person is emotionally or physiologically stressed.

A glucose tolerance test works like this. First, blood is drawn (after an overnight fast) to obtain the fasting glucose level. The person is then given a measured amount of glucose to drink (in the form of a flavored beverage). Blood is drawn again at regular intervals of 30 to 60 minutes (different clinics use different intervals). Table 19–3 lists the upper limits considered normal and the values suggestive of diabetes for each time interval. At least two of the glucose levels should exceed the latter values for diabetes to be diagnosed. A person whose glucose levels fall between the upper limits of normal and the values suggestive of diabetes is diagnosed as having impaired glucose tolerance.

TABLE 19–3. Interpretation of Glucose Tolerance Test Results[a]

Time (minutes)	Upper Limits of Normal (mg/100 ml)	Values Suggestive of Diabetes (mg/100 ml)
0	115	140
60	200	>200
120	140	200

[a]This is one of many variations of the glucose tolerance test.

Urine tests frequently provide the first clue that a person may have diabetes. Urine tests for sugar and ketones are often performed during routine examinations. Although positive tests for these substances do not always mean diabetes (for example, ketones may be present in people who are following low-carbohydrate diets or are fasting), they suggest the need for blood tests. Urine is tested by dipping indicator paper into the urine sample. The paper changes color and is then compared with a color chart to determine the approximate concentration of glucose. The results are read as percentages, indicating how much glucose is present in the urine.

With another method of urine testing, a tablet is dropped into the urine sample; the color of the urine is then compared with a color chart. People can check their urine at home using the methods taught by professionals at the hospital or clinic. This enables them to be sure their insulin and diet are appropriate. Records of urine test results are useful to the health care team to review at medical appointments.

Urine is checked before meals and at bedtime. The double-void method of urine collection is recommended by some practitioners, although its usefulness has been questioned.[2] (To use this method, the person voids once, then voids again one-half hour later, and tests the second sample.) This method ensures that the glucose measurement does not reflect the concentration of urine stored in the bladder for a long time.

Direct monitoring of blood glucose levels at home is preferred to urine testing to help individuals maintain better contol of their glucose levels. More and more people with diabetes are using this system. Blood testing is more sensitive and more accurate than urine testing.[3] To use this method, the person pricks a finger to get a blood sample (the same method used to determine hematocrit). Paper strips (as with urine samples) can be used to determine blood glucose concentrations. Meters that provide a more accurate readout of the actual glucose concentration are also available, although they are more expensive as well.

Ideally, the person performs the test seven times during the day (before each meal, two hours after each meal, and at bedtime) until good blood glucose control is established. However, many practitioners realize the strain this may place on the individual and instead recommend four tests daily. The person can test at any of the seven times listed above, but the times of the tests should vary daily. Once control has been established, testing can be reduced to once or twice daily.

Another test used to monitor control of blood glucose levels is the measurement of *glycosylated hemoglobin* (or hemoglobin A_{lc}). As blood glucose levels rise, small glucose molecules spontaneously attach to an amino acid on each hemoglobin. The altered hemoglobin no longer releases oxygen properly, and it remains in circulation for the life of the red blood cell (approximately 120 days). Normally, only 4 to 8 percent of the hemoglobin is glycosylated, but when blood glucose levels remain high for a period of time, the percentage goes up to 16 percent.

Measurement of glycosylated hemoglobin allows the physician to determine how successful diabetes control has been over the past two to four months. The test has another advantage. Urine and blood glucose tests are a reflection of diabetes control just before the test. A person who has been in poor control can have a normal urine and blood test just by starving or by using extra insulin the day before going to the doctor. But glycosylated hemoglobin reflects control over several months, so the client can't easily outfox the test.

Treatment of the Person with Insulin-Dependent Diabetes

The goals of therapy for diabetes are the same for all:

- Maintain blood glucose levels in an acceptable range.
- Prevent or delay the onset or progression of associated complications.
- Encourage people to resume normal activities.

Diet therapy for all people with diabetes encompasses these goals. Additionally, diet therapy should be designed to help people achieve and maintain optimal nutrition status. The person with diabetes has the same nutrient requirements as any other person of the same age, stature, and activity level. The diet is designed to minimize changes in blood glucose levels and to prevent or treat

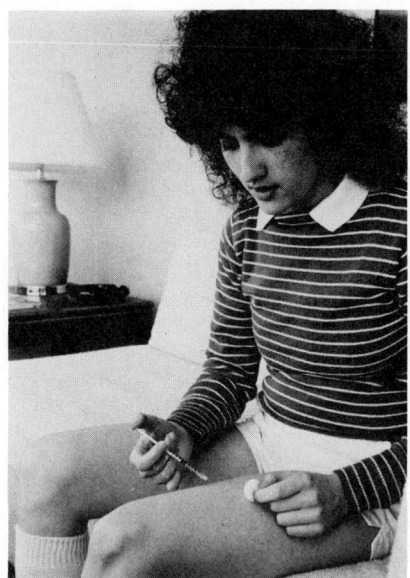

The first dose of human insulin was given to a person in the United Kingdom in 1980. Since then, an estimated 200,000 people in the world have received human insulin. Additional research and refinement of human insulins will generate wider use of these products.

Symptoms of hyperglycemia:
   Glucosuria
   Intense thirst
   Confusion
   Nausea
   Vomiting
   Labored breathing
   Acetone breath

Symptoms of hypoglycemia:
   Nervousness
   Weakness
   Sweating
   Shallow breathing
   Double vision
   Dizziness

One example of the way insulin might be administered:

• 30 to 45 minutes before breakfast—an injection of a mixture of rapid-acting and long-acting insulin.
• 30 minutes before lunch—an injection of rapid-acting insulin.
• 30 minutes before supper—an injection of a mixture of rapid-acting and long-acting insulin.

the complications of diabetes. The means of achieving these goals—that is, the treatment—depends on the type of diabetes.

Insulin

For the person with IDDM, the treatment plan involves coordinating insulin, diet, and exercise. Because persons with type I diabetes can't make insulin, insulin must come from another source. Commercial insulin is commonly extracted from the pancreas of cattle. Insulins made from porcine pancreatic extracts and, more recently, human insulins, are also available. The many types of insulin are described as fast acting, intermediate acting, or long acting, depending on how quickly they begin to work and on how long they remain active. Table 19–4 lists examples of the various types of insulin and their actions. Because insulin is a protein, it would be digested if taken by mouth; therefore, it must be injected.

Normally, people secrete insulin after a meal and have it available to help store energy nutrients when they are plentiful. The person with type I diabetes, however, has to take insulin at a prescribed time and so has to make sure to have nutrients from food available when the insulin is present. The physician prescribes the exact type, dosage, and administration schedule of insulin based on the individual's stage of growth, activity patterns, eating habits, and individual responses.

The person who gets too little insulin or doesn't get insulin when glucose from foods is available risks hyperglycemia and diabetic ketoacidosis. The person who gets too much insulin or has too little glucose available when insulin is high risks severe hypoglycemia. The discovery of insulin has been invaluable, but insulin therapy cannot achieve the same degree of blood glucose control as the body can.

Generally, two or more types of insulin are mixed together and given more than once a day to approximate the times when insulin would normally be present in the bloodstream. Insulin needs rise as body weight increases. Activity reduces insulin needs. Exercise has an insulinlike effect in lowering blood glucose levels. Insulin needs increase during stress, such as pregnancy, surgery, and infection and other illnesses.

To ensure that the insulin schedule, diet, and exercise regimen are coordinated, each client must learn to monitor urine or blood glucose levels at home.

TABLE 19–4. Actions of Some Types of Insulins

Type	Duration of Activity	Peak of Action
Fast acting		
Regular crystalline	5 to 7 hours	2 to 4 hours
Semilente	12 to 16 hours	2 to 8 hours
Intermediate acting		
Globin	12 to 18 hours	6 to 8 hours
NPH/lente	18 to 24 hours	8 to 14 hours
Long acting		
Protamine zinc	24 to 30 hours	16 to 24 hours
Ultralente	30 to 36 hours	18 to 29 hours

Home monitoring of blood glucose levels is gradually replacing urine testing because it is more accurate.

IDDM Diet

The diet for the person with type I diabetes is carefully orchestrated to mesh insulin therapy and exercise. Appropriate control of IDDM necessitates a lifelong commitment on the part of the person with diabetes to a carefully planned diet, exercise, and insulin program. Therefore, a careful and thorough diet history and food preference list should be obtained so that the diet can be planned within the framework of the individual's lifestyle.

food preference list:
a list of a person's likes and dislikes.

The carbohydrate-controlled diet is most frequently planned using the exchange lists in Table 18–2. The first concern is to provide adequate kcalories to maintain or achieve ideal body weight. Of the total kcalories, 55 to 60 percent should come from carbohydrate, and fewer than 30 percent from fat.[4] Protein intake consistent with the RDA is recommended. Nutrients are divided fairly evenly into meals that, in turn, are coordinated with insulin dosage.

In type I diabetes, the timing and composition of meals and snacks must be consistent from day to day and must be eaten at about the same time each day. People with insulin-dependent diabetes may be able to maintain better blood glucose control if they eat smaller meals with two or three snacks. They should include carbohydrate in every meal and snack, roughly in proportion to total kcalories. Each meal usually contains from 20 to 40 percent of the total kcalories and carbohydrate, and each snack contains about 10 percent. The distribution often consists of three meals, a bedtime snack, and sometimes a midafternoon or midmorning snack, depending on the individual's blood glucose levels. Table 19–5 shows how this distribution works for a sample 2,200 kcalorie diet. A sample 2,200-kcalorie diabetic diet menu is also shown so that you can see how this distribution is translated into foods.

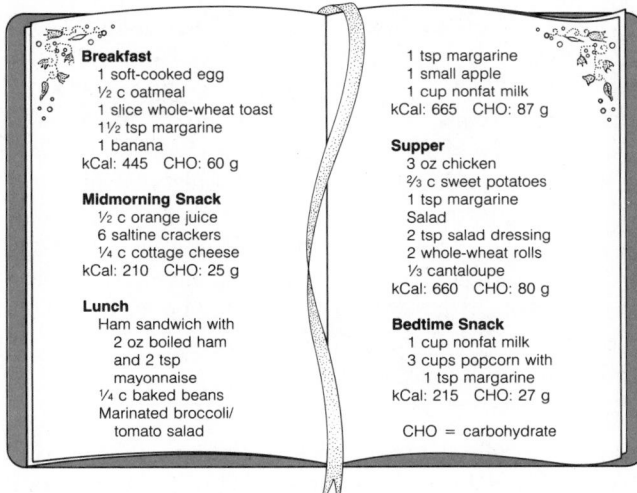

Breakfast
1 soft-cooked egg
½ c oatmeal
1 slice whole-wheat toast
1½ tsp margarine
1 banana
kCal: 445   CHO: 60 g

Midmorning Snack
½ c orange juice
6 saltine crackers
¼ c cottage cheese
kCal: 210   CHO: 25 g

Lunch
Ham sandwich with
    2 oz boiled ham
    and 2 tsp
    mayonnaise
¼ c baked beans
Marinated broccoli/
    tomato salad

1 tsp margarine
1 small apple
1 cup nonfat milk
kCal: 665   CHO: 87 g

Supper
3 oz chicken
⅔ c sweet potatoes
1 tsp margarine
Salad
2 tsp salad dressing
2 whole-wheat rolls
⅓ cantaloupe
kCal: 660   CHO: 80 g

Bedtime Snack
1 cup nonfat milk
3 cups popcorn with
    1 tsp margarine
kCal: 215   CHO: 27 g

CHO = carbohydrate

Sample 2,200 kcalorie diabetic diet

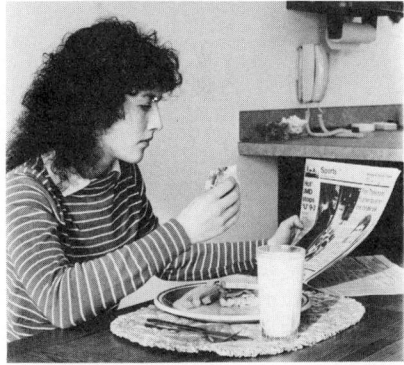

To appreciate the progress made in the treatment of diabetes since insulin became available, contrast this picture with the dietary advice given to the person with diabetes by Dr. John Rollo in 1797: *Breakfast, 1½ pints of milk and ½ pint of lime water mixed together; bread and butter. For noon, plain blood puddings, made of blood and suet only. Dinner, game or old meats which have been long kept; and so far as the stomach may bear, fat and rancid old meats, as pork, to eat in moderation. Supper, the same as breakfast.*

TABLE 19–5. Distribution of Energy and Carbohydrate in a Sample Diabetic Diet

	Breakfast (2/10)	Midmorning Snack (1/10)	Lunch (3/10)	Supper (3/10)	Bedtime Snack (1/10)	Total
Energy (kcal)	440	220	660	660	220	2,200
Carbohydrate (g)	56	28	84	84	28	280

These figures are approximations. Chances are that you will not be able to divide meals so that the kcalories and carbohydrate are distributed exactly as you would wish. (See the sample 2,200-kcal diabetic diet menu.)

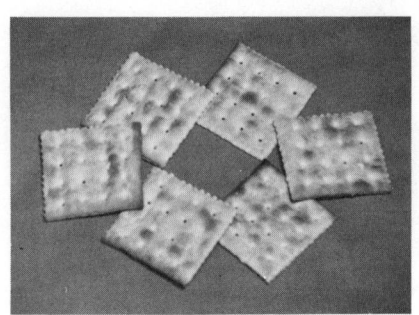

Six saltine crackers = 15 grams carbohydrate.

Note that the carbohydrate-controlled diet is not a low-carbohydrate diet. In fact, the carbohydrate content of the diet is fairly high. Complex carbohydrates that provide fiber are encouraged. In most cases, concentrated sweets are excluded from the diet. However, concentrated sweets (not to exceed five percent of the total kcalories) may be allowed on occasion, particularly for children. Concentrated sweets may also be allowed before vigorous activity or during illness. Encourage the use of low-fat and nonfat milk, lean meats, and polyunsaturated fats to reduce the diet's saturated fat content and help protect against atherosclerosis.

Like all normal persons, the person with type I diabetes must occasionally miss a meal. When this happens, she should take some carbohydrate to protect against hypoglycemia. Usually 15 to 30 grams of complex carbohydrate will forestall hypoglycemia for one to two hours on such occasions.

The person with type I diabetes should carry sugar cubes or hard candy at all times. Why? If he mistakenly takes too much insulin, engages in excessive physical activity, skips meals, or eats too little food, he may develop hypoglycemia. Hypoglycemia can be fatal. As soon as the earliest symptoms appear, he should ingest some form of readily absorbable glucose, such as fruit juice, hard candy, sugar, or glucose solutions.

A tragedy can occur if hypoglycemia isn't recognized. The person suffering from hypoglycemia may appear to be intoxicated and can die. To prevent such a mistake, the person is advised to wear identification in the form of a bracelet or necklace. A card in the wallet may not be adequate, because a wallet might not be checked immediately.

Should a person with diabetes fall unconscious due to hypoglycemia, a would-be rescuer can save his life by turning his head to the side and dripping a concentrated sugar solution (such as honey or syrup) into his cheek. The sugar can be absorbed directly through the cheek epithelium and will raise the blood glucose level.

The person with insulin-dependent diabetes who is in the hospital may have to miss meals to prepare for diagnostic tests, following surgery, or if GI problems prevent food intake. Every hospital should have a standard procedure to deal with the problem. One method is to replace at least half the prescribed carbohydrate and kcalories within three hours after the missed meal. If this cannot be done, the physician is notified and may decide that some other measure is necessary, such as changing the insulin schedule or giving IV dextrose. Sometimes the physician will change the prescription to include more simple carbohydrates, which are easy to eat or drink. Any diet can be modified to include the diabetic diet restrictions. Liquid diets are one example. People with diabetes can also receive tube feedings and total parenteral nutrition.

The person whose blood glucose is well controlled can usually include some alcoholic beverages with the consent of the physician. Since alcohol can cause hypoglycemia in any normal person, the person with diabetes, who is susceptible to hypoglycemia anyway, should be especially careful in using it. Recommend that the person use alcohol only in small quantities and with or shortly before or after meals. Furthermore, of course, everyone should limit alcohol because of its low nutrient density.

People with diabetes often wonder about replacing sugar and foods that contain sugar. In general, special dietetic foods are unnecessary. People often misinterpret *dietetic* to mean *no kcalories,* but this is not the case. Some dietetic foods may be low in sodium instead of sugar, or they may contain reduced but still significant numbers of kcalories.

Some dietetic foods may be helpful, however. They include artificially sweetened soft drinks, artificial sweeteners, and water-packed canned fruits. kCalorie-free soft drinks and beverages, such as artificially sweetened tea, can be used freely and are often well liked. Artificial sweeteners that do not contain significant kcalories can help make the diet acceptable. Nutrition in Practice 19 provides more information about these sweeteners.

Exercise

Exercise is an important consideration in the management of diabetes. For the person with IDDM, regular exercise may lower insulin requirements. For those with NIDDM, exercise can improve glucose tolerance.[5] Strategies for implementing an exercise program were discussed in Chapter 9.

The response of blood glucose levels to exercise in people with IDDM is variable. Those with mild hyperglycemia may experience a fall in blood glucose levels during exercise, whereas those with marked hyperglycemia may experience a greater rise in blood glucose levels. For this reason, exercise should not be undertaken until blood glucose levels fall below 300 mg/ml. During exercise, the person with type I diabetes may need to eat more food or take less insulin. The best way to determine the appropriate course of action is to monitor blood glucose levels before, during, and after exercise. Some general guidelines are provided in Table 19–6. Additional carbohydrate should come from fruits, fruit juices, yogurt, crackers, and other starches.[6]

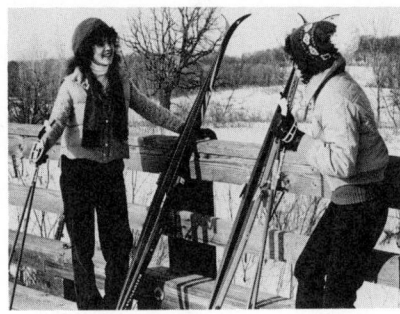

Exercise should be encouraged for the person with diabetes.

Special Concerns for the Child with Diabetes

Diet planning for the child with diabetes involves some special problems. Growth is sporadic, and it is difficult to predict how many kcalories a child will need at any one point in time. Appetite and activity vary widely from day to day. A child might be quite active after school when the sun is shining but

TABLE 19–6. Guidelines for Providing Additional Carbohydrate for Activity for People with Diabetes[a]

Exercise intensity	Blood Glucose Level (mg/ml)	Additional Carbohydrate[b] to Provide (g)
Low intensity	< 100	10–15
	> 100	None
Moderate intensity	< 100	15–20
	100–180	10–15
	180–300	None
Strenuous	< 100	35–40
	100–180	25–50
	180–300	10–15

[a]Adapted from information in M. J. Franz, Exercise and the management of diabetes mellitus, *Journal of the American Dietetic Association* 87 (1987): 872–880.

[b]These values are estimates only. The individual should monitor blood glucose levels to more accurately determine specific needs.

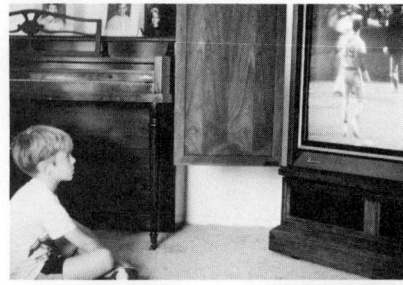

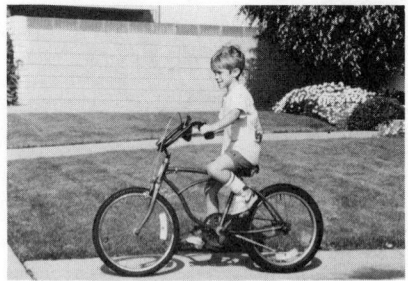

A flexible diet can help meet a child's needs, which vary from day to day.

Hypoglycemia that develops during the night is called **nocturnal hypoglycemia.** It is dangerous, because it can go unrecognized in the sleeping person. Adults as well as children can develop nocturnal hypoglycemia.

The drugs used in NIDDM can be either **oral hypoglycemic agents** (pills that result in lowered blood glucose levels) or insulin. Unlike insulin injections that actually replace the hormone missing from the person with IDDM, oral agents work, in part, by stimulating the release of insulin from the pancreas. Therefore, oral agents are ineffective in IDDM.

may be planted in front of the TV on a rainy day. The level of activity can change the need for food or insulin. For these reasons, it is often recommended that a flexible diet be provided for the child with diabetes. This is not to say, however, that the diet is unrestricted. Meals should be balanced and provide a wide variety of foods. Sweets should be given only at times of vigorous physical activity or to treat hypoglycemia. The child should not be forced to finish a meal but should not skip meals, because hypoglycemia can result. If the child finishes a meal and wants more, he can have more. The child should have his meals at about the same time each day and should eat the same foods as the rest of the family. Many children need to snack two or three times a day.

The possibility that hypoglycemia will develop during the night and go unnoticed is a concern of parents of children with diabetes. Snacks before bedtime may be helpful, particularly if the child is very active late in the day. Additionally, blood glucose can be checked before bedtime (especially in the newly diagnosed child) to help parents protect against hypoglycemia during the night.

Treatment of the Person with Noninsulin-Dependent Diabetes

The goals of treatment for noninsulin-dependent diabetes (NIDDM) are the same as those for insulin-dependent diabetes: control blood glucose levels, minimize complications, encourage activity, and support good nutrition status. But because type II diabetes results from resistance to insulin rather than from lack of insulin, the actual treatment is different. Oftentimes in type II diabetes, blood glucose levels can be controlled by diet alone, although some people need drugs in addition to diet.

TABLE 19–7. Foods to Avoid on a Diet That Excludes Concentrated Sweets

Cakes	Fruit ices	Molasses
Candy	Fruit juices, sweetened	Pastries
Cereals, sweetened	Gelatin, sweetened	Pies
Cookies	Granola	Popsicles
Cranberry sauce	Honey	Puddings
Doughnuts	Ice cream	Sherbert
Frappés	Jam	Soft drinks,
Frosting	Jelly	sweetened
Fruits, canned in syrup,	Marmalade	Sweet rolls
glazed, frozen, or	Milk, chocolate or	Sugar
cooked with sugar	condensed	Sugar
Fruit drinks	Milkshakes	Vegetables, glazed
		Yogurt, fruit-flavored

Dr.'s Order:

Carbohydrate-controlled, weight reduction diet.

The primary goal of diet therapy in NIDDM (type II) is weight reduction (if it is necessary), because the majority of people with type II diabetes are obese, and obesity aggravates insulin resistance.[7] Moderately restricted kcalorie diets that allow a one- to two-pound weight loss per week are recommended. Weight loss in the obese person with diabetes can bring blood glucose levels into the normal range, improve hypertension, and lower levels of fats in the blood (see Chapter 20).

Obese people with severe hyperglycemia are occasionally placed on a medically supervised fast temporarily or on diets very low in kcalories (600 kcal/day) until blood glucose levels are under control. They can then follow less restrictive weight-reduction diets until they reach their desired weights. Although such programs can be successful, often people who lose weight on fasts or very low-kcalorie diets regain all or some of the weight lost. These diets are therefore not generally recommended.

Exercise benefits people with NIDDM in the same ways that it benefits those without diabetes. However, since the risk of heart disease is much higher for people with diabetes, and since those with NIDDM tend to be overweight, an exercise program is strongly encouraged.

The timing and distribution of meals for the person with type II diabetes is not critical, but concentrated sweets are limited, and kcalorie intake must be consistent with the diet plan. Usually, three meals a day with no food between meals is recommended to prevent weight gain. The exchange list system frequently provides the basis for the diet. If the person is already at ideal weight, an ordinary balanced diet that excludes concentrated sweets may be recommended. Table 19–7 lists the foods that should be avoided on such a diet.

In some people with type II diabetes, diet alone is unsuccessful in correcting hyperglycemia. Such people may need to take oral drugs or insulin. Oral hypoglycemic drugs do not replace dieting. Remind your clients who use them to continue their diets.

The Pregnant Woman with Diabetes

Diabetes during pregnancy poses special concerns for both the mother and the infant. The woman may experience episodes of severe hypoglycemia or hyperglycemia. Hypoglycemia can occur early in pregnancy because of transfer of glucose to the fetus, vomiting, or limited food intake resulting from nausea. Therefore, for the woman with IDDM, reduced insulin dosage early in pregnancy may be necessary. Insulin requirements rise in the latter half of pregnancy, however, because the placenta begins secreting hormones that are antagonistic to insulin. The insulin dose may need to be adjusted accordingly.

For the pregnant woman with NIDDM, diet is the major part of therapy. Oral hypoglycemic agents are occasionally given, although insulin may be needed in some cases. When oral agents are used, they are discontinued late in pregnancy and replaced with insulin, because their use is associated with hypoglycemia in the newborn infant.

Gestational diabetes is a type of diabetes that develops during pregnancy, usually in the later part of gestation, in up to three percent of all pregnancies in the United States.[8] The management of gestational diabetes is the same as for the woman with NIDDM.

Blood glucose monitoring is recommended for all pregnant women with any type of diabetes. Careful attention to blood glucose control is essential. In addition to monitoring their blood glucose, pregnant women may also monitor urine ketone levels. Ketosis in early pregnancy is associated with congenital malformations and possibly central nervous system disorders and low intelligence quotients in the offspring.

Education for People with Diabetes

The team approach is most effective in educating people with diabetes. Both group and individual counseling are useful. Each client should understand the objectives of diet (and other) therapy and of how the exchange system works. The teaching-learning process takes time. A person just getting over the shock of being given a diagnosis of diabetes may find the new information difficult to grasp. It is important to take time in explaining the diet without overwhelming the person with information. Plan on spending several sessions when you work with the person with diabetes.

You can help the individual adjust to diet therapy in these ways:

- Encourage the client to be active in the planning process. Adjustment to therapy is better if it fits the individual's lifestyle.
- Explain how to prevent or manage the complications of diabetes and make sure that the client understands you.
- Involve the client's family or companions in the teaching-learning process.

Children can attend summer camps that provide an environment especially designed to offer them a chance to "live" the diabetic lifestyle under supervision until it becomes automatic. Being with counselors and other children who have diabetes helps them to accept and adopt new habits.

Hypoglycemia

Carbohydrate-modified diets are also used in the treatment of hypoglycemia. Strictly speaking, the term *hypoglycemia* simply means low blood glucose. It refers to a symptom, not a disease. More accurately still, it refers to a lab test result (blood glucose below the normal range), and it may or may not have symptoms associated with it.

Dr.'s Order:

Carbohydrate-controlled diet with small, frequent meals.

Hypoglycemia has traditionally been diagnosed when blood glucose levels fall below 50 milligrams per 100 milliliters of blood during a five-hour glucose tolerance test, but it is now considered desirable to make the measurement under conditions of day-to-day life, after a regular meal. In either case, this fall must be accompanied by the symptoms of hypoglycemia—shakiness, weakness, and dizziness—for the diagnosis to be valid.

Hypoglycemia should not occur in the normal person except transiently, because hormones—insulin, glucagon, and others— should continuously adjust blood glucose levels to keep them within the normal range. In some normal individuals, however, hypoglycemia does occur, because their irregular eating habits fail to support steady blood glucose levels. These people may think they have a disease, but in fact they only have symptoms of low blood glucose.

Diagnosed hypoglycemia is of two main types. The first, fasting hypoglycemia, is present after 8 to 12 hours of not eating and frequently signifies a serious problem. The symptoms of this type of hypoglycemia include headache, mental dullness, fatigue, confusion, amnesia, and even seizures and unconsciousness. The treatment is to deal with the underlying medical problem so that the body will again regulate its blood glucose level as it should.

The second main type of hypoglycemia, postprandial or reactive hypoglycemia, occurs several hours after eating. Postprandial hypoglycemia is usually caused by a relative or absolute oversecretion of insulin in response to food. Normally, when carbohydrates are absorbed, blood glucose rises, and insulin is secreted in amounts above the basal level so that blood glucose falls back to normal. In postprandial hypoglycemia, however, insulin is oversecreted and blood glucose falls too low. The typical symptoms—rapid heartbeat, trembling, sweating, weakness, and anxiety—usually are mild, appear suddenly, and resolve fairly quickly. The hypoglycemia associated with dumping syndrome, discussed next, is an example of reactive hypoglycemia.

In true reactive hypoglycemia, diet is the mainstay of therapy. The diet is similar to the diabetic diet, and the exchange lists are often used for instruction. The person is advised to avoid all concentrated sweets and to eat four to six small meals a day. kCalories appropriate to achieve or maintain IBW are given. A survey of teaching hospitals found that 83 percent of the respondents use

People who think they have hypoglycemia when they do not are sometimes said to have **nonhypoglycemia.**

fasting hypoglycemia:
chronic low blood glucose, the symptom of an underlying disorder of the pancreas, liver, pituitary gland, or other body organ or system; it is resolved by treatment of the underlying medical condition.

postprandial or **reactive hypoglycemia:**
low blood glucose within six hours after a meal; an overreaction to the carbohydrate in the meal; often treatable by diet.
post = after
prandium = meal

either a low-carbohydrate diet or a moderately restricted carbohydrate diet for people with hypoglycemia, even though the value of this restriction is disputed.[9] Alcohol should be omitted or restricted if the person with hypoglycemia tolerates it poorly.

Dumping Syndrome

Surgery in which part or all of the stomach has been removed is called a **gastrectomy** or **gastric resection.**

Reactive hypoglycemia can occur in the person who has had a significant portion of the stomach removed. A typical scenario goes something like this: Mr. Fremont had a fairly extensive gastric resection about a week ago and has just begun eating solid foods. He swallows the food; about 15 minutes later, he begins to feel weak and dizzy. He looks pale, his heartbeat is rapid, and he breaks out into a sweat. Shortly thereafter, he develops diarrhea. What causes this sequence of events?

dumping syndrome:
the symptoms that result from the rapid emptying of undigested food into the jejunum: sweating, weakness, diarrhea shortly after eating, and hypoglycemia later.

Dr.'s Order:

Carbohydrate-controlled, postgastrectomy diet.

Mr. Fremont has lost an important function of his stomach. Food no longer empties at a controlled rate into the intestine. Instead, it gets "dumped" rapidly into the jejunum. (Even if the duodenum was not bypassed during surgery, it is so short that food passes quickly into the jejunum.) As the food is digested, the number of particles in the intestinal contents increases. Water from the body moves into the intestinal lumen to dilute the concentration. The volume of circulating blood diminishes rapidly, causing weakness, dizziness, and rapid heartbeat. The large fluid load in the jejunum causes hyperperistalsis, and diarrhea results. Figure 19–2 outlines the sequence of events that occur in dumping syndrome.

After about two to three hours, Mr. Fremont again develops many of the same symptoms: dizziness, fainting, nausea, and sweating. This time the cause is different. Carbohydrates from the meal were rapidly digested and then absorbed, causing blood glucose levels to rise quickly. The pancreas responded by overproducing insulin, making blood glucose levels fall sharply. The symptoms of hypoglycemia now occur.

Not all people who have had gastrectomies develop the diarrhea of dumping syndrome. Even fewer develop hypoglycemia. Many people who initially experience dumping syndrome gradually adapt to a fairly normal diet. However, a special diet is available for the period immediately following surgery or for prolonged or severe cases.

The postgastrectomy diet is a carbohydrate-controlled diet designed to alleviate dumping syndrome. Fluid and electrolyte balances are carefully monitored and imbalances are corrected. Foods containing protein and fat are emphasized. Since these nutrients are digested more slowly than carbohydrate in the intestine, they do not attract fluid into the intestine as rapidly as do carbohydrates. Advise the client to be especially careful not to eat concentrated sweets (sugar, cookies, cakes, pies, soft drinks), because these foods are the most rapidly digested carbohydrates. Recommend small, frequent meals to fit the reduced storage capacity of the stomach. Suggest that a person wait about 45 minutes after each meal before drinking liquids. This helps slow the rate

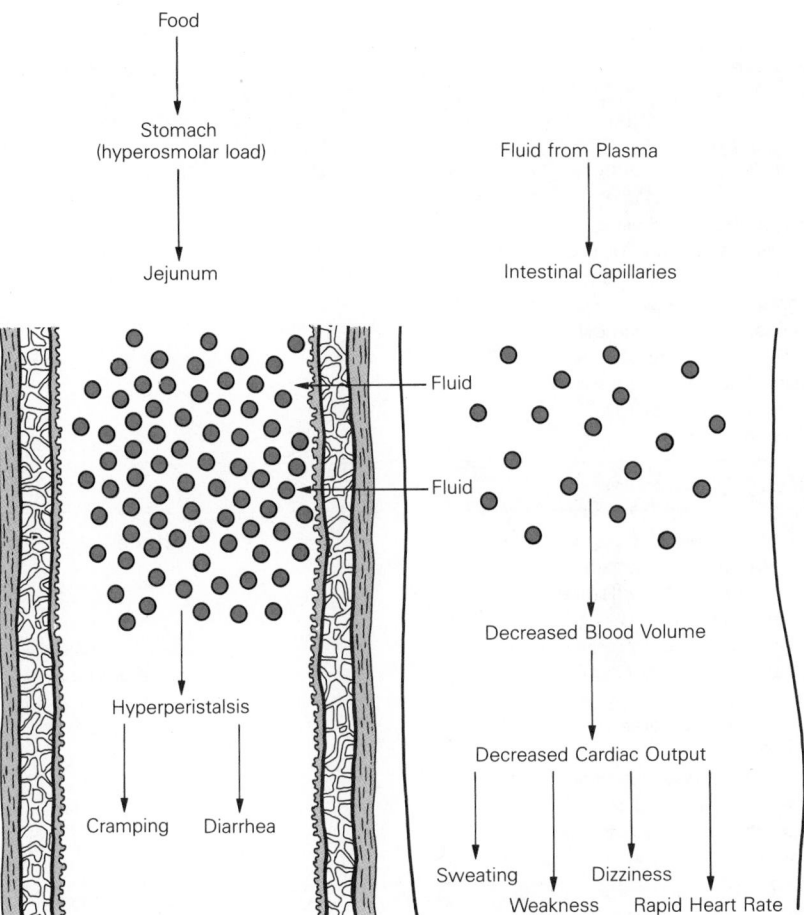

FIGURE 19–2 **Dumping syndrome.**
Dumping syndrome is a physiological
reaction to the presence of highly
concentrated intestinal contents.

at which food passes from the stomach to the intestine. You can also have the
person lie down immediately after eating to help slow down the transit of
food to the intestine. Pectin, a type of dietary fiber, can be added to the diet
to help prevent the symptoms of dumping syndrome. Table 19–8 lists foods
included on and excluded from the postgastrectomy diet. A sample postgastrectomy diet menu is also provided.

The diet planner tailors the diet carefully to meet each person's needs. Initially, visit the client after each meal to uncover food intolerances. For example,
some people develop lactose intolerance and are unable to tolerate any milk
at all (see next section).

Gradually, many people will be able to tolerate small amounts of concentrated
sweets, larger quantities of food, and some liquids with meals. Unfortunately,
diet is not successful in correcting the symptoms of dumping syndrome for
everyone. When all dietary measures fail, additional surgery is sometimes necessary to correct the problem.

TABLE 19–8. Postgastrectomy Diet

Food Item	Allowed	Excluded	Comments
Meats/meat alternates	X		Any type
Grains/starchy vegetables			
Plain breads, crackers, rolls, unsweetened cereal, rice, pasta, corn, lima beans, parsnips, peas, white potatoes, sweet potatoes, pumpkin, yams, winter squash	X		Limit to 5 servings daily
Sweetened cereal; cereal containing dates, raisins, or brown sugar		X	
Nonstarchy vegetables			
Chicory, Chinese cabbage, endive, escarole, lettuce, parsley, radishes, watercress	X		As desired
Asparagus, bean sprouts, beets, broccoli, Brussels sprouts, cabbage, carrots, cauliflower, celery, cucumbers, eggplant, green pepper, greens, mushrooms, okra, onions, rhubarb, sauerkraut, string beans, summer squash, tomatoes, turnips, zucchini	X		Limit to two ½-c servings daily; individual tolerances will vary
Vegetables prepared with sugar		X	
Fruits			
Unsweetened fruits and fruit juices	X		Limit to three servings daily
Sweetened fruits and fruit juices		X	
Fats	X		Any type
Beverages			
Milk (whole milk, nonfat milk, or buttermilk)	X		If tolerated
Coffee, tea, dietetic carbonated beverages	X		
Alcohol, carbonated beverages, sweetened milk, cocoa, fruit drinks		X	
Desserts			
Cakes, cookies, ice cream, sherbet		X	
Other			
Honey, jam, jelly, syrup, sugar		X	

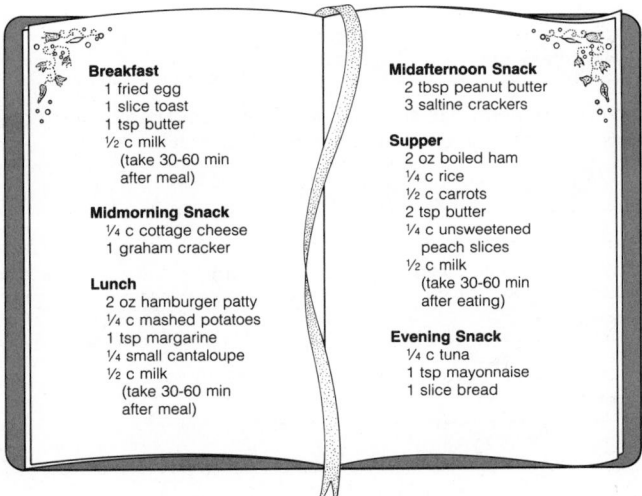

Sample postgastrectomy diet menu.

Other nutrition concerns arise in people with gastrectomies. Iron-deficiency anemia is common; an iron supplement can help correct the deficiency. Anemia also can arise from a deficiency of vitamin B_{12} or folacin. You may recall that vitamin B_{12} cannot be absorbed without the intrinsic factor, which is synthesized in the stomach. Depending on the location and extent of the gastric resection, intrinsic factor production may be reduced or absent and vitamin B_{12} absorption correspondingly impaired. Vitamin B_{12} must then be given by injection to correct the deficiency. Supplemental folacin can be given orally.

Malabsorption of fat and many nutrients can also occur as a consequence of surgery in which a portion of the stomach has been removed. Malabsorption is discussed in Chapter 20.

Diets Restricted in Simple Carbohydrate

In some carbohydrate-controlled diets, certain types of simple sugars are avoided. The most common diet of this kind is the one used to treat lactose intolerance.

A lactose-restricted diet is a highly individualized diet, because people vary widely in the amount of lactose they can tolerate. The person who is sensitive to even small amounts of lactose must follow a lactose-free diet as shown in Table 19–9. A sample menu is also illustrated. As you can see, this diet can be difficult to follow, because lactose is a hidden ingredient in many foods.

The health care team should teach the person on a lactose-free diet to be a label reader. Remind the client to avoid foods that include these ingredients on the label: milk, milk solids, lactose, whey, and casein. Even some drugs contain lactose as fillers; therefore, check all drugs with the pharmacist.

Fortunately, not all people with lactose intolerance must avoid lactose completely. The amount of lactose allowed depends on the client's tolerance. Many times only milk, milk beverages, creamed foods, and ice cream have to be avoided. Cheeses, particularly aged cheeses, often can be tolerated. Some people

Be alert to the presence of lactose in a food whenever the label lists any of these ingredients:

- Milk
- Milk solids
- Lactose
- Whey
- Casein

TABLE 19–9. Foods to Avoid on a Lactose-Free Diet

Meat and meat alternates

Breaded or creamed meats, fish, or poultry; sausage or cold cuts containing nonfat-milk solids; omelets or soufflés made with milk; some peanut butter.

Milk and milk products

Whole, nonfat, evaporated, condensed, or dried milk; yogurt; cheese; ice cream; sherbet; whey and casein milk treated with lactobacillus/acidophilus culture; custard; pudding.

Fruits and vegetables

Any canned or frozen fruit or vegetable processed with lactose; creamed, breaded, or buttered vegetables.

Grains

Breads and rolls made with milk; prepared muffin, biscuit, waffle, pancake, cake, or cookie mixes; some dry cereals; French toast; pie crusts made with butter or margarine.

Other

Some cocoas, instant coffees, margarines, and dressings; butter; cream; creamed soups; chewing gum; chocolate; toffee; peppermint; butterscotch; caramels; some drugs and vitamin-mineral supplements; monosodium glutamate; sugar substitutes containing lactose.

can also drink buttermilk, because it contains less lactose. Yogurt is generally well tolerated, although recent studies suggest that the brand of yogurt is important.[10] Some brands of yogurt are better tolerated than others. Rec-

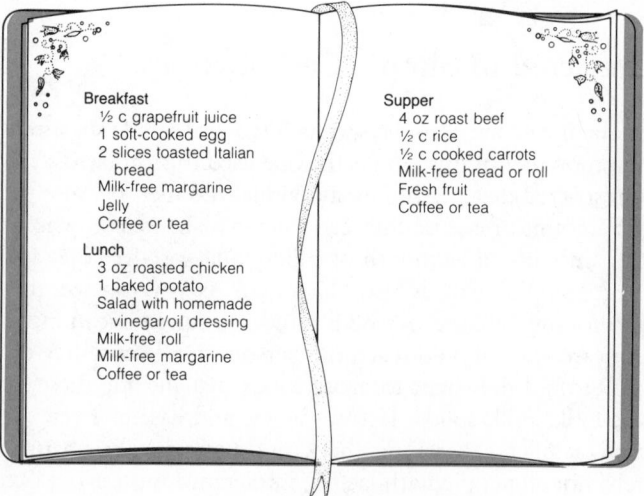

Breakfast
½ c grapefruit juice
1 soft-cooked egg
2 slices toasted Italian
    bread
Milk-free margarine
Jelly
Coffee or tea

Lunch
3 oz roasted chicken
1 baked potato
Salad with homemade
    vinegar/oil dressing
Milk-free roll
Milk-free margarine
Coffee or tea

Supper
4 oz roast beef
½ c rice
½ c cooked carrots
Milk-free bread or roll
Fresh fruit
Coffee or tea

Sample lactose-free diet menu.

ommend that the person try a different brand of yogurt if one brand is not tolerated.

Many people can use commercially prepared products containing lactose without difficulty. Some may even be able to use milk or ice cream in limited quantities. Others can add an enzyme preparation (Lact-Aid) to milk before they drink it. The enzyme splits much of the lactose in milk to glucose and galactose. Milk, ice cream, cottage cheese, and American cheese pretreated with lactase are also available in many areas of the United States.

A word of caution: people who consume no milk or too little milk and milk products often have diets that are calcium deficient. Encourage the use of milk and milk products for those who can tolerate them. Calcium-fortified soy milk can be used as a beverage or in cooking. Other food sources of calcium (see Chapter 8) can be used frequently. In some cases, a calcium supplement may be indicated.

A galactose-free diet is another type of simple carbohydrate-restricted diet. It is similar to a lactose-free diet, because galactose is a part of the lactose molecule. All foods omitted from a lactose-free diet must be strictly excluded from a galactose-free diet. In addition, peas, organ meats, such as liver and brain, and monosodium glutamate must be avoided. The galactose-free diet is used in the treatment of galactosemia. The diet must be followed very carefully.

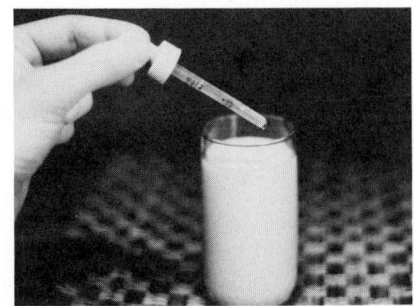

An enzyme preparation added to milk splits lactose into glucose and galactose.

Lactose-restricted diets may be deficient in calcium.

Peas contain galactose, and organ meats and monosodium glutamate can be metabolized to galactose.

Lactose Intolerance

Lactose intolerance results from a deficiency of the digestive enzyme lactase. Lactase is the enzyme that splits lactose to glucose and galactose in the intestine. In rare cases, a person is simply born with a deficiency of lactase. More often, lactase deficiency develops as a consequence of another disease, or lactase levels gradually diminish as the person ages.

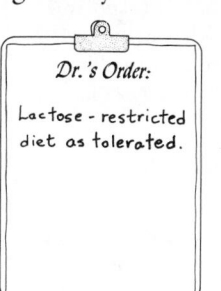

Dr.'s Order:

Lactose - restricted diet as tolerated.

Lactose tolerance is often temporary. It can occur as a consequence of intestinal disorders, surgery of the GI tract, malnutrition, radiation therapy, or chemotherapy. In such cases, lactose can gradually be reintroduced into the diet.

When lactase is deficient, lactose cannot be absorbed, and the intestinal contents become concentrated. Water from the body is drawn into the gut to reduce the high concentration. The result is cramps, distention, and diarrhea. You may recall that this is similar to what happens in dumping syndrome. Furthermore, bacteria in the intestine metabolize the lactose to irritating acids and gases that also contribute to cramping and diarrhea.

The treatment of lactose intolerance is a lactose-restricted diet. Some people may be sensitive to as little as a few grams of lactose, while others can tolerate moderate amounts without ill effects.

A person born with little or no lactase activity has **primary lactose intolerance. Secondary lactose intolerance** is caused by another disease. **Developmental lactose intolerance** describes a lactase deficiency that develops as a person grows older.

Galactosemia

Galactosemia is an inherited disorder caused by a deficiency of any one of four enzymes that normally convert galactose into glucose in the body. Brain

galactosemia (ga-lac-toe-SEE-mee-uh): an inherited disorder characterized by a deficiency of one of several enzymes necessary to convert galactose to glucose in the body.

damage, liver disease, growth failure, cataracts, and mental retardation can result.

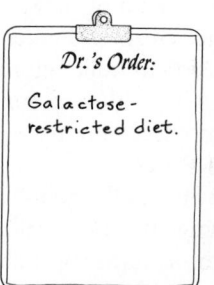

Dr.'s Order:

Galactose-restricted diet.

In several types of the disorder, the galactose-free diet is critical and must be instituted soon after birth. In early infancy, the diet can be lifesaving. Special soy-based formulas replace standard infant formulas. Breastfeeding is contraindicated, because breast milk contains large amounts of galactose. The child's caretakers must fully understand the diet and its role in the disorder. They must understand how to read labels, as discussed earlier.

Carbohydrate-modified diets are very important in controlling symptoms and preventing complications of metabolic disorders. Chapter 21 discusses how fat-modified diets can be used to correct metabolic abnormalities of blood lipid levels. Other fat-modified diets of value in treating disorders of the GI tract are described in Chapter 20.

CASE STUDY

Child with Type I Diabetes

Sam is a 10-year-old boy who was diagnosed as having type I diabetes. His parents had taken him to visit their physician when he began to lose weight, to urinate excessively, and to complain of thirst. Several family members also have diabetes. Recently Sam was admitted to the emergency room because of nausea and vomiting. He complained of intense thirst, was confused, and was breathing hard. The physician could smell acetone on his breath. Urine tests for glycosuria and ketonuria were positive. Blood tests showed that the blood glucose level was 400 milligrams per 100 milliliters. The diagnosis was diabetic ketoacidosis. Sam is 5 feet tall and weighs 80 pounds.

1. Explain the appearance of the symptoms that eventually led to the initial diagnosis of diabetes.

2. Were Sam's physical symptoms and laboratory tests consistent with the diagnosis of diabetic ketoacidosis? How can you distingush between diabetic ketoacidosis and insulin shock?

3. When Sam recovers, what information will he need to prevent future incidents of ketoacidosis?

4. Assume that Sam has never had a diabetic diet instruction. What dietary modifications will be important for him to follow? How do these recommendations contrast with those suggested for a person with type II diabetes?

5. Think about Sam's age and list some special needs of the child with diabetes.

Notes

1. M. J. Franz and coauthors, Exchange lists: Revised 1986, *Journal of the American Dietetic Association* 87 (1987): 28–34.

2. D. W. Guthrie, D. Hinnen, and R. A. Guthrie, Single-voided vs. double-voided urine testing, *Diabetes Care* 2 (1979): 269

3. C. A. Beebe, Self blood glucose monitoring: An adjunct to dietary and insulin management of the patient with diabetes, *Journal of the American Dietetic Association* 87 (1987): 61–65.

4. Franz and coauthors, 1987.

5. M. J. Franz, Exercise and the management of diabetes mellitus, *Journal of the American Dietetic Association* 87 (1987): 28–34.

6. Franz, 1987.

7. M. C. Wheeler, L. Delahanty, and J. Wylie-Rosett, Diet and exercise in noninsulin-dependent diabetes mellitus: Implications for dietitians from the NIH Consensus Development Conference, *Journal of the American Dietetic Association* 87 (1987): 480–485.

8. R. K. Kalkhoff, Medical management of diabetes in pregnancy, in *Clinical Diabetes Mellitus: A Problem Oriented Approach,* ed. J. K. Davison (New York: Thieme, 1986), pp. 472–484.

9. L. S. Bell, L. N. Tiglio, and M. M. Fairchild, Dietary strategies in the treatment of reactive hypoglycemia, *Journal of the American Dietetic Association* 85 (1985): 1141–1143.

10. D. H. Wytock and J. A. DiPalma, All yogurts are not created equal, *American Journal of Clinical Nutrition* 47 (1988): 454–457.

Sugar Substitutes

The person who must avoid concentrated sweets or the person on a weight reduction diet who wishes to avoid sugar often is interested in finding substitutes for refined sugar that satisfy the sweet tooth. However, these people often question the safety and usefulness of sugar substitutes. This Nutrition in Practice discusses several alternative sweeteners and addresses many concerns regarding the safety of sweeteners.

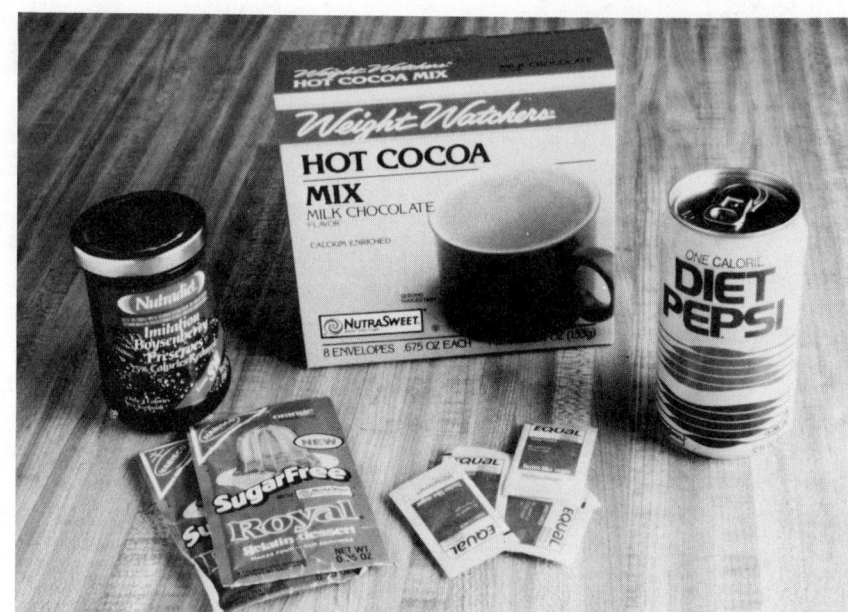

Artificially sweetened products are in wide use.

I'm mixed up about the kcalories in sugar substitutes. In some sugar-free things I use, like soft drinks, the product is also low kcalorie. But when I buy sugar-free gum, the label says that the gum isn't low kcalorie. Why?

The two sugar-free products you mentioned, soft drinks and chewing gum, contain two different kinds of sugar substitutes or alternative sweeteners. Artificial sweeteners (saccharin, aspartame, and cyclamates) do not contain appreciable kcalories in the amounts typically used. On the other hand, nutritive sweeteners (fructose, sorbitol, and xylitol) do contain kcalories. They are used because they are absorbed more slowly than sucrose and do not promote dental caries. People with certain disorders (such as diabetes) who must restrict their intakes of concentrated sweets may also find these products useful. Chapter 2 contains a Miniglossary of Sweeteners.

I'm not sure I understand why someone with diabetes can use nutritive sweeteners and not sucrose. Is that practice safe?

Actually, no one is sure how safe nutritive sweeteners are for the person with diabetes. Before nutritive sweeteners can be widely recommended for these individuals, more research will be needed to see what their longterm metabolic effects are. Presently, it appears that people with diabetes can use them in small quantities if three criteria are met. First, their blood glucose levels should be under control. Second, they should be of normal weight. And third, they should count the sweeteners as part of their carbohydrate allowance.

What about artificial sweeteners? Can people with diabetes use them?

Yes. They can be used in the diabetic diet without counting the kcalories they contribute. So can any person who is trying to lose weight.

Okay. Let me ask you this. I am not diabetic or overweight, but I try to limit the amount of sugar I eat and drink. I have read that saccharin causes cancer and that it was almost banned. Is it safe for me to use?

That's a difficult question to answer. Questions concerning the safety of saccharin have not been fully answered. Saccharin has not been *shown* to cause cancer in human beings. Three large-scale population studies were completed in 1980. One, involving 9,000 people, showed a distinctly greater risk of cancers in some groups, such as women who drank two or more diet sodas a day and people who both smoked heavily and used artificial sweeteners heavily. Another study, involving over 1,000 people, showed little or no excess risk of bladder cancer but could not conclude that there was no risk at all. As of now, two alternative conclusions are possible:

1. Saccharin causes tumors, possibly cancerous, in rats but not in people.
2. Saccharin is a weak carcinogen in people, and its effects will take more years of exposure to become apparent.

What about aspartame? I have also heard that it isn't safe to use.
First of all, before you can understand some of the concerns that have been raised about aspartame, it is important to know what aspartame is. Aspartame is the active ingredient in Nutra Sweet and is composed of two amino acids, phenylalanine and aspartic acid, connected by a single carbon.

One concern regarding aspartame centers around people who cannot metabolize phenylalanine normally. In the extreme case, phenylketonuria (PKU), there is an inherited inability to dispose of excess phenylalanine. An infant with PKU must have some phenylalanine to grow (phenylalanine is an essential amino acid), but too much can lead to severe mental

retardation. For children with PKU, products containing aspartame should be avoided altogether.

In other cases, a person may not have PKU but may carry one defective gene that affects phenylalanine metabolism. As many as 10 percent of the population may carry such altered genes. A theory has been advanced that any of these people or their offspring might be harmed if they eat too much phenylalanine. Logically, then, high levels of aspartame in the diet of the whole population could be a potential health hazard. The fear that a large number of people might be affected or that any unborn children or their mothers might be at risk for serious harm is considered an alarmist view by the originator of the research on the genetics of phenylalanine metabolism. He contends that the interpretation of his work was stretched beyond the scope of the information it legitimately provided.[1]

The Food and Drug Administration has received numerous complaints from consumers who blame aspartame for headaches, dizziness, swelling of the larynx, skin rashes, and nausea.[2] However, investigations into these reports concluded that the complaints were isolated and that any health consequences were minor.

Are there any other concerns about aspartame?
Yes. An expert in the area of hormones and the nervous system has raised another objection to aspartame.[3] He says that because it is a small molecule, it is rapidly digested and absorbed. His theory holds that a sudden rise in phenylalanine could affect the brain's chemical balance. He

considers that aspartame may still be found guilty of causing some of the altered behavior and functional changes that individual people have reported.

In their search for possible negative aspects of aspartame, researchers are also focusing on substances other than the two amino acids. They point to the single carbon that binds the amino acids together. When it is split off during digestion or when aspartame breaks down during product storage, that carbon forms methyl alcohol.

It is true that normal proteins don't contain such single carbons, but many other foods do. Tests have shown that even if someone should eat or drink six times the FDA's maximum projected intake of aspartame, no buildup of methyl alcohol would be seen in the blood. In other words, even if someone were to take in an excessive amount of aspartame, the amount of methyl alcohol produced would not be enough to do any damage.

Why am I seeing so many new products that are sweetened with NutraSweet?
When aspartame first appeared on the market in 1981, it was approved for use only as a tabletop sweetener. In 1983, aspartame was approved for use in carbonated beverages, and in 1986, it could be found in a variety of items such as frozen fruit bars, juice drinks, instant teas, and breath mints. The chemical nature of aspartame was such that it was not stable when exposed to high temperatures, so it could not be used in baked goods. However, a new process has been developed by which aspartame can be protected from high temperatures. The FDA is currently

considering a petition by aspartame's manufacturer to approve its use in baked goods and baking mixes.

Over 160 products available in the United States today are sweetened with aspartame, and this number will increase significantly as additional uses gain approval. The FDA approved aspartame based on the assumption that no one will consume more than 50 milligrams per kilogram of body weight in a day.[4] For a 132-pound person, this adds up to 80 packets of Equal (the tabletop form of NutraSweet) or about 15 soft drinks sweetened with aspartame only. The company that produces aspartame estimates that if all the sugar and saccharin in the U.S. diet were replaced with aspartame, one percent of the population would be consuming the FDA maximum. There is concern, however, that the expanding market of foods sweetened with aspartame increases the likelihood that FDA maximum levels will be exceeded. It is possible that a child who drinks a quart of aspartame-sweetened beverages on a hot day and who has pudding, chewing gum, cereal, and other products sweetened with aspartame could exceed the FDA maximum levels in a day.

From what you've said, I gather that saccharin and aspartame are probably safe, but they could pose some risks. Until more is known, should I use these artificial sweeteners?

To decide whether or not to use artificial sweeteners in your diet you must decide if the benefits you will receive are worth any risks you may be taking. We have just discussed the possible risks. What are the benefits? One is better dental health, because artificial sweeteners—which replace sugar—don't cause tooth decay, while sugar does. Another may be weight loss, because aspartame certainly lowers the kcalorie contents of foods in which it replaces sugar. If you want to lose weight, however, you will find artificial sweeteners useful only if they replace sugar, not if you simply add them to your diet. An additional benefit for people with diabetes or hypoglycemia is taste: they can enjoy the sweet taste of sugar without changing their blood glucose levels.

The most important consideration when using artificial sweeteners is to remember to use them in moderation. Almost every substance, including water, can be harmful if the dose is high enough.

And don't forget: When you want something sweet, your choice is not just between sugar and artificial sweeteners. You can reach for natural foods such as fruits to satisfy your sweet tooth.

Notes

1. A UCLA endocrinologist, William Pardridge, estimated that 10 percent of the U.S. population would be affected this way. The research referred to is by Dr. Harvey L. Levy, director of the PKU program, Children's Hospital, Boston (personal communication), September 1984.
2. M. S. Boyd, Artificial sweeteners: Doubts linger over aspartame while new products await approval, *Environmental Nutrition* 10 (1987): 4–5; Artificial sweeteners—Lingering doubts, *American Institute for Cancer Research*, Winter 1988, p. 11.
3. Richard Wurtman, endocrinologist at the Massachusetts Institute of Technology, in a letter to the editor, *New England Journal of Medicine* 83 (1983): 429–430.
4. *A Health Care Practioner's Guide,* a pamphlet (1987) available from The NutraSweet Company, P.O. Box 111, Skokie, IL 60676.

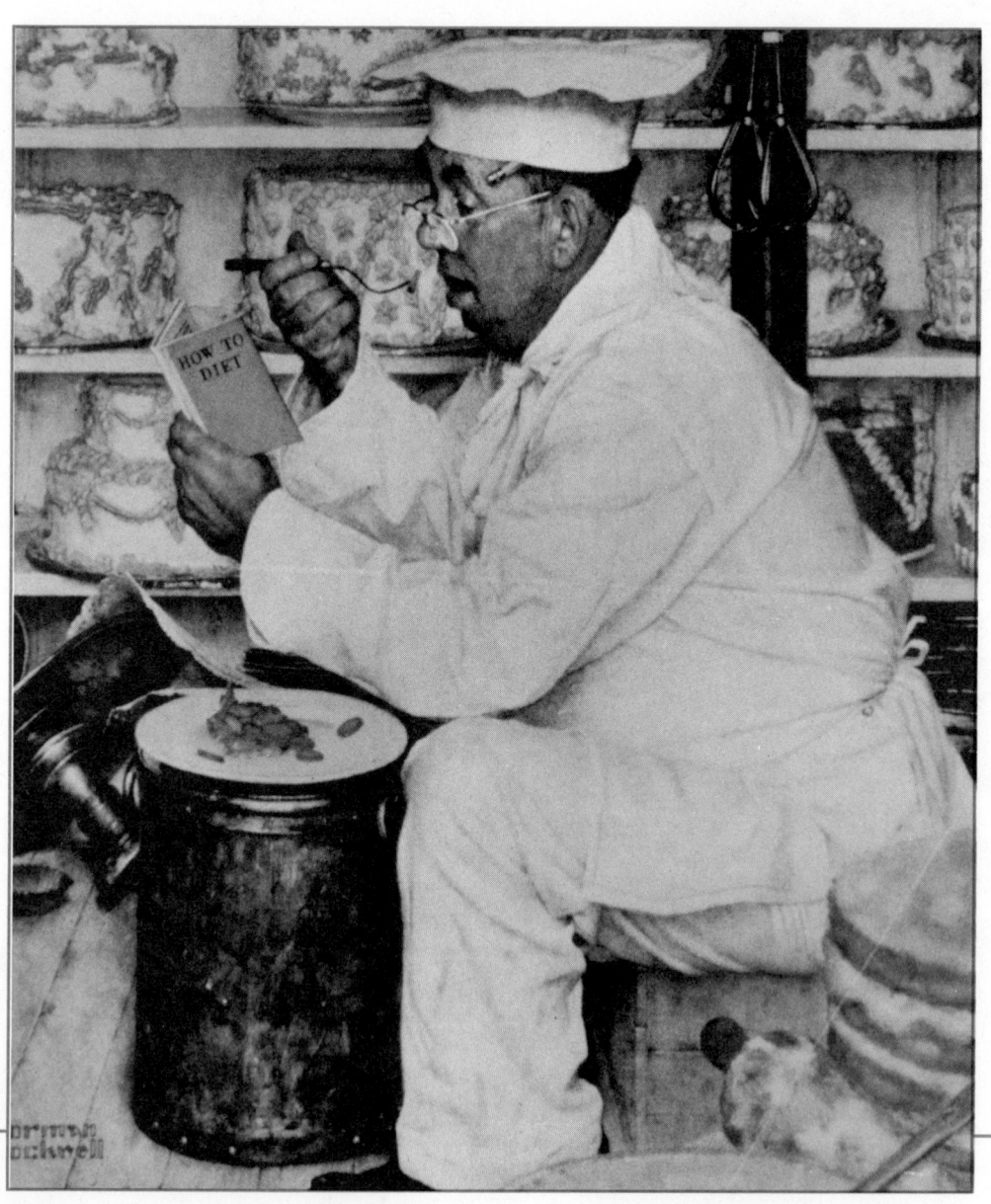

20

Diets Modified in Fat, I: Low-Fat Diets

Diets modified in fat are of two basic types. People on low-fat diets limit the total amount of fat in their diets. People on fat-controlled diets watch not only how much fat they eat but also the types of fats—polyunsaturated and monounsaturated versus saturated. These two diets are frequently confused in the clinical setting even though there is a considerable difference between them. Low-fat diets are used in the treatment of GI disorders that result in malabsorption of fat. Fat-controlled diets are used in treating abnormal blood lipid levels to help prevent or delay the development of coronary heart disease, discussed in Chapter 21. Table 20–1 lists indications for the use of low-fat diets. Table 21–1 (Chapter 21) shows disorders for which fat-controlled diets are used.

Low-Fat Diets

Low-fat diets prevent many of the problems associated with the malabsorption of fat. A low-fat diet limits the total amount of fat to 15 to 35 percent of the total kcalories. An example of a typical low-fat diet is given in Table 20–2. The exchange list system presented in Chapter 18 can also be used to plan a low-fat diet. The client is instructed to use low-fat milk and lean meat exchanges and to limit the total number of fat and meat exchange servings. The exact number of fat servings allowed depends on the diet. For example, on a 30-gram low-fat diet, the client would be allowed five lean meat exchanges (15 grams of fat) and three fat exchanges (15 grams of fat). A sample menu is shown in the text.

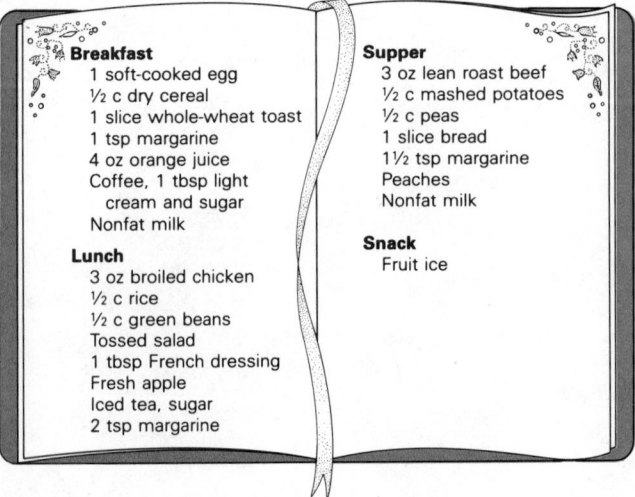

Breakfast
1 soft-cooked egg
½ c dry cereal
1 slice whole-wheat toast
1 tsp margarine
4 oz orange juice
Coffee, 1 tbsp light
   cream and sugar
Nonfat milk

Lunch
3 oz broiled chicken
½ c rice
½ c green beans
Tossed salad
1 tbsp French dressing
Fresh apple
Iced tea, sugar
2 tsp margarine

Supper
3 oz lean roast beef
½ c mashed potatoes
½ c peas
1 slice bread
1½ tsp margarine
Peaches
Nonfat milk

Snack
Fruit ice

Sample low-fat diet menu.

A low-fat diet can be difficult to follow. Fats give flavors to foods—flavors that some people may miss. Low-fat foods can also be difficult to purchase. You can offer a client these suggestions:

TABLE 20–1. Indications for the Use of Low-Fat Diets

Acquired immune deficiency syndrome (AIDS)
Blind-loop syndrome
Cystic fibrosis
Fat malabsorption (steatorrhea)
Gallbladder disease
Hiatal hernia
Inflammatory bowel disease
Liver disease
Pancreatitis
Short-bowel syndrome
Reflux esophagitis

- Purchase low-fat meats. Fish, poultry, and veal are lower in fat than red meats. To be sure that ground meat doesn't have too much fat, buy a lean piece of beef or pork and have the butcher grind it for you. Ground turkey can be an excellent substitute for ground beef or ground pork.

- Tempt your taste buds by cooking meats in mixtures of vegetables such as tomatoes, green peppers, carrots, mushrooms, and onions.

- Remember to use herbs and spices. Unless otherwise indicated, salt is not limited on a low-fat diet.

- Make gravy from bouillon or broth seasoned with wine and herbs and thickened with cornstarch or flour.

- Blenderize low-fat cottage cheese or yogurt made from skim milk with herbs for a zesty salad dressing.

- Substitute reduced-kcalorie margarine for regular margarine, because it has half the fat. Reduced kcalorie mayonnaise and salad dressing also contain less fat.

- Use butter salt or imitation butter flavoring to season food.

- Broil, bake, or steam foods instead of frying whenever possible. To pan fry foods, try vegetable cooking sprays and no-stick pans instead of fat.

- Make homemade stews and soups and refrigerate them overnight. Skim off the excess fat that forms on top before using them the next day.

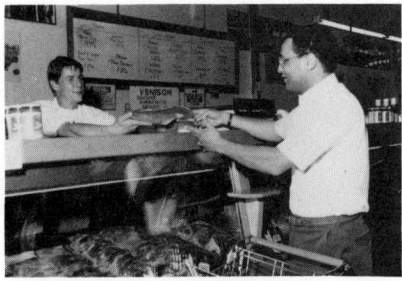

Grocers can trim excess fat from meats before you purchase them.

You can also suggest to your client to check low-kcalorie cookbooks. They often feature recipes low in fat.

Sometimes, a person must be on a very low-fat diet and may have a hard time getting enough kcalories. In such cases, medium-chain triglycerides (MCT) can serve as a source of kcalories. They are available through the pharmacy or dietary department. MCT contain as many kcalories as regular fats, but they are digested and absorbed differently from long-chain triglycerides. MCT oil can be used in place of oil in salad dressings, beverages, desserts, and other dishes. However, when MCT provide a large portion of the fat kcalories in the diet, the diet planner must be careful that the person on a low-fat diet gets adequate amounts of essential fatty acids. Medium-chain triglycerides cannot be used to meet these needs; the regular fat that is used must contain the essential fatty acids.

TABLE 20–2. Low-Fat Diet (50 g fat)

Use

1. Nonfat milk, nonfat-milk cheeses, yogurt made from nonfat milk, sherbet, and fruit ices.
2. Low-fat egg substitutes and up to three regular eggs per week.
3. Up to 6 oz of lean meats and poultry without skin daily.
4. Up to 6 daily servings of fat. One serving is any one of the following:
   - 1 tsp butter, margarine, shortening, oil, or mayonnaise.
   - 1 strip crisp bacon.
   - 1 tbsp heavy cream or Italian or French dressing.
   - ⅛ avocado.
   - 2 tbsp light cream.
   - 6 small nuts.
   - 5 small olives.
   If fat is used to cook or season food, it must be taken from this allowance.
5. All vegetables prepared without fat.
6. All fruits prepared without fat.
7. Plain white or whole-grain bread; nonfat cereals, pasta, rice, noodles, and macaroni.
8. Clear soups and cream soups made with nonfat milk.
9. Angel food cake and fruit whips made with gelatin, sugar, and egg-white meringues.
10. Jelly, jam, honey, gumdrops, jelly beans, and marshmallows.

Do not use

1. Whole milk, chocolate milk, whole-milk cheese, and ice cream.
2. Pastries, cake, pie, sweet rolls, or breads made with fat.
3. More than one egg a day, fried or fatty meats (sausage, luncheon meats, spareribs, frankfurters), duck, goose, or tuna packed in oil (unless well drained).
4. More than six servings of fat.
5. Desserts, candy, or anything made from chocolate or nuts.
6. Creamed soups made with whole milk.

Suggestions

1. To make the diet still lower in fat, reduce the fat and meat (and egg) servings.
2. To increase the fat content, give additional fat or meat servings.
3. To improve acceptance of the diet, check the fat content of a well-liked food and allow that food if posible. Use the exchange system fat list for alternate suggestions for fat servings.

Malabsorption

Many conditions that involve or affect the digestive organs result in the malabsorption of nutrients. Malabsorption arises from either the improper digestion or the improper absorption of nutrients. Table 20–3 highlights the risk factors for poor nutrition status that may occur in people with malabsorption.

Malabsorption of fat, carbohydrate, protein, vitamins, and minerals are all known to occur. Most commonly, it is fat that is malabsorbed. You may recall that fat is digested and absorbed in a different, more complex way than either

TABLE 20–3. Risk Factors for Poor Nutrition Status in Malabsorption Syndromes

Reduced Intake	Increased Nutrient Losses	Increased Nutrient Needs
Abdominal pain	Blind loop syndrome	Drug therapy
Anorexia	Diarrhea	Surgery
Bowel rest	General malabsorption	
Emotional stress	Short-bowel syndrome	
Food intolerance	Steatorrhea	
Indigestion		
Nausea		

carbohydrate or protein (see Chapter 5). Fat not absorbed is excreted from the body in the stools (steatorrhea).

The effects of fat malabsorption can be quite severe (see Figure 20–1). The loss of fat in the stools means that valuable kcalories are also lost. Excreted along with the undigested fat are fat-soluble vitamins. Calcium and magnesium form soaps with unabsorbed fatty acids, so they too are lost in the stools. Vitamin D loss can further add to calcium depletion.

The loss of calcium with fatty acids can cause another problem—enteric hyperoxaluria. Oxalate, present in some foods, normally binds with calcium in the gut, and both are excreted. But when calcium binds instead to unab-

steatorrhea (STEE-at-oh-REE-uh): fatty diarrhea characterized by stools that are foamy, greasy, and malodorous.

enteric hyperoxaluria (en-TER-ick HIGH-per-ox-sa-LOO-reeah): a condition of excess oxalate absorption that comes about because calcium is unable to bind oxalate in the gut. It leads to kidney stone formation.

FIGURE 20–1
Some effects of fat malabsorption.

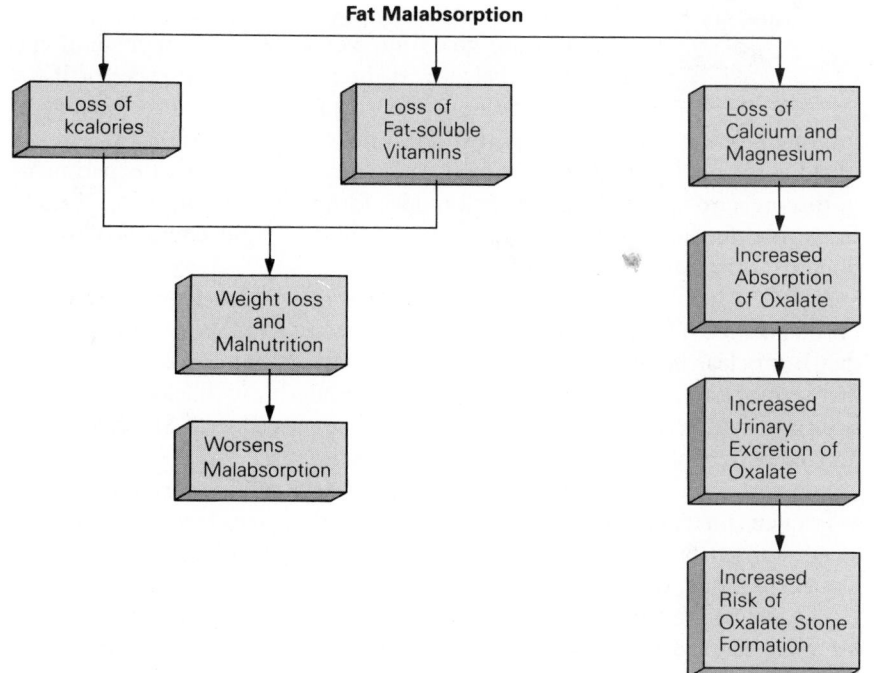

sorbed fatty acids, the oxalate is left unbound and can be absorbed. Because oxalate is not metabolized by the body, its absorption leads to the excretion of oxalate in the urine. High urinary oxalate favors the formation of kidney stones (see Nutrition in Practice 22).

The primary treatment of steatorrhea is to correct the underlying disorder. Along with this treatment, fat is restricted, and fat-soluble vitamins are supplemented in a water-miscible form that is easy to absorb. Medium-chain triglycerides can be used to add kcalories. Often, the person with malabsorption is initially given about 50 grams of fat per day. Gradually, the amount of fat is increased to coincide with the client's tolerance.

water-miscible (MISS-i-bull) **vitamins:** fat-soluble vitamins that readily mix with water and can be absorbed without fat.

Pancreatitis

One disorder that can result in malabsorption is pancreatitis, an inflammation of the pancreas most often caused by biliary tract disease, surgery (often of the stomach or biliary tract), or alcoholism. The damaged pancreas retains pancreatic secretions, including digestive enzymes, that begin to destroy the pancreas itself. The blood picks up some of these enzymes, causing serum amylase and lipase levels to rise. These elevated levels are indicators of pancreatitis. Typical symptoms of pancreatitis include severe abdominal pain and nausea and vomiting.

pancreatitis (PAN-cree-uh-TIE-tis): inflammation of the pancreas.

amylase: a starch-digesting enzyme secreted by the pancreas.

lipase: a lipid-digesting enzyme secreted by the pancreas.

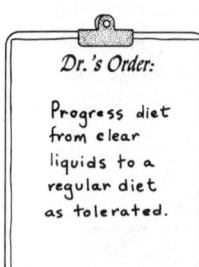

Dr.'s Order:

Progress diet from clear liquids to a regular diet as tolerated.

The goal of therapy for pancreatitis is to reduce the stimulation of pancreatic secretions. No food is given by mouth, since food stimulates bicarbonate and enzyme secretions from the pancreas. A nasogastric tube is inserted, but not for feeding. Instead, the tube is used as a straw to suction out the stomach's contents which further reduces stimulation of the pancreas.

Fluids are given intravenously to maintain fluid and electrolyte balance. If the pancreatitis is severe or if the person is malnourished, total parenteral nutrition may be indicated. Some studies suggest that TPN does not stimulate pancreatic secretions to the degree that an enteral diet would, but results of experiments in this area are unclear.[1] People with milder forms of pancreatitis may benefit from tube feedings of hydrolyzed formulas, although no controlled studies document the benefits of such feedings.[2]

A person who is free of abdominal pain, has active bowel sounds, and has normal or near-normal serum amylase levels can try an oral diet. Progress the diet from clear liquids to a low-fat diet to a regular diet as tolerated. At the first sign of pain, or if serum amylase levels rise, food is withheld. When these signs and symptoms subside again, food can be reintroduced. Six small meals may be better tolerated than larger, less frequent meals.

Sometimes an acute attack of pancreatitis doesn't subside, or attacks occur at frequent intervals. This condition describes chronic pancreatitis, most commonly caused by repeated alcohol abuse. Pancreatic tissue is destroyed and, like nerve tissue, cannot regenerate.

The pancreas normally excretes enzymes far in excess of needs, so even after extensive damage has occurred, digestion may still proceed normally. However, with chronic pancreatitis and extensive degeneration of the pancreas, digestion, expecially of fat, is permanently impaired. A special diet is required. Diet

acute: developing rapidly and lasting for only a short time. Conditions that develop slowly and are of long duration are described as *chronic*.

therapy during active attacks of pancreatitis is the same as for acute pancreatitis. Between attacks, the client should follow a low-fat, bland diet (Chapter 16). Small meals may be easiest to digest. The person with chronic pancreatitis usually tolerates about 50 to 70 grams of fat per day; restricting fat to less than this amount is unnecessary. The client takes enzyme replacements with meals to aid in the digestion and absorption of fat and protein. Absolutely no alcohol is permitted. If steatorrhea persists, fat-soluble vitamins are given in supplement form. Vitamin B_{12} absorption may be reduced, so injections of vitamin B_{12} may be required.

Pancreatitis also may damage the pancreatic cells that produce insulin. In such cases, the individual becomes glucose intolerant as in diabetes and must also follow a diabetic diet (see Chapter 19).

Cystic Fibrosis

Cystic fibrosis (CF) is a hereditary disease that may affect many organs, including the pancreas, lungs, liver, heart, gallbladder, and small intestine. People with CF often have three major symptoms: Pancreatic insufficiency, chronic lung disease, and abnormal electrolyte levels in the sweat. The pancreas is affected in 80 to 85 percent of people with CF. The airways of the lungs also become plugged with mucus, making it difficult for the person to breathe. Lung infections become likely and are the usual cause of death in people with CF.

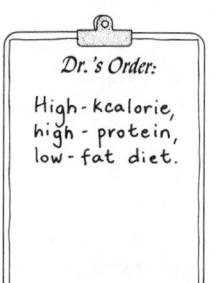

Dr.'s Order:
High-kcalorie, high-protein, low-fat diet.

Cystic fibrosis is characterized by production of a very thick mucus by glands throughout the body. The mucus obstructs the small pancreatic ducts and interferes with the secretion of digestive enzymes and pancreatic juices. Malabsorption results, affecting many nutrients—fat, protein, vitamins, and minerals— and frequently leads to malnutrition. Many young people with CF are short and very thin for their age.

The energy needs of people with CF are about 150 percent of the RDA for their sex and age. These high energy needs reflect the loss of nutrients through malabsorption, frequent infections, and the extra energy required simply to breathe. Children with CF often fail to meet even normal energy requirements, explaining why many of these children fail to grow to their potential.

A high-kcalorie, high-protein, low-fat diet that is nutritionally balanced and carefully tailored to the individual's tolerance is recommended. In the past, diets for people with CF were often severely restricted in fat. However, individuals generally know how much fat they can take before uncomfortable GI symptoms occur. Furthermore, fat is an important source of kcalories and essential fatty acids. Essential fatty acid deficiencies are well documented in children with CF. Therefore, the current trend is to prescribe a liberal fat intake for the person with CF who can tolerate it. For individuals who cannot tolerate fat, MCT oil can provide additional kcalories.

Enzyme replacements play an important part in the therapy of CF by helping to reduce malabsorption considerably. They cannot correct it completely, however. People who have persistent steatorrhea, gas, and abdominal distention may need to have their dosages of enzyme replacements adjusted rather than their fat intakes reduced.

Goals of diet therapy in chronic pancreatitis:
  Maintain optimal nutrition status.
  Reduce steatorrhea, if present.
  Minimize pain as necessary.
  Avoid subsequent attacks of active pancreatitis.

A bland diet eliminates foods that stimulate gastric acid secretion, which in turn stimulate the secretions of the pancreas.

Enzyme replacements are extracts of pork or beef pancreatic enzymes that help with digestion.

cystic fibrosis (CF): a hereditary disorder that affects many organs, including the pancreas, lungs, liver, heart, gallbladder, and small intestine.

Breastfeeding is recommended for the infant with CF, as it is for most infants. Infants who are not breastfed can usually tolerate a regular infant formula taken with enzyme replacements. However, studies have suggested that infants with CF who are fed predigested infant formulas (Pregestimil) are more likely to grow normally than infants with CF who are given standard infant formulas.[3] As the child is weaned from breast milk or formula, fat is restricted only if steatorrhea cannot be controlled by enzyme replacements.

The best way to ensure that people with CF are eating enough is to regularly assess their nutrition status, paying particular attention to monitoring height and weight. Nutrition care plans can then be revised as necessary.

Vitamin-mineral supplements (two tablets daily) are usually given. The fat-soluble vitamins should preferably be given in a water-miscible form that can be absorbed without fat. Zinc supplements may also be needed.

Maintenance of adequate nutrition status for the person with CF is extremely important; nutrition status and the severity of pulmonary disease appear to be related.[4] Several research centers are experimenting with home parenteral and enteral nutrition programs to meet the nutrient needs of people with CF.[5] Children eat a regular diet and are fed by tube or parenteral nutrition during the night to help augment nutrient intake. Such programs are promising, although they present practical and psychological difficulties for the person with CF and their caretakers. One group of practitioners has successfully used high-kcalorie formulas (two kcalories per milliliter) to raise energy intake in a more practical, less intrusive way.[6]

Depletion of electrolytes (sodium and chloride) is another nutrition-related concern. Fever, high environmental temperature, or diarrhea can rapidly precipitate electrolyte depletion. During such times, encourage the person to use extra salt.

Inflammatory Bowel Diseases

Several conditions can cause inflammation of the bowel and result in malabsorption. Two such disorders—Crohn's disease and ulcerative colitis—show similar clinical, pathologic, and biologic features, and both often lead to malnutrition. Their cause or causes remain unknown. In Crohn's disease, inflammation of the bowel is accompanied by cracklike ulcers and many granulomas. Crohn's disease can occur anywhere in the GI tract but most often develops in the ileum and colon. The person with Crohn's disease often reports weight loss, fever, diarrhea, and cramping abdominal pain. The disease may be self-limited and eventually may be cured, but it often recurs. Inflammation and scarring may narrow the intestinal lumen, sometimes causing obstruction.

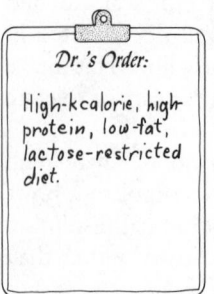

Dr.'s Order:
High-kcalorie, high protein, low-fat, lactose-restricted diet.

The person with Crohn's disease is at high risk for developing nutrient deficiencies for many reasons. For one, malabsorption limits the availability of nutrients. Diarrhea can upset fluid and electrolyte balances. The person usually has lost weight, and during periods when the disease is active, abdominal pain and emotional stress may cause food intake to be reduced considerably. In addition, oral intake may be withheld so that the bowel can rest, particularly when the person has developed an obstruction or when a fistula has formed. Furthermore,

Crohn's disease: inflammation and ulceration along the length of the GI tract, often with granulomas.

granuloma: (gran-you-LOH-mah): a granular tumor or growth.
granulum = little grain
oma = tumor

fistula (FIS-too-lah): an abnormal opening between two organs or from an organ to the skin.
fistula = pipe

drug therapy used to treat the disease can affect nutrition status. If surgery is required, nutrient needs become even greater.

As you can see, restoring and maintaining nutrition status for the person with Crohn's disease can be an extremely difficult task. Multiple nutrient deficiencies can develop that may reduce the effectiveness of drug therapy and threaten immune function.[7] Protein-kcalorie malnutrition and deficiencies of calcium, magnesium, zinc, iron, vitamin B_{12}, folacin, vitamin C, and fat-soluble vitamins are commonly reported.[8]

As mentioned earlier, during the acute stages of the disease, bowel rest is sometimes desirable. Bowel rest may be beneficial whenever food intake significantly aggravates diarrhea, when the bowel is obstructed, or when rest might help a fistula to close. During complete bowel rest, TPN can be used to successfully deliver needed nutrients (see Chapter 15). In some cases, complete bowel rest may eliminate the need for surgery.[9]

Low-fat, low-fiber hydrolyzed and defined formula diets have been used successfully during acute periods of Crohn's disease to provide nutrition without the need for TPN. Since hydrolyzed formulas are easily absorbed in the upper small intestine, they also allow the bowel to rest. Encourage the person to accept the formula by mouth by offering different flavors and serving the formula appropriately. However, recommend tube feeding if the person can't tolerate the formula orally. Although hydrolyzed formulas are hypertonic and may contribute to diarrhea in some people, they can safely be administered at full strength in many people with Crohn's disease.[10] By starting the formula at full strength, unnecessary delays in delivering all needed nutrients can be avoided. The client is gradually progressed to an oral diet as tolerated. A high-kcalorie, high-protein, low-fat, low-fiber diet is recommended. High-fiber foods can cause an obstruction and are avoided. Lactose intolerance frequently develops, and the person is then advised to eliminate milk and milk products. Supplemental vitamins and minerals are often prescribed. Encourage the client to eat a nutrient-rich, well-balanced diet, and reassess nutrition status frequently to ensure that nutrient needs are being met.

> The person with Crohn's disease often needs a lot of emotional support. The incidence of the disease is highest in teenagers; the individual who has it is typically young and often depressed. The disease is highly unpredictable; just when a person feels well, a relapse may occur, necessitating another round of surgery. The person may feel that food itself causes the disease and may react by eating very little.

Unlike Crohn's disease, which can occur anywhere along the GI tract, ulcerative colitis occurs only in the large intestine. It is characterized by severe diarrhea, rectal bleeding, cramping, abdominal pain, anorexia, and weight loss. Diarrhea can be almost continuous, resulting in poor absorption of nutrients and great losses of fluids and electrolytes. Anemia may be present because of blood loss from rectal bleeding.

Many of the dietary principles outlined for Crohn's disease apply to ulcerative colitis. A primary concern is to assure adequate intake of fluid and electrolytes. High-fiber foods are avoided, because they can irritate the colon. High-kcalorie,

Drugs used in the treatment of Crohn's disease include antibiotics (sulfasalazine) and corticosteroids. See Appendix B for possible affects on nutrient status.

High-kcalorie, high-protein diets are discussed in Chapter 17, and lactose intolerance is discussed in Chapter 19.

high-protein foods are recommended. Fat is restricted if the client has symptoms of fat malabsorption. Milk and milk products are frequently eliminated because lactose intolerance is common. Supplemental vitamins or minerals may be necessary.

Blind Loop Syndrome

Another disorder that causes fat malabsorption by interfering with fat digestion occurs in blind loop syndrome. In some types of gastric resections, a portion of the small intestine is bypassed, making that portion nonfunctional. The portion bypassed, but not removed, is called a blind loop. Figure 20–2 illustrates one such gastric resection.

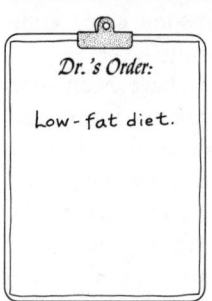

Stasis occurs in the blind loop, and bacteria, normally not present in that part of the intestine, flourish. The bacteria can partly dismantle bile salts, making the bile salts ineffective in fat digestion and absorption. The result is fat malabsorption. Bacteria also compete with the host for vitamin B_{12} and folacin, limiting the supply available to the host. A low-fat diet, parenteral vitamin B_{12}, and/or oral folacin supplements are given to prevent malabsorption and vitamin deficiency. Antibiotics are also prescribed to inhibit bacterial growth. Sometimes the blind loop must be removed surgically.

Short Bowel Syndrome

Pancreatitis, CF, and blind loop syndrome are examples of disorders that can cause malabsorption because they interfere with the digestion of nutrients.

blind loop syndrome:
the problems of fat malabsorption and vitamin B_{12} depletion that can result from the overgrowth of bacteria in a bypassed segment of the intestine.

A **resection** is the removal of a portion of something. Figure 20–2 illustrates gastric resection.

stasis (STAY-sis):
standing still. Normal actions of the intestines keep a steady stream of secretions flowing through them. Stasis in a blind loop allows bacteria to flourish.

FIGURE 20–2
A blind loop resulting from a gastric resection. Note that the segment of the intestine bypassed is no longer flushed by the steady flow of secretions that would normally flow through it.

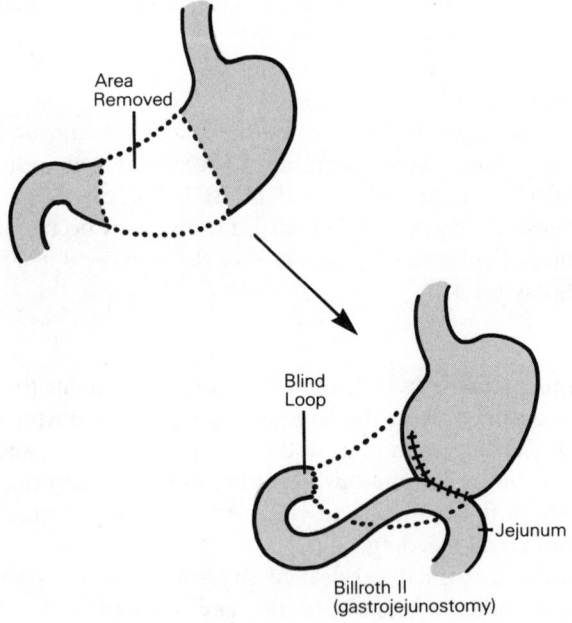

Short bowel syndrome results in malabsorption because the surface area of the intestine normally available for absorbing nutrients is greatly reduced.

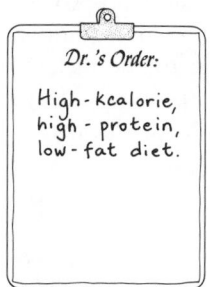

Dr.'s Order:
High-kcalorie, high-protein, low-fat diet.

Short-bowel syndrome may result from surgery in which more than 50 percent of the small intestine is resected. Intestinal resections may be necessary for some people with inflammatory bowel diseases, cancer of the intestine, intestinal obstruction, diverticulitis, or impaired blood supply to the intestine. When a large segment of the small intestine must be resected, the person may experience protein and fat malabsorption, diarrhea, weight loss, muscle wasting, hypocalcemia, hypomagnesemia, and anemia.

People with short bowel syndrome generally absorb carbohydrates and most water-soluble vitamins without difficulty, but their ability to absorb fat, protein, fat-soluble vitamins, calcium, and magnesium is impaired. When the ileum (last portion of the small intestine) has been resected, vitamin B_{12} cannot be absorbed and must be supplemented parenterally. Bile salts are also normally reabsorbed in the ileum also. If they are not reabsorbed, a reduced body pool of bile salts will be available for recycling which will intensify the fat malabsorption. Figure 20–3 shows the site of absorption of different nutrients.

After a small bowel resection, a remarkable adaptive mechanism occurs in the portion of the intestine that remains intact. The bowel becomes longer, thicker, and wider. The result is a greater ability of the remaining bowel to absorb nutrients. The presence of nutrients in the remaining gut appears to stimulate this adaptive response. However, if too much bowel has been resected, even adaptation will fail to compensate for the reduced surface area. In such cases, the person may require permanent support by parenteral means.

short bowel syndrome:
a complex of symptoms that may include malabsorption, diarrhea, weight loss, hypocalcemia, hypomagnesemia, and anemia; it can occur whenever the absorptive surface of the small bowel is reduced.

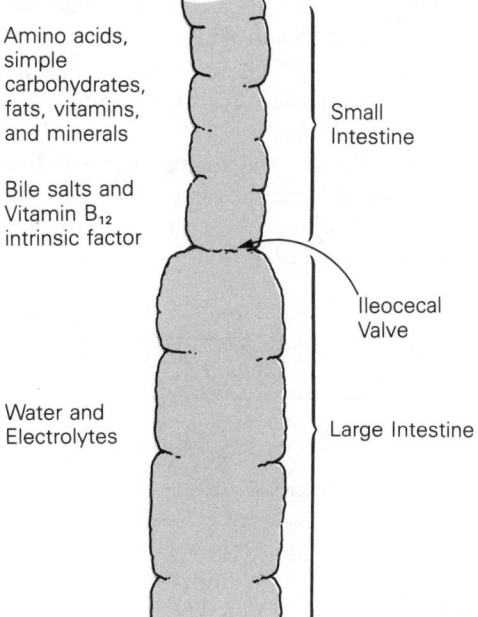

Amino acids, simple carbohydrates, fats, vitamins, and minerals

Bile salts and Vitamin B_{12} intrinsic factor

Water and Electrolytes

Small Intestine

Ileocecal Valve

Large Intestine

FIGURE 20–3
Nutrient absorption in the GI tract.
Absorption of 90 to 95% of nutrients takes place in the first half of the small intestine. After a resection, nutrient absorption is reduced.

Immediately after surgery, the primary nutrition concern is the replacement of fluids and electrolytes. Parenteral feedings are given in the immediate post-operative period. The diet is gradually progressed to a low-fat, high-protein, oral diet, if such a diet can be tolerated. MCT can help provide additional kcalories. Research in animals suggests that adding pectin to the diet can significantly improve adaptation of the bowel following a resection.[11] Further studies will be needed to see if such an effect will occur in human beings.

Gallbladder Disease

cholecystitis (KO-lee-sis-TIE-tis): inflammation of the gallbladder.
chole = bile
cist = sac

The gallbladder stores and concentrates the bile produced in the liver. Some-times the gallbladder becomes inflamed (cholecystitis) or filled with stones.

The symptoms associated with cholecystitis vary. Pain in the area of the gallbladder may occur gradually or suddenly and can be quite severe. Fre-quently nausea, vomiting, and flatulence are present.

Most gallstones form when the cholesterol in the bile gets too concentrated. The cholesterol becomes insoluble in the bile and precipitates, thus causing stones to form. Restricting cholesterol in the diet is unnecessary, because the gallbladder's cholesterol doesn't come from food but from saturated fat and other nutrients made into cholesterol by the liver.

A person with gallstones has **cholelithiasis** (KO-lee-li-THIGH-ah-sis). If the stones obstruct the duct leading to the intestine, **choledocholithiasis** (ko-LED-oh-ko-li-THIGH-ah-sis) is present.
litho = stone
docho = duct

Low-fat diets have traditionally been prescribed for people with gallbladder diseases. The rationale was that fat in the intestine causes the gallbladder to contract, which can cause pain. However, a recent study showed that the gallbladder contracts and ejects bile at the same rate after either a high-fat or a low-fat meal.[12] Thus, the best advice for clients with gallbladder disease is not necessarily to avoid fat but to consume a well-balanced diet and avoid foods, or amounts of food, that cause pain.

Some people with gallbladder disease are intolerant to fat or to particular foods, and their diets should be adjusted accordingly. Obese people should be encouraged to lose weight, especially if surgery is being considered.[13] A high-fiber diet is thought to help prevent gallstone formation, but more research is needed to confirm this possibility.

Often, people with gallstones must have their gallbladders removed (cho-lecystectomy). Following surgery, the same care as outlined in Chapter 16 for other people after surgery is given. When the person advances to an oral diet after surgery, fat is allowed as tolerated.

CASE STUDY

Crohn's Disease

Sara was first diagnosed with Crohn's disease when she was 18 years old. At that time, she weighed 120 lb and was 5′7″ tall. Her normal weight was 130 lb until she began having the symptoms that eventually were found to be caused by Crohn's disease. Since that time, she has been hospitalized several times and has undergone surgery twice to resect portions of the small bowel.

She has an ileostomy. She is now 21, her weight is 123 lb, and she is in the hospital again with a suspected intestinal obstruction. As anticipated from her weight loss history, Sara's nutrition assessment shows that she is suffering from severe PCM. In talking to Sara, you discover that she is very particular about the foods she eats and often simply forgets to eat. She is engaged to be married in 2 months. Sara's physician decided to begin TPN, with strict orders that nothing be given by mouth in the hope that surgery can be avoided.

1. Review Sara's weight history. What is her ideal body weight? What measures could have been taken to avoid weight loss?

2. What are the possible benefits to Sara of TPN?

3. Assume that Sara does well on TPN and is able to avoid surgery. What type of diet will she be placed on when oral intake resumes? Are there any dietary precautions made necessary by the ileostomy (see Chapter 16)? What individual nutrients should be considered?

4. Consider Sara's long-term dietary management. What goals for weight gain should be established? How would you monitor results?

Notes

1. D. F. Kirby and R. M. Craig, The value of intensive nutritional support in pancreatitis, *Journal of Parenteral and Enteral Nutrition* 9 (1985): 353–357.
2. Kirby and Craig, 1985.
3. P. M. Farrell, E. H. Mischler, and S. A. Sondrell, Predigested formula for infants with cystic fibrosis, *Journal of the American Dietetic Association* 87 (1987): 1353–1356.
4. L. A. Lester and coauthors, Supplemental parenteral nutrition in cystic fibrosis, *Journal of Parenteral and Enteral Nutrition* 10 (1986): 289–295.
5. L. D. Levy and coauthors, Effects of long-term nutritional rehabilitation and body composition and clinical status in malnourished children and adolescents with cystic fibrosis, *Journal of Pediatrics* 107 (1986): 225–230; A. L. Mansell and coauthors, Short-term pulmonary effects of total parenteral nutrition in children with cystic fibrosis, *Journal of Pediatrics* 104 (1984): 700–705; R. W. Shepherd and coauthors, Changes in body composition and muscle protein degeneration during nutritional supplementation in nutritionally growth retarded children with cystic fibrosis, *Journal of Pediatric Gastroenterology and Nutrition* 2 (1983): 439–446.
6. S. A. Sondrel and coauthors, Oral nutritional supplementation in cystic fibrosis, *Nutritional Support Services* 7 (April 1987): 20–22.
7. J. B. Kirsner and R. B. Shorter, Recent developments in "nonspecific" inflammatory bowel disease: Part I, *New England Journal of Medicine* 306 (1982): 775–785.
8. M. I. Gee and coauthors, Protein-energy malnutrition in gastroenterology outpatients: Increased risk in Crohn's disease, *Journal of the American Dietetic Association* 84 (1984): 1460–1464.
9. E. Lerebours and coauthors, An evaluation of total parenteral nutrition in the management of steroid-dependent and steroid-resistant patients with Crohn's disease, *Journal of Parenteral and Enteral Nutrition* 10 (1986): 274–278.
10. R. G. Rees and coauthors, Elemental diet administered nasogastrically without starter regimens to patients with inflammatory bowel disease, *Journal of Parenteral and Enteral Nutrition* 10 (1986): 258–262.
11. M. J. Koruda and coauthors, The effect of a pectin-supplemented elemental diet on intestinal adaptation to massive small bowel resection, *Journal of Parenteral and Enteral Nutrition* 10 (1986): 343–350.
12. M. Mogadam and coauthors, Gallbladder dynamics in response to various meals: Is dietary fat restriction necessary in the management of gallstones? *American Journal of Gastroenterology* 79 (1984): 745–747.
13. R. S. Hurley and H. S. Mekhjian, Dietary habits of patients with cholelithiasis: Do we need to instruct? *Journal of the American Dietetic Association* 87 (1987): 209–211.

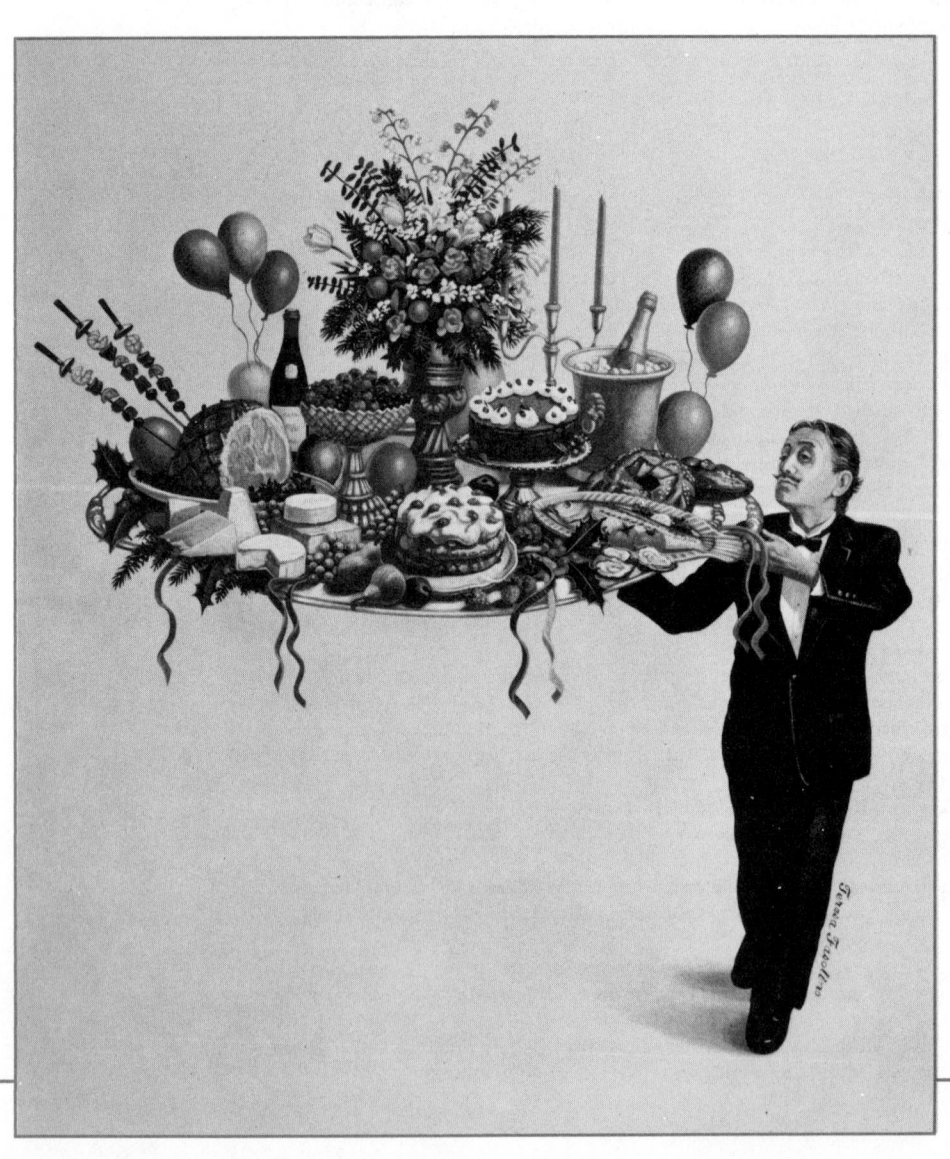

21

Diets Modified in Fat, II: Fat-Controlled, Mineral-Modified Diets

Illustration by Teresa Fasolino.

TABLE 21-1. Indications for the Use of Diets Modified in Fat and Minerals

Atherosclerosis
Diabetes mellitus
Hyperlipidemia
Hypertension
Myocardial infarction
Nephrotic syndrome
Renal failure (chronic)

Saturated fats carry the maximum possible number of hydrogen atoms. **Monosaturated fats** lack two hydrogen atoms and have one double bond between carbons. **Polyunsaturated fats** lack four or more hydrogen atoms and have two or more double bonds between carbons.

Fat-controlled, mineral-modified diets are most frequently prescribed to treat disorders of the cardiovascular system. Table 21–1 lists disorders for which such diets are frequently prescribed. Cardiovascular diseases (CVD) remain the leading cause of adult deaths in the United States.[1] In terms of dollars and cents, it is estimated that the economy has lost 59 billion dollars in productivity because of illness and premature deaths attributed to CVD. Despite these grim statistics, mortality from CVD has been declining by about two percent per year since 1968. Although this news gives us a reason to be optimistic, a good deal still needs to be done.

Fat-Controlled Diets

A fat-controlled diet is a diet in which both the amount and the types of fats are prescribed. It is important for a person on such a diet to pay attention to the amounts of polyunsaturated, monounsaturated, and saturated fats as well as cholesterol. Chapter 3 discusses food sources of the various fats. Table 21–2 shows the fatty acid contents of some common foods. Table 21–3 describes a fat-controlled diet. A sample menu is also provided.

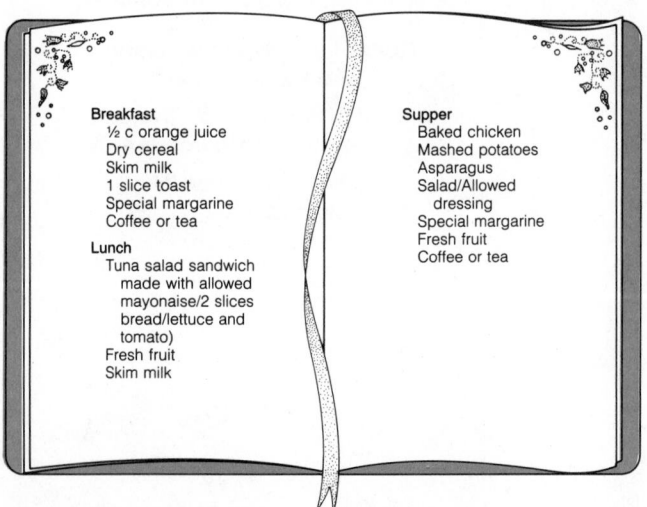

Breakfast
½ c orange juice
Dry cereal
Skim milk
1 slice toast
Special margarine
Coffee or tea

Lunch
Tuna salad sandwich made with allowed mayonaise/2 slices bread/lettuce and tomato)
Fresh fruit
Skim milk

Supper
Baked chicken
Mashed potatoes
Asparagus
Salad/Allowed dressing
Special margarine
Fresh fruit
Coffee or tea

Sample fat-controlled diet menu. All foods are prepared with allowed amounts and types of fats.

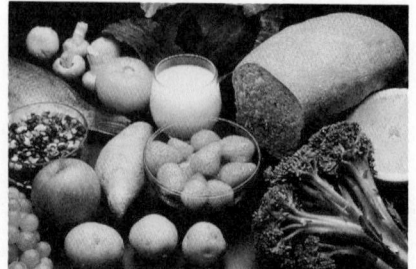

Foods to enjoy on a fat-controlled diet.

The purpose of a fat-controlled diet is to adjust the levels of blood lipids and blood cholesterol to reduce the risk of heart disease. The diet may be difficult for many people to follow, and drastic changes cannot be expected overnight. The development of many new products for use with fat-controlled diets (cholesterol-free eggs, special cheeses, and polyunsaturated margarines) can help considerably. The American Heart Association (AHA) publishes many pamphlets and recipe booklets that are available to both professionals and the

TABLE 21–2. Fatty Acids in Common Fat-containing Foods[a]

Food	Total Fat[b]	Saturated	Monoun-saturated	Polyun-saturated	Linoleic
Animal fat					
Chicken	100	32	45	18	17
Pork (lard)	100	40	44	12	10
Beef (tallow)	100	48	42	4	4
Avocado	15	2	9	2	2
Butter	81	50	23	3	2
Egg yolk	33	10	13	4	4
Margarine, first ingredient					
Safflower (liquid)—tub	80	13	16	48	48
Corn oil (liquid)—tub	80	14	30	32	37
Corn oil (liquid)—stick	80	15	36	24	23
Soybean oil (hydrogenated)—stick	81	15	46	14	10
Nuts					
Walnuts, English	63	7	10	42	35
Walnuts, black	60	5	11	41	37
Brazil nuts	68	17	22	25	25
Pecans	71	6	43	18	17
Peanut butter	52	10	24	15	15
Peanuts	48	9	24	13	13
Salad and cooking oils					
Safflower	100	9	12	74	73
Sunflower	100	10	21	64	64
Wheat germ	100	17	16	61	61
Corn	100	13	25	58	57
Soybean, unhydrogenated	100	14	24	57	50
Cottonseed	100	26	19	51	50
Sesame	100	15	40	40	40
Soybean, hydrogenated[c]	100	15	43	37	22
Peanut	100	17	47	31	30
Palm	100	48	38	9	9
Olive	100	14	72	9	8
Coconut	100	86	6	2	2
Shortening made from vegetable fat	100	25	44	26	23

[a]Within each group, foods highest in polyunsaturated fats are listed first. As you can see, the linoleic acid content closely parallels the polyunsaturated fat content. Fish oils are not shown, because insufficient data were available for this comparison.

[b]The saturated, monounsaturated, and polyunsaturated fatty acids don't add up to 100% of the fat, because there are other, minor fat compounds present.

[c]Common salad and cooking oil for commercial and household use.

Source: Adapted from U.S. Department of Agriculture, Agricultural Research Service, *Fat in Food and Diet,* Agriculture Information Bulletin no. 361 (Washington, D.C.: Government Printing Office, 1977), and H. B. Brown, *Current Focus on Fat in the Diet,* a White Paper (Chicago: American Dietetic Association, 1977).

public to help people make the suggested dietary changes. Recently, the AHA approved a system for identifying foods that meet its dietary recommendations.[2] Processed foods that meet the association's guidelines for fat, cholesterol, and salt will be endorsed as "heart-healthy." Such an endorsement can help people on fat-controlled diets to select processed foods that they can use.

TABLE 21–3. Foods to be Avoided on a Fat-Controlled Diet

Meat and meat alternates
Canned, cured, salted, or smoked meats, including luncheon meats, sausage, ham, bacon, frankfurters; highly marbled and fatty meats; organ meats and sweetbreads; caviar; frozen dinners; egg yolks in excess of two per week.
Milk and milk products
Whole, 2%, and buttermilk; milk products made with more than 1% milk fat, including some yogurts, ice cream; half and half; buttermilk; eggnog; nondairy coffee creamer; high-fat cheeses (containing more than 2 g of fat per ounce) including American, blue, brick, Brie, Camembert, cheddar, Colby, cream, Edam, feta, Gouda, gruyere, Monterey jack, Muenster, provolone, Roquefort, Swiss.
Fruits and vegetables
Any prepared with egg, butter, cream, or cheese sauces; fried vegetables.
Grains
Butter rolls, egg bread, bagels, cheese bread, biscuits, muffins, doughnuts, sweet rolls, pancakes, French toast, cheese crackers, butter crackers, cereal containing coconut, coconut oil, or nuts; potato chips, corn chips, and other fried snacks; grains prepared with eggs, whole milk, cream, fats, or vegetable shortening.
Fats
Butter, meat fat, lard, ham hocks, salt pork, fat back, bacon drippings; gravy or sauce made from fats to be avoided; margarine made from animal fat; salad dressing made from sour cream or cheese; chocolate; coconut or coconut oil; palm or palm kernel oil; cashew, pistachio, and macadamia nuts; nondairy creamer.
Other[a]
Salt, high-salt seasonings or sauces such as Worcestershire or soy; pickles; relish.

[a]Because of the relationship between atherosclerosis and hypertension, a diet moderately restricted in salt is recommended for the individual on a fat-controlled diet. More information on sodium- and salt-restricted diets is given later in this chapter.

Sucrose polyester and Simplesse (see Chapter 3) are fat substitutes that may be available in the future to help those on fat-controlled diets to enjoy the taste of fat without actually consuming it.

The diabetic exchange lists can easily be adapted for use by people with elevated blood lipids. One can carefully adjust the cholesterol and saturated fats in the diet by limiting the use of medium-fat and high-fat meats, whole milk, saturated fats, and bread exchanges high in fat.

Studies of the role of foods in altering blood lipid levels continue to receive high priority. Thus, the advice given today may be outdated tomorrow. Omega-3 fatty acids (found in fish oils) have been associated with reduced serum triglycerides, reduced LDL cholesterol, and slowed progression of atherosclerosis. Including fish in the diet frequently may prove to be beneficial for preventing and treating heart disease. Studies have also suggested that olive oil (a monounsaturated fat) may be as effective as polyunsaturated oils in lowering blood lipids. An added benefit of olive oil is that it does not lower HDL levels, whereas the polyunsaturated oil does.[3] Studies will need to be repeated on a larger number of people to confirm these findings and their potential application.

> The distinction between *blood* cholesterol and the cholesterol in *food* is important here. Everyone agrees that lower blood cholesterol levels are desirable, but whether it helps to reduce cholesterol intake from foods is not clear. We discuss this question more fully in Nutrition in Practice 21A.

Coronary Heart Disease

Diseases of the heart and blood vessels are grouped together and termed cardiovascular disease. When the blood supply to the heart is obstructed, coronary heart disease (CHD) results. When the blood supply to any tissue is cut off, ischemic heart disease (IHD) occurs. The most common cardiovascular disorder is CHD; atherosclerosis is the most common type of CHD.

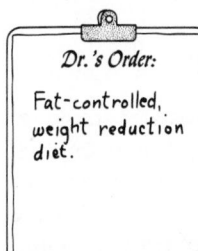

Dr.'s Order:

Fat-controlled, weight reduction diet.

Coronary heart disease is the major cause of death in the United States despite the fact that its prevalence is decreasing. More than one million people suffer heart attacks each year, and half of these people die. Two conditions characterize CHD: Hypertension (high blood pressure—discussed later) and atherosclerosis.

Atherosclerosis

Atherosclerosis is characterized by an accumulation of lipid plaque within the arterial wall. As the plaque enlarges, it narrows the lumen of the artery, raising the pressure of the blood against the wall (much as water pressure increases in a garden hose that has been pinched). The increased pressure can damage the artery wall as well as all organs in the body. Plaque also causes the wall to lose its elasticity so that it cannot expand in response to the beat of the heart; the blood pressure then rises further. This is why atherosclerosis is sometimes called hardening of the arteries. Figure 21–1 illustrates the development of atherosclerosis.

If the plaque narrows the lumen enough, it can completely block the flow of blood within an artery. Death results to all tissues that depend on the artery for nutrients and oxygen. Clots can form and plug the artery. If the blood supply to the heart muscle is cut off, angina or a heart attack can result. When a critical supply of blood to the brain is involved, the result is a stroke. The kidneys, lungs, and peripheral arteries can also be affected. Figure 21–2 shows the interrelationships of various cardiovascular disorders.

A general term used to describe thickening and hardening of the arteries is **arteriosclerosis.** When this process is due to the accumulation of lipid plaque within the arterial wall, the condition is called **atherosclerosis.**

plaque:
mounds of lipid material mixed with smooth muscle cells and calcium that are lodged in artery walls.

gangrene (GANG-green):
death of tissue caused by lack of blood flow to the area.

thrombus:
a stationary clot.

thrombosis:
the blocking off of a blood vessel by a clot.

embolus (EM-boh-luss):
a thrombus that breaks loose.

embolism:
the sudden closure of a blood vessel caused by embolus.

angina (an-JYE-nah or ANN-juh-nuh):
pain in the region of the heart caused by lack of oxygen.

FIGURE 21–1
Development of atherosclerosis.

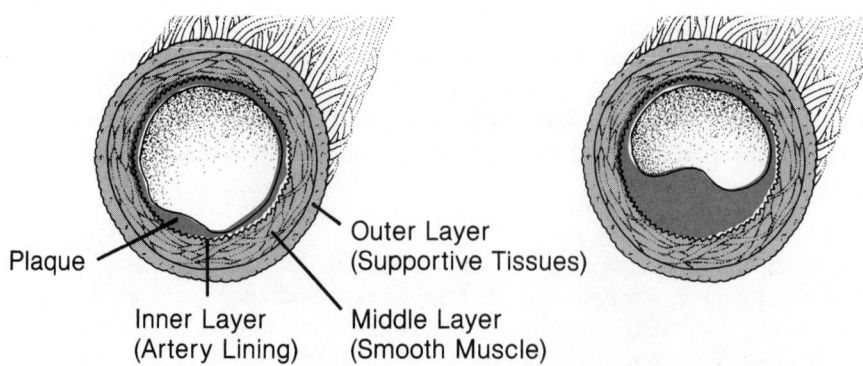

Plaque

Outer Layer
(Supportive Tissues)

Inner Layer
(Artery Lining)

Middle Layer
(Smooth Muscle)

An artery (section) with plaque just beginning to form. Plaques can easily appear in a person as young as 15.

The same artery, years later, half blocked by plaque.

Among the many risk factors associated with atherosclerosis are: smoking, gender (being male), heredity (including diabetes), high blood pressure, lack of exercise, obesity, stress, high blood cholesterol, excesses and deficiencies of many nutrients, and personality characteristics. Not all the risk factors are known, but three have emerged thus far as major predictors of risk: Smoking, high blood cholesterol, and high blood pressure.

The best treatment of atherosclerosis is prevention. All attempts should be made to control the risk factors of atherosclerosis whenever possible. As far as diet is concerned, the AHA recommends that all people (regardless of their blood lipid levels) follow a fat-controlled diet.[4] Specifically, the recommendations include:

- Adjust kcalorie intake to achieve or maintain ideal body weight.
- Limit total fat intake to less than 30 percent of kcalories. Saturated, monosaturated, and polyunsaturated fats should contribute equally to fat kcalories.
- Replace fat kcalories with carbohydrate. Carbohydrates should account for 55 percent of the total kcalories. Complex carbohydrates should provide the majority of these kcalories.
- Limit cholesterol intake to less than 300 milligrams per day.
- Reduce sodium intake to less than three grams per day. (Sodium-restricted diets are discussed later in the chapter.)

Table 21–4 describes ways to achieve these dietary modifications. The recommendation that all people follow a fat-controlled diet is controversial. Nutrition in Practice 21A discusses the controversy and provides additional information about the use of diet in the prevention of atherosclerosis.

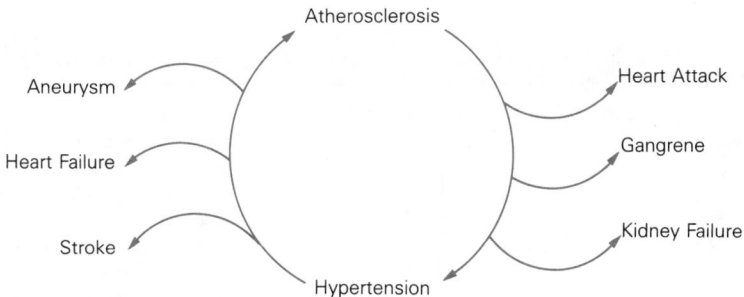

FIGURE 21–2
Interrelationships of various cardivascular disorders.

Far less controversial is the use of fat-controlled diets in the treatment of people who have elevated blood lipids, or hyperlipidemia. Cholesterol, triglycerides, or both may be elevated. Since these lipids are carried through the blood in the lipoproteins (see Chapter 3), different lipoproteins are also elevated. For example, when cholesterol levels are high, low-density lipoproteins (LDL) are elevated; when triglycerides are high, very-low-density lipoproteins (VLDL), or chylomicrons, are elevated. An elevation of any lipid or lipoprotein is called *hyperlipoproteinemia*. Table 21–5 summarizes the dietary modifications useful for controlling various lipid elevations.

One of the most widely used systems for classifying hyperlipidemias is shown in Table 21–6. Using this system, six basic types of hyperlipidemias have been identified. These include types I, IIa, IIb, III, IV, and V. Types II and IV are by far the most common, and they are associated with a high risk of coronary heart disease. Table 21–6 shows which lipoproteins are abnormal in each type of hyperlipidemia. For our purposes here, however, we are not concerned with specific types of hyperlipidemias as much as with how the diet is used to change abnormal lipoprotein patterns.

The AHA recommends a gradual reduction of total fat, saturated fat, and cholesterol for the treatment of elevated serum cholesterol and triglyceride levels.[5] Weight reduction is important for the person who is overweight. Com-

hyperlipidemia (HIGH-per-LIP-ih-DEE-mee-ah):
elevated blood lipids.

hyperlipoproteinemia (HIGH-per-LIP-oh-PRO-teen-EE-mee-ah):
elevated blood lipoproteins; often used interchangeably with hyperlipidemia.

TABLE 21–4. The American Heart Association Diet

To control the amount and kind of fat you eat:
- Limit your intake of meat, seafood, and poultry to no more than 6 ounces per day.
- Use chicken or turkey (without skin) or fish in most of your main meals.
- Choose lean cuts of meat, trim all the fat you can see, and throw away the fat that cooks out of the meat.
- Substitute meatless or "low-meat" main dishes for regular entrees.
- Use no more than a total of 5 to 8 teaspoons of fats and oils per day for cooking, baking, and salads.

To control your intake of cholesterol-rich foods:
- Use no more than three egg yolks a week, including those used in cooking.
- Limit your use of shrimp, lobster, and organ meats.

Source: Reproduced with permission from *The American Heart Association Diet,* American Heart Association.

TABLE 21–5. Dietary Approaches for Lowering Blood Lipids[a]

Elevated Lipid	Major Lipoprotein Involved	Dietary Approach
Dietary triglycerides	Chylomicrons	Total fat restriction
Triglycerides	VLDL	Weight reduction
		Restriction of total fat to less than 20 to 30% of total kcalories
Cholesterol	LDL	Restriction of saturated fat to 10% of fat kcalories
		Restriction of cholesterol to 100 to 300 mg/day

[a]The dietary approach to raising HDL would include weight reduction, correction of elevated triglycerides, and a moderate consumption of alcohol.

plex carbohydrates are recommended. The use of oat products along with a fat-controlled diet can help lower serum cholesterol levels.[6]

The first phase of treatment is the diet described in Table 21–3. After the client has instituted and adjusted to the first phase of the diet, the diet is further restricted as follows:

- 25 percent of kcalories from fat, with equal amounts of the three types of fats.
- 60 percent of kcalories from carbohydrate, emphasizing complex carbohydrates.
- Cholesterol intake of 200 to 250 milligrams per day.

In the final phase, the diet is restricted even further:

- 20 percent of kcalories from fat, with equal amounts of the three types of fats.
- 65 percent of kcalories from carbohydrate, emphasizing complex carbohydrate.
- Cholesterol intake of 100 to 150 milligrams per day.

The client's response to the diet in terms of both blood lipid levels and compliance determines which level of restriction is appropriate. Drug therapy is recommended only if diet therapy fails to bring lipids to normal levels, if

TABLE 21–6. The Hyperlipidemias

Type	Lipoprotein Abnormality
I	Elevated chylomicrons, triglycerides, and cholesterol
IIa	Elevated LDL and cholesterol
IIb	ELevated LDL, VLDL, cholesterol, and triglycerides
III	Elevated VLDL, cholesterol, and triglycerides
IV	Elevated VLDL; normal or elevated cholesterol and triglycerides
V	Elevated chylomicrons, VLDL, triglycerides, and cholesterol

TABLE 21–7. Drug Therapy in Hyperlipidemias

Drug	Lipid Lowered	Nutrition-related Side Effects
Cholestyramine	Cholesterol	Nausea, vomiting, abdominal discomfort, constipation; reduced vitamin B_{12} absorption; malabsorption of fat-soluble vitamins and calcium.
Colestipol	Cholesterol	Same as above.
Clofibrate	Triglycerides, cholesterol	Nausea, vomiting, abdominal discomfort, loose stools; reduced absorption of carotene, glucose, iron, vitamin B_{12}, and electrolytes.
Gemfibrozil	Triglycerides, cholesterol	Nausea, vomiting, abdominal discomfort.
Lovastatin	Cholesterol	Diarrhea, flatulence, altered taste perceptions.
Nicotinic acid	Triglycerides, cholesterol	Nausea, vomiting, abdominal discomfort; decreased glucose tolerance.
Probucol	Cholesterol	Nausea, vomiting, abdominal discomfort, diarrhea.

blood lipid levels are markedly elevated, or if the risk of CHD is especially high because of other risk factors. Drugs useful in the treatment of hyperlipidemias and their nutrition-related side effects are shown in Table 21–7.

Elevated chylomicrons (as in types I and V hyperlipidemia) are treated with a low-fat diet. Instruct the client to limit the amount rather than the type of fat. MCT oil may be used as a source of fat in type I hyperlipidemia, because MCT are not transported in the chylomicron. However, MCT oil is not used in type V, because it can cause an even greater elevation in VLDL, which are already elevated.

Encourage the people with type I or type V hyperlipidemia to avoid alcohol, which can cause elevated serum triglyceride levels. Furthermore, types I and V hyperlipidemia can occur secondary to alcohol abuse or pancreatitis, both of which require that alcohol be avoided.

Evidence is mounting that low serum levels of HDL may be a significant risk factor for the development of CHD. Dietary measures aimed at raising HDL levels include weight reduction (if necessary), correction of hypertriglyceridemia, and a moderate consumption of alcohol. Additionally, frequent and vigorous exercise and abstinence from cigarette smoking are encouraged.

People with hyperlipidemia are frequently advised to follow a sodium-restricted diet in addition to the fat-controlled diet. This recommendation is made because hypertension and hyperlipidemia are frequently found in the same individual. Furthermore, since hypertension is another risk factor for the development of atherosclerosis, any measure that might prevent hypertension is warranted. Hyperlipidemia often occurs along with other disorders, including diabetes (Chapter 19), renal disease (Chapter 22), and nephrotic syndrome (discussed later in this chapter). When these disorders are present in tandem, the diet is adjusted accordingly.

Sodium-Restricted or Low-Salt Diets

1 tsp of salt contains about 2 g of sodium.

Sodium-restricted diets are recommended for people with a variety of disorders, including hypertension, congestive heart failure, some kidney diseases, and cirrhosis, and for people who have suffered heart attacks. People who have diabetes or coronary heart disease (CHD) or who are on corticosteroids may also be advised to follow sodium-restricted or low-salt diets. A sample of a low-sodium diet menu is shown in the text.

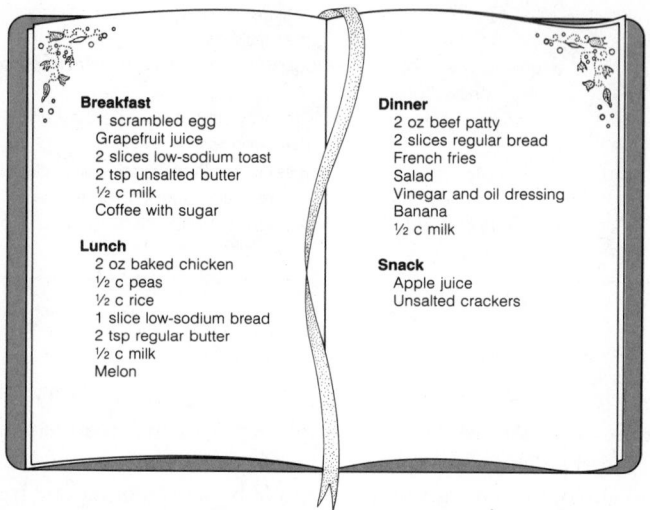

Breakfast
1 scrambled egg
Grapefruit juice
2 slices low-sodium toast
2 tsp unsalted butter
½ c milk
Coffee with sugar

Lunch
2 oz baked chicken
½ c peas
½ c rice
1 slice low-sodium bread
2 tsp regular butter
½ c milk
Melon

Dinner
2 oz beef patty
2 slices regular bread
French fries
Salad
Vinegar and oil dressing
Banana
½ c milk

Snack
Apple juice
Unsalted crackers

Sample 1 mg low-sodium diet menu.

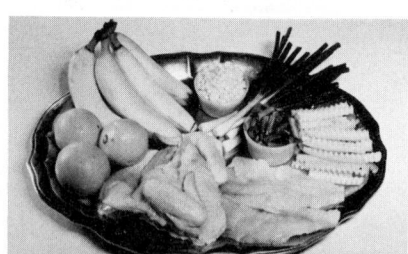

Foods to enjoy on a sodium-restricted diet.

The actual foods that must be restricted vary greatly, depending on the level of sodium prescribed. The diet may contain from 250 milligrams to about four grams of sodium daily. Table 21–8 shows the foods allowed on several different sodium-restricted diets. Table 21–9 describes a no-added-salt or 4-grams sodium diet.

People may find it difficult to drastically change their sodium intakes. Foods eaten without salt may taste unpalatable to the person who normally uses salt liberally. Diet compliance will probably be poor if the person is handed an instruction sheet with no additional encouragement or guidance. You can take several measures to help your client:

- Reduce your client's sodium gradually so that the person can adjust to the flavor of unsalted foods. (People who must be on very low sodium diets, however, usually cannot gradually reduce their sodium intakes.)

- See the person regularly to adjust the sodium level, give encouragement, and help with questions.

- Recommend the use of spices and herbs as shown in Table 21–10 to replace salt in cooking. Cookbooks with low-sodium recipes can be a big help.

TABLE 21–8. Low-Sodium Diets

Foods	Number of Servings Allowed on Various Levels of Sodium Restriction				Serving Size	Sodium per Serving (mg)
	250 Mg	500 Mg	1,000 Mg	2,000 Mg		
Nonfat, whole, and evaporated milk	0	2	2	2	8 oz	120
Low-sodium milk	2	Not restricted	Not restricted	Not restricted	8 oz	7
Meat, fish, poultry, and unsalted cheese	4	4	4	6	1 oz	25
Egg	1	1	1	1	1	60
Bread and allowed ready-to-eat cereal	0	0	2	5	1 slice or ¾ oz	200
Low-sodium bread, cereal, and cereal products	7	7	7	4 or more	Varies	5
Fresh, frozen, or canned without salt: asparagus, bean sprouts, broccoli, Brussels sprouts, cabbage, cauliflower, cucumbers, eggplant, endive, escarole, green pepper, collard and turnip greens, lettuce, mushrooms, okra, onions, radishes, rhubarb, rutabaga, string beans, summer squash, tomatoes, watercress, zucchini, and low-sodium tomato and vegetable juices	2	2	2	Not restricted	½ c	9
Fresh, frozen, or canned without salt: corn, lima beans, parsnips, peas, potatoes, pumpkin, sweet potatoes, winter squash, and yams	1	1	1	Not restricted	½ c	5
Canned vegetables and vegetables frozen with salt	0	0	0	1	½ c	200
Salted butter and margarine	0	0	2	6	1 tsp	50
Regular mayonnaise	0	0	2	6	1½ tsp	50

General diet guidelines:
The foods listed below cannot be used unless they have been calculated into the diet. However, allowances can be made, particularly when the higher levels of sodium are allowed. For example, a person on a 2-g sodium diet who does not drink milk can have 240 mg of sodium from any other food source (see Appendix C). With this in mind, the following foods should be avoided:
1. Salt used in cooking or at the table.
2. Highly salted snacks, such as potato chips, corn chips, tortilla chips, salted popcorn, and pretzels.
3. Barbeque sauce; bouillon cubes (except low sodium); catsup; celery salt, seeds, or leaves; chili sauce; garlic salt; horseradish made with salt; meat extracts, sauces, and tenderizers; monosodium glutamate; prepared mustard; olives; onion salt; pickles; relishes; saccharin; soy sauce; and Worcestershire sauce.
4. Commercial foods made with milk: Ice cream, sherbet, malted milk, milk mixes, and milk shakes.
5. Artichokes, beets, carrots, Chinese or red cabbage, greens (except those listed with vegetables in table above), sauerkraut, and spinach.
6. Maraschino cherries, crystallized or glazed fruits, and dried fruit with sodium sulfite added.
7. Brains; kidneys; canned, salted, or smoked meats; bacon; luncheon meats; chopped or corned beef; kosher meats; shellfish; regular cheeses; egg substitutes; and regular peanut butter.
8. Salted butter or margarine, salt pork, commercial salad dressing (except low sodium), and salted nuts.
9. Leavening agents, such as baking powder and baking soda; rennet tablets; pudding mixes; and molasses.
10. Fountain beverages; instant cocoa mixes; prepared beverage mixes (including fruit-flavored powders); and commercial candy, cakes, cookies, sweetened gelatin mixes, pastries, puddings, cakes, and biscuit mixes.
11. Most commercial dry cereals or instant hot cereals; puffed wheat, puffed rice, and shredded wheat are allowed.

Source: Adapted from American Dietetic Association, *Handbook of Clinical Dietetics* (New Haven, Conn.: Yale University Press, 1981).

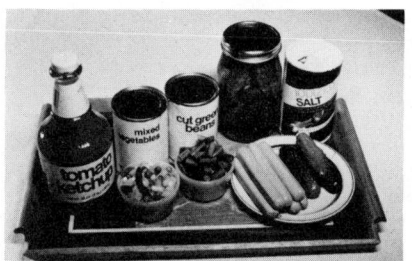

These foods are high in sodium.

TABLE 21–9. No-Added-Salt Diet

- You may lightly salt foods during cooking, but do not add salt at the table.
- Avoid foods high in sodium, including:

Meats—bacon; bologna; cold cuts; chipped or corned beef; frankfurters; smoked meats; sausage; salt pork or codfish; canned, salted, or smoked fish.

Sauces, seasonings, and condiments—regular catsup; celery, garlic, and onion salt; regular chili sauce; commercial meat extracts; meat tenderizers; monosodium glutamate; olives; pickles; prepared mustard; soy and Worcestershire sauce.

Other—regular canned or frozen soups; regular bouillon; soup mixes; pretzels, popcorn, crackers, salted nuts, potato chips, or other salted snack foods; sauerkraut; regular cheese; regular peanut butter.

- Low-sodium products can be substituted for regular foods.

Read labels. You may be surprised to learn that some processed foods that contain no table salt and don't taste salty have lots of sodium. Look for the word *soda* or *sodium* or the symbol *Na* on labels. Examples are *sodium* bicarbonate (baking *soda*), mono*sodium* glutamate, most baking powders, di*sodium* phosphate, *sodium* alginate, *sodium* benzoate, *sodium* hydroxide, *sodium* proprionate, *sodium* sulfite, and *sodium* saccharin.

TABLE 21–10. Sodium-Free Spices and Flavorings

Allspice	Onion powder
Almond extract	Paprika
Bay leaves	Parsley
Caraway seeds	Pepper
Cinnamon	Peppermint extract
Curry powder	Pimiento
Garlic	Rosemary
Garlic powder	Sage
Ginger	Sesame seeds
Lemon extract	Thyme
Mace	Turmeric
Maple extract	Vanilla extract
Marjoram	Vinegar
Mustard powder	Walnut extract
Nutmeg	

The person who must limit potassium should not use potassium-containing salt substitutes.

- Teach your client to read labels. Some words to look out for besides *salt* are given in the margin.

Help people to realize that table salt is not the only source of sodium. Processed foods, milk, and dairy products are high in sodium. Most people are surprised to learn that a serving of cornflakes contains more sodium than a similar weight serving of potato or corn chips.[7] Even some local water supplies have a high sodium content, and when the water is used for preparing and cooking foods, it can significantly contribute to sodium intake. You can check with the local health department for information on the sodium content of the water in your area. Medications, such as antacids, antibiotics, cough medicines, laxatives, pain relievers, and sedatives, may contain sodium. Some toothpastes and mouthwashes also contain large amounts of sodium. Dentists frequently prescribe salt water solutions to irrigate the mouth of the person with gum disease. A significant amount of sodium can be absorbed through the gums this way.[8]

Many low-sodium products are available for use with low-sodium diets. In general, you can plan a palatable diet without the use of these products. Some people, however, particularly those on diets very low in sodium, like to use low-sodium items to add variety. It is important for you and your client to recognize that many of these products are not sodium free, so the amount of sodium they contain must be calculated into the diet.

The sodium in salt substitutes is generally replaced by potassium. Many people don't like the taste of salt substitutes but may find them acceptable if they use them sparingly. Salt substitutes should not be heated, however, because they turn bitter. Some people find food more acceptable without any salt at all. Potassium-containing salt substitutes increase potassium intake. Although this may be good in the treatment of some disorders, in others, such as renal disease, potassium must be restricted, and salt substitutes with potassium are contraindicated. Thus, a physician should be consulted before a salt substitute is used. Other products contain a combination of half regular table salt and half salt substitute. Such products may be more palatable, but they also can contribute significant amounts of salt to the diet.

Hypertension

The body has to maintain a certain blood pressure to sustain the lives of its cells. The pressure of the blood against the walls of the arteries ensures that fluids carrying nutrients and oxygen move out of the arteries into the tissues to deliver their cargo. The blood pressure also helps ensure efficient filtration of wastes into the urine as blood passes through the kidneys.

Dr.'s Order:

No-added-salt, high-potassium, weight-loss diet.

When the blood pressure falls, the life of all the body's cells are threatened. The kidneys detect the lowered pressure and immediately set in motion a mechanism to raise the blood pressure again.

Sometimes, however, the kidneys are fooled. They experience a "water deficiency" when there is none. They then raise the blood pressure with harmful effects. Most often, the cause is atherosclerosis (hardening of the arteries), which deprives the kidneys of water just as if the body had a water deficiency. In response to poor circulation of blood fluid, the kidneys raise the blood pressure, and the heart has to pump extra hard to push the fluid around against resistant arteries. Added body weight (obesity) raises the pressure further, and surplus adipose tissue means miles of additional capillaries through which the blood must be pumped. The combination of high blood pressure, obesity, and atherosclerosis is deadly.

In 10 percent of the cases, hypertension is caused by recognized kidney disease and is called secondary hypertension. The other 90 percent of hypertension cases may also be caused by kidney disease, but the cause is unknown. The vast majority of cases are called *essential* hypertension, meaning that the disease process is primary.

The role of diet in the prevention of hypertension has been debated extensively. Most of the controversy centers on whether a high-sodium diet causes hypertension and, conversely, whether a sodium-restricted diet can prevent it. Additionally, the idea that sodium is a major factor responsible for people's high blood pressure has recently been yielding to the idea that it is salt (sodium chloride) rather than sodium itself that is responsible for the effects seen. Overwhelmingly, sodium's accompanying anion in foods and in body fluids is chloride. Thus, much of the early research that implicated sodium in hypertension's causation may have unwittingly uncovered the effects of sodium's silent partner, chloride. The controversy about sodium and other minerals implicated in hypertension is discussed in Nutrition in Practice 21B. However, it is clear that some people are sensitive to sodium or salt and tend to have high blood pressure that they can lower by reducing their sodium or salt intakes. Many professionals and agencies (including the FDA) recommend that the general public restrict salt intake. They reason that at worst, such a diet cannot be harmful.

The value of incorporating a salt-restricted diet in the treatment of established hypertension is far less controversial. The person with hypertension is often treated with a combination of diet and drugs. A no-added-salt diet is generally advised. Even a mild sodium restriction can result in a modest fall in blood pressure. Weight is also important in the control of hypertension.

hypertension:
chronic elevated blood pressure.

Secondary hypertension is caused by kidney disease. **Primary** or **essential hypertension** is of unknown origin.

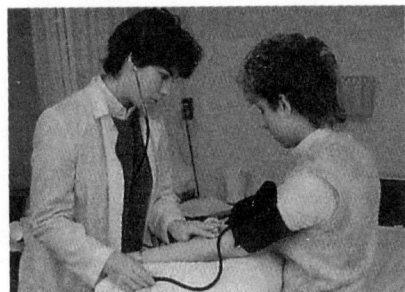

Health care professionals measure blood pressure to identify people with hypertension.

Drugs used to treat hypertension include diuretics and adrenergic blockers. Diuretics work by increasing fluid loss, thus lowering blood pressure. Adrenergic blockers interfere with a neurotransmitter to alter blood pressure. Side effects including fatigue, sexual complaints, and sleep disturbances are commonly reported.

The overweight person with hypertension can also reduce blood pressure simply by losing weight. Although most people who take medication for hypertension will need to take it for the rest of their lives, a small percentage of people may be able to stop taking medication for four or more years if they adhere to a sodium-restricted, weight-loss diet.[9] For those who must continue drug therapy, following the diet along with limiting alcohol consumption may help reduce drug-related side effects.[10]

The diet that is currently recommended for the treatment of people with hypertension restricts all sources of sodium. However, this advice may change if additional research shows that salt rather than sodium is the culprit in hypertension. The rationale for restricting sources of sodium other than salt, such as sodium bicarbonate or sodium proprionate, would not be valid.

When sodium is retained in the body, potassium is excreted. For this reason, many practitioners recommend that good sources of potassium be included in the daily diet. In such a case, salt substitutes containing potassium may be useful. If fed large quantities of sodium, even subjects with normal blood pressure ultimately show a rise in blood pressure—and at the same time, their potassium excretion increases. If fed potassium simultaneously with the sodium, they do not have a rise in blood pressure.[11] Additionally, some diuretics used in the treatment of hypertension can lead to a potassium deficiency. People on these drugs should be encouraged to include good sources of potassium

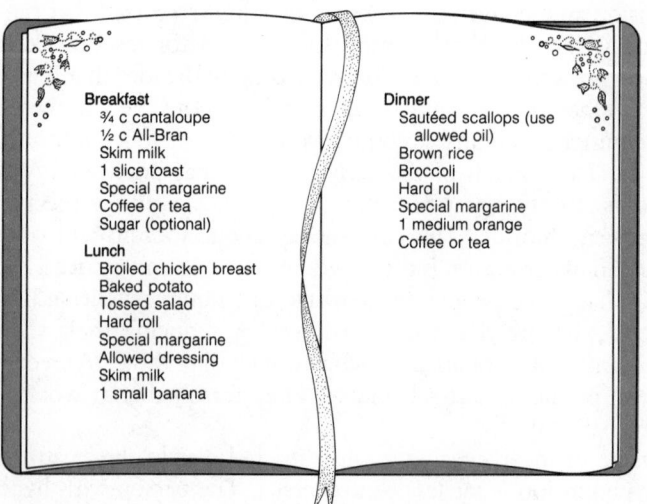

Breakfast
¾ c cantaloupe
½ c All-Bran
Skim milk
1 slice toast
Special margarine
Coffee or tea
Sugar (optional)

Lunch
Broiled chicken breast
Baked potato
Tossed salad
Hard roll
Special margarine
Allowed dressing
Skim milk
1 small banana

Dinner
Sautéed scallops (use allowed oil)
Brown rice
Broccoli
Hard roll
Special margarine
1 medium orange
Coffee or tea

Sample no-added salt, fat-controlled, high-potassium diet menu. Foods for this menu are prepared with little or no salt and minimal amounts of fat. The fats used for cooking or for flavor are monounsaturated or polyunsaturated.

daily; they may be advised to use potassium supplements. Table 21–11 lists foods high in potassium, and Appendix C shows the sodium and potassium contents of foods. Watch for signs of hypokalemia, such as weakness (particularly of the legs), unexplained numbness or tingling sensation, cramps, irregular heartbeat, and excessive thirst and urination. Blood levels of potassium should be monitored regularly to prevent hypokalemia.

Many professionals also advise hypertensive clients to follow a fat-controlled diets. This measure is taken partly because hypertensive people are at greater than normal risk for developing atherosclerosis and partly because polyunsaturated fat may help reduce blood pressure.[12] A sample no-added-salt, fat-controlled, high-potassium menu is shown in the text.

TABLE 21–11. Foods High in Potassium

Vegetables	
Artichokes	Potatoes, baked or pared and boiled
Asparagus	Potatoes, sweet
Beets	Pumpkins
Broccoli	Rutabagas
Brussels sprouts	Spinach
Cabbage, common varieties and Chinese	Squash
Dried beans and peas	Tomatoes
Green beans	Tomato juice
Kale	Turnip greens
Mixed vegetables	Vegetable juice
Parsnips	Winter squash
Pinto beans	Yams

Fruits	
Apricots	Oranges
Apricot nectar	Papayas
Avocados	Peaches
Bananas	Pears
Cantaloupes	Pineapple juice
Dates	Pineapples
Figs	Prune juice
Grapefruit juice	Prunes
Grapefruits	Raisins
Honeydew melons	Rhubarb
Kiwi fruit	Strawberries
Nectarines	Tangerines
Orange juice	

Other	
Chocolate	Molasses, dark and light
Cocoa	Peanuts
Meat	Walnuts
Milk	Wheat germ

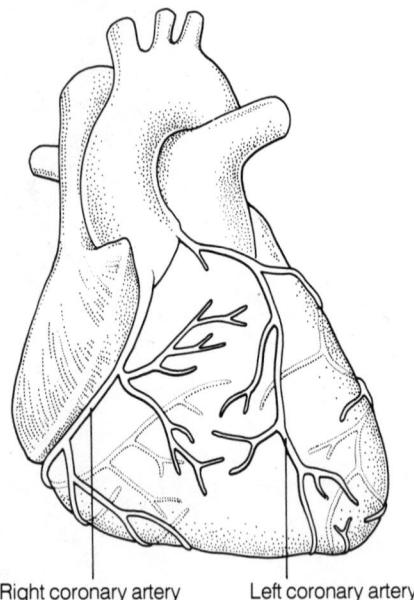

Right coronary artery   Left coronary artery

The **coronary arteries** that lie on the heart's surface supply the heart muscle with nutrients and oxygen.

rheumatic (roo-MAT-ick) **heart disease:**
a general term used to describe heart damage (often affecting the heart valves) that occurs due to rheumatic fever (caused by a bacterial infection).

shock:
sudden, dramatic shift of fluid from the blood to the interstitial space.

Heart Attacks

The heart gets its nutrients and oxygen not from inside its chambers but from arteries that lie on its surface. A myocardial infarction (MI), or heart attack, occurs when the supply of blood to the heart muscle is cut off, resulting in tissue death. Atherosclerosis is a common contributor to heart attacks; some other contributors are abnormal blood clotting, hypertension, spasms of the coronary arteries, infection of the membrane covering the heart, and rheumatic heart disease. As an area of heart tissue dies, enzymes associated with heart cells leak out into the general circulation in a manner similar to the leaking out of digestive enzymes in people with pancreatitis. An elevated level of these enzymes in the blood is often used to diagnose heart attacks.

Dr.'s Order:

Progress diet from a liquid, 2 g sodium diet to a bland, fat-controlled, no-added-salt diet as tolerated.

The heart attack victim, like an accident victim, is in shock at first. In shock, fluid leaves the vascular compartment and moves temporarily to the interstitial space. The person experiences this fluid shift as if it came from dehydration and complains of extreme thirst. The body does not need water when this occurs, however, and increasing its fluid load at such a time would be unwise.

Do not offer food to an individual immediately after an MI; nausea is common. If, as shock resolves, the person remains nauseated, IV infusions are started to prevent dehydration.

After several hours of observation, the person can usually begin to eat. At this time, provide foods that minimize the work of the heart. The diet is moderately restricted in sodium (about two grams) and is low in kcalories (1,000–1,200). Begin with liquid or soft, bland foods given in frequent, small feedings. Such foods are easier to eat and may reduce gas formation and abdominal distension. Abdominal distention pushes the diaphragm up toward the heart, thus placing additional stress on the heart muscle. Temperature extremes can stimulate nerves that slow the heart rate. Many physicians also restrict caffeinated coffee and tea during the first few days after an MI, but this measure is controversial.

After the person is out of immediate danger (in about five to ten days), tailor the diet to meet individual needs—for example, to deal with such conditions as hyperlipidemia, hypertension, obesity, or diabetes. Often, a diet to reduce weight (Chapter 18), control fat, and moderately restrict sodium is appropriate and can be planned to include only three meals a day.

People who continue to have chest pain after an MI may benefit from eating small, frequent meals. Advise them to eat slowly and to rest before and after meals.

Probably all of us know at least one person who seems destined to have a heart attack. He is the overweight, hard-driving executive with hypertension who jokes about exercising and dieting. Then one day it happens. When you visit him in the hospital, you can hardly believe your ears.

Overnight, it seems, your friend's attitude has changed dramatically. He now realizes that he is mortal and begins to value his life. He suddenly respects any advice the health care team can offer. He wants to take positive steps toward changing his lifestyle and improving his chances for survival.

Your friend is a typical MI victim. He is like a sponge trying to soak up any advice that may help him. It is a pleasure to work with a person who listens to what you say and does his best to follow your advice. Be sure to seize the opportunity afforded to you by giving sound and useful counsel. Your friend will benefit from your suggestions, and you will be rewarded by his interest and appreciation.

Congestive Heart Failure

Many diseases—CHD, hypertension, and kidney disease—can lead to congestive heart failure (CHF). In CHF, the heart can no longer pump enough blood through the circulatory system. Because the heart is not adequately pumping, blood flow to the kidneys is reduced. This change signals the kidneys to retain fluid. The retained fluid increases the load on the heart and further weakens it. Since blood entering the heart from the veins cannot be pumped out effectively, peripheral, and sometimes pulmonary edema results. The person becomes "congested" with excess fluids. The heart enlarges and begins to beat more rapidly to try to compensate for its inability to pump. CHF is life threatening, particularly when it is accompanied by pulmonary edema.

congestive heart failure:
a syndrome in which the heart can no longer adequately pump blood through the circulatory system.

pulmonary edema:
accumulation of fluid in the lungs.

Dr.'s Order:

Bland, sodium-restricted, fluid-restricted, diet given in small, frequent meals.

Another complication occurs because of the heart's inadequate pumping ability. The supply of nutrients and oxygen normally carried in the blood to the peripheral tissues is disrupted. Malnutrition can result, particularly as the disorder progresses. Other factors intensify the risk of malnutrition, including anorexia, altered taste sensitivity, intolerance to food odors, physical exhaustion precipitated simply by the act of eating, the diet used for treatment (some people find the diet unappealing), and the long-term use of medications that interfere with nutrition status. Undernutrition in people with CHF often goes unnoticed, because edema masks these people's underweight condition. Malnutrition, in turn, can precipitate or aggravate heart failure.[13]

Diuretics and drugs that increase the strength of heart muscle contractions are important in the treatment of CHF. Bed rest helps to reduce the workload on the heart. Diet therapy includes measures to reduce the work required of the damaged heart and to alleviate edema. A sodium- and fluid-restricted diet (see Chapter 22) tailored to the individual's needs is recommended. Generally, a two-gram sodium diet and a fluid restriction of about 1 ½ to 2 liters of fluid are provided daily. Such a diet can help prevent fluid overload and reduce diurectic needs.[14]

The person with CHF is often underweight and malnourished, as previously mentioned. However, if the person is overweight, weight reduction is very important in relieving additional stress to the heart.

People suffering from CHF can easily become exhausted when eating and may benefit from frequent small meals and snacks. As in MI, small feedings of foods least likely to form gas will reduce the abdominal distension that displaces the diaphragm toward the heart. Liquid formulas of high-nutrient density may be useful. Tube feedings may be necessary to prevent or correct malnutrition when the person cannot take adequate foods by mouth. If a tube feeding is necessary, the feeding should be delivered with the person in a sitting or only slightly reclining position to reduce the risk of aspiration. In some cases, TPN may be indicated. When liquid formulas, tube feedings, or parenteral solutions are given, the amount of fluid must be carefully monitored. kCalorically dense enteral and parenteral solutions can be useful in CHF.

Although it is important to provide adequate nutrients to the person with CHF, overfeeding the severely malnourished person is also a concern. Too rapid refeeding may increase the blood volume and metabolic rate and overload the already taxed heart. A gradual return to optimal intake is a wiser course.

Nephrotic Syndrome

The loss of protein in the urine is **proteinuria.**

Nephrotic syndrome is not a disease but rather a combination of symptoms caused by the loss of plasma protein into the urine. Normally, only small plasma proteins pass through the nephrons (the functional units of the kidney); these proteins are then reabsorbed and returned to the blood. In nephrotic syndrome, this mechanism is defective and plasma proteins are lost in the urine. Because albumin is the major plasma protein, it is also the major protein lost.

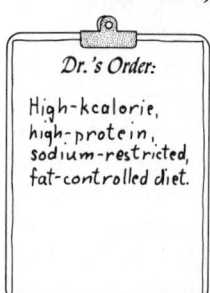

Dr.'s Order:

High-kcalorie, high-protein, sodium-restricted, fat-controlled diet.

As plasma proteins are lost, the blood levels of proteins fall sharply. Together with other factors, low blood protein levels cause fluid to move into the interstitial space, and edema develops. As protein loss continues, lean body mass breaks down. Losses of other plasma proteins, such as immunoglobulins, render the person with nephrotic syndrome prone to infections, which can further compromise nutrition status. The loss of transferrin, the iron-carrying protein, can lead to anemia (see Figure 21–3). Serum lipid levels rise markedly for unknown reasons.

Treatment of nephrotic syndrome depends largely on the underlying cause. Diet is always important in preventing protein malnutrition and alleviating edema. A diet high in kcalories (50 to 60 kcalories per kilogram of body weight) and high in protein (about 120 grams per day) is prescribed. Sodium restriction is important, because the body avidly retains sodium in nephrotic syndrome. In the early treatment, a diet very low in sodium (250 milligrams) is used to help mobilize the fluid that has accumulated in the interstitial space. Diuretics also are used for this purpose. Once the person is free of edema and sodium balance has been achieved, the sodium restriction is liberalized to about 1,500 milligrams per day, which is still a fairly low sodium intake. If potassium-wasting diuretics are prescribed, foods high in potassium (see Table 21–11) become important in the diet.

People with nephrotic syndrome often have hyperlipidemia, most commonly type II or type V. Because such individuals are also at high risk for atherosclerosis, it is often recommended that they follow the appropriate fat-controlled diet.

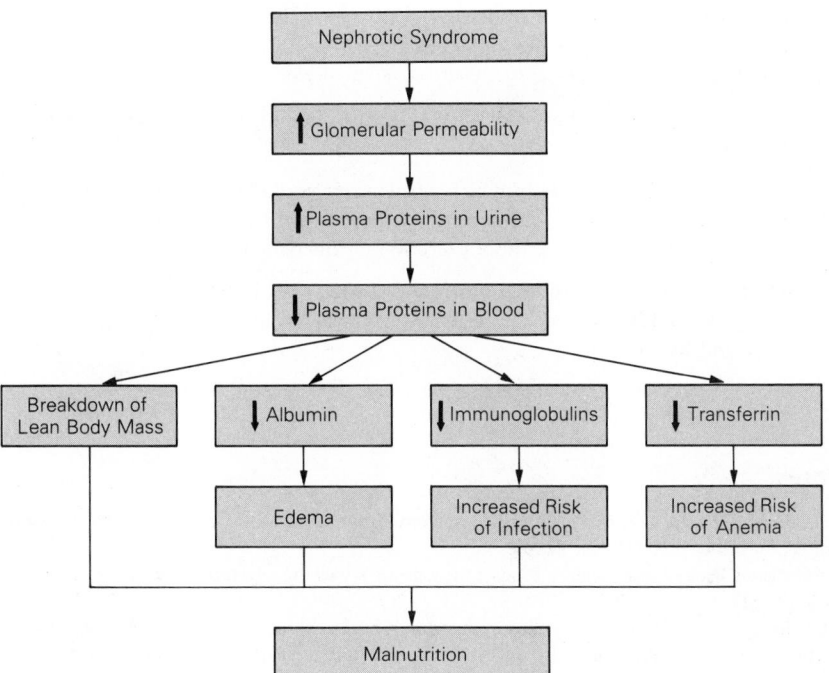

FIGURE 21–3
Consequences of nephrotic syndrome.

CASE STUDY

Hyperlipidemia and Hypertension

Mr. Garrett, age 45, has just been diagnosed to have type IV hyperlipidemia. He is 5′7″ tall and weighs 200 lbs. Mr. Garrett has a family history of CHD. His diet is high in kcalories, cholesterol, total fat, saturated fat, and sodium. He smokes a pack of cigarettes a day. Mr. Garrett runs a family-owned video rental business and his lifestyle leaves little room for exercise. About once a month Mr. Garrett enjoys playing golf with a group of friends. His wife cherishes her role as homemaker, and Mr. Garrett boasts that she is the best cook in town. Mr. Garrett also has hypertension, for which diuretics have been prescribed. He frequently forgets to take his pills, though, and his blood pressure is often quite high.

1. Name the risk factors for CHD in Mr. Garrett's history. Which of them can he control? Which can be helped by diet? What complications can result from CHD?

2. What type of diet, if any, would you recommend for Mr. Garrett's type of hyperlipidemia? Explain the rationale for each diet change. How will his current diet change? What types of foods should he eat?

3. What type of diet, if any, would you recommend for Mr. Garrett's hypertension? What suggestions might you offer to help him make the necessary

diet changes? Are these diet changes consistent with those you would recommend for type IV hyperlipidemia? What blood value should be monitored regularly? Why?

4. How can you enlist the aid of Mrs. Garrett in helping Mr. Garrett improve his diet?

5. Name at least three ways in which Mr. Garrett could benefit from losing weight. How can exercise fit into a weight loss plan? Describe ways Mr. Garrett could incorporate more exercise into his daily routine.

6. Describe nutrition considerations if Mr. Garrett should have a heart attack or develop CHF. Discuss the relationship of these disorders to hyperlipidemia and hypertension.

Notes

1. Centers for Disease Control, Years of life lost from cardiovascular disease, *Journal of the American Medical Association* 256 (1986): 2794.

2. Associated Press, Heart-healthy foods to get group's backing, *Atlanta Constitution,* June 27, 1988, p. 15D.

3. C. Sirtori and coauthors, Controlled evaluation of fat intake in the Mediterranean diet: Comparative activities of olive oil and corn oil on plasma lipids and platelets in high-risk patients, *American Journal of Clinical Nutrition* 44 (1986): 635–642.

4. American Heart Association, The American Heart Association Diet. An eating plan for healthy Americans, American Heart Association National Center, Dallas, Texas, 1985.

5. American Heart Association, Recommendations for treatment of hyperlipidemia in adults, *Circulation* 69 (1984): 1065A–1090A.

6. L. V. Van Horn and coauthors, Serum lipid response to oat product intake with a fat-modified diet, *Journal of the American Dietetic Association* 86 (1986): 759–764.

7. S. W. Lugar and E. McCormick, Letter to the editor: Breakfast of champions or of hypertensives? *New England Journal of Medicine* 314 (1986): 1052–1053.

8. S. B. Kaminsky, W. B. Gillette, and T. J. O'Leary, Sodium absorption with oral hygiene procedures, *Journal of the American Dental Association* 114 (1987): 644–646.

9. A. L. Dannenberg and W. B. Kannel, Remission of hypertension: The 'natural' history of blood pressure treatment in the Framingham study, *Journal of the American Medical Association* 257 (1987): 1477–1483.

10. R. S. Stamler and coauthors, Nutritional therapy for high blood pressure: Final report of a four-year randomized controlled trial—The Hypertension Control Program, *Journal of the American Medical Association* 257 (1987): 1484–1490.

11. A. W. Caggiula, R. R. Wing, and R. G. Jacob, An apple a day: The role of potassium in the treatment of mild hypertension, *Behavioral Medicine Abstracts* 4, Summer 1983, p. 137.

12. P. Puska and coauthors, Controlled, randomised trial of the effect of dietary fat on blood pressure, *Lancet,* January 18, 1983, pp. 1–5.

13. S. M. Poindexter, W. E. Dear, and S. J. Dudrick, Nutrition in congestive heart failure, *Nutrition in Clinical Practice* 1 (1986): 83–88.

14. R. W. Hamilton and V. M. Buckalew, Sodium, water and congestive heart failure, *Annals of Internal Medicine* 100 (1984): 902–903.

Diet and the Prevention of Atherosclerosis

More than half the people who die in the United States each year die of heart and blood vessel disease, mostly by way of heart attacks and strokes. The underlying condition that contributes to most of these deaths is coronary heart disease (CHD). There is little wonder, then, that much effort has been focused on preventing CHD. Nutrition in Practice 21A discusses whether people can prevent atherosclerosis by following special diet guidelines.

I'm very concerned about preventing atherosclerosis. Several members of my family have hyperlipidemia, and others have died from CHD. What are my chances of having the same problem?

First of all, it's important for you to remember that no one knows the causes of atherosclerosis. The risk factors for CHD that have been identified are correlations only. Smoking, high blood cholesterol, and high blood pressure seem to be the most important of these, but clearly there are others, still unknown.

Table NP21A–1 shows one way of calculating your risk score based on present knowledge. Such a quiz helps you look not only at what your risks may be but also points out areas that you can change to reduce your risk. From statistics pooled from many studies on risk factors, the AHA has published the *Coronary Risk Handbook*. The small portion dealing with six-year predictions for a 45-year-old man is shown in Table NP21A–2. The table illustrates dramatically that the

chances of having a healthy heart and arteries are much greater if you don't smoke and your blood cholesterol and blood pressure are low.[1]

Well, after taking the quiz, I see there are some areas that I can change to improve my risk score. I can't help but wonder if it will really help.

Many people, of course, would like to know the answer to your question. Again, there are no absolutes, but many studies are being conducted to try to find out.

In some massive studies conducted during the 1970s, thousands of men were persuaded to give up smoking, take medication to reduce their blood pressure if it was high, and alter their diets to reduce their blood cholesterol levels. These studies were complicated by a curious situation, however: everyone else was doing those same things. Word had gotten around to the whole U.S. population that these measures were beneficial. The studies failed to show significant improvement of the experimental groups over controls, perhaps because there *were* no good controls. An analysis of the impressive downturn in the rate of deaths from CHD between the late 1960s and the late 1970s suggests that a large-scale prevention effort may have been spontaneously mounted by the entire U.S. population.

In any case, something certainly seems to have happened in that 10-year period in which 200,000 lives were saved.[2] At a major conference held in 1979, the experts who had

been following the lifestyle changes and trends among people in the United States reported four significant events:

1. We are smoking less.
2. We are controlling our blood pressure better.
3. Our blood cholesterol levels have fallen slightly.
4. We are exercising more.

In other words, independently of the research studies, people have been taking measures that are lowering mortality. The evidence from review of the effect of taking these measures suggests that reduction of risk factors is advisable for all members of the population, not just for those most prone to heart attacks.

Fortunately, I don't have high blood pressure and I quit smoking years ago. Tell me more about blood cholesterol levels.

Let's first clarify one point: We are talking about *blood* cholesterol, not the cholesterol in foods. In the blood, cholesterol is carried in LDL and HDL. It is the LDL that are associated with heart disease. Changes in diet that reduce serum cholesterol concentrations mostly do so by reducing LDL. The most important dietary factor affecting blood cholesterol is saturated fat, not the cholesterol in foods. The most effective dietary measures to lower blood cholesterol are these:

NUTRITION IN PRACTICE 21A

TABLE NP21A–1. Your Risk of Heart Disease

	H	E	A	R	T

Everyone plays the game of health whether he wants to or not. What is your score? Add up the numbers in each category that most nearly describe you.

	1	2	3	4	6
Heredity[a]	No known history of heart disease	One relative with heart disease over 60 years	Two relatives with heart disease over 60 years	One relative with heart disease under 60 years	Two relatives with heart disease under 60 years
Exercise	1 Intensive exercise, work, and recreation	2 Moderate exercise, work, and recreation	3 Sedentary work and intensive recreational exercise	5 Sedentary work and moderate recreational exercise	6 Sedentary work and light recreational exercise
Age	1 10–20	2 21–30	3 31–40	4 41–50	6 51–65
Lbs.	0 More than 5 lb below standard weight	1 ± 5 lb standard weight	2 6–20 lb overweight	4 21–35 lb overweight	6 36–50 lb overweight
Tobacco	0 Nonuser	1 Cigar or pipe	2 10 cigarettes or fewer per day	4 20 cigarettes or more per day	6 30 cigarettes or more per day
Habits of eating fat[b]	1 0%: No animal or solid fats	2 10%: Very little animal or solid fats	3 20%: Little animal or solid fats	4 30%: Much animal or solid fats	6 40%: Very much animal or solid fats

[a]Diabetes and hypertension in the family are also predictors.

[b]If you know your blood cholesterol, use it instead. Below 180 = 0 points. 180–200 = 1 point. 201–235 = 2 points. 236–260 = 4 points. 261–300 = 5 points. Over 300 = 6 points.

Your risk of heart attack:
  4–9 Very remote.
10–15 Below average.
16–20 Average.
21–25 Moderate.
26–30 Dangerous.
31–35 Urgent danger—reduce score!
Other conditions—such as stress, high blood pressure, and increased blood cholesterol—detract from heart health and should be evaluated by your physician.

Source: Courtesy of Loma Linda University.

TABLE NP21A–2. Risk of Developing CHD Within Six Years (The effect of the three major risk factors are shown alone and in combination for a 45-year-old man.)

Smoker	Cholesterol (mg/100 ml[a])	Blood Pressure (mm mercury[b])	Risk (per 100)
No	185	105	1.5
No	185	195	4.4
No	335	195	16.7
Yes	335	195	23.9

[a]Milligrams of cholesterol per 100 ml blood.

[b]The first of the two numbers recorded (for example, *120* in 120/70). The silver column that rises on a blood-pressure instrument is a column of mercury; the height to which it is pushed is marked off in millimeters.

Source: U.S. Senate, Select Committee on Nutrition and Human Needs, *Diet Related to Killer Diseases II, Part 1, Cardiovascular Disease* (hearings), (Washington, D.C.: U.S. Government Printing Office), 1977.

* Lower your saturated fat intake to 10 percent of total kcalories or less.
* Partially substitute monounsaturated and polyunsaturated fats for saturated fats.
* Limit your cholesterol intake to 300 mg a day or less.

There is less agreement about the third of these than about the other two.

A factor that complicates the question of whether we should reduce our intakes of cholesterol from food is an accident that has occurred repeatedly in research on this question. When purified cholesterol sits in a jar on a laboratory shelf, it changes chemically to a variety of oxidation products. When experimental animals are fed diets containing this product, they aren't actually being fed cholesterol. The researchers may therefore report that cholesterol is responsible for the results of the study when in fact it is not.

The fact that cholesterol oxidizes readily on exposure to air is of great concern to researchers, because it happens that the oxidation products are highly toxic to the arteries. Researchers are concerned, too, because oxidation of cholesterol may occur not only in bottles in the laboratory but also in meats, eggs, and milk products that are exposed to air—especially those that are highly processed.[3] The question of whether or not we should attempt to reduce our intake of dietary cholesterol is thus still open.

What can I do to reduce my blood cholesterol levels while waiting for the answers to these questions?
A host of studies has produced a host of possible answers to your question. Many foods and nutrients have been studied to see if they raise or lower blood cholesterol levels, and some of the findings are surprising and interesting. It appears as if the person who wishes to use every possible dietary means to lower blood cholesterol would do all of the following:

* Eat fish, especially fatty fish such as mackerel and salmon, often.
* Use nonfat milk and nonfat milk products, especially fermented products such as yogurt, freely.
* Consume abundant legumes of many varieties, including soybeans and chickpeas.
* Eat generous amounts of fiber-rich fruits and vegetables, including many raw ones.
* Use whole grains (especially oats, and not especially wheat) and sprouts (especially alfalfa sprouts) often.
* Flavor foods liberally with garlic and hot peppers.

Of particular interest are the new findings on fish and fiber. As mentioned in Chapter 3, fish oils contain EPA and other omega-3 fatty acids, which lower blood cholesterol and triglycerides and reduce the tendency of blood to clot.[4] One or two fish dishes a week are all it takes to exert a significant effect,[5] and the fattiest cold-water fish are the most effective: Mackerel, herring, sardines, bluefish, salmon, tuna, Pacific oysters, European anchovies, squid, and others.

Dietary fiber may also confer benefits. Persons on high-fiber diets have been shown to excrete more bile acids, sterols, and fat than persons on low-fiber diets. One reason for the lowered blood cholesterol levels following a high-fiber regimen is a faster transit time for materials through the GI tract which allows less time for cholesterol absorption. Also, if the body is losing bile acids bound to fiber components, it must simultaneously synthesize new bile acids from its stores of cholesterol, and some of these will then be excreted, reducing body cholesterol further. Diets high in fiber are typically low in fat and cholesterol anyway—another advantage to emphasizing fiber.

The various dietary fibers have varying effects on blood cholesterol. The soluble fibers pectin and guar gum have greater cholesterol-lowering effects than the insoluble fibers cellulose and lignin. Indeed, rolled oats and oat bran, rich in soluble fiber, have favorable effects on blood cholesterol, whereas wheat bran, high in cellulose, is far less effective. Apples, pears, peaches, oranges, and grapes are good sources of pectin.

In addition to taking these positive measures, concentrate on obtaining adequate nutrients from food without eating excessive kcalories and go easy on protein-rich foods. These food choices resemble those advocated by the *Dietary Guidelines*, which thus seem to have mounting evidence in their favor.

Earlier you mentioned that cholesterol is carried in the blood in LDL and HDL. I have heard of HDL in the news and am wondering if they are related to CHD risk.

Yes, they are, but in a different way. While most of the blood cholesterol is carried in the LDL and correlates *directly* with CHD risk, some is carried in the HDL and correlates *inversely* with risk. In fact, for men over 50, the most potent single predictor of heart-attack risk may be the HDL level—the higher, the better. A word of caution: As with other risk factors, we don't know for sure if raising HDL will have a beneficial effect on reducing CHD risk.

How can I raise my HDL levels?

One way to have higher HDL levels is to be female. Women have higher HDL levels than men. Another, interestingly, seems to be to stop smoking. Nonsmokers have uniformly higher HDL levels than smokers. Still another is to be in the process of losing weight.

A few investigators have reported that the consumption of moderate amounts of alcohol appeared to raise HDL levels; however, it is becoming apparent that there is more than one kind of HDL and that the kind of HDL affected by alcohol may not be the "good" kind. But by far the most powerful influence on HDL levels is exercise—prolonged, intense, and frequent. Evidence suggests that HDL levels can be improved in very sedentary people who become only moderately active.[6]

Is there anything else I should know about reducing my risk of heart disease?

Remember that even if you religiously take all the steps discussed here, there is no 100 percent guarantee that you will never have heart trouble. We'd encourage you to do them anyway, though, because they are good health practices.

Although diet and nutrition have been the focus of attention here, it seems important to conclude by taking a broader view of the problem of CHD. Nutrition is obviously not the only factor involved. The lifestyle of our whole society is an urbanized, competitive, industrial society with built-in stresses that have a major impact on health. Society itself may need to change in fundamental ways before we can arrive at ultimate solutions to some health problems.

Notes

1. M. F. Oliver, Diet and coronary heart disease, *British Medical Bulletin* 37 (1981): 49–58.
2. R. Levy, Introduction, in *Proceedings of the Conference on the Decline in Coronary Heart Disease Mortality*, ed. R. J. Havlik and M. Feinleib, U.S. Department of Health, Education, and Welfare, Public Health Service, National Institutes of Health, NIH publication no. 79–1610, May 1979, p. 1.
3. F. A. Kummerow, Nutrition imbalance and angiotoxins as dietary risk factors in coronary heart disease, *American Journal of Clinical Nutrition* 32 (1979): 58–83.
4. A. M. Fehily and coauthors, The effect of fatty fish on plasma lipid and lipoprotein concentrations, *The American Journal of Clinical Nutrition* 38 (1983): 349–351; W. S. Harris and coauthors, in *Nutrition and Heart Disease* (London: Churchill Livingston, 1983) as cited by Fish oils, serum lipids and platelet aggregation, *Nutrition and the MD*, January 1985.
5. D. Kromhout, E. B. Bosschieter, and C. D. Coulander, The inverse relation between fish consumption and 20-year mortality from coronary heart disease, *New England Journal of Medicine* 312 (1985): 1205–1209.
6. Dozens of research articles now support this finding. A typical one is J. G. Brook and coauthors, High-density lipoprotein subfractions in normolipemic patients with coronary atherosclerosis, *Circulation* 66 (1982): 923–926.

Minerals and Hypertension

The role of diet in preventing hypertension has been much debated. Most of the controversy centers on whether a high-salt diet causes hypertension and, conversely, on whether a salt-restricted diet can prevent it. Studies on the roles of other minerals and their effects on blood pressure have also been in the news.

I have heard it said so many times that cutting down on sodium is a good idea for everyone. Is it?
Sodium clearly has something to do with blood pressure. In fact, for years, research on populations has seemed to indicate that high sodium intakes were a major factor responsible for people's high blood pressure; but recently that idea has been yielding to the idea that it is salt (sodium chloride) that is responsible for the effects seen. As mentioned in Chapter 21, sodium's accompanying anion in foods and in the body fluids is chloride. Early research that implicated sodium in hypertension's causation may have unwittingly uncovered the effects of sodium's silent partner, chloride. Apparently, sodium in combination with other negative ions causes water retention and certain hormonal responses, but sodium chloride, uniquely, seems to raise blood pressure.[1]

The sodium (and chloride) concentration in the blood and other body tissues is maintained through an elaborate regulatory mechanism involving the kidneys, the adrenal glands, the pituitary gland, and other glands. Most people can therefore safely consume more salt than they need, and rely on these control mechanisms to regulate the excretion and retention of sodium as needed. Genetically salt-sensitive individuals, however, experience high blood pressure from excesses in salt intake.

How dietary salt contributes to hypertension in those who are salt-sensitive is unknown, but recent research suggests a chain of events that leads to contraction of the small arteries, increasing peripheral resistance. The chain begins with an inherited or acquired defect in the kidneys.

When salt intake exceeds what the kidneys can excrete, sodium, chloride, and other negative ions are retained in the blood, water accompanies them, and the blood volume expands. The extra fluid volume is thought to help bring about the secretion of a hormone (natriuretic hormone) not normally active, that enables the kidneys to excrete some of the excess. However, the same hormone moves sodium (and chloride and other negative ions) into the smooth muscle cells that line the arteries, and affects their membranes so that they bring in too much calcium, too. The more calcium, the more these muscle cells contract, the more peripheral resistance increases and the higher the blood pressure rises.[2] In short, the hormone trades a wrong for a right: It reduces the blood volume, but it increases peripheral resistance so that blood pressure stays high.

For salt-sensitive individuals, then, eating a diet low in salt is a wise idea. But for others—the majority of people with hypertension—this may not be an effective diet strategy. Salt restriction does not lower blood pressure in half of the hypertensive people in whom it is tried.[3]

However, because not all those who are salt-sensitive know who they are and no one can tell by "feel" when blood pressure is high, some authorities contend that the whole population should be encouraged to reduce salt intake. The U.S. government's *Dietary Guidelines for Americans* and the Canadian government's guidelines both recommend a moderate reduction in salt intake. Clearly it is important to see what other dietary factors are important in hypertension.

Earlier you mentioned that other minerals might be involved. Which ones are they?
Several minerals have been linked to hypertension, most notably potassium, calcium, and magnesium. It is difficult to look at any of these minerals (including sodium) individually, because a change in one nutrient generally means that the intake or availability of other nutrients will be modified.

Potassium and sodium provide a good example. As discussed in Chapter 21, when sodium is retained in the body, potassium is excreted. Population studies reveal another interrelationship between sodium and potassium. People who eat many foods high in sodium—processed foods, for example—necessarily eat fewer potassium-containing foods, such as fruits and whole vegetables, at the same time (see Table NP21B–1). So it is difficult to pinpoint whether an increased availability of sodium or a decreased availability of potassium or both are related to blood pressure.

How do calcium and magnesium fit into the picture?
Calcium and magnesium are implicated because of the observation that people who drink hard water have a lower incidence of hypertension and heart disease than those who drink soft water. Hard water contains more calcium and magnesium, whereas soft water contains more sodium and chloride. Is it the higher sodium content of soft water that contributes to hypertension or the calcium and magnesium in hard water that protect against it? Other evidence also suggests that calcium prevents hypertension.

I'd like to know more about this evidence.
An excellent review of the subject has been published.[4] Although it is beyond the scope of this discussion to mention all of the studies cited in the review, we list a synopsis from the review:

- Several dietary surveys suggest that people with high blood pressure eat

TABLE NP21B–1. Whole Unprocessed Foods Versus Processed Foods—Potassium and Sodium Content

Food	Amount	Potassium (mg)	Sodium (mg)	Potassium-to-Sodium Ratio
Milk Foods				
Milk	1 c	370	122	3:1
Chocolate pudding (cooked from mix)	1 c	354	343	1:1
Chocolate pudding (instant)	1 c	335	820	1:2
Meats				
Beef roast (cooked)	3 oz	279	42	7:1
Corned beef (canned)	3 oz	51	803	1:16
Chipped beef	3 oz	170	3660	1:22
Vegetables				
Corn (cooked)	1 c	304	71	4:1
Creamed corn (canned)	1 c	248	671	1:3
Sugar-coated cornflakes	1 c	27	262	1:10
Fruits				
Peaches (fresh)	1 peach	202	1	202:1
Peaches (canned)	1 peach	333	5	67:1
Peach pie	1 piece	201	201	1:1
Grains				
Whole-wheat flour	1 c	444	4	100:1
Whole-wheat bread	1 slice	68	132	1:2
Doughnut, snack cake	1	23	125	1:5

less calcium (as a group) than do people with normal blood pressure.

- In a double-blind, placebo-controlled study, blood pressure was reduced in 45 percent of hypertensive subjects who took calcium supplements.

- The same study also suggested that people with hypertension may have an altered calcium balance. Although those with hypertension reported eating less calcium than normal subjects, they excreted more calcium in the urine. When given calcium supplements, the normal subjects

showed an increased urinary excretion of calcium as expected. Surprisingly, though, those with hypertension showed no increase in urinary excretion.

Is there more evidence about magnesium and hypertension?
Magnesium accompanies calcium in many foods, and also in hard water, and hard water has long been known to be geographically associated with lower blood pressure than soft water. More direct evidence favoring adequate magnesium intakes as

protective against hypertension comes from a study showing that magnesium deficiency causes visible changes in the walls of arteries and capillaries and makes them tend to constrict, a possible mechanism for its hypertensive effect.

I see: It's a complicated story. How can I translate all these findings into an eating plan to guard against hypertension?

Of course, as you can see, no one really knows the answer to that question. But it probably can't hurt to:

• Keep your intake of sodium at a moderate level (about four grams of sodium a day).

• Eat good sources of potassium daily—lots of fresh, whole foods.

• Be sure to meet your calcium needs daily. Dairy products have advantages over calcium supplements, because they provide fair amounts of potassium and magnesium as well.

Don't forget that we've been talking only about minerals. It's also a necessity to keep your weight under control and to pay attention to your fat intake, because atherosclerosis and hypertension are often found together.

Notes

1. T. W. Kurtz, H. A. Al-Bander, and C. Morris, "Salt-sensitive" essential hypertension in men: Is the sodium ion alone important? *New England Journal of Medicine* 317 (1987): 1043–1048.

2. M. P. Blaustein and J. M. Hamlyn, Sodium transport inhibition, cell calcium, and hypertension: The natriuretic hormone/Na-Ca exhcange/hypertension hypothesis, *American Journal of Medicine* 77 (4A) (1984): 45–59.

3. J. K. Huttunen and coauthors, Dietary factors and hypertension, *Acta Medica Scandinavica* (Supplement) 701 (1985): 72–82.

4. H. J. Henry and coauthors, Increasing calcium intake lowers blood pressure? The literature reviewed, *Journal of the American Dietetic Association* 85 (1985): 182–185.

5. M. R. Joffres, D. M. Reed, and K. Yano, Relationship of magnesium intake and other dietary factors to blood pressure: The Honolulu heart study, *American Journal of Clinical Nutrition* 45 (1987): 469–475.

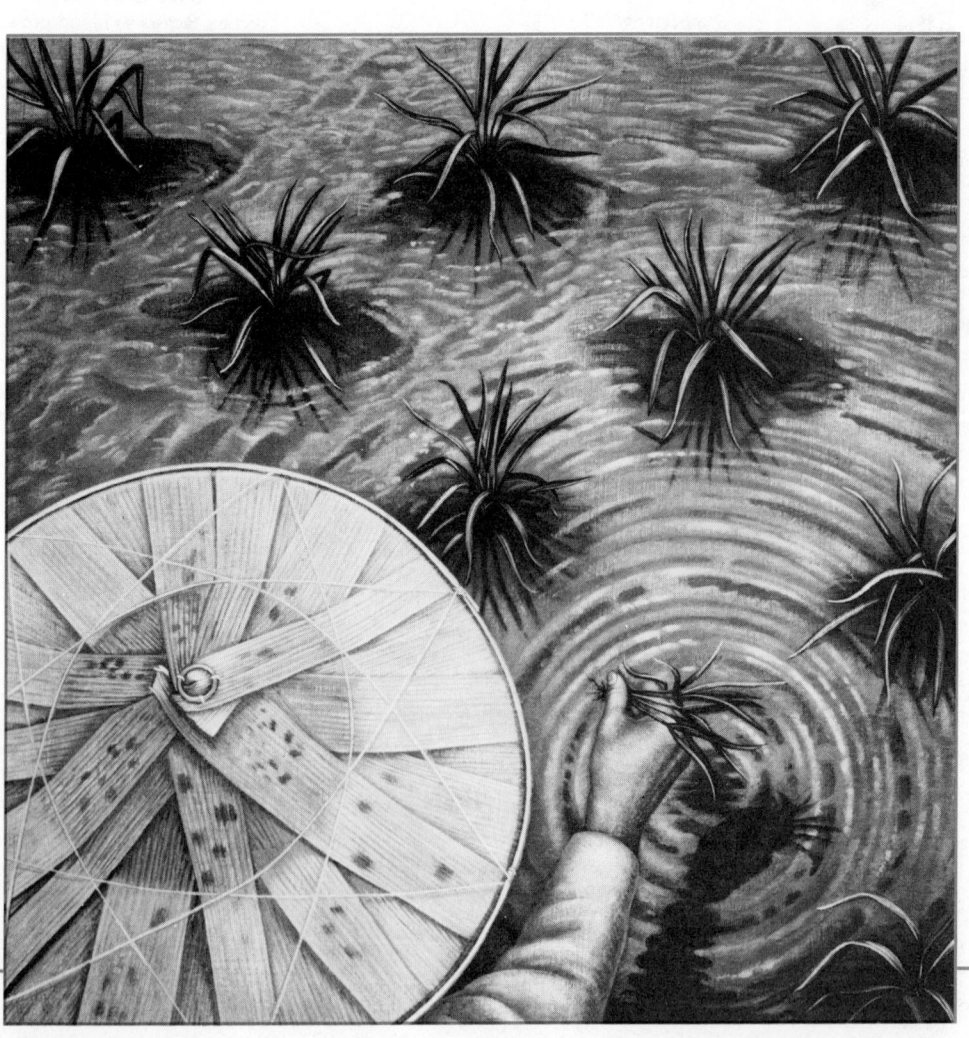

CHAPTER

22

Diets Modified in Protein, Minerals, and Water

DIETS DISCUSSED

Protein-Restricted Diets

Fluid-Restricted Diets

Gluten-Restricted Diets

Phenylalanine-Restricted Diets

Case Study: Renal Failure

Nutrition in Practice:
Nutrition in the Prevention
and Treatment of
Kidney Stones

CONDITIONS DISCUSSED

Hepatitus

Cirrhosis

Dietary Treatment

Hepatic Coma

Chronic Renal Disease

Acute Renal Failure

Celiac Disease

PKU

Illustration by Teresa Fasolino.

Diets modified in protein and amino acids are among the most difficult to plan and follow. Likewise, the disorders they are used to treat are complicated and hard to manage. Yet, most of these diets are critical, and failure to follow them can have adverse and sometimes fatal consequences. Table 22–1 shows some disorders for which protein-modified diets are indicated.

In most cases, protein- and amino acid-restricted diets are carefully prescribed by physicians and translated into actual foods by a trained dietitian. Although you may not be the diet planner, you may need to answer questions or communicate information about the diet to the client or the client's family.

Protein-Restricted Diets

Protein-restricted diets generally provide the amounts of protein necessary to maintain nutrition status but not enough to allow the buildup of waste products from protein metabolism that can be toxic to the tissues when they accumulate. Protein-restricted diets contain from no protein (for temporary use only) to about 60 grams of protein daily. A sample 60-gram protein-restricted diet is shown in the text.

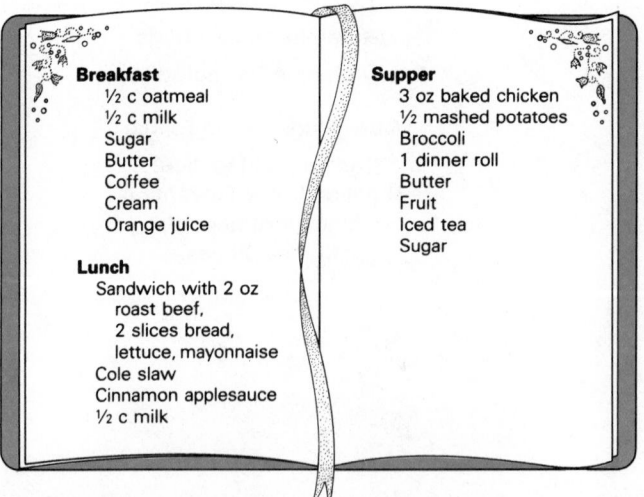

Breakfast
½ c oatmeal
½ c milk
Sugar
Butter
Coffee
Cream
Orange juice

Lunch
Sandwich with 2 oz roast beef, 2 slices bread, lettuce, mayonnaise
Cole slaw
Cinnamon applesauce
½ c milk

Supper
3 oz baked chicken
½ mashed potatoes
Broccoli
1 dinner roll
Butter
Fruit
Iced tea
Sugar

Sample 60-gram protein-restricted diet menu.

Foods from the milk, meat, and bread exchanges must be carefully controlled. Vegetables and fruits also contain some protein, and for very low-protein diets, even these foods must be calculated into the diet. The lower the amount of protein allowed, the more important it becomes that all the protein included in the diet be of high quality. Milk and eggs are used preferentially for this purpose unless contraindicated for other reasons.

The lower the protein content of the diet, the more difficult it is to ensure that the total kcalorie intake is adequate. Furthermore, it is critical that kcalories be adequate; otherwise the protein available will be used for energy rather than in protein synthesis. Whenever possible, encourage the client on a low-protein diet to use many fats (margarine, cream, butter) and concentrated sweets (hard candy, jelly, sugar), which provide high amounts of kcalories. Special low-protein products (pastas, bread, cookies, wafers, and gelatin) made with wheat starch can improve energy intake and add variety to the diet. The taste of many of these products is acceptable.[1] Carbohydrate supplements in powdered and liquid forms are also available.

Often, people on a protein-restriced diet must also be on other restrictive diets. For example, those with renal failure may also need to restrict sodium and potassium, follow a fat-controlled diet for hyperlipidemia, and limit concentrated sweets because of diabetes. This presents further challenges to the individual and the diet planner to assure adequate intake of nutrients.

Imagine what a protein-restricted diet is really like. Consider, for example, what the person on a 30-gram protein diet is actually getting. On such a diet, the total protein allowance would be spent on just one egg, two ounces of meat, half a cup of milk, and one serving each of a vegetable and bread. You can probably already see some problems. The amounts of foods allowed from the major food groups are very small. The kcalorie and nutrient content of the diet is inadequate. You may be able to see why fat is not restricted unless necessary, because adding fat wherever possible can help boost kcalorie intake considerably. If the type of fat must be restricted, fewer food choices are available. Other foods that do not contain protein, such as candy, jelly, and sugar, can also help. However, in some cases, even concentrated sweets must be limited. Obviously, protein-restricted diets are among the most difficult diets to plan and follow.

Liver Disease

Protein-restricted diets are used for two major disorders of the liver: cirrhosis and hepatic coma. A liver disorder in which a protein-restricted diet is not indicated is hepatitis, because in this case the liver can handle a normal protein intake and needs this protein to repair itself. Provide a well-balanced, normal diet to the person with hepatitis who is in good nutrition status. The malnourished person with hepatitis, like any malnourished person, needs a high-kcalorie, high-protein diet (see Chapter 17). People with alcohol-related hepatitis are at high risk for poor nutrition status; malnutrition is a common complication of alcohol abuse, and hepatitis further taxes nutrient stores.

Anorexia, nausea, vomiting, and fever are common symptoms of hepatitis. The person with malnutrition, unable to take foods orally, may be given IV

TABLE 22–1. Indications for the Use of Diets Modified in Protein and Fluid

Protein-restricted diets

Acute renal disease
Chronic renal disease
Cirrhosis
Hepatic coma

Gluten-restricted diets

Celiac disease

Phenylalanine-restricted diets

Phenylketonuria

Fluid-restricted diets

Acute renal disease (oliguric phase)
Chronic renal disease
Cirrhosis
Hepatic coma

hepatitis (HEP-ah-TIE-tis): inflammation of the liver caused by a virus, alcohol, or drugs. Hepatitis can progress to cirrhosis.
hepat = liver
itis = inflammation

The impact of alcohol abuse on nutrition status is the subject of Nutrition in Practice 6.

glucose solutions temporarily. Suggest small, frequent meals, liquid supplements, or both for the person who experiences difficulty eating. Tube feedings should be considered if anorexia and nausea persist. Parenteral nutrition may be necessary if vomiting becomes a problem.

Cirrhosis

Cirrhosis is a serious liver disorder. In cirrhosis, liver cells filled with fat or damaged by inflammation die, and scar tissue invades the liver. Chronic alcohol abuse is the most common cause of cirrhosis in the United States. Keep in mind, however, that not all people with cirrhosis are alcohol abusers and not all alcohol abusers develop cirrhosis. Cirrhosis can result from congenital causes, toxic chemicals, infections, biliary obstructions, heart disease, or unknown causes.

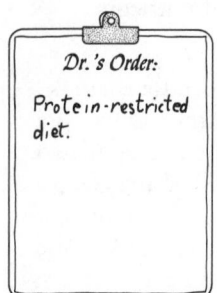

Dr.'s Order:

Protein-restricted diet.

Normal liver tissue is soft and flexible, but scars are unyielding. The portal vein and the hepatic artery carry 1½ quarts of blood every minute through the miles of intermeshed capillaries in the liver. Because this huge volume of blood cannot pulse easily through the mass of scar tissue in the cirrhotic liver, it backs up into the portal vein. Blood pressure in the vein consequently rises sharply, causing portal hypertension. A diagram of the liver's circulatory system is shown in Figure 22–1.

As pressure rises, plasma is forced from the liver's blood vessels into the abdominal cavity, and the belly swells. The accumulation of fluid in the abdominal cavity is a type of edema called ascites, a self-aggravating condition. Because the volume of blood in the circulatory system is now reduced, less blood reaches the kidneys. The kidneys respond by setting in motion a chain of events involving the hormone aldosterone, which triggers the body's retention of sodium and water. Edema now spreads to all body compartments. To make matters worse, the diseased liver cannot dispose of aldosterone as it normally does, so aldosterone levels remain high.

Normal blood flow through the liver is blocked, so some of the blood takes a detour through smaller blood vessels around the liver and out to the rest of the body. These blood vessels, known as shunts or collaterals, often develop in the area of the esophagus. Frequently, the increased pressure enlarges the collateral blood vessels until they bulge into the lumen of the esophagus, as varicose veins do in the legs, creating esophageal varices. The lining of the esophagus on top of the varices eventually erodes. Many times the erosion penetrates into the varices themselves and massive bleeding follows.

Under normal circumstances, the liver removes ammonia—a waste product of amino acid metabolism—from the circulation and converts it to urea. A seriously diseased liver can't synthesize urea, so it can't clean up the ammonia from the blood. The problem is further aggravated, because some blood that is carrying ammonia is not even reaching the liver; instead, it is shunted by way of the collaterals. High blood ammonia levels impair functioning of the central nervous system, compounding the risk of hepatic coma (discussed later in the chapter).

cirrhosis (sih-ROW-sis):
a disease of the liver characterized by scarring. *Laennec's cirrhosis* is the type associated with alcohol abuse and malnutrition.

The **portal vein** carries nutrients from the digestive organs to the liver; the **hepatic artery** brings oxygen-rich blood from the heart to the liver; the **hepatic vein** returns blood from the liver to the heart.

portal hypertension:
elevated blood pressure in the portal vein caused by obstructed blood flow through the liver.

Bile pigments from the diseased liver spill into the blood and accumulate, causing the skin, whites of the eyes, and mucous membranes to become yellow, a condition known as **jaundice.**

ascites (uh-SITE-eez):
a type of edema characterized by the accumulation of fluid in the abdominal cavity.

collaterals:
small blood vessels that develop to divert blood flow away from an obstructed organ. These blood vessels are also called **shunts.**

esophageal varices (ee-SOF-ah-GEE-al VAIR-ih-seez):
tangles of distended blood vessels that protrude into the esophagus.

hyperammonemia (HIGH-per-am-moe-KNEE-mee-uh):
elevated blood ammonia levels.

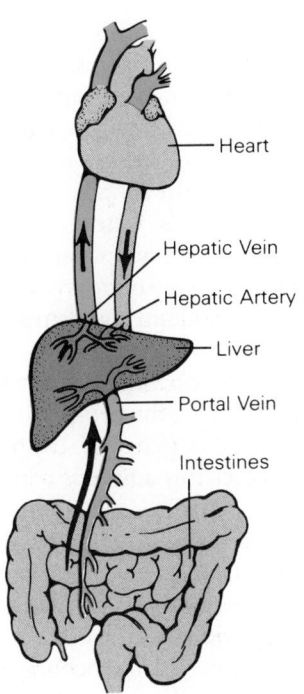

FIGURE 22–1
The liver's circulatory system. Note that poor circulation in the liver can cause high blood pressure in the portal vein. Back pressure can also enlarge veins surrounding the intestinal system, including the esophagus.

Dietary Treatment

A protein-restricted diet is a cornerstone of therapy in cirrhosis. A daily intake of 35 to 45 kcalories per kilogram of actual body weight (about 2,000 to 3,000 kcalories) is recommended to maintain the person in positive nitrogen balance.[2] Enough protein should be given so that liver cells can regenerate, but too much protein will result in more ammonia buildup, which can lead to hepatic coma. In the absence of hepatic coma, the diet should be adequate in kcalories and should meet the RDA for protein (1.0 to 1.5 grams per kilogram of body weight).[3]

Total abstinence from alcohol is necessary to protect the cirrhotic liver from further injury. Fat is not restricted unless the client develops steatorrhea (see Chapter 20), a clear sign that fat absorption has failed. If fat must be restricted, MCT can be used as a source of kcalories.

The diet is usually supplemented with large amounts of water-soluble vitamins (up to five times more than the RDA). Remember that the B vitamins are necessary coenzymes for the liver's many metabolic reactions and repair work. In malnutrition, the water-soluble vitamins are among the first to be depleted. A person with a prolonged prothrombin time should be offered vitamin K supplements. Otherwise, fat-soluble vitamins are provided only if a deficiency has been identified. Frequently, the RDA amounts of these vitamins are adequate.

prothrombin time:
the time it takes for the blood to clot. Both vitamin K deficiency and liver disease can prolong this time.

For people with ascites, fluids (see Fluid-Restricted Diets) and sodium (see Chapter 21) are restricted. The level of the restriction varies with the severity of the ascites. Sodium amounts may range from 250 to 2,000 milligrams per day; fluids from 1,500 to 2,000 milliliters per day. Weigh the person *daily*. Weight fluctuations are used to assess changes in fluid balance. If weight gain is rapid, the person is gaining fluid. In contrast, sudden weight loss indicates that the person is successfully excreting water.

To provide a diet low in sodium that will stimulate the appetite and provide adequate protein is a difficult task. Many high-protein foods contain significant amounts of sodium. Special low-sodium supplements and milk products are available to circumvent this problem.

The person who has bleeding esophageal varices will be unable to take food by mouth. When there is no bleeding, the person with esophageal varices may be advised to follow a low-fiber diet (Chapter 16) to avoid irritation, painful swallowing, or bleeding; however this advice is controversial and its benefits are unclear.[4]

The person with anorexia may accept food more willingly in small, frequent meals than in fewer large ones. Diet is vital to recovery from cirrhosis. Therefore, every effort must be made to ensure its acceptance. Work closely with the person and the family to individualize the diet, and serve foods attractively. Try the tactics suggested in Chapter 14 to encourage the client to eat.

Hepatic Coma

hepatic coma:
a state of unconsciousness that results from severe liver disease; also called *portal systemic encephalopathy.*

Hepatic coma is a dangerous complication of liver disease. Typically, the person with impending hepatic coma exhibits mental disturbances, such as changes in judgment, personality, or mood, and sometimes sleep patterns. The exact mechanisms causing hepatic coma are unknown, but rising blood ammonia levels play an important role. Most people in hepatic coma have elevated blood ammonia levels, although the degree of the elevation does not correlate with the severity of coma.

Phenylalanine and tyrosine are the aromatic amino acids; they are characterized by a ringlike structure.

Leucine, isoleucine, and valine are the branched-chain amino acids; they are characterized by a branched structure.

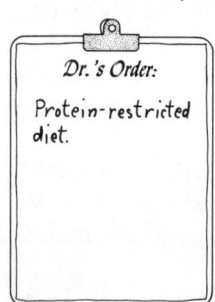

Dr.'s Order:
Protein-restricted diet.

Blood amino acid patterns also change in hepatic coma. Aromatic amino acids normally are catabolized by the liver, and this catabolism is impaired in liver disease. Consequently, aromatic amino acid levels rise. Hormonal changes that occur in liver disease result in the uptake of branched-chain amino acids by muscle cells. Therefore, circulating branched-chain amino acid levels fall. The high ratio of aromatic to branched-chain amino acids in the blood may cause the production of substances that act like neurotransmitters, and these substances may, in turn, contribute to hepatic coma.[5]

Two enteral formulas that are low in aromatic amino acids and high in branched-chain amino acids are Hepatic-Aid II and Travasorb-Hepatic. These formulas can be given orally or by tube. Parenteral solutions of similar amino acid composition are also available.

When a person shows signs of impending coma, protein intake is restricted to 40 to 60 grams per day. Drug therapy is given simultaneously to rid the body of excess ammonia. If protein restriction and drug therapy fail to improve the person's neurological status, special enteral or parenteral formulations that are low in aromatic amino acids and high in branched-chain amino acids may be tried. If coma ensues, both total protein and special formulas must be limited.[6] As improvement becomes evident, protein can gradually be added in 10- to 15-gram increments per day for five to seven days until the RDA for protein is reached. People should not be kept on zero-protein diets for more than a few days. Such diets cause breakdown of body proteins which can make matters worse.

Vegetable protein and dairy protein may be better tolerated than meat protein, perhaps because vegetable protein has fewer amino acids that readily form ammonia. Vegetable and dairy proteins also have a lower content of aromatic amino acids than do meats. In addition, diets high in plant foods contain more fiber, which prevents constipation, thereby reducing the time available for the production and absorption of ammonia in the gut. Such diets have been shown to reduce both urea nitrogen production and urinary nitrogen excretion.[7]

Fluid-Restricted Diets

The purpose of a fluid-restricted diet is to prevent overhydration in people with disorders that cause fluid to be retained abnormally by the body. Some of these disorders are liver disease, renal disease, myocardial infarction, and congestive heart failure.

All beverages and foods contain some water. Although liquids are carefully calculated and controlled on a fluid-restricted diet, generally the only foods that are controlled are those composed largely of water. Table 22–2 lists foods that must be calculated as part of the fluid allowance.

Many people on fluid-restricted diets experience extreme thirst. Some suggestions can help relieve this thirst:

TABLE 22–2. Substances Controlled on Fluid-Restricted Diets

Beverages	
Alcoholic beverages	Milk
Carbonated beverages	Tea
Coffee	Water
Juices	Any other
Foods[a]	
Ice cream (melts to ½ initial volume)	Popsicles
Ice milk (melts to ½ initial volume)	Sherbet (melts to ⅔ initial volume)
Jello	Soup
Other	
Cream	Ice (melts to 9/10 initial volume)

[a]Although all foods contain some water, these are the foods considered part of the fluid allowance on a fluid-restricted diet.

- Chew gum or suck hard candy.
- Freeze fluids so that they take longer to consume.
- Add lemon juice to water to make the water more refreshing.
- Gargle with refrigerated mouthwash.

Fluid restriction is a temporary measure most of the time. Sometimes, though, as in renal disease, the diet is long term. When long-term fluid restriction is necessary, watching fluid intake may be difficult. One method to help monitor fluid intake is to fill a container of water with the total fluid allowance at the start of each day. For example, a person can fill a jar with 1,500 milliliters of water if this is the fluid allowance. After taking each liquid food or drink, the person can discard an equivalent amount of water from the container and can look at the jar to get an idea of how much fluid is left for the day. Remind the person to save some of the fluid allowance for taking medications, if necessary.

Renal Disease

The kidneys:
  Maintain fluid, electrolyte, and acid-base balance.
  Eliminate metabolic waste products.
  Help regulate blood pressure.
  Produce a hormone that stimulates red blood cell production.
  Activate Vitamin D.

The **nephron** (NEF-ron), the working unit of the kidney, consists of the glomerulus and a tubule. The **glomerulus** (glow-MARE-you-lus) is a cup-shaped membrane enclosing a tuft of capillaries. The first part of the **tubule** surrounds the glomerulus. A pressure gradient between the glomerulus and the tubule returns needed materials to the blood and sends the wastes to the bladder.

renal failure:
failure of the nephrons to maintain normal function.

Like the liver, the kidneys play a vital role in the maintenance of the body's homeostasis. The kidneys filter out substances that the body doesn't need and eliminate these waste products in the urine. In so doing, these organs serve many important homeostatic functions: They maintain fluid, electrolyte, and acid-base balance, and they rid the body of metabolic waste products. Figure 22–2 shows a nephron, the working unit of the kidney, and illustrates how nephrons work.

The kidneys also help regulate blood pressure and produce a hormone, erythropoietin, which stimulates red blood cell production. Vitamin D is converted to its final, most active form in the kidneys so that it can perform its vital functions.

With all the tasks the kidneys perform, there is little doubt that serious consequences result when the kidneys fail. Renal disease can be caused by damage to the kidneys themselves or by other diseases, such as diabetic nephropathy (Chapter 19), hypertension (Chapter 21), or atherosclerosis (Chapter 21). Renal failure can occur suddenly (acute renal failure) or over a period of time (chronic renal failure). Acute renal failure may be temporary; chronic renal failure is irreversible.

In the early stages of renal disease, the nephrons get bigger in an attempt to maintain normal function. The hypertrophied nephrons work so efficiently that about 80 percent of them can be destroyed before renal function is seriously affected.

As more nephrons fail, normal blood and urine composition is altered. Blood urea nitrogen (BUN), creatinine, and uric acid are the body's principal nitrogen-containing metabolic waste products. They accumulate in the blood when renal function is impaired, and high levels of BUN, creatinine, and uric acid are seen in the person with renal failure.

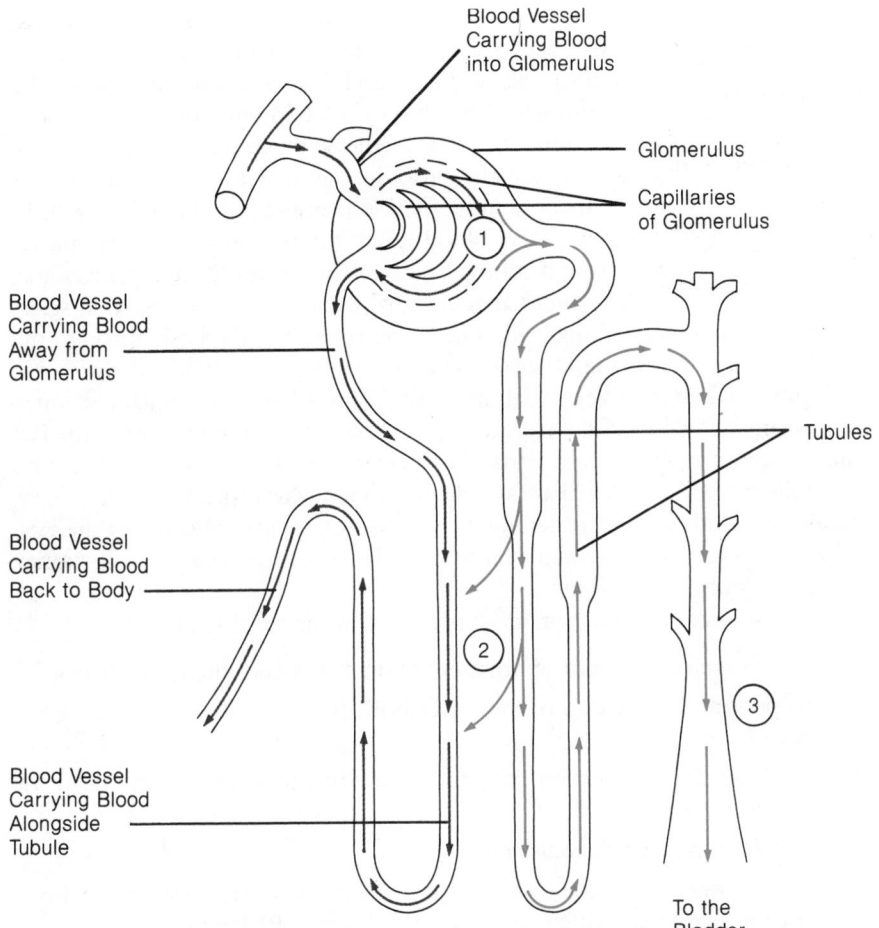

Blood Vessel Carrying Blood into Glomerulus

Glomerulus

Capillaries of Glomerulus

Blood Vessel Carrying Blood Away from Glomerulus

Tubules

Blood Vessel Carrying Blood Back to Body

Blood Vessel Carrying Blood Alongside Tubule

To the Bladder

FIGURE 22–2

One of the kidney's many functioning nephrons. Blood flows into the glomerulus, and some of its fluid is filtered into the tubules (1). Then the blood passes alongside the tubules, which return fluid and substances needed by the body (2). The waste materials that remain pass from the tubules on to the bladder (3).

As renal failure progresses to a severe stage, the buildup of toxic waste products in the blood (uremia) can precipitate a complex of symptoms known as the uremic syndrome. The person with uremia experiences a wide array of symptoms in virtually every body system. Fatigue, weakness, diminished mental alertness, muscular twitches, muscle cramps, anorexia, nausea, vomiting, stomatitis, and an unpleasant taste in the mouth are some of the symptoms. The skin may itch uncomfortably. In later stages, GI ulcers and bleeding are common.

uremic (you-REE-mic) **syndrome:** a complex of symptoms seen late in renal failure, caused by the buildup of toxic waste products in the blood.

Chronic Renal Disease

The early stages of renal disease generally involve no dietary restrictions. As renal function declines, the diet is carefully adjusted. Eventually, diet alone can no longer prevent uremia, and the person must begin dialysis or receive a kidney transplant to survive. This stage of renal disease is known as end-stage renal disease (ESRD).

end-stage renal disease (ESRD): The severe state of renal disease in which diet alone is no longer effective in maintaining normal kidney function.

diffusion and osmosis:
the movement of water across a membrane to equalize the concentration of particles on both sides of the membrane. Water moves from the less concentrated to the more concentrated side.

peritoneal (PERR-ee-toe-NEE-al) **dialysis:**
removal of wastes from the blood using the peritoneum as a semipermeable membrane.

hemodialysis (HE-mow-die-AL-ih-sis):
removal of wastes from the blood by passing the blood outside the body through tubes made of semipermeable membranes submerged in a water solution.

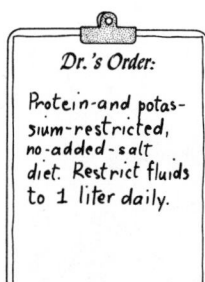

Dr.'s Order:

Protein-and potassium-restricted, no-added-salt diet. Restrict fluids to 1 liter daily.

Dialysis works on the principles of diffusion and osmosis across a semipermeable membrane and is used to remove excess fluids and wastes from the blood. The membrane that covers the abdominal organs (the peritoneum) can serve as the semipermeable membrane, in which case the procedure is called *peritoneal dialysis*. A synthetic semipermeable membrane can also be used. In such a case, blood leaves the person's artery and passes through tubing made of the semipermeable membrane. The tubes are continually bathed by solutions that selectively remove unwanted material. The blood returns to the body through the person's veins after being cleansed. This procedure is called *hemodialysis*.

A preferred alternative to dialysis in ESRD is a kidney transplant. Kidney transplants can successfully restore kidney function and normal growth. For this reason, transplants are particularly desirable for children. People who generally are not considered as candidates for kidney transplants are the elderly, people with other life-threatening conditions, or people who prefer dialysis. Given a choice, many would prefer transplants; however, a suitable kidney donor can't always be found.

The objectives of dietary management of chronic renal failure are:

- To achieve or maintain optimal nutrition status and nitrogen balance.
- To prevent the buildup of toxic metabolic products, thus minimizing the risk of uremia.
- To delay the progression of renal failure and to postpone the need for dialysis.
- To foster the client's well-being.
- To prevent complications, such as growth failure, wasting syndrome, bone disease, hypertension, edema, and congestive heart failure.

wasting syndrome:
the pattern of failure to grow in children and reduced muscle mass, fat tissue, and blood protein levels in people of any age that frequently develop as a consequence of renal disease.

The actual diet is highly individualized. The one most often prescribed is a protein-restricted diet in which total kcalories, sodium, potassium, phosphorus, and fluids are carefully controlled.

In both liver disease and renal disease, protein-restricted diets help prevent the buildup of toxins that result from amino acid metabolism—with one important distinction. In liver disease, blood ammonia levels rise, because the liver cannot convert ammonia to urea. Thus, ammonia is the toxin. In kidney disease, the liver does make urea, but the kidneys can't excrete it in the urine. Blood ammonia levels are normal, blood urea levels rise, and urea is the toxin of concern.

The ideal renal diet provides enough protein to support normal nitrogen balance without an elevation of BUN. Diet prescriptions may range from as low as 20 grams of protein to as high as 70 grams. A more liberal protein allowance is given to the person on dialysis, because the dialysis procedure results in protein loss. Table 22–3 summarizes nutrient needs of people with

TABLE 22–3. Typical Nutrient Needs in Chronic Renal Failure[a]

	Predialysis	Hemodialysis	Peritoneal Dialysis
Energy (kcal/kg)	35–50	35–50	35–50
Protein (g/kg)	0.55–0.60	1.0–1.2	1.2–1.5
Fluid (ml)	1,500–3,000	750–1,500	750–1,500
Sodium (g)	1.0–3.0	1.0–1.5	1.0–1.5
Potassium (g)	1.5–2.8	1.5–2.8	3.0–3.5
Phosphorus (mg)	600–1,200	600–1,200	600–1,200
Supplements			
Calcium (mg)	1,200–1,600	1,000	1,200–1,600
Folacin (mg)	1	1	1
Vitamin B$_6$ (mg)	5	10	10
Vitamin C (mg)	70–100	100	100
Other water-soluble vitamins	RDA	RDA	RDA
Vitamin D	As appropriate	As appropriate	As appropriate

[a]The actual amounts of these nutrients in the diet must be highly individualized based on each person's responses.

Source: Adapted from J. D. Kopple, Nutritional therapy in kidney failure, *Nutrition Reviews* 39 (1981): 193–206; D. J. Rodriguez and V. M. Hunter, Nutritional intervention in chronic renal failure, *Nursing Clinics of North America* 16 (1981): 573–585.

chronic renal failure and shows how these needs change for the person on hemodialysis or peritoneal dialysis.

Regardless of the protein allowance, all people with renal failure need adequate kcalories to achieve or maintain ideal body weight and to prevent protein breakdown. Children with renal disease often fail to grow normally, and people of any age with renal disease may have the wasting syndrome—reduced muscle mass, depleted fat stores, and lowered blood protein levels. Special attention to the nutrient needs of people with renal disease can help prevent wasting syndrome.

The little girl beams with pleasure when Charlie, the nurse, comes into the room. This is one of the high points of her day. "Do you have a lollipop for me?" she asks.

"Yep," says Charlie, reaching into his pocket. "Your favorite color, red. Eat it all up and I'll bring you another one."

Why is this nurse feeding the child candy? Because the child has renal disease and has a hard time getting enough kcalories to protect the protein she eats, the staff has been instructed to keep giving her sugar in whatever form she will accept it. A lollipop is like a clear liquid, because it melts in the mouth. It contains no protein or electrolytes to burden the kidney, but it offers sugar to help spare protein. Nothing could be more appropriate for this growing child's health.

Renal disease causes disturbances in the sea of fluid and electrolytes that bathes the cells. Sodium is one electrolyte that is affected. Early in renal failure, the person can maintain sodium balance with a moderate sodium intake. As renal disease progresses, however, both sodium and water must be restricted to prevent hypertension, edema, and heart failure. A typical diet will contain from one to four grams of sodium and from 500 to 3,000 milliliters of fluid daily.

Because individual needs vary, each person's weight, blood pressure, and urine output are carefully monitored to determine exact needs. Body weight and blood pressure will increase if the person is retaining sodium (and fluid). The person's weight and blood pressure will fall if sodium intake is too low. Urine output is also useful as a basis for estimating daily fluid needs. Simply add 500 milliliters for insensible water loss to 24-hour urine output. Potassium is often moderately restricted to 1½ to 3 grams per day. Table 21–11 lists foods high in potassium. A sample renal diet menu is illustrated in the text.

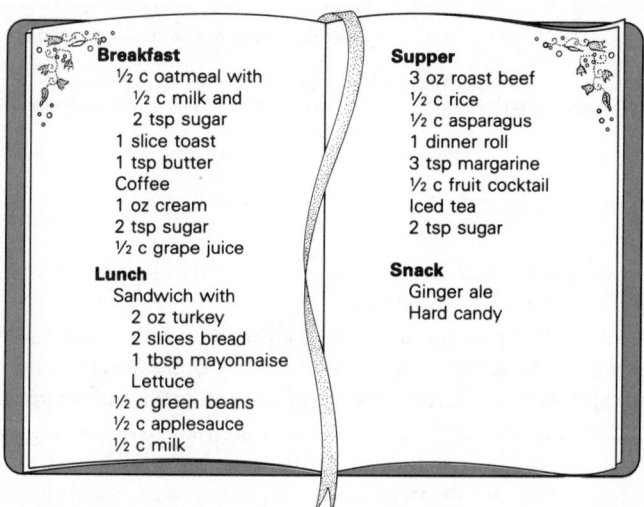

Breakfast
½ c oatmeal with
½ c milk and
2 tsp sugar
1 slice toast
1 tsp butter
Coffee
1 oz cream
2 tsp sugar
½ c grape juice

Lunch
Sandwich with
2 oz turkey
2 slices bread
1 tbsp mayonnaise
Lettuce
½ c green beans
½ c applesauce
½ c milk

Supper
3 oz roast beef
½ c rice
½ c asparagus
1 dinner roll
3 tsp margarine
½ c fruit cocktail
Iced tea
2 tsp sugar

Snack
Ginger ale
Hard candy

Sample renal diet menu (60 grams of protein and sodium- and potassium-controlled). Add kcalories to this diet by preparing food with oil or unsalted margarine (regular margarine, if allowed) and using additional sugar or syrup whenever possible. For example, eating canned fruit packed in heavy syrup, rather than juice, adds kcalories.

When urine volume is reduced, **oliguria** exists; **anuria** means that no urine is being excreted.

A person on dialysis who is excreting little or no urine will need to be extremely careful not to exceed the prescribed sodium, potassium, and fluid allowances. This person will need the lower range of intakes for these nutrients.

Bone disease frequently occurs in people with chronic renal failure, because the normal ratio of calcium to phosphorus in the blood is upset. Dietary control can help prevent the problem. The person is advised to restrict phosphorus intake by avoiding foods high in phosphorus, such as those shown in Table 22–4. Since most foods high in phosphorus are also high in protein, it is not difficult to manage this restriction. Most people with renal disease also receive

TABLE 22–4. Foods High in Phosphorus

Chocolate	Milk and milk products
Cocoa	Nuts
Dried beans and peas	Organ meats
Dried fruit	Peanut butter
Fish, canned	Whole-grain breads
Game meats	Whole-grain cereals

calcium supplements to help prevent bone disease. Large doses of vitamin D or smaller doses of the active form of vitamin D can be given to improve the absorption and utilization of calcium.

Vitamin deficiencies frequently develop in people with renal failure. The restrictive diet is partly responsible, since diets low in potassium are also low in water-soluble vitamins. Vitamins can be lost in dialysis, and drug therapy can change nutrient needs. Uremia can affect the metabolism of nutrients. For these reasons, generous amounts of vitamin B_6, vitamin C, and folacin are given, along with the RDA of the remaining water-soluble vitamins. Other than vitamin D, supplementation of the fat-soluble vitamins is usually not necessary. Iron and zinc supplements may also be prescribed.

Lastly, many people with chronic renal failure develop type IV hyperlipo-proteinemia and atherosclerosis. Some are also diabetic. In such cases, further dietary restrictions are made as appropriate (see Chapters 19 and 21).

No doubt you have long since arrived at the conclusion that designing renal diets is a task for a specialist. The complexities pile up, and the diet planner must carefully adjust intakes of sodium, potassium, protein, kcalories, liquids, lipids, vitamins, and minerals. He also must find food combinations that will deliver the necessary amounts of these nutrients. To deliver these nutrients, he must find foods that *the individual on the diet will accept and enjoy*. The renal dietitian faces these challenges every day.

With all that hard work to do, the diet planner has still another task—communicating with, especially listening to, the client. Inside that tangled web of grossly altered metabolic processes, dialysis lines, and toxic products is a person, often a frightened or discouraged one. One individual will say she dreams of ice cream sodas, forbidden because of their high-sodium content. She needs to feel understood, at least. Another says he feels guilty because his mother spends so much time preparing special foods for him. He too needs support. Another is fighting guilt and resentment because she repeatedly sneaks forbidden foods high in protein in spite of the rules she knows she should follow. If you have ever been "on a diet," even though it wasn't a renal diet, you will appreciate some of the problems these people face.

The person with renal disease has to live a life that involves many frustrations. Successful treatment often hinges on compliance with diet and drug orders. All the members of the health care team need to know what is involved if they are to offer the most effective support possible.

Acute Renal Failure

Acute renal failure occurs suddenly and is the consequence of another medical condition. The typical victim of acute renal failure is hypercatabolic and has a major illness, such as an infection or a burn, or has suffered cardiac arrest. Suddenly, the GFR drops, urine output decreases, blood pressure shoots up, and toxic waste products begin to build in the blood. As the body's cells break down, potassium is released from the intracellular fluid, and the kidneys are unable to excrete it. Blood potassium levels rise sharply. Hiccups, anorexia, nausea, and vomiting are common clinical symptoms of acute renal failure. GI bleeding and diarrhea sometimes occur. Drowsiness, agitation, and confusion are frequently seen.

The early phase of acute renal failure—when urine volume is reduced—is the **oliguric phase;** the phase characterized by large fluid and electrolyte losses in the urine is the **diuretic phase;** the gradual return of renal function marks the **recovery phase.**

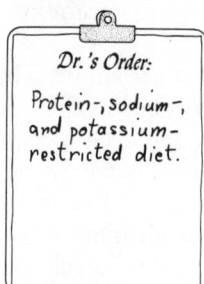

Dr.'s Order:

Protein-, sodium-, and potassium- restricted diet.

In the early stages of acute renal failure, urine volume often diminishes markedly. Sometimes, though, too much urine is produced. Later, the kidneys are unable to conserve water, and the person begins excreting large amounts of urine. In some cases, acute renal failure is reversible. In others, it progresses into chronic renal failure. About half of all people with acute renal failure die.

The primary concern in acute renal failure is to treat the underlying disorder in order to prevent permanent or further damage to the kidneys. For example, if severe blood loss is the problem, a blood transfusion is given to restore blood volume. Other measures must be taken to restore fluid and electrolyte balance and minimize levels of toxic products. In addition to the nutrition factors discussed in the following paragraphs, diurectics are often used to mobilize fluids in the oliguric phase of acute renal failure. Dialysis (either peritoneal or hemodialysis) is necessary when blood urea, creatinine, or potassium is high.

As mentioned, the person in acute renal failure is often hypercatabolic and suffering from another major illness. Add to these conditions nausea, vomiting, and confusion, and you have a person who really needs kcalories but is unable to eat. The person's actual energy needs depend on the rate of catabolism; usually 35 to 50 kcalories per kilogram of body weight are needed.

Protein needs also vary, depending on catabolic rate. Generally, protein is restricted to 30 to 40 grams per day. Some practitioners prefer to provide a higher protein intake, even if dialysis might be necessary, to prevent negative nitrogen balance and its possible consequences (see Chapter 13). If dialysis is instituted, a more liberal protein intake of 70 to 85 grams may be allowed.

Fluid and electrolyte restrictions are also warranted. Sodium may be restricted (500 to 1,000 milligrams) in the oliguric phase, but this may change as the person enters the diurectic phase. Likewise, potassium is often restricted to less than two grams per day in the oliguric phase but may need to be supplemented in the diuretic phase.

The total amount of fluid is carefully adjusted to avoid overhydration or dehydration. Fluid requirements can be calculated by measuring urine output. To the volume of urine, add about 400 to 500 milliliters for water lost through the skin, lungs, and perspiration. Additional fluid is given if the person experiences vomiting, diarrhea, or high fever. In the oliguric phase, the person will need small volumes of fluids. In the diuretic phase, up to three liters of urine may be lost daily, and large amounts of fluids will have to be provided.

Celiac Disease and the Gluten-Restricted Diet

Celiac disease, a hereditary disease with an incidence of about one in every 2,000 to 3,000 births, is characterized by malabsorption resulting from a sensitivity to gluten. Gluten is a protein found in wheat, oats, rye, and barley. A fraction of the gluten protein, gliaden, acts as a toxic substance. It causes the intestinal villi to atrophy, seriously reducing the absorptive surface of the intestinal tract. The disaccharidases and carrier molecules normally found on the villi become deficient. Malabsorption of many nutrients, including fat, protein, carbohydrate, fat-soluble vitamins, iron, calcium, magnesium, zinc, and some water-soluble vitamins, results.

The person with celiac disease often experiences steatorrhea, diarrhea, weight loss, and malnutrition. Anemia may occur as a result of iron, folacin, or vitamin B_{12} deficiency. Because protein is malabsorbed, serum protein levels can fall dramatically and edema and swelling result. The individual may bleed easily because of clotting abnormalities precipitated by a vitamin K deficiency. Calcium deficiency can result in tetany and bone pain.

Fortunately, the intestine can recover almost completely when gluten is removed from the diet. However, lactase deficiency and lactose intolerance may be permanent. If the person does not follow the diet, symptoms return.

The treatment for celiac disease sounds deceptively simple: Eliminate gluten. Unfortunately, gluten is found in many common foods. As you can see from Table 22–5, many foods contain wheat, oats, rye, or barley in some form. Wheat flour is used as an extender in many processed foods (ice cream, salad dressings, canned foods).

Help the person with celiac disease to understand what food to avoid. Be sure the individual and the family understand how to read food labels. Suggest the use of arrowroot, cornmeal, and potato, rice, and soybean flours as substitutes for wheat flour in recipes. Support groups of people with celiac disease and their families are organized in some parts of the country. They can be a great source of help for the individual with celiac disease.

celiac (SEE-lee-ack) **disease:**
a sensitivity to gliadin that causes flattening of the intestinal villi and generalized malabsorption; also called *gluten-sensitive enteropathy* (EN-ter-OP-ah-thee) or *celiac sprue.*

gluten (GLUE-ten):
a vegetable protein found in wheat, oats, rye and barley.

gliadin (GLIGH-ah-din):
a fraction of the gluten protein.

An easy way to remember the grains that must be restricted in celiac disease is to remember **WORB** (wheat, oats, rye, and barley).

PKU and the Phenylalanine-Restricted Diet

Phenylketonuria (PKU) is an inherited disorder of metabolism involving the essential amino acid, phenylalanine. In PKU there is an absence of the enzyme that normally converts excess phenylalanine to another amino acid, tyrosine. Phenylalanine and its metabolites build up to toxic levels in the blood. If left untreated, an infant with PKU will suffer severe mental retardation and abnormal growth and development.

The treatment of PKU is the phenylalanine-restricted diet. It must be started very early in life to prevent mental retardation. In most states, infants receive a test for PKU shortly after birth. Again, early diagnosis and early dietary treatment are critical.

The purpose of a phenylalanine-restricted diet is to limit phenylalanine in order to prevent the accumulation of excessive levels in the blood. At the same

phenylketonuria (FEN-ill-KEY-toe-NEW-ree-ah) **(PKU):**
an inborn error of metabolism in which phenylalanine cannot be converted to tyrosine. Alternative metabolites of phenylalanine accumulate in the tissues, causing damage, and overflow into the urine.

TABLE 22–5. Gluten-Restricted Diet

Meat and meat alternates
Any allowed except those that are breaded, prepared with bread crumbs, or creamed.

Milk and milk products
Any allowed except milk mixed with Ovaltine, commercial chocolate milk with a cereal additive, pudding thickened with wheat flour, ice cream or sherbet containing gluten stabilizers.

Fruits and vegetables
Any allowed except those that are breaded, prepared with bread crumbs, or creamed.

Grains
Allowed: Bread, cereal, or dessert products made from arrowroot, cornmeal, soybean flour, rice flour, potato flour or gluten-free starch; gluten-free macaroni or porridge; tapioca; cornmeal, cornflakes, popcorn, hominy; rice, cream of rice, puffed rice, rice flakes; potato chips.   Not allowed: Bread, cereal, or dessert products made from wheat, rye, oats, or barley; commercially prepared mixes for biscuits, cornbread, muffins, pancakes, buckwheat pancakes, cakes, cookies, and waffles; bran; pasta, macaroni, and noodles; malt; pretzels; wheat germ; doughnuts; ice cream cones.

Other (not allowed)
Beer; ale; certain whiskeys (Canadian rye); cereal beverages (Postum); root beer; commercial salad dressings that contain gluten stabilizers; soups containing any ingredient not allowed (barley, noodles, etc.).

Lofenalac is a special formula used in the treatment of PKU that is low in phenylalanine. Another formula, Phenyl-Free, contains no phenylalanine.

time, enough phenylalanine must be provided to promote normal growth and development. The diet planner, usually a specialist, determines the right amount of phenylalanine by monitoring the blood phenylalanine levels.

The diet must also provide ample kcalories, protein, and essential nutrients. Since tyrosine is not made from phenylalanine in PKU, adequate tyrosine must be given in the diet. Infants are given special formulas low in phenylalanine, and later, solids are gradually introduced. The diet planner uses special lists of foods to plan the diet. A sample menu is shown in the text.

There is some controversy about whether or not the diet can be discontinued as the child gets older. However, a woman with PKU who is pregnant must follow the diet or her unborn infant can be seriously affected. Congenital malformations and mental and physical retardation are likely when the fetus is exposed to high phenylalanine levels.

The successful treatment of PKU depends on the parents. They must understand the diet and the consequences of poor compliance. As the child grows, he must grasp these important concepts. The health care team must provide the parents and child with the help, support, and understanding they need to cope with the disorder and to alter their lifestyles appropriately.

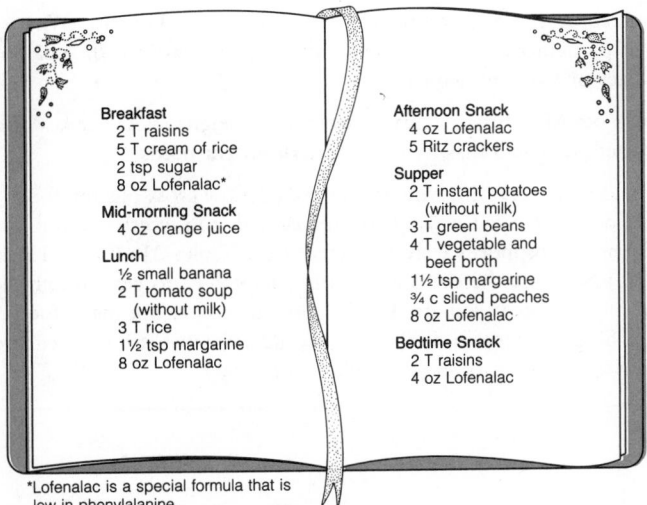

Breakfast
  2 T raisins
  5 T cream of rice
  2 tsp sugar
  8 oz Lofenalac*

Mid-morning Snack
  4 oz orange juice

Lunch
  ½ small banana
  2 T tomato soup
    (without milk)
  3 T rice
  1½ tsp margarine
  8 oz Lofenalac

Afternoon Snack
  4 oz Lofenalac
  5 Ritz crackers

Supper
  2 T instant potatoes
    (without milk)
  3 T green beans
  4 T vegetable and
    beef broth
  1½ tsp margarine
  ¾ c sliced peaches
  8 oz Lofenalac

Bedtime Snack
  2 T raisins
  4 oz Lofenalac

*Lofenalac is a special formula that is
low in phenylalanine.

Sample phenylalanine-restricted menu for a child with PKU.

Diet compliance is critical in the treatment of diseases discussed in this chapter. In the case of cirrhosis, failure to adhere to the diet can sometimes lead to hepatic coma and death. In the final stages of renal disease, the consequences of poor dietary compliance are the early appearance of the uremic syndrome or else the need for almost continuous dialysis. Failure to adhere to the gluten-restricted diet in celiac disease leads to serious nutrient deficiencies and wasting. In PKU, poor dietary compliance, although not fatal, results in otherwise avoidable mental and physical retardation. Although diets restricted in protein and amino acids are complicated and difficult for clients to understand and follow, adherence to these diets can make a lifesaving difference.

CASE STUDY

Renal Failure

Mrs. Ethan was 42 when she began to have kidney problems. While she was being treated in the hospital for a major burn, she developed acute renal failure. Gradually, the acute renal failure progressed to chronic renal failure. At 5 feet 3 inches tall, she weighs 100 pounds. Up to this point, she has been able to avoid dialysis by following a 50-gram protein, fluid- and electrolyte-restricted diet. Mrs. Ethan has been married for 17 years and has two teenage children. She works as a bank teller and spends time each weekend doing hospital volunteer work.

1. Describe the two stages of acute renal failure. What nutrients are of concern in each stage? What factors would the physician keep in mind when prescribing Mrs. Ethan's kcalorie, protein, and electrolyte needs during the episode of acute renal failure?

2. Think about the diet of a person with chronic renal disease. What nutrients are of particular concern? How would the diet change if the person had diabetes or hyperlipidemia?

3. How does Mrs. Ethan's current weight for height affect her kcalorie needs? What effect would dialysis have on her nutrient needs?

4. Write down everything you ate yesterday. Now cross out the foods you could not have eaten if you had been on a diet in which sodium, potassium, and phosphorus were restricted. (Use Tables 21–9, 21–11 and 22–4.) Now use the exchange lists in Chapter 18 to get a rough idea of how much protein you ate. Would you have to cut out many foods to follow a 50-gram protein diet? If yes, would your diet still be adequate in kcalories? Would it be easy to follow every day?

Notes

1. M. A. S. Van Duyn, Acceptability of selected low-protein products for use in a potential diet therapy for chronic renal failure, *Journal of the American Dietetic Association* 87 (1987): 909–914.
2. E. P. Shronts, Nutritional assessment of adults with end-stage hepatic failure, *Nutrition in Clinical Practice* 3 (1988): 113–119.
3. E. P. Shronts, 1988; N. H. Mezitis, Nutritional management in liver disease, *Nutrition in Clinical Practice* 3 (1988): 108–112.
4. B. J. Visocan, Nutritional management of alcoholism, *Journal of the American Dietetic Association* 83 (1983): 693–696.
5. D. T. Hiyama and J. E. Fischer, Nutritional support in hepatic failure: Current thought in practice, *Nutrition in Clinical Practice* 3 (1988): 96–105.
6. E. P. Shronts and coauthors, Nutrition support of the adult liver transplant candidate, *Journal of the American Dietetic Association* 87 (1987): 441–451.
7. F. L. Weber and coauthors, Effects of vegetable diets on nitrogen metabolism in cirrhotic subjects, *Gastroenterology* 89 (1985): 538–544.

Nutrition in the Prevention and Treatment of Kidney Stones

Chapter 22 discussed renal disease and its dietary treatment. A far more common kidney disorder is kidney stones. In the United States, about one in every 500 adults suffers from kidney stones, a painful and potentially dangerous condition. The person who has experienced a kidney stone may have a recurrence, but a large percentage of people with kidney stones report only a single episode. This suggests that with proper treatment, a recurrence of kidney stones may be preventable. The purpose of this Nutrition in Practice is to review some of the information that has been learned regarding the role of diet in the prevention and treatment of kidney stones. Much of the information is controversial, and research is still necessary to delineate the facts more fully.

What are kidney stones?
Kidney stones are masses of varying composition that form in the kidney. Most kidney stones contain calcium oxalate (60 percent of all stones), calcium phosphate (9 percent), or a combination of the two (11 percent). Less common stones are composed of uric acid, cystine, or magnesium ammonium phosphate.

What causes kidney stones to form?
Calcium stones may form in response to a variety of underlying medical conditions that cause either elevated serum calcium levels, excessive urinary excretion of calcium, or deficiencies of substances in the urine that normally inhibit stone formation. Most frequently, calcium stones are associated with excessive urinary calcium excretion for which no cause can be identified (idiopathic hypercalciuria). Uric acid stones are associated with the excessive urinary excretion of uric acid, an acid urine, and a small urine volume. Cystine stones occur as the result of a metabolic disorder that is characterized by the abnormal excretion of cystine in the urine (cystinuria). Table NP22–1 summarizes some of the disorders that are associated with stone formation.

TABLE NP22–1. Disorders Associated with Kidney Stones

Cystinuria
Glucocorticoid excess
Gout
Hyperparathyroidism
Hyperthyroidism
Immobilization
Malabsorption
Malignancies (some types)
Osteoporosis
Paget's disease
Recurrent urinary tract infections
Renal tubular acidosis
Vitamin D intoxication

The exact mechanisms by which kidney stones form are not clearly understood. Why is it, for example, that nearly all of us pass crystals in the urine, whereas only 10 percent of us actually develop kidney stones?[1] Three theories that help explain how kidney stones form are widely accepted by practitioners. These theories form the basis for the current treatment and prevention of kidney stones.

One mechanism thought to be important in stone formation is called *supersaturation*. Stone constituents are relatively insoluble in urine. When their concentrations get high, they form crystals that eventually precipitate and get larger. The more concentrated a mineral is in the urine, the greater the likelihood that a stone will form.

Another mechanism that may be important in the development of some stones is the formation of a small seed (sometimes called a *nucleus* or *nidus*) composed of a mineral different from that found in the remainder of the stone. The seed is formed from the crystallization of a mineral that is supersaturated in the urine. The crystalline structure then provides a matrix upon which a less saturated mineral can attach. In some cases, calcium oxalate stones have been found to form around a uric acid seed. The treatment of a stone of this type would involve the mineral found in the seed rather than the minerals that make up most of the stone.

Finally, it is widely believed that a deficiency of one or more naturally occurring stone inhibitors in the urine may contribute to stone formation. Citrate (a type of phosphate) and a type of polysaccharide are probable inhibitors.[2] Magnesium, zinc, and ribonucleic acid (RNA) might also have this effect. All of these substances have been identified as inhibitors of calcium oxalate stone formation.[3] What is not known is how important they are in the clinical situation. More research is needed to answer this question.

What happens to the stones once they form?

Stones that are small (less than five millimeters, or one fifth of an inch in diameter) may pass through the ureters and be excreted in the urine. Larger stones cannot exit the body in this way. If only a few small stones are formed, the stones do not cause any problems. However, if a larger stone enters a ureter (see Figure NP22–1), a severe, stabbing pain, called *renal colic,* results. Pain can also occur when small pieces of the stone break off and travel down the ureters with urine. The pain normally starts in the back, just above the ribs, and follows the course of the stone. Once the stone reaches the bladder, the pain usually subsides. If a stone blocks the flow of urine or causes an infection, it must be removed either surgically or by newer techniques that use sound waves or shock waves to break up the stone so that it can be passed.

How does diet fit into the picture?

The answer to this question is complicated, because so many

FIGURE NP22–1
The urinary tract.

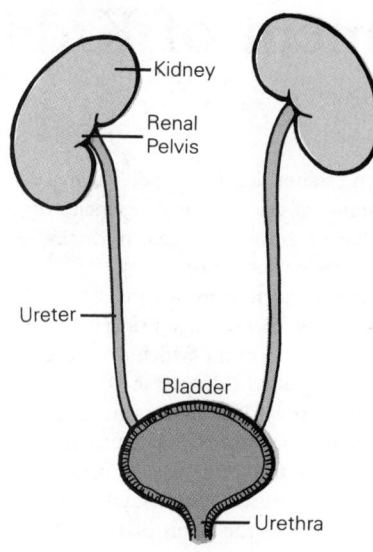

disorders can result in stone formation (see Table NP22–1). Studies have shown differences between the diets of people with kidney stones and those without them.[4] In one study, the diets of males with stones were significantly lower in thiamin than the diets of those in the control group. People with stones took vitamin C supplements more than twice as frequently as people in the control group. The same researchers then subdivided the group of stone formers further, based on the type of stone (calcium, oxalate, and uric acid).[5] They found that people with calcium oxalate stones without an identifiable underlying cause had lower intakes of dietary fiber, phytate, magnesium, phosphate, and thiamin than the control group. All the study group participants who excreted excessive

urinary oxalate had a significantly higher intake of vitamin C than the control group. Although the significance of these findings is unclear at this time, the studies suggest that differences in diet may play a role in the development of kidney stones.

Universal agreement does exist on one aspect of diet in the prevention and treatment of kidney stone formation: a high fluid intake is encouraged. The person with a kidney stone is advised to drink enough fluid so that a urine volume of at least two liters per day is maintained. Furthermore, fluid intake should be spread out regularly throughout the day. Maintenance of a large urine volume ensures that the concentration of minerals in the urine will be diluted, and the risk of stone formation is thus reduced. Other aspects of diet in the treatment of kidney stones have been far more controversial and have changed dramatically in recent years.

What are some of the controversies?

One of the most controversial topics in the treatment of stones concerns the role of calcium restriction for the person with a calcium-containing stone. On the surface, it appears reasonable that the diet of a person who is excreting large amounts of calcium in the urine should be restricted in calcium. For years, people with calcium stones were routinely instructed to follow a low-calcium diet (400 to 600 milligrams of calcium). However, evidence suggests that a calcium restriction is indicated in only one type of kidney stone former—the person who regularly ingests high amounts of calcium. Even in this case, calcium intake is restricted to an average (not a low) calcium intake. The diet should meet, but not exceed, the RDA for calcium.

To restrict the calcium intakes of other types of stone formers may actually be harmful. One ill effect is obvious—a calcium deficiency can lead to bone disorders. Studies of people with excessive urinary calcium levels have suggested that these individuals lose more calcium from their bones than normal subjects, which raises urinary calcium, obviously making stone formation more, not less, likely. Such individuals also excrete more calcium than they ingest, which indicates that they are in negative calcium balance.[6]

Calcium restriction could cause other harmful effects for the person with a calcium oxalate stone. You may recall that calcium normally binds to oxalate in the intestine. It is possible that if dietary calcium is severely limited, oxalate absorption may increase, resulting in enteric hyperoxaluria. This actually increases the likelihood that a calcium oxalate stone will form.[7] Rather than restrict calcium, people with calcium oxalate stones are advised to restrict their intakes of foods high in oxalate. Table NP22–2 shows foods that contain considerable amounts of oxalate. Supplemental vitamin-mineral preparations and medicines containing calcium are discouraged. Vitamin D can increase calcium absorption from the GI tract, a problem for the person who forms calcium stones due to excessive absorption of calcium. Megadoses of vitamin C also have been reported to cause hyperoxaluria. Some people metabolize vitamin C to oxalate; therefore, people with hyperoxaluria should avoid vitamin C

TABLE NP22–2. Foods High in Oxalate

Vegetables

Baked beans canned in tomato sauce	Leeks
Beans (green, wax, or dried)	Mustard greens
Beets	Okra
Celery	Parsley
Chard, Swiss	Peppers, green
Chives	Potatoes, sweet
Collards	Rutabagas
Dandelion greens	Spinach
Eggplant	Summer squash
Escarole	Watercress
Kale	

Fruits

Blackberries	Lemon peel
Blueberries	Lime peel
Currants, red	Orange peel
Dewberries	Raspberries
Fruit cocktail	Rhubarb
Gooseberries	Strawberries
Grapes, Concord	Tangerines

Other

Chocolate	Pepper (more than 1 tsp/day)
Cocoa	Soybean crackers
Cola beverages	Soybean curd (tofu)
Draft beer	Tea
Fruit cake	Tomato soup
Grits	Vegetable soup
Peanut butter	Wheat germ

Source: Adapted from D. M. Ney and coauthors, *The Low Oxalate Diet Book* (San Diego: University of California, 1981).

supplements. Calcium-containing antacids must also be avoided.

Thiazide diuretics are frequently prescribed for the person with calcium stones that are not associated with another medical condition. However, since these diuretics can cause a deficiency of potassium, they are sometimes given along with another

type of diuretic that conserves potassium. People on thiazide diuretics are advised to follow a moderately restricted sodium diet, because a high sodium intake can offset the beneficial effects of the diuretic and can cause potassium to be excreted excessively.[8] Therefore, potassium levels are monitored closely, and potassium supplements are given, if necessary.

Sodium restriction may have another benefit: Some evidence suggests that calcium excretion is linked to sodium excretion.[9] Therefore, a moderately restricted sodium diet might reduce excessive calcium levels in the urine, even for calcium stone formers not taking thiazide diuretics. Other studies have shown that a high protein intake increases the urinary excretion of calcium also. However, no studies have demonstrated a beneficial effect of protein restriction on calcium stone formation.

In summary, the calcium in the diet of a person with calcium stones who consumes excessive amounts of calcium is restricted to the RDA level. People with calcium oxalate stones are cautioned to limit their intakes of foods high in oxalate. Those on thiazide diuretics may benefit from a moderately restricted sodium intake and possibly a potassium supplement, if potassium becomes deficient. Of course, fluid intake is encouraged.

Can diet be of value in treating or preventing other types of stones?
Another common practice in the treatment of many types of kidney stones has been to prescribe diets that were meant to change the acidity of the urine. An acid ash diet, intended to make the urine more acid, centers on meat, cheese, eggs, whole grains, and some fruits. An alkaline ash diet, intended to reduce the acidity of the urine, emphasizes milk, vegetables, and most fruits. Diet can affect the acidity of the urine. However, current methods used to calculate the effect of different foods on the acidity of the

urine are difficult to use, and they are inaccurate.[10] Until a better estimate of the effect of dietary components on urine acidity is available, drug therapy for this purpose will be more reliable; indeed, it is more frequently used today.

Uric acid stones can form when the urine is consistently acid and when excess uric acid is present in the urine.

A metabolic disorder, gout, is frequently associated with uric acid stones. A generous fluid intake is encouraged. At one time, low-purine diets were commonly prescribed to reduce uric acid levels in the urine. A low-purine diet is restricted in red meats, particularly organ meats, anchovies, sardines, and meat extracts. The diet is restrictive, and benefits of

Miniglossary

cystinuria (SIS-te-NEW-ree-ah) a metabolic disorder in which large amounts of the amino acids cystine, lysine, arginine, and ornithine are excreted in the urine.

enteric hyperoxaluria excessive urinary excretion of oxalate caused by excess oxalate absorption in the intestine; it occurs because calcium is unable to bind to oxalate in the intestine, thus allowing oxalate absorption.

gout a metabolic disorder characterized by acute arthritis and inflammation of the joints that results in excess uric acid in the blood and sometimes in the urine.

hyperparathyroidism (HIGH-per-para-THIGH-roy-dizm) a condition characterized by the excessive secretion of parathyroid hormone, which generally results in elevated serum calcium levels, low serum phosphorus levels, and abnormal bone metabolism.

hyperthyroidism a condition characterized by the excessive secretion of thyroid hormones, which results in an accelerated metabolic rate.

idiopathic hypercalciuria (HIGH-per-kal-see-YOU-ree-ah) excessive urinary excretion of calcium not related to a known underlying medical condition.

nidus (NIGH-dus), **nucleus** a small bit of crystallized mineral that serves as a matrix for further crystallization.

Paget's (PAJ-ets) **disease** a chronic inflammatory disease of the bones that may occur in elderly people, named for Sir James Paget, an English surgeon.

pH see p. 54.

renal colic the severe pain that accompanies the movement of a kidney stone through the ureter.

renal tubular acidosis a condition in which the nephron cannot maintain acid-base balance; it can lead to potassium depletion, rickets, or osteomalacia.

struvite another name for magnesium ammonium phosphate.

supersaturation a term that describes the concentration of a substance in a liquid at the point where it is too concentrated to stay in solution and instead precipitates.

such a diet have not been proven. Furthermore, drug therapy is now available that is effective in reducing uric acid levels. However, it may be useful to limit excessive protein, and a diet containing no more than 120 grams of protein per day is advisable.[11] Drug therapy may be prescribed to reduce the acidity of the urine.

Magnesium ammonium phosphate (struvite) stones can precipitate when the urine becomes alkaline. This most often occurs when the urinary tract becomes infected with microorganisms that release ammonia. No specific diet therapy other than a well-balanced diet is recommended for this type of kidney stone.

As previously mentioned, cystine stones form as a result of a metabolic disorder called cystinuria. In cystinuria, large amounts of the amino acid cystine (in addition to other amino acids) are excreted in the urine. A diet low in the amino acid methionine is prescribed, because methionine produces the nonessential amino acid cystine. Drug therapy to reduce the acidity of the urine may also be beneficial.

As you can see, many connections between diet and kidney stones have been explored. Dramatic advances in the nonsurgical treatment of kidney stones have no doubt triggered a renewed interest in this area. A health care professional has an important responsibility to keep up with changes such as these so as to provide the best possible care for clients.

Notes

1. B. Goldwasser, J. L. Weinerth, and C. C. Carson, Calcium stone disease: An overview, *Journal of Urology* 135 (1986): 1–9.
2. S. P. Kanig and R. L. Conn, Kidney stones: Medical management and newer options for stone removal, *Postgraduate Medicine* 78, no. 6 (1985): 38–51.
3. Goldwasser, Weinerth, and Carson, 1986.
4. H. M. Griffith and coauthors, A case-controlled study of dietary intake of renal stone patients: 1. Preliminary analysis, *Urology Research* 14 (1986): 67–74.
5. H. M. Griffith and coauthors, A case-controlled study of dietary intake of renal stone patients: 2. Urine biochemistry and stone analysis, *Urology Research* 14 (1986): 75–82.
6. F. L. Coe and J. H. Parks, Recurrent renal calculi: Causes and prevention, *Hospital Practice* 21, no. 3A (1986): 49–57.
7. P. Bataille and coauthors, Effect of calcium restriction on renal excretion of oxalate and the probability of stones in the various pathophysiological groups with calcium stones, *Journal of Urology* 130 (1983): 218–223.
8. Coe and Parks, 1986.
9. Kanig and Conn, 1985.
10. J. Dwyer and coauthors, Acid/alkaline ash diets: Time for assessment and change, *Journal of the American Dietetic Association* 85 (1985): 841–845.
11. Goldwasser, Weinerth, and Carson, 1986.

APPENDIXES

A

Recommended Nutrient Intakes (RDA, RNI)

Some of the U.S. recommendations appear in the RDA table on the inside front cover. The remaining RDA are here, in Tables A–1 and A–2. The U.S. RDA used on food labels are on the inside back cover. The Canadian recommendations are in Tables A–3 and A–4.

TABLE A-1 Estimated Safe and Adequate Daily Dietary Intakes of Additional Selected Nutrients (United States)[a]

	Vitamins			**Electrolytes**		
Age (years)	Vitamin K (µg)	Biotin (µg)	Pantothenic Acid (mg)	Sodium (mg)	Potassium (mg)	Chloride
0–0.5	12	35	2	115–350	350–925	275–700
0.5–1.0	10–20	50	3	250–750	425–1275	400–1200
1–3	15–30	65	3	325–975	550–1650	500–1500
4–6	20–40	85	3–4	450–1350	775–2325	700–2100
7–10	30–60	120	4–5	600–1800	1000–3000	925–2775
11+	50–100	100–200	4–7	900–2700	1525–4565	1400–4200
Adults	70–140	100–200	4–7	1100–3300	1875–5625	1700–5100

	Trace Elements[b]					
Age (years)	Chromium (mg)	Selenium (mg)	Molybdenum (mg)	Copper (mg)	Manganese (mg)	Fluoride (mg)
0–0.5	0.01–0.04	0.01–0.04	0.03–0.06	0.5–0.7	0.5–0.7	0.1–0.5
0.5–1.0	0.02–0.06	0.02–0.06	0.04–0.08	0.7–1.0	0.7–1.0	0.2–1.0
1–3	0.02–0.08	0.02–0.08	0.05–0.10	1.0–1.5	1.0–1.5	0.5–1.5
4–6	0.03–0.12	0.03–0.12	0.06–0.15	1.5–2.0	1.5–2.0	1.0–2.5
7–10	0.05–0.20	0.05–0.20	0.10–0.30	2.0–2.5	2.0–3.0	1.5–2.5
11+	0.05–0.20	0.05–0.20	0.15–0.50	2.0–3.0	2.5–5.0	1.5–2.5
Adults	0.05–0.20	0.05–0.20	0.15–0.50	2.0–3.0	2.5–5.0	1.5–4.0

[a]Because there is less information on which to base allowances, these figures are not given in the main table of the RDA and are provided here in the form of ranges of recommended intakes.
[b]Since the toxic levels for many trace elements may be only several times usual intakes, the upper levels for the trace elements given in this table should not habitually be exceeded.

TABLE A-2 Recommended Energy Intakes for Individuals of Average Height, Weight, and Activity Levels

Age	Weight		Height		Energy Needs[a]	
(years)	(kg)	(lb)	(cm)	(inches)	(cal)	(MJ)[b]
Infants						
0–0.5	6	13	60	24	kg × 115(95–145)	kg × 0.48
0.5–1.0	9	20	71	28	kg × 105(80–135)	kg × 0.44
Children						
1–3	13	29	90	35	1300 (900–1800)	5.5
4–6	20	44	112	44	1700 (1300–2300)	7.1
7–10	28	62	132	52	2400 (1650–3300)	10.1
Males						
11–14	45	99	157	62	2700 (2000–3700)	11.3
15–18	66	145	176	69	2800 (2100–3900)	11.8
19–22	70	154	177	70	2900 (2500–3300)	12.2
23–50	70	154	178	70	2700 (2300–3100)	11.3
51–75	70	154	178	70	2400 (2000–2800)	10.1
76+	70	154	178	70	2050 (1650–2450)	8.6
Females						
11–14	46	101	157	62	2200 (1500–3000)	9.2
15–18	55	120	163	64	2100 (1200–3000)	8.8
19–22	55	120	163	64	2100 (1700–2500)	8.8
23–50	55	120	163	64	2000 (1600–2400)	8.4
51–75	55	120	163	64	1800 (1400–2200)	7.6
76+	55	120	163	64	1600 (1200–2000)	6.7
Pregnant					+300	
Lactating					+500	

[a]The energy allowances for the young adults are for men and women doing light work. The allowances for the two older age groups represent mean energy needs over these age spans, allowing for a 2% decrease in basal (resting) metabolic rate per decade and a reduction in activity of 200 cal/day for men and women between 51 and 75 years, 500 cal for men over 75, and 400 cal for women over 75. The customary range of daily energy output, shown in parentheses, is based on a variation in energy needs of ±400 cal at any one age, emphasizing the wide range of energy intakes appropriate for any group of people. Energy allowances for children through age 18 are based on median energy intakes of children of these ages followed in longitudinal growth studies. The values in parentheses are 10th and 90th percentiles of energy intake, to indicate the range of energy consumption among children of these ages.
[b]MJ stands for megajoules (1 MJ = 1000 kJ).

TABLE A–3 Recommended Nutrient Intakes for Canadians

Age	Sex	Weight (kg)	Protein (g/day)[a]	Fat-Soluble Vitamins		
				Vitamin A (RE/day)[b]	Vitamin D (µg/day)[c]	Vitamin E (mg/day)[d]
Months						
0–2	Both	4.5	11[f]	400	10	3
3–5	Both	7.0	14[f]	400	10	3
6–8	Both	8.5	17[f]	400	10	3
9–11	Both	9.5	18	400	10	3
Years						
1	Both	11	19	400	10	3
2–3	Both	14	22	400	5	4
4–6	Both	18	26	500	5	5
7–9	M	25	30	700	2.5	7
	F	25	30	700	2.5	6
10–12	M	34	38	800	2.5	8
	F	36	40	800	2.5	7
13–15	M	50	50	900	2.5	9
	F	48	42	800	2.5	7
16–18	M	62	55	1000	2.5	10
	F	53	43	800	2.5	7
19–24	M	71	58	1000	2.5	10
	F	58	43	800	2.5	7
25–49	M	74	61	1000	2.5	9
	F	59	44	800	2.5	6
50–74	M	73	60	1000	2.5	7
	F	63	47	800	2.5	6
75+	M	69	57	1000	2.5	6
	F	64	47	800	2.5	5
Pregnancy (additional)						
First trimester			15	100	2.5	2
Second trimester			20	100	2.5	2
Third trimester			25	100	2.5	2
Lactation (additional)			20	400	2.5	3

Note: Recommended intakes of energy and of certain nutrients are not listed in this table because of the nature of the variables upon which they are based. The figures for energy are estimates of average requirements for expected patterns of activity. For nutrients not shown, the following amounts are recommended: **thiamin,** 0.4 mg/1000 cal (0.48 mg/5000 kJ); **riboflavin,** 0.5 mg/1000 cal (0.6 mg/5000 kJ); **niacin,** 7.2 niacin equivalents/1000 cal (8.6 NE/5000 kJ); **vitamin B₆,** 15 µg (as pyridoxine)/g protein; **phosphorus,** same as calcium.

Recommended intakes during periods of growth are taken as appropriate for individuals representative of the midpoint in each age group. All recommended intakes are designed to cover individual variations in essentially all of a healthy population subsisting upon a variety of common foods available in Canada.

TABLE A–3 (continued)

Water-Soluble Vitamins			Minerals				
Vitamin C (mg/day)	Folacin (μg/day)[e]	Vitamin B_{12} (μg/day)	Calcium (mg/day)	Magnesium (mg/day)	Iron (mg/day)	Iodine (μg/day)	Zinc (mg/day)
20	50	0.3	350	30	0.4[g]	25	2[h]
20	50	0.3	350	40	5	35	3
20	50	0.3	400	45	7	40	3
20	55	0.3	400	50	7	45	3
20	65	0.3	500	55	6	55	4
20	80	0.4	500	65	6	65	4
25	90	0.5	600	90	6	85	5
35	125	0.8	700	110	7	110	6
30	125	0.8	700	110	7	95	6
40	170	1.0	900	150	10	125	7
40	170	1.0	1000	160	10	110	7
50	160	1.5	1100	220	12	160	9
45	160	1.5	800	190	13	160	8
55	190	1.9	900	240	10	160	9
45	160	1.9	700	220	14	160	8
60	210	2.0	800	240	8	160	9
45	165	2.0	700	190	14	160	8
60	210	2.0	800	240	8	160	9
45	165	2.0	700	190	14[i]	160	8
60	210	2.0	800	240	8	160	9
45	165	2.0	800	190	7	160	8
60	210	2.0	800	240	8	160	9
45	165	2.0	800	190	7	160	8
0	305	1.0	500	15	6	25	0
20	305	1.0	500	20	6	25	1
20	305	1.0	500	25	6	25	2
30	120	0.5	500	80	0	50	6

[a]The primary units are grams per kilogram of body weight. The figures shown here are examples.
[b]One retinol equivalent (RE) corresponds to the biological activity of 1 μg of retinol, 6 μg of β-carotene, or 12 μg of other carotenes.
[c]Expressed as cholecalciferol or ergocalciferol.
[d]Expressed as d-α-tocopherol equivalents, relative to which β- and γ-tocopherol and α-tocotrienol have activities of 0.5, 0.1, and 0.3, respectively.
[e]Expressed as total folate.
[f]The assumption is made that the protein is from breast milk or is of the same biological value as that of breast milk at first, and that between three and nine months the child is weaned. Adjustments for the changing quality of protein have been made accordingly.
[g]It is assumed that breast milk is the source of iron up to two months of age.
[h]Based on the assumption that breast milk is the source of zinc for the first two months.
[i]After menopause the recommended intake is 7 mg/day.

Source: Health and Welfare Canada, *Recommended Nutrient Intakes for Canadians* (Ottawa: Canadian Government Publishing Centre, 1983), Table X.1, pp. 179–180, as revised in the second printing.

TABLE A–4 Average Energy Requirements (Canada)

Age	Sex	Average Height (cm)	Average Weight (kg)	Requirements[a]					
				Cal/Kg	MJ/Kg	Cal/Day	MJ/Day	Cal/Cm	MJ/Cm
Months									
0–2	Both	55	4.5	120–100[b]	0.50–0.42[b]	500	2.0	9.0	0.04
3–5	Both	63	7.0	100– 95[b]	0.42–0.40[b]	700	2.8	11.0	0.05
6–8	Both	69	8.5	95– 97[b]	0.40–0.41[b]	800	3.4	11.5	0.05
9–11	Both	73	9.5	97– 99[b]	0.41	950	3.8	12.5	0.05
Years									
1	Both	82	11	101	0.42	1110	4.8	3.5	0.06
2–3	Both	95	14	94	0.39	1300	5.6	13.5	0.06
4–6	Both	107	18	100	0.42	1800	7.6	17.0	0.07
7–9	M	126	25	88	0.37	2200	9.2	17.5	0.07
	F	125	25	76	0.32	1900	8.0	15.0	0.06
10–12	M	141	34	73	0.30	2500	10.4	17.5	0.07
	F	143	36	61	0.25	2200	9.2	15.5	0.06
13–15	M	159	50	57	0.24	2800	12.0	17.5	0.07
	F	157	48	46	0.19	2200	9.2	14.0	0.06
16–18	M	172	62	51	0.21	3200	13.2	18.5	0.08
	F	160	53	40	0.17	2100	8.8	13.0	0.05
19–24	M	175	71	42	0.18	3000	12.4		
	F	160	58	36	0.15	2100	8.8		
25–49	M	172	74	36	0.15	2700	111.2		
	F	160	59	32	0.13	1900	8.0		
50–74	M	170	73	31	0.13	2300	9.6		
	F	158	63	29	0.12	1800	7.6		
75;	M	168	69	29	0.12	2000	8.4		
	F	155	64	23	0.10	1500	6.0		

[a]Requirements can be expected to vary within a range of ± 30%.
[b]First and last figures are averages at the beginning and at the end of the three-month period.
Source: Health and Welfare Canada, *Recommended Nutrient Intakes for Canadians* (Ottawa: Canadian Government Publishing Centre, 1983), Table II.1, pp. 22–23, as revised in the second printing.

B

Nutrition Assessment

Competent medical care includes attention to nutrition. A client's nutrition status can be evaluated by a dietitian or other qualified health care professional using the information gathered from several nutrition assessment sources. The accurate gathering of this information and its careful interpretation are the basis for a meaningful evaluation. This appendix provides a sample of the procedures, standards, charts, and other forms commonly used in nutrition assessment.

Nutrition assessment involves four techniques:

- History taking.
- Anthropometric measures.
- Physical examination.
- Biochemical analysis (clinical or lab tests).

Each of these techniques involves collecting data in a variety of ways and interpreting the findings in relation to the total picture.

Historical Data

Many clues about a person's present nutrition status are revealed in the person's historical data. A client's history is explored from several angles: medical, social, and drug as well as diet. Table 13–2 lists risk factors associated with poor nutrition status that might be identified in a history, and Form 13–1 shows how such information might be collected. As you can see, many circumstances in a person's life have an impact on nutrition status and provide the assessor with clues to possible problems. Forms 13–2, 13–3, and 13–4 help the assessor uncover specific information about each client's dietary habits.

Medical and social histories can often be obtained from records completed by the attending physician, nurse, or other health care worker. Additional information can be gathered through an interview.

The drug history requires special attention. Hundreds of drugs interact with nutrients, creating the possibility of imbalances or deficiencies. They must not be overlooked in assessing a person's nutrition status. Form B–1 elicits the necessary information regarding drugs, and Table B–1 identifies commonly used drugs and their effects on nutrition. Table B–2 shows specific nutrients and some drugs that can affect these nutrients. Table 14–2 provides examples of drugs that affect food intake and Table 14–3 shows how drugs should be given with respect to food.

FORM B–1. Drug History

1a. Do you have any health problems for which you are taking prescription medications at the present time? Yes _____ No _____
If yes:

Health problem	Proprietary name of drug	Generic name of drug	Dose frequency	Duration of intake

1b. Are you taking any other medication a doctor has prescribed (name of drug unknown, reason for taking unknown)? Yes _____ No _____
If yes:

Description of drug	Dose	Frequency	Duration of intake

2a. Have you taken prescription medication for any of the health problems listed below within the past three months? Yes _____ No _____
If yes:

Health problem	Drug name	Duration of intake	When discontinued	Reason for stopping	Still taking[a]
Asthma					
Arthritis					

[a]Check (√) if still taking.

Infection (specify)
Tuberculosis
Malaria
High blood pressure
Fluid retention
Psoriasis
Colitis
High cholesterol
Parkinson's disease
Liver disease
Kidney disease
Blood disease
Bone disease
Gout
Blood clots
Diabetes
Other (specify)

2b. Have you taken any other medication within the past three months that a doctor has prescribed (name of drug unknown, reason for taking unknown)? Yes ____ No ____

Description	Dose	Frequency	Duration of intake

3a. Do you take medications, self-prescribed, for any reason? Yes ____ No ____
If yes:

Complaint	Constantly	Frequently	Occasionally
Constipation			
Indigestion			
Headache			
Nervousness			
Insomnia			
Pain			
Menstrual cramps			
Colds and sinus trouble			
Other (state)			

3b. If response to 3a is positive in one or more categories, what medication do you take to relieve these complaints, and how much do you need to gain relief?

Complaint	Drug	Dose	Frequency	Duration
Constipation				
Indigestion				
Headache				
Nervousness				
Insomnia				
Pain				
Menstrual cramps				
Colds and sinus trouble				
Other (state)				

4. Are you taking birth control pills now? Yes ____ No ____
If yes:
  Name:
  Duration of intake:

Have you taken birth control pills within the past six months? Yes ____ No ____
If yes:
  Name:
  Duration of intake:
  Date discontinued:
  Reason for stopping:

Source: Adapted from D. Roe, *Drug-Induced Nutritional Deficiencies* (Westport, Conn.: AVI Publishing Company, 1976), Table 4.2, pp. 106–108.

TABLE B–1. Selected Drug-Nutrient Interactions

Drug	Nutrient	Effect on Nutrition
Alcohol	Energy	↓ intake
	Protein	↓ intake
	Fat	↑ buildup in liver
		↓ absorption
	Thiamin	↓ absorption ↓ storage
	Vitamin B$_6$	↓ activation
	Folacin	↓ absorption, utilization
	Vitamin B$_{12}$	↓ absorption
	Magnesium	↑ urinary excretion
	Zinc	↑ urinary excretion
Amphetamines	↓ Nutrient intake	causes anorexia, dry mouth, metallic taste, nausea, vomiting
Analgesics	Folacin	↓ serum levels; altered transport
Aspirin	Vitamin C	↑ urinary excretion
	Thiamin	↑ urinary excretion
	Vitamin K	↑ urinary excretion
	Iron	may cause blood loss
Antacids		
Aluminum hydroxide	Phosphorus	↓ absorption
Other types	Thiamin	↑ destruction
Anticoagulants	Vitamin K	↓ conversion to active form
Anticonvulsants	Folacin	↓ serum levels
	Vitamin B$_6$	↓ serum levels
	Vitamin B$_{12}$	↓ serum levels
	Vitamin D	↓ conversion to active forms
	Vitamin K	↑ requirement
Antimicrobials		
Chloramphenicol	Riboflavin	↑ requirement (?)
	Vitamin B$_6$	↑ requirement (?)
	Vitamin B$_{12}$	↑ requirement (?)
Neomycin	Fats	↓ absorption
	Nitrogen	↓ absorption
	Carbohydrates	↓ absorption
	Folacin	↓ absorption
	Vitamin B$_{12}$	↓ absorption
	Fat-soluble vitamins	↓ absorption
	Calcium	↓ absorption
	Iron	↓ absorption
	Potassium	↓ absorption
	Vitamin K	↓ intestinal synthesis
Penicillin	Potassium	↑ urinary excretion
Tetracycline	Fat	↓ absorption
	Amino acids	↓ absorption
	Calcium	↓ absorption
	Iron	↓ absorption
	Magnesium	↓ absorption
	Zinc	↓ absorption
	Niacin	↑ urinary excretion
	Riboflavin	↑ urinary excretion

TABLE B–1. (continued)

Drug	Nutrient	Effect on Nutrition
	Folacin	↑ urinary excretion
	Vitamin C	↑ urinary excretion
Antineoplastic agents		
Methotrexate and pyrimethamine	Folacin	folacin antagonist
	Vitamin B$_{12}$	↓ absorption
	Fat	↓ absorption
	↓ Nutrient; intake and general malabsorption	anorexia, nausea, vomiting, mouth sores
5-Fluorouracil	Protein	↓ absorption and synthesis
Antitubercular drugs		
Cycloserine	Vitamin B$_6$	Vitamin B$_6$ antagonist
	Protein	↓ synthesis
	Calcium	↓ absorption (?)
	Magnesium	↓ absorption (?)
	Vitamin B$_6$	↓ serum levels (?)
	Folacin	↓ serum levels (?)
	Vitamin B$_{12}$	↓ serum levels (?)
Isonicotinic acid hydrazide (INH)	Vitamin B$_6$	Vitamin B$_6$ antagonist
		↑ urinary excretion
		causes deficiency
	Niacin	causes deficiency
	Vitamin B$_{12}$	↓ absorption
		↓ serum levels
Para-aminosalicylic acid	Folacin	↓ absorption
	Vitamin B$_{12}$	↓ absorption
	Fat	↓ absorption
	Iron	↓ absorption
Chelating agents		
Penicillamine	Vitamin B$_6$	↑ requirement
		↑ urinary excretion
	Zinc	↑ urinary excretion
	Iron	↑ urinary excretion
	Copper	↑ urinary excretion
	↓ Nutrient intake	alters taste; causes anorexia, nausea, vomiting
Cholesterol-lowering agents		
Cholestyramine	Fat and cholesterol	↓ absorption
	Fat-soluble vitamins	↓ absorption
	Folacin	↓ absorption
	Iron	↓ absorption
	Vitamin B$_{12}$	↓ absorption
		↓ blood levels
	Calcium	↑ urinary excretion
		↓ blood levels
Clofibrate	Vitamin B$_{12}$	↓ absorption
	Iron	↓ absorption
	↓ Nutrient intake	alters taste; causes nausea and GI irritation

TABLE B–1. (continued)

Drug	Nutrient	Effect on Nutrition
Colchicine	Fat	↓ absorption
	Nitrogen	↓ absorption
	Folacin	↓ absorption
	Vitamin B$_{12}$	↓ absorption
	Sodium	↓ absorption
	Potassium	↓ absorption
Corticosteirods	Vitamin D	↑ metabolism
		↑ requirement
	Vitamin B$_6$	↑ requirement
	Vitamin C	↑ requirement
		↑ urinary excretion
	Calcium	↓ absorption
		↑ urinary excretion
	Phosphorus	↓ absorption
	Zinc	↑ urinary excretion
		↓ serum levels
	Glucose	↑ serum levels
	Triglycerides	↑ serum levels
	Cholesterol	↑ serum levels
	Potassium	↑ urinary excretion
	Nitrogen	↑ urinary excretion
Diuretics		
Furosemide	Calcium	↑ urinary excretion
	Sodium	↑ urinary excretion
	Potassium	↓ serum levels
	Chloride	↓ serum levels
	Magnesium	↓ serum levels
	Zinc	↑ serum levels
		↓ storage in liver
Mercurials	Thiamin	↑ urinary excretion
	Calcium	↑ urinary excretion
	Sodium	↑ urinary excretion
	Potassium	↑ urinary excretion
	Chloride	↑ urinary excretion
	Magnesium	↑ urinary excretion
Thiazides	Sodium	↑ urinary excretion
	Potassium	↓ blood levels
	Chloride	↓ blood levels
	Calcium	↑ urinary excretion
		↑ blood levels
	Magnesium	↑ urinary excretion
	Phosphorus	↓ blood levels
	Glucose	↑ blood levels(?)
Triamterene	Sodium	↑ urinary excretion
	Folacin	↓ serum levels
	Vitamin B$_{12}$	↓ serum levels
Glutethimide	Vitamin D	↑ metabolism
Hydralazine	Vitamin B$_6$	↑ urinary excretion
Hypoglycemics Phenformin and metformin	Vitamin B$_{12}$	↓ absorption

TABLE B–1. (continued)

Drug	Nutrient	Effect on Nutrition
Laxatives		
Cathartics	Fat	↓ absorption
	Glucose	↓ absorption
	Vitamin D	↓ absorption
	Calcium	↓ absorption
	Potassium	↓ absorption
Mineral oil	Fat-soluble vitamins	↓ absorption
	Calcium	↓ absorption
	Phosphates	↓ absorption
Levodopa	Amino acids	↑ requirement
	Vitamin B_6	↑ requirement
	Vitamin C	↑ requirement
	Sodium	↓ urinary excretion
	Potassium	↓ urinary excretion
Oral contraceptives	Vitamin B_6	↑ requirement
		↓ blood levels
	Riboflavin	↑ requirement
		↓ blood levels
	Folacin	↓ absorption
		↓ blood levels
	Vitamin B_{12}	↓ blood levels
	Vitamin C	↓ blood levels
	Vitamin A	↑ blood levels
	Calcium	↑ absorption
	Iron	↑ serum levels
	Copper	↑ serum levels
	Magnesium	↓ blood levels(?)
	Zinc	↓ blood levels(?)
Potassium salts	Vitamin B_{12}	↓ absorption
Sulfonamides		
Salicylazosulfapyridine	Folacin	↓ absorption
	Iron	↓ blood levels
		↓ blood levels
Others	Folacin	↓ intestinal synthesis
	Vitamin K	↓ intestinal synthesis
	B vitamins	↓ intestinal synthesis

↑ increases
↓ decreases
(?) possible effect

Sources: Data from R. E. Hodges, Drug-nutrient interactions, in *Nutrition in Medical Practice* (Philadelphia: Saunders, 1980), pp. 323–331; R. C. Theuer and J. J. Vitale, Drug and nutrient interactions, in *Nutritional Support of Medical Practice,* eds. H. A. Schneider, C. E. Anderson, and D. B. Coursin (Hagerstown, Md.: Harper & Row, 1977), pp. 297–305; A. O. Moore and D. E. Powers, *Food-Medication Interactions,* ed. C. H. Smith (Tempe, Ariz.: A. O. Moore and D. E. Powers, 1981); A. Grant, *Nutritional Assessment Guidelines* (Seattle: A. Grant, 1979), pp. 63–96; D. C. March, *Handbook: Interactions of Selected Drugs with Nutritional Status in Man* (Chicago: American Dietetic Association, 1978).

TABLE B–2. Nutrients That May Be Affected by Drugs

Nutrient	Agents That Affect Nutrient Status
Protein	5-Fluorouracil, neomycin
Carbohydrates	Metformin, phenformin, corticosteroids, chlorothiazide
Fats and fatty acids	Neomycin, cholestyramine, clofibrate
Thiamin	Antacids, ethanol, carbohydrates
Riboflavin	Boric acid, oral contraceptive steroids
Niacin	Isoniazid, 6-mercaptopurine, 5-fluorouracil
Vitamin B_6	Isoniazid, ethanol, oral contraceptive steroids, penicillamine, hydralazine, cycloserine, levodopa
Folates	Diphenylhydantoin, methotrexate, pyrimethamine, ethanol, oral contraceptive steroids, phenylbutazone
Vitamin B_{12}	Para-aminosalicylic acid, barbiturates, colchicine, cholestyramine, phenformin, oral contraceptive steroids
Vitamin C	Aminopyrine, cigarettes, diphenylhydantoin, oral contraceptive steroids, paraldehyde, salicylates
Vitamin A	Mineral oil (disputed), cholestyramine, oral contraceptive steroids
Vitamin D	Phenobarbital, diphenylhydantoin, cholestyramine, mineral oil
Vitamin E	Mineral oil, iron, polyunsaturated fatty acids, cholestyramine
Vitamin K	Sodium warfarin (Coumadin), barbiturates, ascorbic acid, mineral oil
Essential fatty acids	Continuous infusions of glucose
Sodium	Thiazides, ethacrynic acid, spironolactone (Aldactone)
Potassium	Thiazides, cathartics
Calcium	Oxalates, fatty acids, phytates, phosphates
Phosphorus	Aluminum hydroxide, total parenteral nutrition
Magnesium	Ethanol, ethacrynic acid
Iron	Phytic acid, oxalates, phosphates, ascorbic acid
Zinc	Ethanol, penicillamine, oral contraceptive steroids
Copper	Ethanol, penicillamine, phytates, corticosteroids

Source: R. E. Hodges, *Nutrition in Medical Practice* (Philadelphia: Saunders, 1980), p. 328. Reprinted with permission.

Anthropometric Measures

One use of anthropometric measures is to assess growth in children. Although special equipment is available to measure an infant's length (see Figure B–1), in many settings a less accurate method is used: with the infant lying on a flat surface, a measuring tape is run along the side of the baby from the top of the head to the heel of the foot. Care is taken to

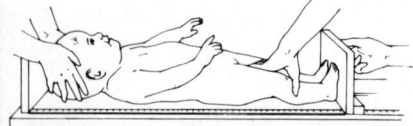

FIGURE B–1

Measurement of an infant. An infant is measured lying down by use of a length measuring device with a fixed headboard and movable footboard. Note that two people are needed to measure the infant's length. Illustration courtesy Ross Laboratories.

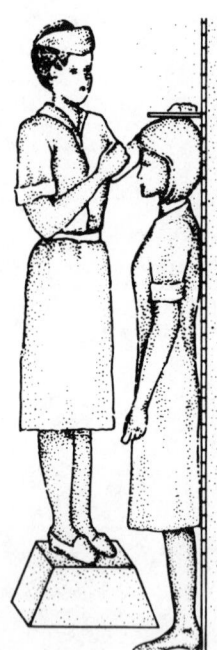

FIGURE B–2

Measurement of an adult. Height is measured most accurately when the person stands against a flat wall to which a measuring tape has been affixed. When the person is taller than the measurer, the measurer can stand on a stool to help ensure that the proper height measurement is obtained.

ensure that the infant's legs and body are straight. Since this is difficult to accomplish, it requires two people to obtain an accurate measurement.

A child that can stand erect and cooperate can be measured in the same manner as an adult. The best way to measure height is to have the person being measured stand against a flat wall to which a measuring tape or stick has been affixed (see Figure B–2). The person should not be wearing shoes and should stand erect with heels together. The person's line of sight should be horizontal, and the heels, buttocks, shoulders, and head should be touching the wall. After carefully checking the height measurement, the assessor should record the result immediately to avoid misplacing or forgetting the measurement. Height is recorded in either inches or centimeters, depending on the policy of the institution.

Although less desirable, the measuring rod of a scale can be used to measure height by using the same general procedure. The person should be facing away from the scale, and extra care should be

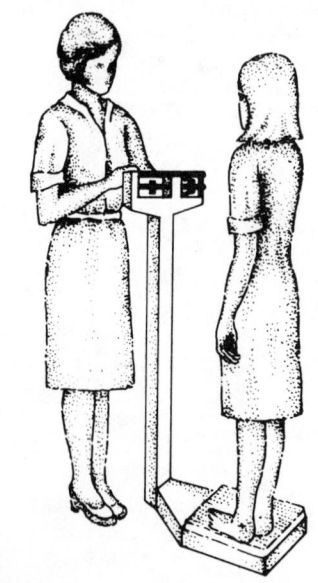

FIGURE B–3

Weighing an adult. Whenever possible, subjects are measured on beam balance scales to ensure accuracy.

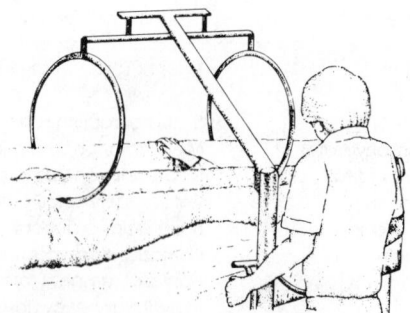

FIGURE B–4

Weighing an adult using metabolic scales. Metabolic bed scales are used to measure patients who cannot get out of bed.

taken to ensure that the person is standing as straight as possible.

Unfortunately, it is a common practice in many health care institutions to ask clients how tall they are rather than measuring their height. Self-reported height should be used only as a last resort when measurement is not practical (for example, in the case of an uncooperative patient or an emergency admission).

In adults, weight measurements should be taken on a beam balance that frequently is checked for accuracy (see Figure B–3). Standardized conditions under which people are weighed increase the usability of repeated weight measurements. Whenever possible, a person should be weighed at the same time of day (preferably before breakfast), in the same amount of clothing (hospital gown, without shoes), after having voided, and on the same scale. Bedridden patients can be measured with metabolic scales (see Figure B–4). Bathroom scales are not accurate and should not be used. Like all measurements, observed weight should be recorded immediately. Weight is recorded in either pounds or kilograms, depending on the policy of the institution.

To assess growth in infants and children, use Figures B–5a and B–5b, B–6a and B–6b, B–7a and B–7b, and B–8a and B–8b. Follow these steps:

- Select the appropriate figure based on age and sex. For example, for a 3-month-old female infant weighing 12 pounds with a length of 23 inches, you would use the chart for girls, birth to 36 months (Figure B–5a).

- Locate the child's age on the bottom or top of the chart (in our example, 3 months).
- Locate the child's weight in pounds or kilograms on the lower left or right side of the chart (in our example, 12 pounds).
- Mark the chart where the age and weight lines intersect. (In our example, this is just above the 50th percentile. Note where the chart is marked.)
- To find the child's percentile for length or height and age, start by locating the child's age on the top of the chart and the length on the upper right or left side. Proceed as you did when you were comparing age and weight. (Note the mark on the chart for the baby in the example.)

In pregnancy, satisfactory growth of the fetus is normally assumed if the pregnant woman's weight gain is normal. Figure B–9 is a weight-gain grid used for assessment purposes.

Among the standards used for anthropometric measures are several already presented. A table of average weights for height is often used as a standard for individual people's weight. To use the height-weight table, the assessor refers to a table of frame sizes such as the one based on elbow breadth (see inside back cover) or the one that compares wrist circumference to height (see Figure B–10 and Table B–3). The table of average weights for height may not be useful in cases where a person has weighed much more or much less than the average throughout life. To assess such a person's weight, it may be more informative to compare the present weight, not with an "ideal" body weight, but with the usual body weight. The percentages of a person's actual weight compared with ideal or usual body weight are useful indicators of malnutrition (Table B–4).

The triceps fatfold measurement provides an estimate of body fat (see Figure B–11). Triceps fatfold percentiles are given in Table B–5. The midarm circumference (MAC) provides an index of the arm's total area (see Figure B–12 and Table B–6); and an arithmetical calculation subtracts the fat from the total area, leaving an estimate of the lean tissue in the arm—the mid-arm muscle circumference (MAMC). The MAMC (see Figure B–13 and Table B–7) reflects the body's total skeletal muscle mass.

To assess protein-kcalorie malnutrition, several lab tests are used in conjunction with these anthropometric measures. Table B–8 shows that different compartments are depleted, depending on whether the person has kwashiorkor (from protein deficiency as reflected in skeletal muscle and visceral protein), marasmus (from kcalorie deficiency as reflected in body fat), or a mixture of the two.

Physical Examination

Chapters 7 and 8 discuss some symptoms of vitamin and mineral deficiencies and toxicities, revealing that many tissues and organs reflect signs of malnutrition. Table B–9 presents some of the signs of vitamin/mineral malnutrition, body system by body system.

Biochemical (Lab) Tests

Biochemical or clinical lab tests help to determine what is really happening inside the body. Blood and urine samples are most often used to directly measure nutrients or metabolites that are affected by poor nutrition. Table B–10 summarizes the biochemical tests used to assess vitamin-mineral status.

Standards for determining the severity of depletion of serum albumin and transferrin are given in Table B–11. Creatinine-height index standards are given in Tables B–12a and B–12b.

*This factor converts the fatfold measurement and also converts millimeters to centimeters.

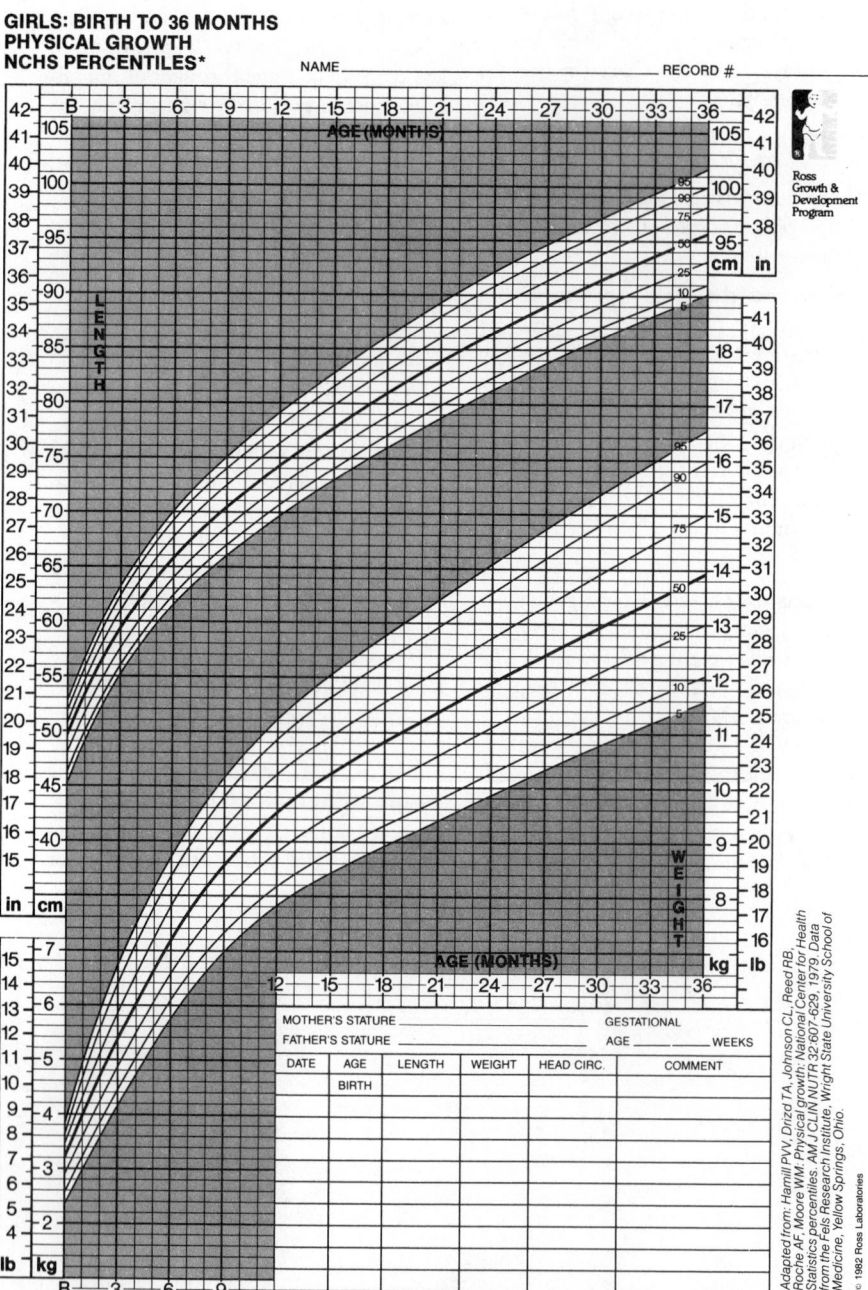

FIGURE B–5a

Girls: Birth to 36 Months Physical Growth NCHS Percentiles—Length and Weight for Age.

BOYS: BIRTH TO 36 MONTHS
PHYSICAL GROWTH
NCHS PERCENTILES*

NAME_____ RECORD #_____

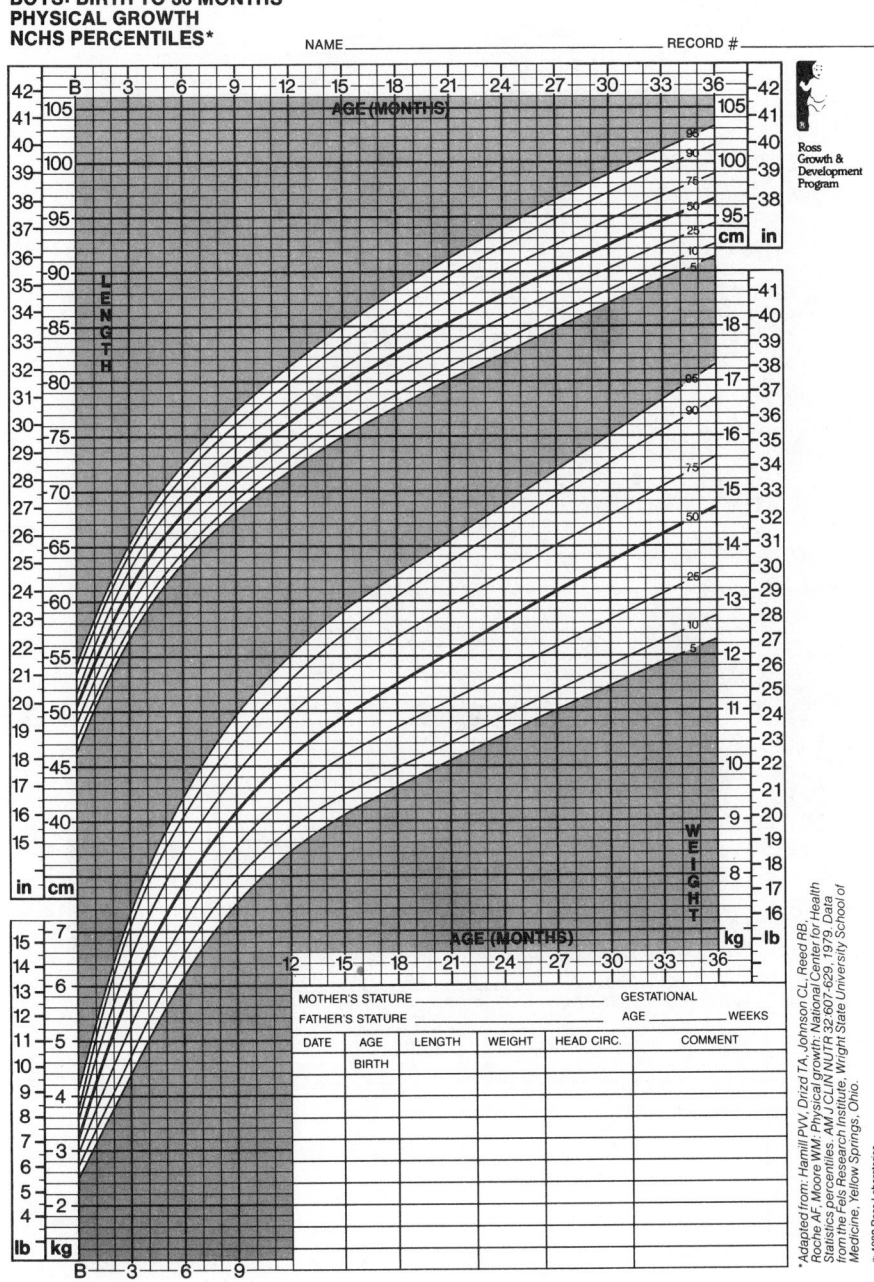

Ross
Growth &
Development
Program

*Adapted from: Hamill PVV, Drizd TA, Johnson CL, Reed RB,
Roche AF, Moore WM. Physical growth: National Center for Health
Statistics percentiles. AM J CLIN NUTR 32:607-629, 1979. Data
from the Fels Research Institute, Wright State University School of
Medicine, Yellow Springs, Ohio.
© 1982 Ross Laboratories

FIGURE B–5b

Boys: Birth to 36 Months Physical Growth NCHS Percentiles—Length and Weight for Age.

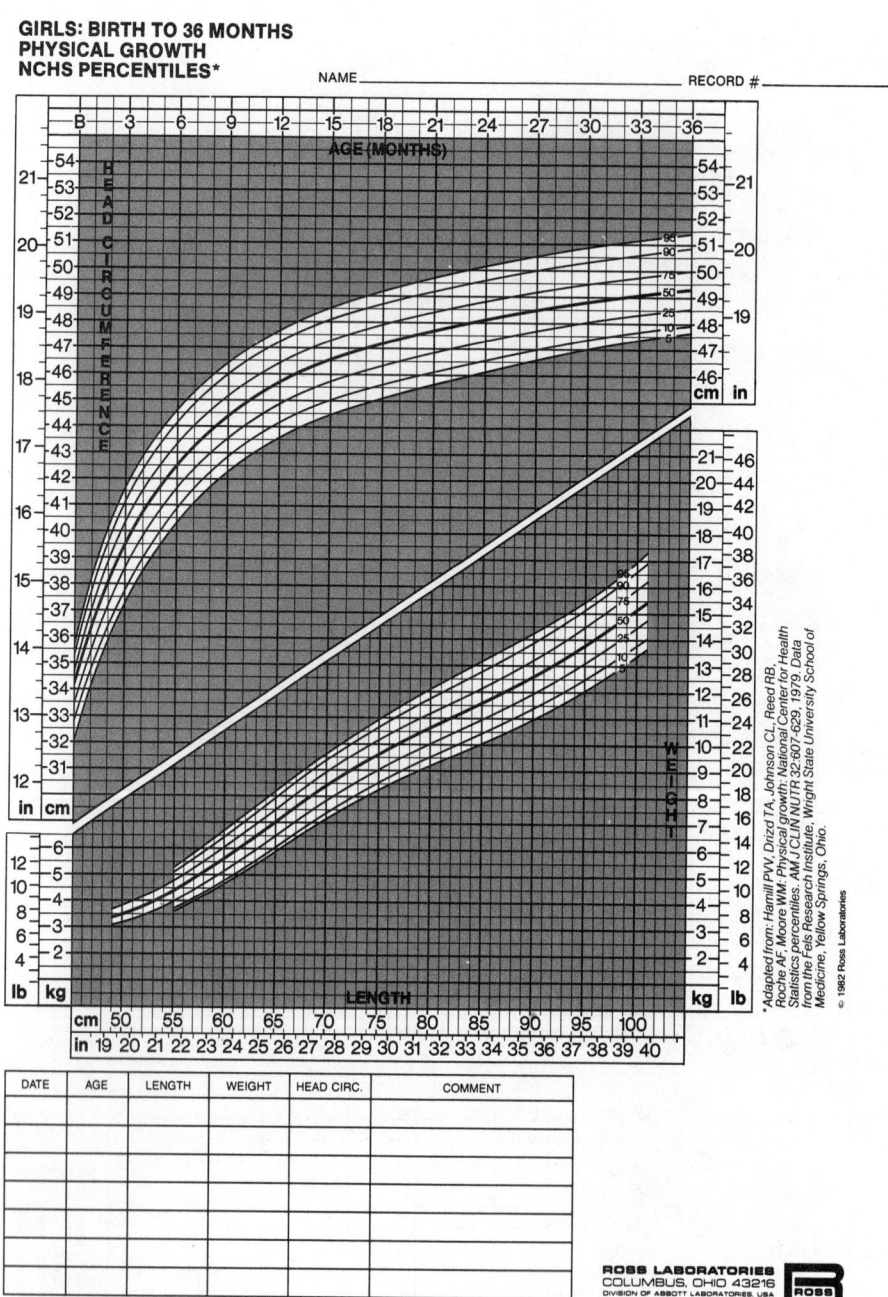

*Adapted from: Hamill PVV, Drizd TA, Johnson CL, Reed RB, Roche AF, Moore WM: Physical growth: National Center for Health Statistics percentiles. AM J CLIN NUTR 32:607–629, 1979. Data from the Fels Research Institute, Wright State University School of Medicine, Yellow Springs, Ohio.

© 1982 Ross Laboratories*

GIRLS: BIRTH TO 36 MONTHS PHYSICAL GROWTH NCHS PERCENTILES*

DATE	AGE	LENGTH	WEIGHT	HEAD CIRC.	COMMENT

ROSS LABORATORIES
COLUMBUS, OHIO 43216
DIVISION OF ABBOTT LABORATORIES, USA

G106 (0.05)/JUNE 1985   LITHO IN USA

FIGURE B–6a

Girls: Birth to 36 Months Physical Growth NCHS Percentiles—Head Circumference for Age and Weight for Length.

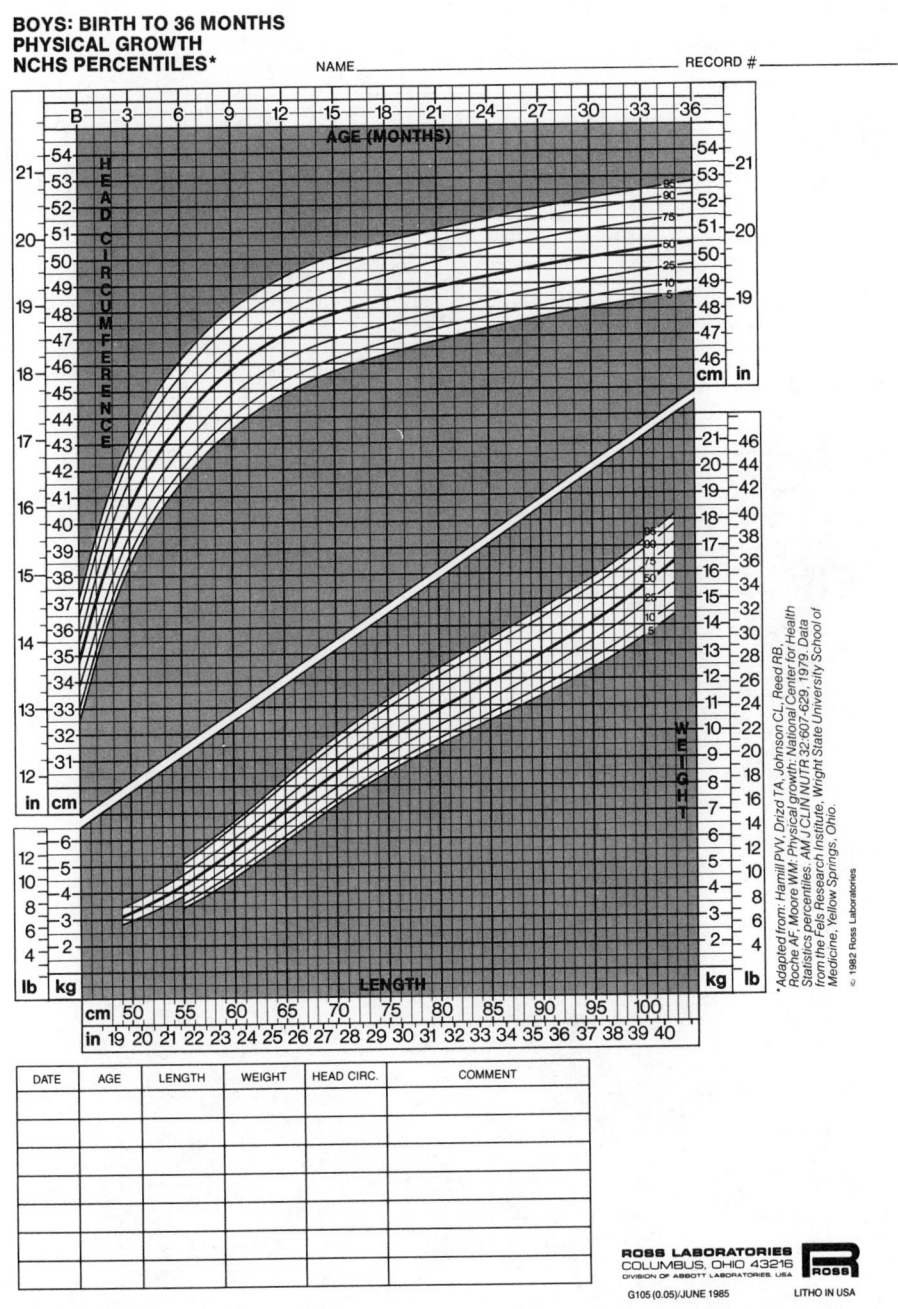

**BOYS: BIRTH TO 36 MONTHS
PHYSICAL GROWTH
NCHS PERCENTILES***

NAME_____ RECORD #_____

FIGURE B—6b

Boys: Birth to 36 Months Physical Growth NCHS Percentiles—Head Circumference
for Age and Weight for Length.

ROSS LABORATORIES
COLUMBUS, OHIO 43216
DIVISION OF ABBOTT LABORATORIES, USA

G105 (0.05)/JUNE 1985   LITHO IN USA

*Adapted from: Hamill PVV, Drizd TA, Johnson CL, Reed RB,
Roche AF, Moore WM: Physical growth: National Center for Health
Statistics percentiles. AM J CLIN NUTR 32:607–629, 1979. Data
from the Fels Research Institute, Wright State University School of
Medicine, Yellow Springs, Ohio.

© 1982 Ross Laboratories

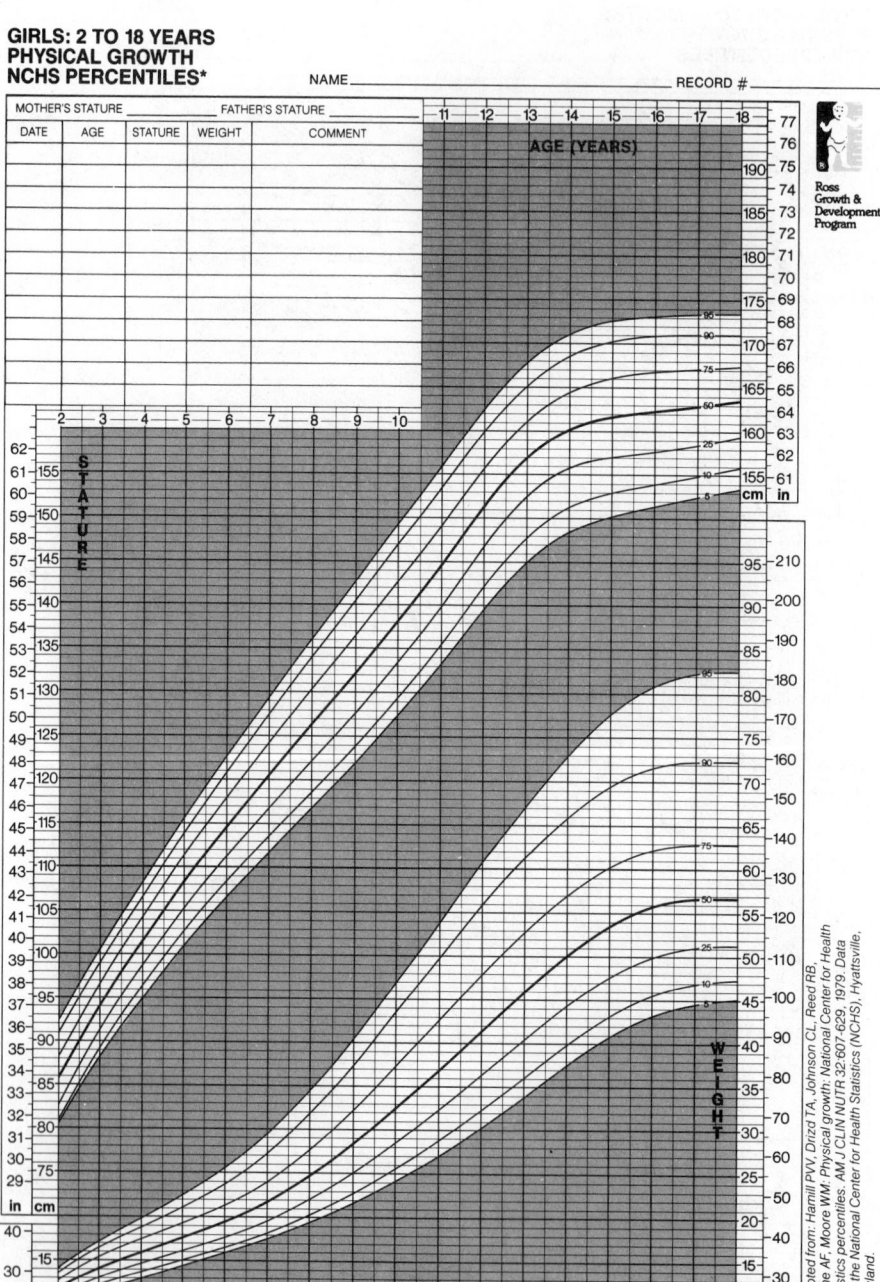

FIGURE B–7a

Girls: 2 to 18 Years Physical Growth NCHS Percentiles—Height and Weight for Age.

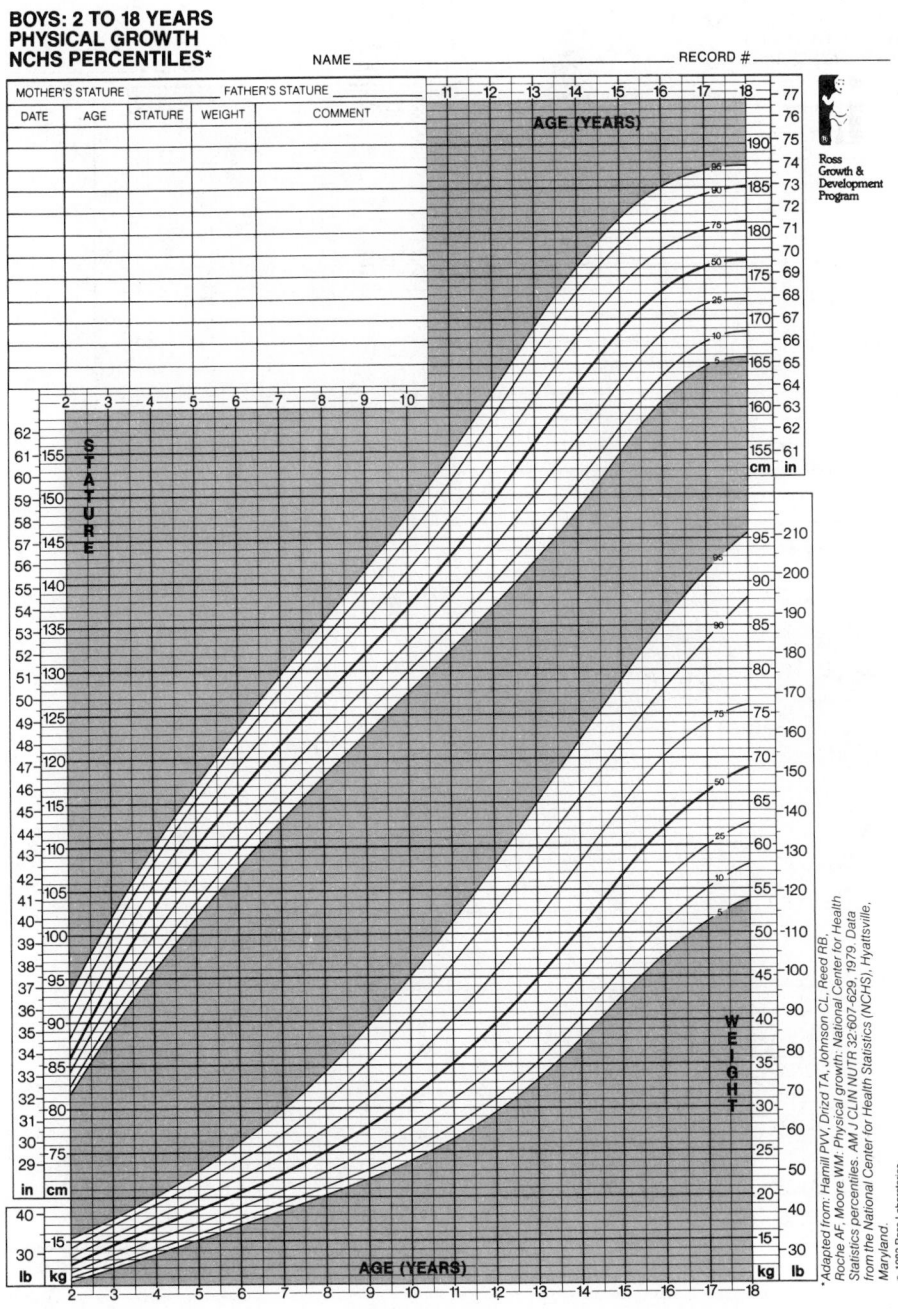

FIGURE B–7b

Boys: 2 to 18 Years Physical Growth NCHS Percentiles—Height and Weight for Age.

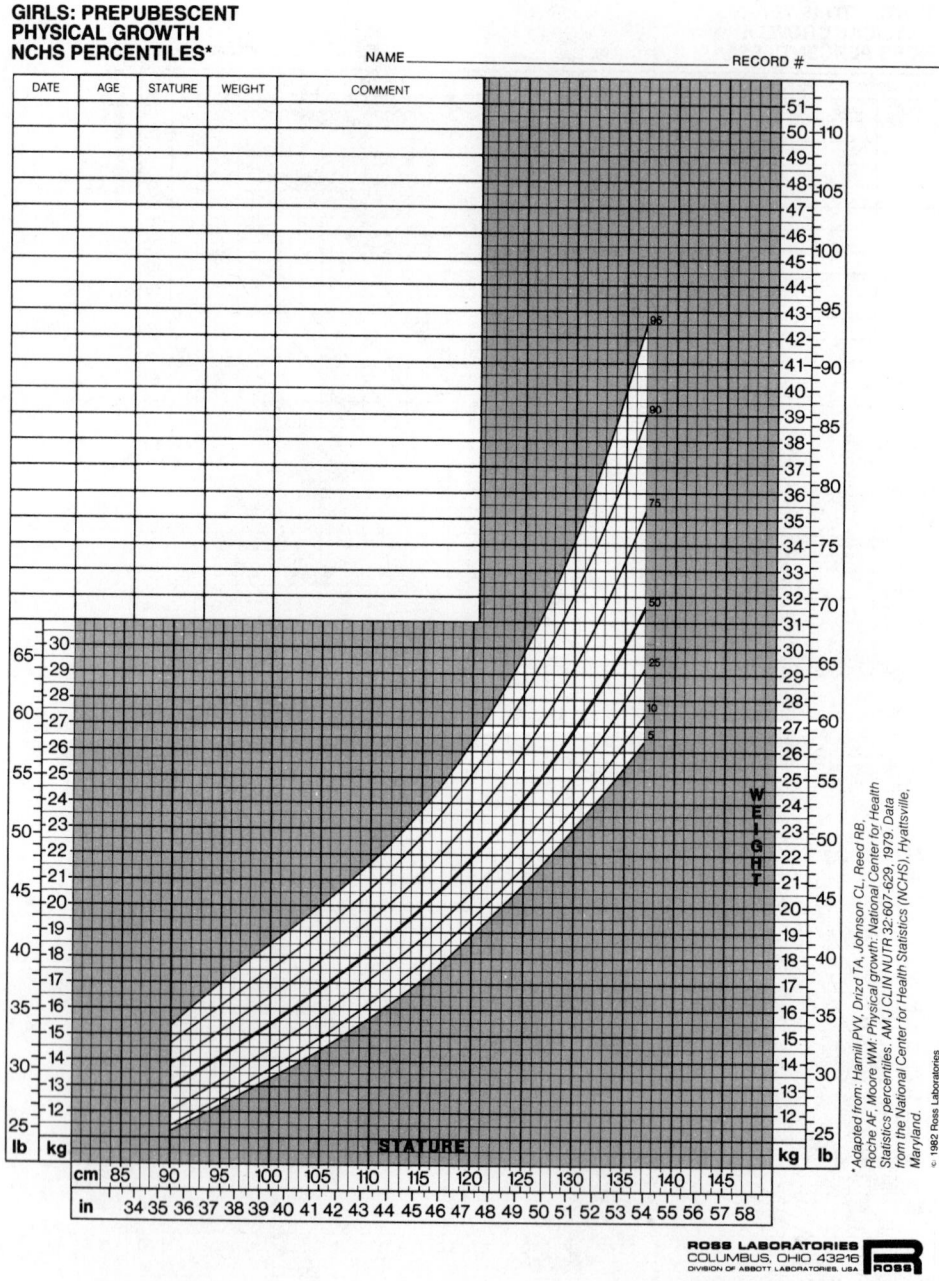

GIRLS: PREPUBESCENT PHYSICAL GROWTH NCHS PERCENTILES*

Adapted from: Hamill PVV, Drizd TA, Johnson CL, Reed RB, Roche AF, Moore WM: Physical growth: National Center for Health Statistics percentiles. AM J CLIN NUTR 32:607-629, 1979. Data from the National Center for Health Statistics (NCHS), Hyattsville, Maryland.

ROSS LABORATORIES
COLUMBUS, OHIO 43216
DIVISION OF ABBOTT LABORATORIES, USA

G108 (0.05)/JUNE 1985   LITHO IN USA

FIGURE B—8a

Girls: Prepubescent Physical Growth NCHS Percentiles—Weight for Height.

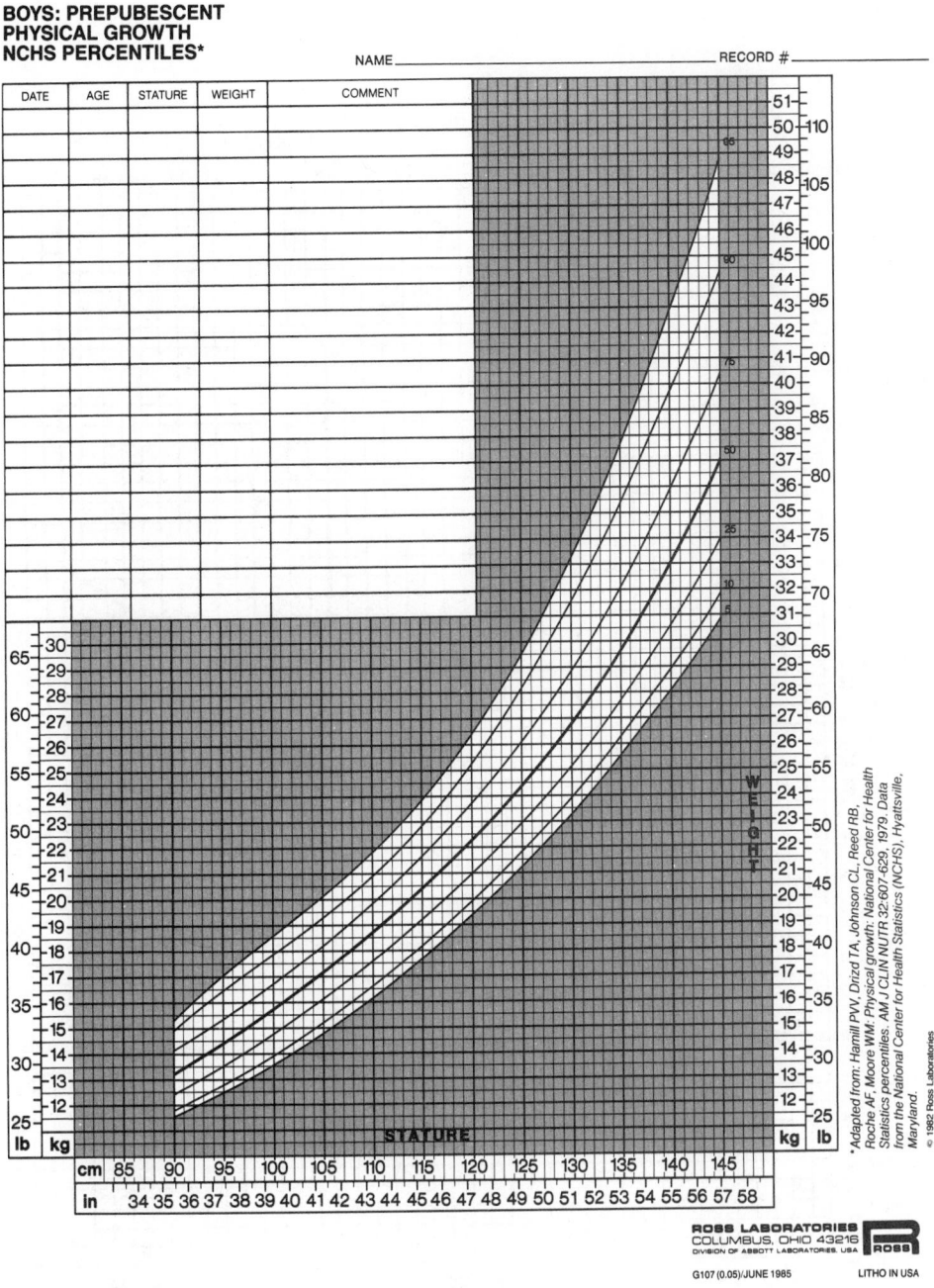

*Adapted from: Hamill PVV, Drizd TA, Johnson CL, Reed RB, Roche AF, Moore WM: Physical growth: National Center for Health Statistics percentiles. AM J CLIN NUTR 32:607-629, 1979. Data from the National Center for Health Statistics (NCHS), Hyattsville, Maryland.

© 1982 Ross Laboratories

ROSS LABORATORIES
COLUMBUS, OHIO 43216
DIVISION OF ABBOTT LABORATORIES, USA

G107 (0.05)/JUNE 1985   LITHO IN USA

FIGURE B—8b

Boys: Prepubescent Physical Growth NCHS Percentiles—Weight for Height.

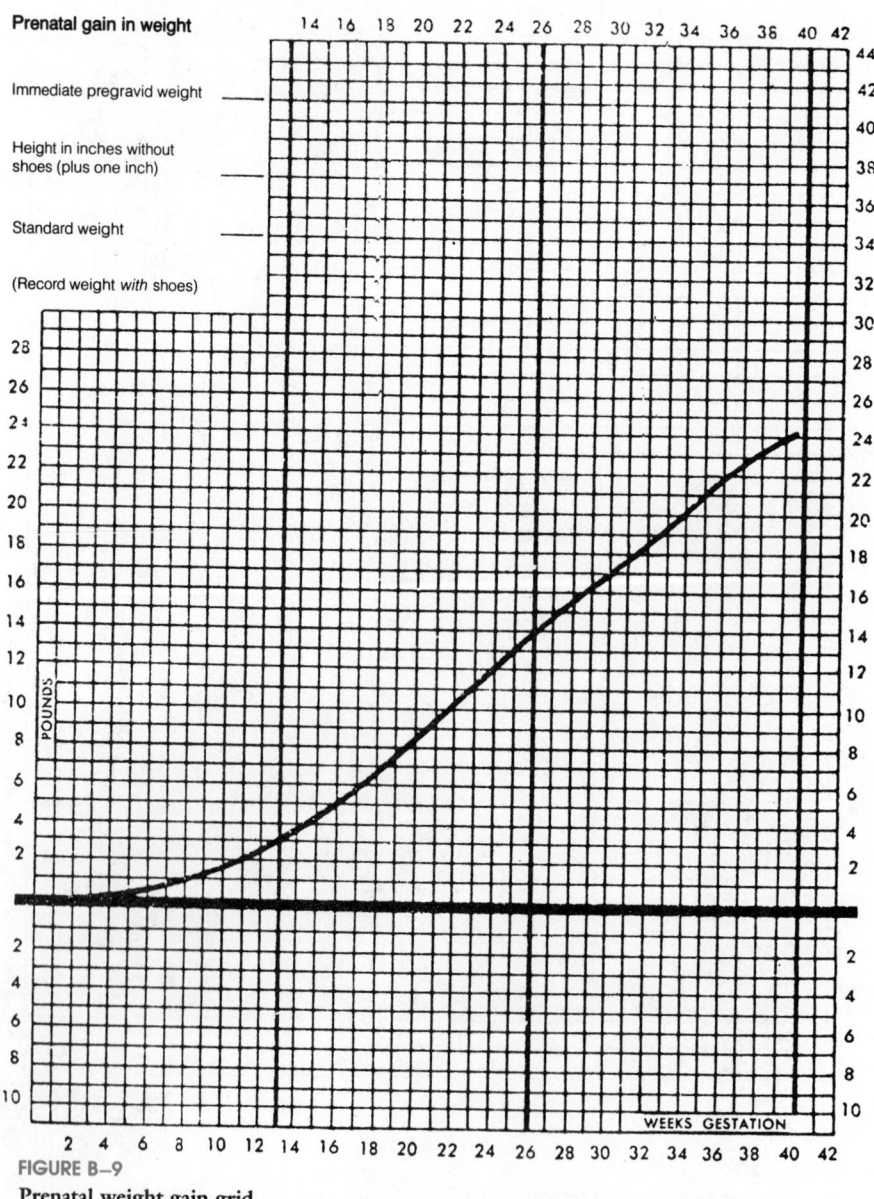

Prenatal gain in weight

Immediate pregravid weight _____

Height in inches without
shoes (plus one inch) _____

Standard weight _____

(Record weight *with* shoes)

FIGURE B–9

Prenatal weight gain grid.

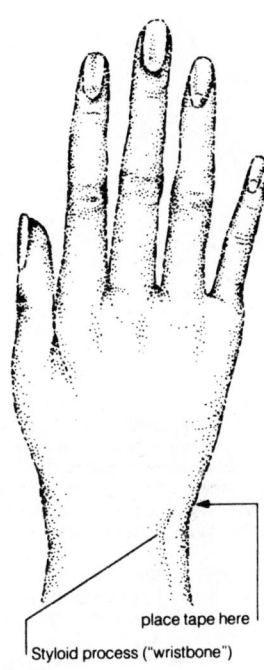

place tape here

Styloid process ("wristbone")

FIGURE B–10

Wrist circumference. The wrist circumference is measured as shown above.

TABLE B–3. Frame Size from Height-Wrist Circumference Ratios (r)

	Male r Values[a]	Female r Values[a]
Small	>10.4	>11.0
Medium	9.6–10.4	10.1–11.0
Large	<9.6	<10.1

[a]$r = \dfrac{\text{Height (cm)}}{\text{Wrist circumference (cm)}^{b}}$

[b]The wrist is measured where it bends (distal to the styloid process), on the right arm.

Source: Adapted from J. P. Grant, Patient selection, *Handbook of Total Parenteral Nutrition* (Philadelphia: Saunders, 1980), p. 15.

TABLE B–4. Weight as an Indicator of Malnutrition

%IBW[a]	%UBW[b]	Degree of Undernutrition
80–90%	85–95%	Mildly depleted
70–79%	75–84%	Moderately depleted
<70%	<75%	Severely depleted

[a]Percent ideal body weight.
[b]Percent usual body weight.

Source: Adapted from J. P. Grant, Patient selection, *Handbook of Total Parenteral Nutrition* (Philadelphia: Saunders, 1980), p. 11.

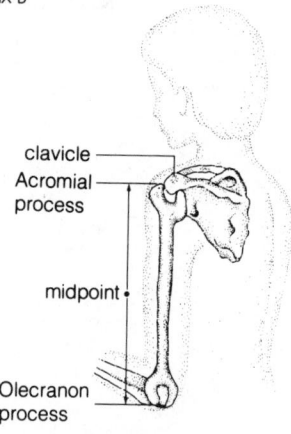

clavicle
Acromial
process

midpoint

Olecranon
process

FIGURE B–11

How to measure the triceps fatfold.

A. Find the midpoint of the arm:
1. Ask the subject to bend his arm at the elbow and lay his hand across his stomach. (If he is right-handed, measure the left arm, and vice versa.)
2. Feel the shoulder to locate the acromial process. It helps to slide your fingers along the clavicle to find the acromial process. The olecranon process is the tip of the elbow.
3. Place a measuring tape from the acromial process to the tip of the elbow. Divide this measurement by 2 and mark the midpoint of the arm with a pen.

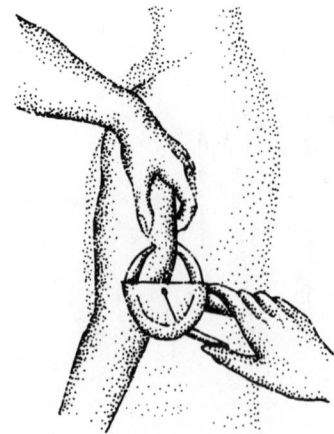

B. Measure the fatfold:
1. Ask the subject to let his arm hang loosely at his side.
2. Grasp a fold of skin and subcutaneous fat between the thumb and forefinger slightly above the midpoint mark. Gently pull the skin away from the underlying muscle. (This step takes a lot of practice. If you want to be sure you don't have muscle as well as fat, ask the subject to contract and relax his muscle. You should be able to feel if you are pinching muscle.)
3. Place the calipers over the fatfold at the midpoint mark and read the measurement to the nearest 10 mm in two to three seconds. (If using plastic calipers, align pressure lines and read measurement to the nearest 1.0 mm in two to three seconds.)
4. Repeat steps 2 and 3 twice more. Add the three readings and then divide by 3 to find the average.

TABLE B–5. Triceps Fatfold Percentiles (millimeters)

Age	Male					Female				
	5th	25th	50th	75th	95th	5th	25th	50th	75th	95th
1–1.9	6	8	10	12	16	6	8	10	12	16
2–2.9	6	8	10	12	15	6	9	10	12	16
3–3.9	6	8	10	11	15	7	9	11	12	15
4–4.9	6	8	9	11	14	7	8	10	12	16
5–5.9	6	8	9	11	15	6	8	10	12	18
6–6.9	5	7	8	10	16	6	8	10	12	16
7–7.9	5	7	9	12	17	6	9	11	13	18
8–8.9	5	7	8	10	16	6	9	12	15	24
9–9.9	6	7	10	13	18	8	10	13	16	22
10–10.9	6	8	10	14	21	7	10	12	17	27
11–11.9	6	8	11	16	24	7	10	13	18	28
12–12.9	6	8	11	14	28	8	11	14	18	27
13–13.9	5	7	10	14	26	8	12	15	21	30
14–14.9	4	7	9	14	24	9	13	16	21	28
15–15.9	4	6	8	11	24	8	12	17	21	32
16–16.9	4	6	8	12	22	10	15	18	22	31
17–17.9	5	6	8	12	19	10	13	19	24	37
18–18.9	4	6	9	13	24	10	15	18	22	30
19–24.9	4	7	10	15	22	10	14	18	24	34
25–34.9	5	8	12	16	24	10	16	21	27	37
35–44.9	5	8	12	16	23	12	18	23	29	38
45–54.9	6	8	12	15	25	12	20	25	30	40
55–64.9	5	8	11	14	22	12	20	25	31	38
65–74.9	4	8	11	15	22	12	18	24	29	36

Source: Adapted from A. R. Frisancho, New norms of upper limb fat and muscle areas for assessment of nutritional status, *American Journal of Clinical Nutrition* 34 (1981): 2540–2545.

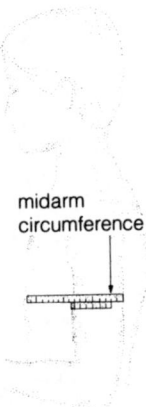

midarm
circumference

FIGURE B–12

How to measure the midarm circumference. Ask the subject to let his arm hang loosely at his side. Place the measuring tape horizontally around the arm at the midpoint mark. This measurement is the midarm circumference.

TABLE B–6. Midarm Circumference (MAC) Percentiles (centimeters)

Age	Male					Female				
	5th	25th	50th	75th	95th	5th	25th	50th	75th	95th
1–1.9	14.2	15.0	15.9	17.0	18.3	13.8	14.8	15.6	16.4	17.7
2–2.9	14.1	15.3	16.2	17.0	18.5	14.2	15.2	16.0	16.7	18.4
3–3.9	15.0	16.0	16.7	17.5	19.0	14.3	15.8	16.7	17.5	18.9
4–4.9	14.9	16.2	17.1	18.0	19.2	14.9	16.0	16.9	17.7	19.1
5–5.9	15.3	16.7	17.5	18.5	20.4	15.3	16.5	17.5	18.5	21.1
6–6.9	15.5	16.7	17.9	18.8	22.8	15.6	17.0	17.6	18.7	21.1
7–7.9	16.2	17.7	18.7	20.1	23.0	16.4	17.4	18.3	19.9	23.1
8–8.9	16.2	17.7	19.0	20.2	24.5	16.8	18.3	19.5	21.4	26.1
9–9.9	17.5	18.7	20.0	21.7	25.7	17.8	19.4	21.1	22.4	26.0
10–10.9	18.1	19.6	21.0	23.1	27.4	17.4	19.3	21.0	22.8	26.5
11–11.9	18.6	20.2	22.3	24.4	28.0	18.5	20.8	22.4	24.8	30.3
12–12.9	19.3	21.4	23.2	25.4	30.3	19.4	21.6	23.7	25.6	29.4
13–13.9	19.4	22.8	24.7	26.3	30.1	20.2	22.3	24.3	27.1	33.8
14–14.9	22.0	23.7	25.3	28.3	32.3	21.4	23.7	25.2	27.2	32.2
15–15.9	22.2	24.4	26.4	28.4	32.0	20.8	23.9	25.4	27.9	32.2
16–16.9	24.4	26.2	27.8	30.3	34.3	21.8	24.1	25.8	28.3	33.4
17–17.9	24.6	26.7	28.5	30.8	34.7	22.0	24.1	26.4	29.5	35.0
18–18.9	24.5	27.6	29.7	32.1	37.9	22.2	24.1	25.8	28.1	32.5
19–24.9	26.2	28.8	30.8	33.1	37.2	21.1	24.7	26.5	29.0	34.5
25–34.9	27.1	30.0	31.9	34.2	37.5	23.3	25.6	27.7	30.4	36.8
35–44.9	27.8	30.5	32.6	34.5	37.4	24.1	26.7	29.0	31.7	37.8
45–54.9	26.7	30.1	32.2	34.2	37.6	24.2	27.4	29.9	32.8	38.4
55–64.9	25.8	29.6	31.7	33.6	36.9	24.3	28.0	30.3	33.5	38.5
65–74.9	24.8	28.5	30.7	32.5	35.5	24.0	27.4	29.9	32.6	37.3

Source: Adapted from A. R. Frisancho, New norms of upper limb fat and muscle areas for assessment of nutritional status, *American Journal of Clinical Nutrition* 34 (1981): 2540–2545.

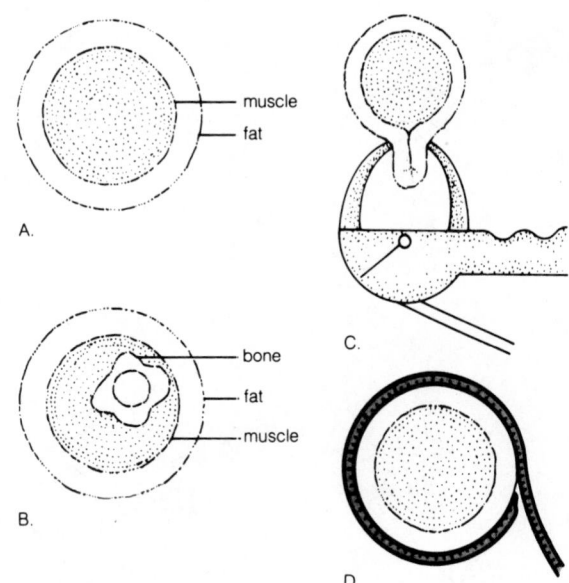

A.

B.

C.

D.

FIGURE B–13

How the midarm muscle circumference is derived.
A. The arm is visualized as an inner circle of muscle surrounded by an outer circle of fat.
B. In reality, the arm is not circular, and there is some bone, but the simplified picture is approximately correct.
C. This measurement (the fatfold) gives you two times the thickness of the fat.
D. This measurement (the tape-measured outer circumference of the arm) gives you the outer circumference (muscle plus fat).
E. An equation then derives the *circumference of the muscle,* an index of the body's total skeletal muscle mass. The equation is:

midarm muscle circumference(cm) =
midarm circumference(cm) − [0.314* × triceps fatfold(mm)]

TABLE B–7. Midarm Muscle Circumference (MAMC) (centimeters)

Age	Male					Female				
	5th	25th	50th	75th	95th	5th	25th	50th	75th	95th
1–1.9	11.0	11.9	12.7	13.5	14.7	10.5	11.7	12.4	13.9	14.3
2–2.9	11.1	12.2	13.0	14.0	15.0	11.1	11.9	12.6	13.3	14.7
3–3.9	11.7	13.1	13.7	14.3	15.3	11.3	12.4	13.2	14.0	15.2
4–4.9	12.3	13.3	14.1	14.8	15.9	11.5	12.8	13.6	14.4	15.7
5–5.9	12.8	14.0	14.7	15.4	16.9	12.5	13.4	14.2	15.1	16.5
6–6.9	13.1	14.2	15.1	16.1	17.7	13.0	13.8	14.5	15.4	17.1
7–7.9	13.7	15.1	16.0	16.8	19.0	12.9	14.2	15.1	16.0	17.6
8–8.9	14.0	15.4	16.2	17.0	18.7	13.8	15.1	16.0	17.1	19.4
9–9.9	15.1	16.1	17.0	18.3	20.2	14.7	15.8	16.7	18.0	19.8
10–10.9	15.6	16.6	18.0	19.1	22.1	14.8	15.9	17.0	18.0	19.7
11–11.9	15.9	17.3	18.3	19.5	23.0	15.0	17.1	18.1	19.6	22.3
12–12.9	16.7	18.2	19.5	21.0	24.1	16.2	18.0	19.1	20.1	22.0
13–13.9	17.2	19.6	21.1	22.6	24.5	16.9	18.3	19.8	21.1	24.0
14–14.9	18.9	21.2	22.3	24.0	26.4	17.4	19.0	20.1	21.6	24.7
15–15.9	19.9	21.8	23.7	25.4	27.2	17.5	18.9	20.2	21.5	24.4
16–16.9	21.3	23.4	24.9	26.9	29.6	17.0	19.0	20.2	21.6	24.9
17–17.9	22.4	24.5	25.8	27.3	31.2	17.5	19.4	20.5	22.1	25.7
18–18.9	22.6	25.2	26.4	28.3	32.4	17.4	19.1	20.2	21.5	24.5
19–24.9	23.8	25.7	27.3	28.9	32.1	17.9	19.5	20.7	22.1	24.9
25–34.9	24.3	26.4	27.9	29.8	32.6	18.3	19.9	21.2	22.8	26.4
35–44.9	24.7	26.9	28.6	30.2	32.7	18.6	20.5	21.8	23.6	27.2
45–54.9	23.9	26.5	28.1	30.0	32.6	18.7	20.6	22.0	23.8	27.4
55–64.9	23.6	26.0	27.8	29.5	32.0	18.7	20.9	22.5	24.4	28.0
65–74.9	22.3	25.1	26.8	28.4	30.6	18.5	20.8	22.5	24.4	27.9

Source: Adapted from A. R. Frisancho, New norms of upper limb fat and muscle areas for assessment of nutritional status, *American Journal of Clinical Nutrition* 34 (1981): 2540–2545.

TABLE B–8. Anthropometric and Biochemical Measures Used to Assess Protein-kCalorie Malnutrition (PCM)

	Body Compartment Measured		
Measure	Body Fat	Skeletal Muscle	Visceral Protein
Anthropometrics			
Weight[a]	X	X	
Triceps fatfold	X		
Midarm circumference	X	X	
Midarm muscle circumference		X	
Lab tests			
Serum albumin			X
Serum transferrin			X
Total lymphocyte count			X
Creatinine-height index[b]		X	

[a]A standard table of weight for height appears on the inside back cover.
[b]The amount of cretinine excreted is thought to reflect total skeletal mass. It therefore should be proportional to height. If creatinine excreted (for a person of a given height) is low, this reflects depleted skeletal muscle. Table B–12 presents standards.

TABLE B–9. Physical Findings Associated with Various Nutrient Imbalances

Physical Finding	Protein-kcalorie	Vitamin A	B Vitamins	Vitamin C	Vitamin D	Iron	Other
Hair							
Dull, dry, sparse, readily plucked, lighter and darker bands (flag sign), depigmented	X						
Face							
Swollen	X						
Dark areas of skin over eyes and under cheeks, flaky skin around nose		X					
Pale		X			X		
Eyes							
Night blindness		X					Zinc
Triangular, shiny gray spots on exposed portion of conjunctiva (mucous membrane lining eyelid)		X					
Dull, opaque, or dry cornea		X					
Softening of cornea, inner eyelids		X					
Inner eyelids and whites dry and pigmented		X					
Cracked and red at corners			X				
Pale conjunctiva			X			X	
White ring around iris							Elevated blood lipids
Raised yellow spots on eye							Elevated blood lipids
Lips							
Bilateral redness, cracking, scaling, or scarring at corners of mouth			X				
Swollen, red lips with vertical cracks			X				

(continued)

TABLE B–9. (continued)

Physical Finding	Protein-kcalorie	Vitamin A	B Vitamins	Vitamin C	Vitamin D	Iron	Other
Tongue							
Swollen, magenta colored			X				
Smooth surface			X				
Atrophy of the surface structures			X				
Bright red, painful			X				
Teeth							
Caries							Excess sugar
Mottled enamel							Excess flouride
Gums							
Bleeding, spongy, receding				X			
Glands							
Enlarged thyroid gland (located at front of neck)							Iodine
Enlarged parotid gland (located just below earlobes	X						General undernutrition
Skin							
Depigmentation, patches of hyperpigmented skin that peels off (flaky-paint dermatosis)	X						
Dry, scaling, rough (skin may appear to have permanent goosebumps)		X					Essential fatty acids
Bilateral hyperpigmentation with redness and swelling on body areas exposed to sunlight; scrotal or vulval dermtosis			X				
Small red or purple skin hemorrhages				X			
Nails							
Spoon-shaped, brittle, ridged						X	
Pale nail bed						X	
Subcutaneous tissue							
Edematous (swollen)	X						
Reduced fat stores	X						
Excessive fat stores							Obesity

TABLE B–10. Laboratory Tests Useful for Assessing Some Vitamin and Mineral Deficiencies

Vitamin	Test
Vitamin A	Serum vitamin A, serum carotene, retinol binding protein
Thiamin	Erythrocyte transketolase
Riboflavin	Erythrocyte glutathione reductase
Niacin	Urinary N-methylnicotinamide, urinary 2-pyridone
Vitamin B_6	Tryptophan load test, serum Vitamin B_6
Folacin	Erythrocyte folate, vitamin B_{12} status, serum free folate
Vitamin B_{12}	Deoxyuridine suppression test
Vitamin C	Leukocyte vitamin C, serum vitamin C
Vitamin D	Serum alkaline phosphatase
Vitamin E	Erythrocyte hemolysis test, plasma or serum tocopherol
Vitamin K	Prothrombin time

Mineral	Test
Calcium	Serum calcium; bone tests under development
Potassium	Serum potassium
Magnesium	Serum magnesium
Iron	Hemoglobin, hematocrit, total iron-binding capacity (TIBC), transferrin saturation, erythrocyte protoporphyrin, leukocyte ferritin
Iodine	Serum protein-bound iodine, radioiodine uptake
Zinc	Serum or plasma zinc, hair zinc

TABLE B–11. Relationship Between Degree of Undernutrition and Serum Proteins

Degree of Depletion	Indicator	
	Albumin (g/100 ml)	Transferrin (mg/100 ml)
Mild	2.8–3.4	150–200
Moderate	2.1–2.7	100–149
Severe	<2.1	<100

TABLE B–12a. Creatinine-Height Index Standards for Men

Height		Small Frame		Medium Frame		Large Frame	
in	cm	Ideal Weight (kg)	Creatinine (mg per 24 hr)	Ideal Weight (kg)	Creatinine (mg per 24 hr)	Ideal Weight (kg)	Creatinine (mg per 24 hr)
61	154.9	52.7	1,212	56.1	1,290	60.7	1,396
62	157.5	54.1	1,244	57.7	1,327	62.0	1,426
63	160.0	55.4	1,274	59.1	1,359	63.6	1,463
64	162.5	56.8	1,306	60.4	1,389	65.2	1,500
65	165.1	58.4	1,343	62.0	1,426	66.8	1,536
66	167.6	60.2	1,385	63.9	1,470	68.9	1,585
67	170.2	62.0	1,426	65.9	1,516	71.1	1,635
68	172.7	63.9	1,470	67.7	1,557	72.9	1,677
69	175.3	65.9	1,516	69.5	1,598	74.8	1,720
70	177.8	67.7	1,557	71.6	1,647	76.8	1,766
71	180.3	69.5	1,599	73.6	1,693	79.1	1,819
72	182.9	71.4	1,642	75.7	1,741	81.1	1,865
73	185.4	73.4	1,688	77.7	1,787	83.4	1,918
74	187.9	75.2	1,730	80.0	1,846	85.7	1,971
75	190.5	77.0	1,771	82.3	1,893	87.7	2,017

TABLE B–12b. Creatinine-Height Index Standards for Women

Height		Small Frame		Medium Frame		Large Frame	
in	cm	Ideal Weight (kg)	Creatinine (mg per 24 hr)	Ideal Weight (kg)	Creatinine (mg per 24 hr)	Ideal Weight (kg)	Creatinine (mg per 24 hr)
56	142.2	43.2	778	46.1	830	50.7	913
57	144.8	44.3	797	47.3	851	51.8	932
58	147.3	45.4	817	48.6	875	53.2	958
59	149.8	46.8	842	50.0	900	54.5	981
60	152.4	48.2	868	51.4	925	55.9	1,006
61	154.9	49.5	891	52.7	949	57.3	1,031
62	157.5	50.9	916	54.3	977	58.9	1,060
63	160.0	52.3	941	55.9	1,006	60.6	1,091
64	162.5	53.9	970	57.9	1,042	62.5	1,125
65	165.1	55.7	1,003	59.8	1,076	64.3	1,157
66	167.6	57.5	1,035	61.6	1,109	66.1	1,190
67	170.2	59.3	1,067	63.4	1,141	67.9	1,222
68	172.7	61.4	1,105	65.2	1,174	70.0	1,260
69	175.2	63.2	1,138	67.0	1,206	72.0	1,296
70	177.8	65.0	1,170	68.9	1,240	74.1	1,334

Source: A. Grant, *Nutritional Assessment Guidelines,* 2nd ed., 1979 (available from P.O. Box 25057, Northgate Station, Seattle, WA 98125).

C

Table of Food Composition

This table of food composition is not the standard table found in most nutrition textbooks. The list of foods chosen is an expanded version of that presented in the 1985 edition of the USDA *Home and Garden Bulletin Number 72, Nutritive Value of Foods.* The *Bulletin,* however, does not contain all the foods listed here nor the values for dietary fiber, vitamin B_6, folacin, magnesium, or zinc.

To achieve a complete and reliable listing of nutrients for all the foods, many sources of information had to be researched. Government sources of information are the primary base for the data: USDA *Handbooks 8–1* through *8–16* and the 1986 release of the USDA's *Home and Garden Bulletin Number 72, Nutritive Value of Foods.* In addition, provisional USDA information of nutrient values—both published and unpublished—and many conversations with the staff members at the USDA Human Nutrition Information Service in Hyattsville, Maryland, have provided professional assistance to refine the data.

Even with all the government sources available, there are still many missing nutrient values, and as the various government data are updated, conflicting values are reported from the USDA for the same items. To fill in the missing values and resolve discrepancies, other sources of information were used. These reliable sources include refereed journal articles, food composition tables from Canada and England, information from other nutrient data banks and publications, unpublished scientific data, and manufacturers' data.

Estimates of nutrient amounts for foods and nutrients include all possible adjustments in the interest of accuracy. When multiple values were reported for a nutrient, the numbers were averaged and weighted with consideration of the original number of samples in the separate sources. Whenever water percentages were available, estimates of nutrient amounts were adjusted for water content. When no water percentage was given, it was assumed to be that shown in the table. Whenever a reported weight appeared inconsistent (cooked eggplant and collards), many kitchen tests were made, and the average weight of the typical product was given as tested.

When estimates of nutrient amounts in cooked foods were derived from reported amounts in raw foods, published retention factors were applied. Some reported data for combination foods were modified in this table to include newer data available for major ingredients. For example, since the "pies" were analyzed and reported, newer data on fruits have been published. Older reported data on certain bakery items were updated for the new enrichment levels for certain nutrients. Furthermore, you may notice that the kcalories from protein, carbohydrates, and fats do not always add up to

the exact number of total kcalories. This is because the kcalories per gram are approximations.

At the end of this table is a list of food items from major fast food chains. The major nutrient quantities given are from available information from manufacturers, and other nutrient quantities are estimates calculated from known values of major ingredients. These values are representative of the products offered at this time, but may change as manufacturers modify the recipes, modify the amount of sodium, change suppliers, and so forth.

Considerable effort has been made to report the most accurate data available and to eliminate missing values. There will always be changes in the future, and the authors* welcome any suggestions or comments.

It is important to know that there can be many different nutrient values reported for foods. Many factors influence the amounts of nutrients in foods, including the mineral content of the soil,

---

*This table has been prepared for West Publishing Company and is copyrighted by ESHA Research in Salem, Oregon—the developer and publisher of "The Food Processor®" computerized nutrition systems. The major sources for the data from the U.S. Department of Agriculture are supplemented by more than 400 additional sources of information. Because the list of references is so extensive, it is not provided here, but it is available from the publisher.

the method of processing, genetics, diet of the animal or fertilizer of the plant, season of the year, methods of analysis, difference in moisture content of the samples analyzed, length and method of storage, and methods of cooking the food.

As a result, different nutrient values for the same food item are reported, even by reliable sources. Although each nutrient from USDA government data is presented as a single number in some USDA publications, it is actually an average of a range of data. In the more detailed reports (Handbook 8 series), the number of samples is identified, and the standard deviation of the data is also noted. USDA data will have different reported values for foods as well, as older information is replaced with newer data in the more recent publications. Therefore, nutrient data should be viewed and used only as a guide, a close approximation of nutrient content.

Dietary fiber deserves a special word. Estimates of dietary fiber are included for all the foods in this table. The sources of this information are primarily from Southgate (England), many journal articles, some of the latest published data from the USDA, and extensive unpublished information from the USDA Human Nutrition Information Service in Hyattsville, Maryland.

This emerging data and additional research and refinement of analytical techniques will modify the data in the future. Dietary fiber is composed of cellulose, hemicellulose, pectin, gums, and mucilages. Very little data is yet available on the gum and mucilage components in foods, but there is considerable data on the other components.

Many different analytical techniques are used to measure various components of fiber, and these methods are undergoing their own review of accuracy in the scientific community. In this table, either an estimate of the total dietary fiber (a specific analytical technique) or a combination of measures for the insoluble components and pectin, when available, is used.

Vitamin A is reported in retinol equivalents. The amount of this vitamin can vary by the season of the year. Reported values in both dairy products and plants are higher in summer and early fall than in winter. The values reported here represent year-round averages. Vitamin A quantity varies widely in the organ meats of all animal products (liver especially) depending on the background of the animal. Vitamin A is also present in very small amounts in regular meat and is often reported as a trace.

Newer reported vitamin A values for some plant foods have increased significantly due to additional information and sometimes to newer plant genetics. New vitamin A values for canned pumpkin are 3.5 times greater than the previously reported values. This information was used to modify the vitamin A value of pumpkin pie, which was not yet updated.

The energy and nutrients in recipes and combination foods vary widely, depending on the ingredients. The various fatty acids and cholesterol are influenced by the type of fat used (the specific type of oil, vegetable shortening, butter, margarine, etc.) during preparation.

Total fats, as well as the breakdown of total fats to saturated, monounsaturated, and polyunsaturated fats, are listed in the table. The fatty acids seldom add up exactly to the total. This is due to rounding and to the existence of small amounts of other fatty acid components that are not included in the basic three categories.

Niacin values are for preformed niacin and do not include additional niacin that may form in the body from the conversion of tryptophan.

Table C–1   Food Composition

Grp	Ref	Food Description	Measure	Wt (g)	H₂O (%)	Ener (kcal)	Prot (g)	Carb (g)	Dietary Fiber (g)	Fat (g)	Fat Breakdown (g) Sat	Mono	Poly
BEVERAGES													
		Alcoholic:											
		Beer:											
1	1	Regular (12 fl oz)	1½ c	356	92	146	1	13	1	0	0	0	0
1	2	Light (12 fl oz)	1½ c	354	95	100[1]	1	5	1	0	0	0	0
		Gin, rum, vodka, whiskey:											
1	3	80 proof	1½ fl oz	42	67	97	0	<.1	0	0	0	0	0
1	4	86 proof	1½ fl oz	42	64	105	0	<.1	0	0	0	0	0
1	5	90 proof	1½ fl oz	42	62	110	0	<.1	0	0	0	0	0
		Liqueur:											
1	1359	Coffee Liqueur, 53 proof	1½ fl oz	52	31	174	0	24	0	<1	.1	t	.1
1	1360	Coffee & cream liqueur, 34 proof	1½ fl oz	47	47	154	1	10	0	7	4.5	2.1	.3
1	1361	Creme de menthe, 72 proof	1½ fl oz	50	28	186	0	21	0	<1	t	t	.1
		Wine:											
1	6	Dessert (4 fl oz)	½ c	118	72	181[2]	<1	14[2]	0	0	0	0	0
1	7	Red	3½ fl oz	103	88	74	<1	2	0	0	0	0	0
1	8	Rosé	3½ fl oz	103	89	73	<1	2	0	0	0	0	0
1	9	White medium	3½ fl oz	103	90	70	<1	1	0	0	0	0	0
		Carbonated:[3]											
1	10	Club soda (12 fl oz)	1½ c	355	100	0	0	0	0	0	0	0	0
1	11	Cola beverage (12 fl oz)	1½ c	370	89	151	0	39	0	0	0	0	0
1	12	Diet cola (12 fl oz)	1½ c	355	100	2	0	<1	0	0	0	0	0
1	13	Diet soda pop–average (12 fl oz)	1½ c	355	100	2	0	<1	0	0	0	0	0
1	14	Ginger ale (12 fl oz)	1½ c	366	91	124	0	32	0	0	0	0	0
1	15	Grape soda (12 fl oz)	1½ c	372	89	161	0	42	0	0	0	0	0
1	16	Lemon-lime (12 fl oz)	1½ c	368	90	149	0	38	0	0	0	0	0
1	17	Orange (12 fl oz)	1½ c	372	88	177	0	46	0	0	0	0	0
1	18	Pepper-type soda (12 fl oz)	1½ c	368	89	151	0	38	0	0	0	0	0
1	19	Root beer (12 fl oz)	1½ c	370	89	152	<1	39	0	0	0	0	0
		Coffee:[3]											
1	20	Brewed	1 c	240	99	2[5]	<1	1	<1	0	0	0	0
1	21	Prepared from instant	1 c	240	99	2[5]	<1	1	0	0	0	0	0
		Fruit drinks, noncarbonated:[6]											
1	22	Fruit punch drink, canned	1 c	253	88	118	<1	30	0	<1	t	t	t
1	1358	Gatorade	1 c	230	99	39	0	11	0	0	0	0	0
1	23	Grape drink, canned	1 c	250	88	112	0	35	<1	<1	t	t	t
1	1304	Koolade, sweetened with sugar	1 c	240	100	100	0	25	0	0	0	0	0
1	1356	Koolade, sweetened with nutrasweet	1 c	240	100	4	0	0	0	0	0	0	0
		Lemonade, frozen:											
1	26	Concentrate (6-oz can)	¾ c	219	52	397	1	103	1	<1	.1	t	.1
1	27	Lemonade prepared from frozen concentrate	1 c	248	89	100	<1	26	<1	<1	t	t	t
		Limeade, frozen:											
1	28	Concentrate (6-oz can)	¾ c	218	50	408	<1	108	1[8]	<1	t	t	.1
1	29	Limeade prepared from frozen concentrate	1 c	247	89	102	<1	27	<1[8]	<1	t	t	t
1	24	Pineapple grapefruit, canned	1 c	250	88	117	1	29	0	<1	t	t	.1
1	25	Pineapple orange, canned	1 c	250	87	125	3	29	0	<1	t	t	.1

[1]kCalories can vary from 78 to 131 for 12 fl oz.

[2]Values for sweet dessert wine. Dry dessert wines contain 149 kcal and 5 g of carbohydrate.

[3]Mineral content varies depending on water source.

[5]kCalorie values from USDA vary from 1 to 4 kcalories per cup.

[6]Usually less than 10% fruit juice.

[8]Dietary fiber values are estimated from values for lemonade.

Chol (mg)	Calc (mg)	Iron (mg)	Magn (mg)	Phos (mg)	Pota (mg)	Sodi (mg)	Zinc (mg)	VT-A (RE)	Thia (mg)	Ribo (mg)	Niac (mg)	V-B6 (mg)	Fola (µg)	VT-C (mg)
0	18	.11	23	44	89	19	.07	0	.02	.09	1.61	.18	21	0
0	18	.14	18	43	64	10	.11	0	.03	.11	1.39	.12	15	0
0	0	.02	0	2	1	<1	.02	0	<.01	<.01	<.01	t	0	0
0	0	.02	0	2	1	<1	.02	0	<.01	<.01	<.01	0	0	0
0	0	.02	0	2	1	<1	.02	0	<.01	<.01	<.01	0	0	0
0	1	.03	1	3	15	4	.01	0	<.01	.01	.08	—	0	0
—	7	.06	1	23	15	43	.08	—	0	.03	.04	—	0	0
0	0	.04	0	0	0	3	—	0	0	0	<.01	0	0	—
0	9	.24	11	11	109	11	.08	0	.02	.02	.25	0	<1	0
0	8	.44	13	14	115	6	.10	0	<.01	.03	.08	.04	2	0
0	9	.39	10	15	102	5	.06	0	<.01	.02	.08	.03	1	0
0	9	.33	11	14	82	5	.07	0	<.01	<.01	.07	.01	<1	0
0	17	.15	4	0	6	75	.36	0	0	0	0	0	0	0
0	9	.12	3	46	4	15	.05	0	0	0	0	0	0	0
0	12	.11	4	30	0	21[4]	.28	0	.02	.08	0	0	0	0
0	14	.14	3	38	7	21[4]	.10	0	0	0	0	0	0	0
0	12	.66	3	1	5	25	.18	0	0	0	0	0	0	0
0	12	.31	4	0	3	57	.26	0	0	0	0	0	0	0
0	9	.25	2	1	4	41	.18	0	0	0	.06	0	0	0
0	19	.23	4	4	9	46	.38	0	0	0	0	0	0	0
0	12	.14	1	41	2	38	.15	0	0	0	0	0	0	0
0	19	.19	4	2	3	49	.26	0	0	0	0	0	0	0
0	4	.96	14	3	130	5	.08	0	0	.02	.53	0	<1	0
0	8	.12	9	8	87	8	.07	0	0	<.01	.69	0	0	0
0	19	.52	5	3	64	56	.31	4	.06	.06	.05	0	3	75
0	23	—	—	0	23	123	—	0	—	—	—	—	—	—
0	3	.41	5	3	13	16	.28	<1	.08	.02	.07	.02	1	85
0	0	0	0	0	0	0	0	0	0	0	0	0	0	6
0	0	0	0	0	0	0	0	0	0	0	0	0	0	6
0	15	1.58	11	19	148	8	.17	21	.06	.21	.16	.06	22	39[7]
0	4	.41	3	5	38	8	.05	5	.02	.05	.04	.02	6	10[7]
0	11	.22	60	13	129	<1	.11	<1	.02	.02	.22	.11	25	26
0	3	.06	15	3	33	<1	.03	<1	<.01	<.01	.05	.03	6	7
0	18	.77	15	14	154	34	.15	9	.08	.04	.67	.10	26	115
0	13	.67	14	10	116	9	.14	133	.08	.05	.52	.12	27	56

[4]Value for product sweetened with aspartame only; sodium is 32 mg if a blend of aspartame and sodium saccharin is used; 75 mg if just sodium saccharin is used.

[7]Vitamin C can range from 5 to 72 mg in a small can of frozen concentrate, and from 1 to 18 mg in 1 c lemonade.

(For purposes of calculations, use "0" for t, <1, <.1, <.01, etc.)

Table C–1 Food Composition

Grp	Ref	Food Description	Measure	Wt (g)	H₂O (%)	Ener (kcal)	Prot (g)	Carb (g)	Dietary Fiber (g)	Fat (g)	Sat	Mono	Poly
											Fat Breakdown (g)		

BEVERAGES—Con.

Fruit and vegetable juices: see Fruit and Vegetable sections

Grp	Ref	Food Description	Measure	Wt (g)	H₂O (%)	Ener (kcal)	Prot (g)	Carb (g)	Dietary Fiber (g)	Fat (g)	Sat	Mono	Poly
1	1357	Perrier,® bottled water, 6.5 fl oz bottle	1 ea	192	100	0	0	0	0	0	0	0	0
		Tea:[3]											
1	30	Brewed	1 c	240	100	2	<.01	1	0	0	0	0	0
1	31	From instant, unsweetened	1 c	237	100	2	0	<1	0	0	0	0	0
1	32	From instant, sweetened	1 c	262	91	86	0	22	0	0	0	0	0

DAIRY

Butter: see Fats and Oils, #158, 159, 160
Cheese, natural:

Grp	Ref	Food Description	Measure	Wt (g)	H₂O (%)	Ener (kcal)	Prot (g)	Carb (g)	Dietary Fiber (g)	Fat (g)	Sat	Mono	Poly
2	33	Blue	1 oz	28	42	100	6	1	0	8	5.3	2.2	.2
2	34	Brick	1 oz	28	41	105	6	1	0	8	5.3	2.4	.2
2	35	Brie	1 oz	28	48	95	6	<1	0	8	5.0	2.3	.3
2	36	Camembert	1 oz	28	52	85	6	<1	0	7	4.3	2.0	.2
		Cheddar:											
2	37	Cut pieces	1 oz	28	37	114	7	<1	0	9	6.0	2.7	.3
2	38	1″ cube	1 ea	17	37	69	4	<1	0	6	3.6	1.6	.2
2	39	Shredded	1 c	113	37	455	28	1	0	37	24	11	1
		Cottage:											
2	40	Creamed, large curd	1 c	225	79	235	28	6	0	10	6.4	3.0	.3
2	41	Creamed, small curd	1 c	210	79	215	26	6	0	9	6.0	2.7	.3
2	42	With fruit	1 c	226	72	279	22	30	0	8	4.9	2.2	.3
2	43	Low fat 2%	1 c	226	79	205	31	8	0	4	2.8	1.2	.1
2	44	Low fat 1%	1 c	226	82	164	28	6	0	2	1.5	.7	.1
2	45	Dry curd	1 c	145	80	123	25	3	0	1	.4	.2	<.1
2	46	Cream	1 oz	28	54	99	2	1	0	10	6.2	2.8	.4
2	47	Edam	1 oz	28	42	101	7	<1	0	8	5.0	2.3	.2
2	48	Feta	1 oz	28	55	75	5	1	0	6	4.2	1.3	.2
2	49	Gouda	1 oz	28	42	101	7	1	0	8	5.0	2.2	.2
2	50	Gruyère	1 oz	28	33	117	8	<1	0	9	5.4	2.9	.5
2	51	Gorgonzola	1 oz	28	39	111	7	0	0	9	5.5	2.4	.5
2	52	Liederkranz	1 oz	28	53	87	5	0	0	8	5.3	2.2	.2
2	53	Monterey jack	1 oz	28	41	106	7	<1	0	9	5.4	2.4	.2
		Mozzarella, made with:											
2	54	Whole milk	1 oz	28	54	80	5	1	0	6	3.7	1.9	.2
2	55	Park skim milk, low moisture	1 oz	28	49	80	8	1	0	5	3.1	1.4	.1
2	56	Muenster	1 oz	28	42	104	6	<1	0	8	5.4	2.5	.2
		Parmesan, grated:											
2	57	Cup, not pressed down	1 c	100	18	455	42	4	0	30	19	8.7	.7
2	58	Tablespoon	1 tbsp	5	18	23	2	<1	0	2	1	.4	<.1
2	59	Ounce	1 oz	28	18	129	12	1	0	9	5.4	2.5	.2
2	60	Provolone	1 oz	28	41	100	7	1	0	8	4.8	2.1	.2
		Ricotta, made with:											
2	61	Whole milk	1 c	246	72	428	28	7	0	32	20	8.9	1
2	62	Part skim milk	1 c	246	74	340	28	13	0	19	12	5.7	.6
2	63	Romano	1 oz	28	31	110	9	1	0	8	4.9	2.2	.2
2	64	Swiss	1 oz	28	37	107	8	1	0	8	5.0	2.1	.3

[3]Mineral content varies depending on water source.

GRP KEY: 1 = BEV 2 = DAIRY 3 = EGGS 4 = FAT/OIL 5 = FRUIT 6 = BAKERY 7 = GRAIN 8 = FISH 9 = BEEF 10 = POULTRY
11 = SAUSAGE 12 = MIXED/FAST 13 = NUTS/SEEDS 14 = SWEETS 15 = VEG/LEG 16 = MISC 22 = SOUP/SAUCE

Chol (mg)	Calc (mg)	Iron (mg)	Magn (mg)	Phos (mg)	Pota (mg)	Sodi (mg)	Zinc (mg)	VT-A (RE)	Thia (mg)	Ribo (mg)	Niac (mg)	V-B6 (mg)	Fola (μg)	VT-C (mg)
0	26	0	1	0	0	3	0	0	0	0	0	0	0	0
0	0	.05	7	1	89	7	.05	0	0	.03	.1	0	12	0
0	5	.05	5	3	47	8	.07	0	0	<.01	<.01	<.09	1	0
0	1	.04	3	3	49	1	.06	0	0	.04	.09	0	5	0
21	150	.09	7	110	73	396	.75	65	.01	.11	.29	.05	10	0
27	191	.13	7	128	38	159	.73	86	<.01	.1	.03	.02	6	0
28	52	.14	6	53	43	178	.7	57	.02	.15	.11	.07	18	0
20	110	.09	6	98	53	236	.68	71	.01	.14	.18	.06	18	0
30	204	.20	8	146	28	176	.92	86	.01	.11	.02	.02	5	0
18	124	.12	5	88	17	107	.54	52	<.01	.07	.01	.01	3	0
119	815	.77	31	579	111	701	3.51	342	.03	.42	.09	.08	21	0
34	135	.26	11	297	190	911	.8	108	.05	.37	.30	.14	27	<1
31	126	.30	11	277	177	850	.8	101	.04	.34	.27	.14	26	<1
25	108	.25	9	236	151	915	.66	81	.04	.29	.23	.12	22	<1
19	155	.36	14	340	217	918	.95	45	.05	.42	.33	.17	30	0
10	138	.32	12	302	193	918	.86	25	.05	.37	.29	.15	28	t
10	46	.33	6	151	47	19	.68	12	.04	.21	.23	.12	21	0
31	23	.34	2	30	34	84	.33	124	<.01	.06	.03	.01	4	0
25	207	.13	8	152	53	274	1.06	72	.01	.11	.02	.02	5	0
25	140	.18	5	96	18	316	.81	36	.04	.23	.29	.02	3	0
32	198	.07	8	155	34	232	1.1	49	<.01	.10	.02	.02	6	0
31	287	.06	4	172	23	95	1	98	.02	.08	.03	.02	3	0
25	149	.12	8	121	26	513	.57	103	.01	.09	.2	.04	9	0
21	110	.12	7	100	68	390	.7	91	.01	.18	.1	.04	34	0
26	212	.2	8	126	23	152	.85	81	<.01	.11	.02	.02	3	0
22	147	.05	5	105	19	106	.7	68	<.01	.07	.02	.02	2	0
15	207	.08	8	149	27	150	.83	54	<.01	.1	.03	.02	3	0
27	203	.13	8	133	38	178	.84	90	<.01	.09	.03	.02	3	0
79	1376	.95	51	807	107	1862	3.19	173	.04	.39	.32	.11	8	0
4	69	.05	3	40	5	93	.16	9	<.01	.02	.02	<.01	<1	0
22	390	.27	14	229	30	528	1	49	.01	.11	.09	.03	2	0
20	214	.15	8	141	39	248	.89	75	<.01	.09	.04	.02	3	0
124	509	.94	28	389	257	207	2.85	330	.03	.48	.26	.11	14	0
76	669	1.09	4	449	307	307	3.29	278	.05	.46	.19	.05	14	0
29	302	.23	12	215	26	340	1	40	.01	.11	.02	.03	2	0
26	272	.05	10	171	31	74	1.1	72	<.01	.1	.03	.02	2	0

(For purposes of calculations, use "0" for t, <1, <.1, <.01, etc.)

Table C–1   Food Composition

Grp	Ref	Food Description	Measure	Wt (g)	H₂O (%)	Ener (kcal)	Prot (g)	Carb (g)	Dietary Fiber (g)	Fat (g)	Sat	Mono	Poly
												Fat Breakdown (g)	

Grp	Ref	Food Description	Measure	Wt (g)	H₂O (%)	Ener (kcal)	Prot (g)	Carb (g)	Dietary Fiber (g)	Fat (g)	Sat	Mono	Poly
DAIRY—Con.													
		Pasteurized processed cheese products:											
2	65	American	1 oz	28	39	106	6	<1	0	9	5.6	2.5	.3
2	66	Swiss	1 oz	28	42	95	7	1	0	7	4.6	2.0	.2
2	67	American cheese food	1 oz	28	44	93	6	2	0	7	4.4	2.0	.2
2	68	American cheese spread	1 oz	28	48	82	5	2	0	6	3.8	1.8	.2
		Cream, sweet:											
		Half and half (cream and milk):											
2	69	Cup	1 c	242	81	315	7	10	0	28	17	8	1
2	70	Tablespoon	1 tbsp	15	81	20	<1	1	0	2	1.1	.5	.1
		Light, coffee or table:											
2	71	Cup	1 c	240	74	469	6	9	0	46	29	13	1.7
2	72	Tablespoon	1 tbsp	15	74	30	<1	1	0	3	1.8	.8	.1
		Light whipping cream, liquid:											
2	73	Cup	1 c	239	64	699	5	7	0	74	46	22	2.1
2	74	Tablespoon	1 tbsp	15	64	44	<1	<1	0	5	2.9	1.4	.1
		Heavy whipping cream, liquid:											
2	75	Cup	1 c	238	58	821	5	7	0	88	55	25	3.3
2	76	Tablespoon	1 tbsp	15	58	51	<1	<1	0	6	3.5	1.6	.2
		Whipped cream, pressurized:											
2	77	Cup	1 c	60	61	154	2	7	0	13	8.3	3.9	.5
2	78	Tablespoon	1 tbsp	4	61	10	<1	<1	0	1	.5	.2	<.1
		Cream, sour, cultured:											
2	79	Cup	1 c	230	71	493	7	10	0	48	30	14	1.8
2	80	Tablespoon	1 tbsp	14	71	30	<1	1	0	3	1.8	.9	.1
		Cream products—imitation and part dairy:											
		Coffee whitener:											
2	81	Frozen or liquid	1 tbsp	15	77	20	<1	2	0	2	1.4	t	t
2	82	Powdered	1 tsp	2	2	11	<1	1	0	1	.6	t	t
		Dessert topping, frozen:											
2	83	Cup	1 c	75	50	239	1	17	0	19	16	1.2	.4
2	84	Tablespoon	1 tbsp	5	50	15	<1	1	0	1	1.0	.1	t
		Dessert topping from mix:											
2	85	Cup	1 c	80	67	151	3	13	0	10	8.6	.7	.2
2	86	Tablespoon	1 tbsp	5	67	9	<1	1	0	1	.5	<.1	t
		Dessert topping, pressurized:											
2	87	Cup	1 c	70	60	185	1	11	0	16	13	1.4	.2
2	88	Tablespoon	1 tbsp	4	60	11	<1	1	0	1	.8	.1	t
		Sour dressing, part dairy:											
2	89	Cup	1 c	235	75	416	8	11	0	39	31	4.6	1.1
2	90	Tablespoon	1 tbsp	15	75	25	<1	1	0	2	2.0	.3	.1
		Imitation sour cream:											
2	91	Cup	1 c	230	71	479	6	15	0	45	41	1.4	.1
2	92	Tablespoon	1 tbsp	14	71	29	<1	1	0	3	2.5	.1	t
		Milk fluid:											
2	93	Whole Milk	1 c	244	88	150	8	11	0	8	5.1	2.4	.3
2	94	2% low-fat milk	1 c	244	89	121	8	12	0	5	2.9	1.4	.2
2	95	2% milk solids added[10]	1 c	245	89	125	9	12	0	5	2.9	1.4	.2
2	96	1% low-fat milk	1 c	244	90	102	8	12	0	3	1.6	.8	.1
2	97	1% milk solids added[10]	1 c	245	90	105	9	12	0	2	1.5	.7	.1
2	98	Skim milk	1 c	245	91	86	8	12	0	<1	.3	.1	t
2	99	Skim milk solids added[10]	1 c	245	90	91	9	12	0	1	.4	.2	t
2	100	Buttermilk	1 c	245	90	99	8	12	0	2	1.3	.6	.1

[10]Milk solids added, label claims less than 10 g protein per cup.

Chol (mg)	Calc (mg)	Iron (mg)	Magn (mg)	Phos (mg)	Pota (mg)	Sodi (mg)	Zinc (mg)	VT-A (RE)	Thia (mg)	Ribo (mg)	Niac (mg)	V-B6 (mg)	Fola (µg)	VT-C (mg)
27	174	.11	6	211	46	406	.93	82	.01	.1	.02	.02	2	0
24	219	.17	8	216	61	388	1.02	65	<.01	.08	.01	.01	2	0
18	163	.24	9	130	79	337	.85	62	.01	.13	.04	.02	2	0
16	159	.09	8	201	69	381	.78	54	.01	.12	.04	.03	2	0
89	254	.17	25	230	314	98	1.23	259	.09	.36	.19	.09	6	2
6	16	.01	2	14	20	6	.08	16	.01	.02	.01	<.01	<1	<1
159	231	.1	21	192	292	95	.65	437	.08	.36	.14	.08	6	2
10	14	.01	1	12	18	6	.04	27	<.01	.02	.01	<.01	<1	<1
265	166	.07	17	146	231	82	.60	705	.06	.30	.1	.07	9	1
17	10	<.01	1	9	15	5	.04	44	<.01	.02	.01	<.01	1	<1
326	154	.07	17	149	179	89	.55	1002	.05	.26	.09	.06	10	1
20	10	<.01	1	9	11	6	.03	63	<.01	.02	.01	<.01	1	<1
46	61	.03	6	54	88	78	.22	124	.02	.04	.04	.03	1	0
3	4	<.01	<1	3	5	5	.01	8	<.01	<.01	<.01	<.01	<1	0
102	268	.14	26	195	331	123	.69	448	.08	.34	.15	.04	25	2
6	16	.01	2	12	20	7	.04	27	<.01	.02	.01	<.01	2	<1
0	1	<.01	<1	10	29	12	<.01	1[9]	0	0	0	0	0	0
0	<1	.02	<1	8	16	4	.01	<1[9]	0	<.01	0	0	0	0
0	5	.09	1	6	14	19	.03	65[9]	0	0	0	0	0	0
0	<1	.01	<1	<1	1	1	<.01	4[9]	0	0	0	0	0	0
8	72	.03	8	69	121	53	.22	39[9]	.02	.09	.05	.02	3	1
<1	5	<.01	<1	4	8	3	.14	3[9]	<.01	<.01	<.01	<.01	<1	<1
0	4	.01	1	13	13	43	.01	33[9]	0	0	0	0	0	0
0	<1	<.01	<1	1	1	3	<.01	2[9]	0	0	0	0	0	0
13	266	.07	23	205	381	113	.87	5[9]	.09	.38	.17	.04	28	2
1	17	<.01	2	13	24	7	.05	<1[9]	.01	.02	.01	<.01	2	<1
0	6	.01	—	102	369	235	0	0	0	0	0	0	0	0
0	<1	<.01	—	6	23	14	0	0	0	0	0	0	0	0
33	291	.12	33	228	370	120	.94	76	.09	.4	.2	.1	12	2
22	297	.12	33	232	377	122	.96	140	.1	.4	.21	.1	12	2
18	314	.12	35	245	397	128	.98	140	.1	.42	.22	.11	12	2
10	300	.12	34	235	381	123	.96	145	.1	.41	.21	.11	12	2
10	314	.12	35	245	397	128	.98	145	.1	.42	.22	.11	12	2
4	302	.1	28	247	406	126	.92	149	.09	.34	.22	.1	14	2
5	316	.12	37	255	419	130	1	149	.1	.43	.22	.11	12	2
9	285	.12	26	219	371	257	1.03	20	.08	.38	.14	.08	12	2

[9]Vitamin A value is largely from beta-carotene used for coloring.

(For purposes of calculations, use "0" for t, <1, <.1, <.01, etc.)

Table C–1 Food Composition

Grp	Ref	Food Description	Measure	Wt (g)	H₂O (%)	Ener (kcal)	Prot (g)	Carb (g)	Dietary Fiber (g)	Fat (g)	Fat Breakdown (g)		
											Sat	Mono	Poly
DAIRY—Con.													
		Milk, canned:											
2	101	Sweetened condensed	1 c	306	27	982	24	166	0	27	17	7.4	1
2	102	Evaporated, whole	1 c	252	74	340	17	25	0	20	12	5.9	.6
2	103	Evaporated, skim	1 c	255	79	200	19	29	0	1	.3	.2	t
		Milk, dried:											
2	104	Buttermilk	1 c	120	3	464	41	59	0	7	4.3	2.0	.3
		Instant, nonfat:											
2	105	Envelope[11]	1 ea	91	4	326	32	48	0	1	.4	.2	t
2	106	Cup	1 c	68	4	244	24	36	0	1	.3	.1	t
2	107	Goat milk	1 c	244	87	168	9	11	0	10	6.5	2.7	.4
2	108	Kefir[13]	1 c	233	82	160	9	9	0	5	2.9	1.2	.1
		Milk beverages and powdered mixes:											
		Chocolate:											
2	109	Whole	1 c	250	82	210	8	26	4	8	5.3	2.5	.3
2	110	2% fat	1 c	250	84	180	8	26	4	5	3.1	1.5	.2
2	111	1% fat	1 c	250	84	160	8	26	4	3	1.5	.8	.1
		Chocolate-flavored beverages:											
2	112	Powder containing nonfat dry milk:	1 oz	28	1	100	4	23	<1	1	.7	.4	t
2	113	Choc drink prepared with water	¾ c	206	86	100	4	23	<1	1	.7	.4	t
2	114	Powder without nonfat dry milk:	¾ oz	22	<1	75	1	20	<1	1	.4	.2	t
2	115	Choc drink prepared with whole milk	1 c	266	81	226	9	31	<1	9	5.5	2.6	.3
2	116	Eggnog, commercial	1 c	254	74	342	10	34	0	19	11	5.7	.9
		Instant Breakfast:											
2	1027	Envelope, dry powder only	1 ea	37	3	130	7	23	0	0	0	0	0
2	1028	Prepared with whole milk	1 c	281	87	280	15	34	0	8	5.1	2.4	.3
2	1029	Prepared with 2% milk	1 c	281	88	251	15	35	0	5	2.9	1.4	.2
2	1283	Prepared with 1% milk	1 c	281	89	232	15	35	0	3	1.5	.7	.1
2	1284	Prepared with skim milk	1 c	282	89	216	15	35	0	<1	.3	.1	t
		Malted milk, chocolate flavor:											
2	117	Powder[14], 3 heaping tsp:	¾ oz	21	1	79	1	18	<1	1	.5	.2	.1
2	118	Malted milk prepared with whole milk	1 c	265	81	229	9	30	<1	9	5.2	2.6	.4
		Malted milk, natural flavor:											
2	119	Powder[14], 3 heaping tsp:	¾ oz	21	2	87	2	16	<1	2	.9	.4	.3
2	120	Malted milk prepared with whole milk	1 c	265	81	237	10	27	<1	10	6.0	2.8	.6
		Milk shakes:											
2	121	Chocolate (10 fl oz)	1¼ c	283	72	360	10	58	<1	11	6.6	3.0	.4
2	122	Vanilla (10 fl oz)	1¼ c	283	75	314	10	51	<1	8	5.3	2.4	.3
		Milk desserts, frozen:											
		Ice cream, regular vanilla (about 11% fat):											
		Hardened:											
2	123	½ gallon	½ gal	1064	61	2153	38	254	0	115	71	33	4
2	124	Cup	1 c	133	61	269	5	32	0	14	8.3	4.1	.5
2	125	Fluid ounces	3 oz	50	61	101	2	12	0	5	3.3	1.6	.2
2	126	Soft serve	1 c	173	60	377	7	38	0	22	14	6.7	1.0

[11] Yields 1 qt fluid milk when reconstituted according to package directions.
[13] Most values provided by product labeling.
[14] The latest USDA data from *Handbook 8–14* on beverages updates previous USDA data.

GRP KEY: 1 = BEV 2 = DAIRY 3 = EGGS 4 = FAT/OIL 5 = FRUIT 6 = BAKERY 7 = GRAIN 8 = FISH 9 = BEEF 10 = POULTRY
11 = SAUSAGE 12 = MIXED/FAST 13 = NUTS/SEEDS 14 = SWEETS 15 = VEG/LEG 16 = MISC 22 = SOUP/SAUCE

Chol (mg)	Calc (mg)	Iron (mg)	Magn (mg)	Phos (mg)	Pota (mg)	Sodi (mg)	Zinc (mg)	VT-A (RE)	Thia (mg)	Ribo (mg)	Niac (mg)	V-B6 (mg)	Fola (µg)	VT-C (mg)
104	868	.58	78	775	1136	389	2.88	248	.28	1.27	.64	.16	34	8
74	657	.48	60	510	764	267	1.94	136	.12	.8	.49	.13	18	5
10	738	.7	68	497	845	293	2.18	300	.11	.8	.4	.14	22	3
83	1421	.36	131	1119	1910	621	4.82	65	.47	1.9	1.05	.41	57	7
16	1120	.28	107	896	1552	500	4.01	646[12]	.38	1.59	.81	.31	45	5
12	837	.21	80	670	1160	373	3.06	483[12]	.28	1.19	.61	.24	34	4
28	326	.12	34	270	499	122	.73	137	.12	.34	.68	.11	2	3
10	350	.5	28	319	205	50	.9	155	.45	.44	.3	.09	20	6
31	280	.6	33	251	417	149	1.02	73	.09	.41	.31	.1	12	2
17	284	.6	33	254	422	151	.91	143	.09	.41	.32	.1	12	2
7	287	.6	33	256	425	152	1.02	148	.1	.42	.32	.1	12	2
1	89	.29	23	88	223	139	1.26	1	.03	.17	.18	.04	3	1
1	89	.29	23	88	223	139	1.26	1	.03	.17	.18	.04	3	1
0	8	.68	21	28	128	45	.33	1	.01	.03	.11	<.01	4	<1
33	300	.8	54	256	498	165	1.26	76	.1	.43	.32	.1	12	3
149	330	.51	47	278	420	138	1.17	203	.09	.48	.27	.13	2	4
0	10	7.9	80	15	0	166	3.00	175	.30	.07	5.00	.40	100	27
33	301	8.0	113	243	370	286	3.95	251	.39	.46	5.20	.50	112	29
18	307	8.0	113	247	377	289	3.96	315	.40	.47	5.21	.51	112	29
10	310	8.0	124	250	381	289	3.96	315	.40	.48	5.21	.51	112	29
4	312	8.0	108	262	406	292	3.96	327	.39	.41	5.22	.50	113	29
1	13	.48	15	37	130	53	.17	4	.04	.04	.42	.03	4	<1
34	304	.6	47	265	499	172	1.09	80	.13	.44	.63	.14	16	3
4	63	.16	20	75	159	103	.21	19	.11	.19	1.1	.09	10	1
37	354	.27	52	303	529	223	1.14	94	.2	.59	1.31	.19	22	3
37	319	.88	47	288	567	273	1.15	64	.16	.69	.46	.14	10	1
32	344	.26	35	289	492	232	1.01	90	.13	.52	.52	.15	9	2
478	1405	.96	149	1075	2053	926	11.3	1064	.42	2.63	1.08	.49	22	6
59	176	.12	18	134	257	116	1.41	133	.05	.33	.13	.06	3	1
23	66	.05	7	50	97	44	.53	50	.02	.12	.05	.02	1	<1
153	236	.43	25	199	338	153	1.99	199	.08	.45	.18	.1	9	1

(12)With added vitamin A.

(For purposes of calculations, use "0" for t, <1, <.1, <.01, etc.)

Table C–1 Food Composition

Grp	Ref	Food Description	Measure	Wt (g)	H₂O (%)	Ener (kcal)	Prot (g)	Carb (g)	Dietary Fiber (g)	Fat (g)	Fat Breakdown (g) Sat	Mono	Poly
DAIRY–Con.													
		Milk desserts, frozen—con.											
		Ice cream, rich vanilla (about 16% fat), hardened:											
2	127	½ gallon	½ gal	1188	59	2805	33	256	0	190	118	55	7
2	128	Cup	1 c	148	59	349	4	32	0	24	15	6.8	.9
		Ice milk, vanilla (about 4% fat):											
		Hardened:											
2	129	½ gallon	½ gal	1048	69	1467	41	232	0	45	28	13	1.7
2	130	Cup	1 c	131	69	184	5	29	0	6	3.5	1.6	.2
2	131	Soft serve (about 3% fat)	1 c	175	70	223	8	38	0	5	2.9	1.3	.2
		Sherbet (2% fat):											
2	132	½ gallon	½ gal	1542	66	2158	17	469	0	31	19	8.8	1.1
2	133	Cup	1 c	193	66	270	2	59	0	4	2.4	1.1	.1
		Milk desserts, other:											
2	134	Custard, baked	1 c	265	77	305	14	29	0	15	6.8	5.4	.7
		Pudding, canned:											
2	135	Chocolate	5 oz	142	68	205	3	30	<1	11	9.5	.5	.1
2	136	Tapioca	5 oz	142	74	160	3	28	0	5	4.8	t	t
2	137	Vanilla	5 oz	142	69	220	2	33	0	10	9.5	.3	.1
		Puddings, prepared from dry mix with whole milk:											
2	138	Chocolate, instant	1 c	260	71	310	8	54	<1	8	4.6	2.2	.4
2	139	Chocolate, regular, cooked	½ c	130	73	150	4	25	<1	4	2.4	1.1	.1
2	140	Rice	½ c	132	73	155	4	27	<1	4	2.3	1.1	.1
2	141	Tapioca	½ c	130	75	145	4	25	0	4	2.3	1.1	.1
2	142	Vanilla, instant	½ c	130	73	150	4	27	0	4	2.2	1.1	.2
2	143	Vanilla, regular, cooked	½ c	130	74	145	4	25	0	4	2.3	1	.1
2	144	Soybean milk	1 c	240	93	79	7	4	0	5	.5	.8	2.0
		Yogurt, low fat:											
2	145	Fruit added[15]	1 c	227	74	231	10	43	<1	2	1.6	.7	.1
2	146	Plain	1 c	227	85	144	12	16	0	3	2.3	1.0	.1
2	147	Vanilla or coffee flavor	1 c	227	79	193	11	31	0	3	1.8	.8	.1
2	148	Yogurt, made with nonfat milk	1 c	227	85	127	13	17	0	<1	.3	.1	t
2	149	Yogurt, made with whole milk	1 c	227	88	138	8	11	0	7	4.8	2.0	.2
EGGS[15a]													
		Raw, large:											
3	150	Whole, without shell	1 ea	52	76	74	6	1	0	5	1.7	2.1	.8
3	151	White	1 ea	35.4	88	16	3	<1	0	<1	0	0	0
3	152	Yolk	1 ea	16.6	49	63	3	<1	0	5	1.7	2.1	.8
		Cooked:											
3	153	Fried in butter	1 ea	46	72	90	6	1	0	6	2.0	2.2	.8
3	154	Hard-cooked, shell removed	1 ea	52	76	74	6	1	0	5	1.7	2.1	.8
3	155	Hard-cooked, chopped	1 c	136	76	194	17	2	0	13	4.4	5.4	2.0
3	156	Poached	1 ea	52	76	74	6	1	0	5	1.7	2.1	.8
3	157	Scrambled with milk and butter (also omelet)	1 ea	64	73	90	7	1	0	6	2.4	2.4	.8
FATS and OILS													
		Butter:											
4	158	Stick	½ c	113	16	813	1	<1	0	92	57	27	3.4
4	159	Tablespoon	1 tbsp	14	16	100	<1	<1	0	12	7.2	3.3	.4

[15]Carbohydrate and kcalories vary widely—consult label if more precise values are needed.

[15a]This data is newest revised information from Hazelton Laboratories, with **24%** less cholesterol.

Chol (mg)	Calc (mg)	Iron (mg)	Magn (mg)	Phos (mg)	Pota (mg)	Sodi (mg)	Zinc (mg)	VT-A (RE)	Thia (mg)	Ribo (mg)	Niac (mg)	V-B6 (mg)	Fola (µg)	VT-C (mg)
701	1212	.83	131	927	1770	867	9.74	1758	.36	2.27	.93	.43	23	5
88	151	.1	16	115	221	108	1.21	219	.04	.28	.12	.05	2	1
146	1404	1.47	147	1035	2117	838	4.40	419	.61	2.78	.94	.68	21	6
18	176	.18	19	129	265	105	.55	52	.08	.35	.12	.09	3	1
13	274	.28	29	202	412	163	.86	44	.12	.54	.18	.13	5	1
113	827	2.47	124	594	1588	709	10.6	308	.26	.71	1.05	.2	108	31
14	103	.31	15	74	198	88	1.33	39	.03	.09	.13	.03	14	4
278	297	1.1	37	310	387	209	1.53	146	.11	.5	.3	.13	24	1
1	74	1.2	24	117	254	285	.70	31	.04	.17	.6	.03	3	<1
1	119	.3	24	113	212	252	.70	<1	.03	.14	.4	.03	3	<1
1	79	.2	24	94	155	305	.70	<1	.03	.12	.6	.03	3	<1
28	260	.6	48	658	352	880	1.18	66	.08	.36	.22	.13	10	2
15	146	.2	24	120	190	167	.59	34	.05	.2	.13	.06	4	1
15	133	.5	16	110	165	140	.60	33	.10	.18	.6	.05	6	1
15	131	.1	16	103	167	152	.50	34	.04	.18	.1	.05	6	1
15	129	.1	16	273	164	375	.50	33	.04	.17	.1	.05	6	1
15	132	.1	16	102	166	178	.50	34	.04	.18	.1	.05	6	1
0	10	1.38	45	117	338	30	.54	8	.39	.17	.35	.10	4	0
10	345	.16	31	325	442	125	1.68	25	.08	.4	.22	.09	21	2
14	415	.18	40	326	531	159	2.02	36	.10	.49	.26	.11	25	2
11	388	.16	36	306	497	150	1.88	30	.10	.46	.24	.1	23	2
4	452	.2	43	354	579	173	2.20	5	.11	.53	.28	.12	28	2
30	275	.11	27	216	352	104	1.34	68	.07	.32	.17	.07	16	1
208	25	.87	6	96	58	67	.61	97	.03	.26	.04	.08	23	0
0	4	.01	3	4	45	50	.06	0	<.01	.09	.03	<.01	5	0
208	26	.95	3	86	15	8	.55	97	.03	.07	.01	.05	26	0
210	25	.87	6	96	58	67	.61	97	.03	.24	.04	.07	17	0
208	25	.87	6	96	58	67	.61	97	.03	.24	.04	.07	17	0
544	66	2.28	15	251	152	175	1.60	254	.07	.64	.09	.19	46	0
208	25	.87	6	96	58	67	.61	47	.03	.24	.04	.07	17	0
212	54	.93	6	115	85	112	.78	105	.03	.24	.04	.07	17	0
247	27	.18	2	26	29	933[16]	.06	852[17]	.01	.04	.05	<.01	3	0
31	3	.02	<1	3	4	116[16]	.01	106[17]	<.01	<.01	.01	t	<1	0

[16] For salted butter; unsalted butter contains 12 mg sodium per stick, or ½ c, 1.5 mg/tbsp, or .5 mg/pat.

[17] Values for vitamin A are a year-round average.

(For purposes of calculations, use "0" for t, <1, <.1, <.01, etc.)

Table C–1 Food Composition

Grp	Ref	Food Description	Measure	Wt (g)	H₂O (%)	Ener (kcal)	Prot (g)	Carb (g)	Dietary Fiber (g)	Fat (g)	Fat Breakdown (g)		
											Sat	Mono	Poly
FATS and OILS—Con.													
		Butter—con.											
4	160	Pat (about 1 tsp)[18]	1 ea	5	16	34	<1	<1	0	4	2.5	1.2	.2
		Fats, cooking:											
4	1363	Bacon fat	1 tbsp	14	<1	126	0	0	0	14	5.0	6.7	1.7
4	1362	Beef fat/tallow	1 c	205	0	1837	0	0	0	205	102	85.6	8.2
4	1364	Chicken fat	1 c	205	<1	1846	0	0	0	205	61.2	92.0	43.0
		Vegetable shortening											
4	161	Cup	1 c	205	0	1812	0	0	0	205	51	91	54
4	162	Tablespoon	1 tbsp	13	0	15	0	0	0	13	3.3	5.8	3.4
		Lard:											
4	163	Cup	1 c	205	0	1849	0	0	0	205	80	93	23
4	164	Tablespoon	1 tbsp	13	0	115	0	0	0	13	5.1	5.9	1.5
		Margarine:											
		Imitation (about 40% fat), soft:											
4	165	8-oz container	8 oz	227	58	785	1	1	0	88	18	36	31
4	166	Tablespoon	1 tbsp	14	58	50	<.1	<.1	0	6	1.1	2.2	2.0
		Regular, hard (about 80% fat):											
4	167	Cup	½ c	113	16	812	1	1	0	91	18	41	29
4	168	Tablespoon	1 tbsp	14	16	100	<1	<1	0	11	2.3	5.1	3.6
4	169	Pat[18]	1 ea	5	16	36	<.1	<.1	0	4	.8	1.8	1.3
		Regular, soft (about 80% fat):											
4	170	8-oz container	8 oz	227	16	1626	2	1	0	183	31	65	79
4	171	Tablespoon	1 tbsp	14	16	100	1	<.1	0	11	2.0	4.0	4.9
		Spread (about 60% fat), hard:											
4	172	Cup	½ c	113	37	610	1	0	0	69	16	29	20
4	173	Tablespoon	1 tbsp	14	37	75	<.1	0	0	9	2.0	3.6	2.5
4	174	Pat[18]	1 ea	5	37	25	<.1	0	0	3	.7	1.3	.9
		Spread (about 60% fat), soft:											
4	175	8 oz container	8 oz	227	37	1225	1	0	0	138	29	72	31
4	176	Tablespoon	1 tbsp	14	37	75	<.1	0	0	9	1.8	4.4	1.9
		Oils:											
		Corn:											
4	177	Cup	1 c	218	0	1927	0	0	0	218	28	53	128
4	178	Tablespoon	1 tbsp	14	0	125	0	0	0	14	1.8	3.4	8.2
		Olive:											
4	179	Cup	1 c	216	0	1909	0	0	0	216	29	159	18
4	180	Tablespoon	1 tbsp	14	0	125	0	0	0	14	1.9	10	1.2
		Peanut:											
4	181	Cup	1 c	216	0	1909	0	0	0	216	36	100	69
4	182	Tablespoon	1 tbsp	14	0	125	0	0	0	14	2.4	6.5	4.5
		Safflower:											
4	183	Cup	1 c	218	0	1927	0	0	0	218	20	26	162
4	184	Tablespoon	1 tbsp	14	0	125	0	0	0	14	1.3	1.7	10
		Soybean:											
4	185	Cup	1 c	218	0	1927	0	0	0	218	33	94	82
4	186	Tablespoon	1 tbsp	14	0	125	0	0	0	14	2	6	5
		Soybean/cottonseed:											
4	187	Cup	1 c	218	0	1927	0	0	0	218	39	64	105
4	188	Tablespoon	1 tbsp	14	0	125	0	0	0	14	2.5	4	7

[18]Pat is 1″ square, ⅓″ high; about 1 tsp; 90 per lb.

Chol (mg)	Calc (mg)	Iron (mg)	Magn (mg)	Phos (mg)	Pota (mg)	Sodi (mg)	Zinc (mg)	VT-A (RE)	Thia (mg)	Ribo (mg)	Niac (mg)	V-B6 (mg)	Fola (μg)	VT-C (mg)
11	1	.01	<1	1	1	41[16]	<.01	38[17]	t	<.01	<.01	t	<1	0
84	—	—	—	—	—	140	—	<1	—	—	—	0	—	—
223	2	.41	—	27	0	0	—	<1	<.01	<.01	<.01	<.01	<1	0
174	—	—	—	—	—	—	—	350	—	—	—	0	0	0
0	0	0	0	0	0	0	.10	0	0	0	0	0	0	0
0	0	0	0	0	0	0	0	0	0	0	0	0	0	0
195	<1	0	<1	6	<1	<1	.23	0	0	0	0	0	0	0
12	<1	0	<1	<1	<1	<1	.01	0	0	0	0	0	0	0
0	40	0	3	31	57	2178[19]	.23	2254[20]	.01	.05	.03	.01	2	<1
0	3	0	<1	2	4	136[19]	.03	141[20]	<.01	<.01	<.01	<.01	<1	<1
0	34	.07	3	26	48	1066[19]	.23	1122[20]	.01	.04	.03	.01	1	<1
0	4	.01	<1	3	6	133[19]	.03	139[20]	<.01	<.01	<.01	<.01	<1	<1
0	2	.01	<1	1	2	47[19]	.01	50[20]	t	<.01	<.01	t	<1	<1
0	60	0	5	46	86	2448[19]	.46	2254[20]	.02	.07	.05	.02	2	<1
0	4	0	<1	3	5	153[19]	.03	140[20]	<.01	<.01	<.01	<.01	<1	<1
0	24	0	2	18	34	1123[19]	.17	1122[20]	<.01	.03	.02	.01	1	<1
0	3	0	<1	2	4	139[19]	.02	139[20]	<.01	<.01	<.01	<.01	<1	<1
0	1	0	<1	1	2	50[20]	.01	50[20]	t	<.01	<.01	t	<1	<1
0	47	0	4	37	68	2256[19]	.35	2254[20]	.16	.06	.04	.01	2	<1
0	3	0	<1	2	4	139[19]	.02	139[20]	.01	<.01	<.01	<.01	<1	<1
0	0	.01	0	2	0	0	.02	0	0	0	0	0	<1	0
0	0	0	0	0	0	0	.03	0	0	0	0	0	0	0
0	<1	.83	<1	3	0	0	.13	0	0	0	0	0	<1	0
0	<1	.05	<1	<1	0	0	.01	0	0	0	0	0	0	0
0	t	.06	<1	0	0	0	.02	t	0	0	0	0	<1	0
0	t	<.01	<1	0	0	0	<.01	t	0	0	0	0	0	0
0	0	0	—	0	0	0	.41	0	0	0	0	0	0	0
0	0	0	—	0	0	0	.03	0	0	0	0	0	0	0
0	<1	.05	<1	1	0	0	.4	0	0	0	0	0	<1	0
0	t	0	<1	t	0	0	.03	0	0	0	0	0	t	0
0	0	0	—	0	0	0	.4	0	0	0	0	0	<1	0
0	0	0	—	0	0	0	.03	0	0	0	0	0	0	0

[16] For salted butter; unsalted butter contains 12 mg sodium per stick, or ½ c, 1.5 mg/tbsp, or .5 mg/pat.

[17] Values for vitamin A are a year-round average.

[19] For salted margarine.

[20] Based on average vitamin A content of fortified margarine. Federal specifications require a minimum of 15,000 IU/lb.

(For purposes of calculations, use "0" for t, <1, <.1, <.01, etc.)

Table C–1   Food Composition

Grp	Ref	Food Description	Measure	Wt (g)	H₂O (%)	Ener (kcal)	Prot (g)	Carb (g)	Dietary Fiber (g)	Fat (g)	Fat Breakdown (g)		
											Sat	Mono	Poly
FATS and OILS—Con.													
		Oils—con.											
		Sunflower:											
4	189	Cup	1 c	218	0	1927	0	0	0	218	23	43	143
4	190	Tablespoon	1 tbsp	14	0	125	0	0	0	14	1.4	2.7	9.2
		Salad dressings/ sandwich spreads:											
4	191	Blue cheese:	1 tbsp	15	32	75	1	1	<1	8	1.5	1.9	4.3
		French:											
4	192	Regular	1 tbsp	16	35	85	<.1	1	<1	9	1.4	4	3.5
4	193	Low calorie	1 tbsp	16	75	24	<.1	2	<1	2	.2	.3	1
		Italian:											
4	194	Regular	1 tbsp	14	34	80	<1	1	<1	9	1.3	3.7	3.2
4	195	Low calorie	1 tbsp	15	86	5	<.1	1	<1	t	t	t	t
		Mayonnaise:											
4	196	Regular	1 tbsp	14	15	100	<1	<1	0	11	1.7	3.2	5.8
4	197	Imitation	1 tbsp	15	63	35	0	2	0	3	.5	.7	1.6
4	198	Ranch style	½ c	119	35	435	4	6	0	45	6.7	19	17
		Mayo type salad dressing:											
4	199	Regular	1 tbsp	15	40	58	<1	4	0	5	.7	1.4	2.7
4	1030	Low calorie	1 tbsp	15	63	35	<1	2	0	3	.5	.8	1.4
4	200	Tartar sauce	1 tbsp	14	34	74	<1	1	<1	8	1.2	2.6	3.9
		Thousand Island:											
4	201	Regular	1 tbsp	16	46	60	<1	2	<1	6	1.0	1.3	3.2
4	202	Low calorie	1 tbsp	15	69	25	<1	2	<1	2	.2	.4	.9
		Salad dressings, prepared from home recipe:											
4	203	Cooked type[21]	1 tbsp	16	69	25	1	2	0	2	.5	.6	.3
4	204	Vinegar and oil	1 tbsp	16	47	70	0	0	0	8	1.5	2.4	3.9
FRUITS and FRUIT JUICES													
		Apples:											
		Raw, with peel:											
5	205	2¾″ diam (about 3 per lb with cores)	1 ea	138	84	80	<1	21	3	<1	.1	t	.1
5	206	3¼″ diam (about 2 per lb with cores)	1 ea	212	84	125	<1	32	5	1	.1	t	.2
5	207	Raw, peeled slices	1 c	110	84	65	<1	16	3	<1	.1	t	.1
5	208	Dried, sulfured	10 ea	64	32	155	1	42	8	<1	t	t	.1
5	209	Apple juice, bottled or canned[23]	1 c	248	88	116	<1	29	<1	<1	.1	t	.1
		Applesauce:											
5	210	Sweetened	1 c	255	80	195	<1	51	4	<1	<.1	t	.1
5	211	Unsweetened	1 c	244	88	106	<1	28	4	<1	<.1	t	<.1
		Apricots:											
5	212	Raw, without pits (about 12 per lb with pits)	3 ea	106	86	51	1	12	2	<1	t	.2	.1
		Canned (fruit and liquid):											
5	213	Heavy syrup	1 c	258	78	214	1	55	4	<1	t	.1	t
5	214	Halves	3 ea	85	78	70	<1	18	1	<.1	t	t	t
5	215	Juice pack	1 c	248	87	119	2	31	4	<.1	t	t	t
5	216	Halves	3 ea	84	87	40	1	10	1	<.1	t	t	t
		Dried:											
5	217	Dried halves	10 ea	35	31	83	1	22	3	<1	t	.1	t
5	218	Cooked, unsweetened, with liquid	1 c	250	75	210	3	55	7	<1	t	.2	.1
5	219	Apricot nectar, canned	1 c	251	85	141	1	36	2	<1	t	.1	t
		Avocados, raw, edible part only:											
5	220	California (½ lb with refuse)	1 ea	173	73	305	4	12	17	30	4.5	19	3.5

[21]Fatty acid values apply to product made with regular margarine.
[23]Also applies to pasteurized apple cider.

Chol (mg)	Calc (mg)	Iron (mg)	Magn (mg)	Phos (mg)	Pota (mg)	Sodi (mg)	Zinc (mg)	VT-A (RE)	Thia (mg)	Ribo (mg)	Niac (mg)	V-B6 (mg)	Fola (µg)	VT-C (mg)
0	0	0	0	0	0	0	—	0	0	0	0	0	0	0
0	0	0	0	0	0	0	—	0	0	0	0	0	0	0
3	12	.03	<1	11	6	<1	.28	10	<.01	.02	.01	<.01	8	t
0	2	.06	<1	1	2	188	.01	t	t	t	t	<.01	0	t
0	6	.07	—	5	3	306	.03	t	t	t	t	0	t	t
0	1	.03	<1	1	5	162	.02	3	t	t	t	.03	0	t
0	1	.03	<1	1	4	136	0	t	t	t	t	0	t	t
8	2	.07	<1	4	5	80	.02	12	<.01	<.01	<.01	<.01	<1	0
4	0	0	—	0	2	75	—	0	0	0	0	0	t	0
47	119	.31	12	100	158	522	.43	86	.04	.17	08	.05	6	1
4	2	.03	<1	4	1	105	0	13	<.01	<.01	t	<.01	t	0
4	3	.03	—	4	1	75	.02	10	.03	t	t	—	t	—
4	3	.1	<1	4	11	182	.02	9	<.01	<.01	<.01	<.01	<1	t
4	2	.09	<1	3	18	110	.03	15	<.01	<.01	.03	<.01	6	t
2	2	.09	<1	3	17	153	0	14	<.01	<.01	.03	<.01	<1	t
9	13	.08	—	14	19	117	0	20	.01	.02	.04	0	<1	t
0	0	0	—	0	1	0	—	0	0	0	0	0	—	0
0	10	.25	6	10	159	1	.05	7	.02	.02	.11	.07	4	8
0	15	.38	9	23	244	1	.08	11	.04	.03	.16	.1	6	12
0	4	.1	3	8	124	1	.04	5	.02	.01	.1	.05	<1	4
0	9	.9	10	24	288	56[22]	.13	0	0	.1	.59	.08	1	3
0	17	.92	8	17	295	7	.07	<1	.05	.04	.25	.07	1	2[24]
0	10	1	7	18	156	8	.1	3	.03	.07	.50	.07	2	4[24]
0	7	.29	7	18	183	5	.06	7	.03	.06	.46	.06	2	3[24]
0	15	.58	8	21	313	1	.28	166	.03	.04	.64	.06	9	11
0	23	.77	18	33	361	10	.27	317	.05	.06	.97	.14	4	8
0	7	.26	6	10	119	3	.09	105	.02	.02	.32	.05	1	3
0	30	.74	24	50	409	9	.27	419	.05	.05	.85	.18	5	12
0	10	.25	8	17	139	3	.1	142	.02	.02	.29	.06	2	4
0	16	1.65	16	41	482	4	.26	253	<.01	.05	1.05	.06	4	1
0	40	4.2	42	103	1222	8	.66	591	.02	.08	2.36	.28	0	4
0	18	.96	13	23	286	8	.23	330	.02	.04	.65	.16	3	2[25]
0	19	2.04	70	73	1097	21	.73	106	.19	.21	3.32	.48	113	14

[22]Sodium bisulfite used to preserve color; unsulfured product would contain lower levels of sodium.

[24]Value based on products without added ascorbic acid. Bottled apple juice with added ascorbic acid usually contains 41.6 mg/100 g, or 103 mg per cup. Check label for specific vitamin C values.

[25]Without added ascorbic acid. Products with added ascorbic acid contain 136 mg per cup. Check label.

(For purposes of calculations, use "0" for t, <1, <.1, <.01, etc.)

Table C–1 Food Composition

Grp	Ref	Food Description	Measure	Wt (g)	H₂O (%)	Ener (kcal)	Prot (g)	Carb (g)	Dietary Fiber (g)	Fat (g)	Fat Breakdown (g)		
											Sat	Mono	Poly
		FRUITS and JUICES—Con.											
		Avacados—con.											
5	221	Florida (1 lb with refuse)	1 ea	304	80	340	5	27	29	27	5	15	5
5	222	Mashed, fresh, average	1 c	230	74	370	5	17	22	35	6	22	5
		Bananas, raw, without peel:											
5	223	Whole, 8¾″ long (weighs 175 g w/peel)	1 ea	114	74	105	1	27	2	1	.2	<.1	.1
5	224	Slices	1 c	150	74	138	2	35	3	1	.3	.1	.1
5	1285	Bananas, dehydrated slices	1 c	100	3	346	4	88	8	2	.7	.2	.3
5	225	Blackberries, raw	1 c	144	86	74	1	18	10	1	.3	.1	.1
		Blueberries:											
5	226	Raw	1 c	145	85	82	1	21	4	1	<.1	.2	.3
		Frozen, sweetened:											
5	227	10-oz container	10 oz	284	77	230	1	62	7	<1	.1	.1	.2
5	228	Cup	1 c	230	77	185	1	51	5	<1	.1	.1	.2
		Cherries:											
5	229	Sour, red pitted, canned water pack	1 c	244	90	90	2	22	3	<1	.1	.1	.1
5	230	Sweet, raw, without pits	10 ea	68	81	49	1	11	1	1	.1	.2	.2
		Cranberry juices:											
5	231	Cranberry juice cocktail[26]	1 c	253	85	145	<1[27]	36	1	<1	t	t	.1
5	232	Cranberry-apple juice	1 c	253	86	169	<1	43	1	1[29]	.2	.1	.4
5	233	Cranberry sauce, canned, strained	1 c	277	61	419	1	108	6	<1	<.1	.1	.2
		Dates:											
5	234	Whole, without pits	10 ea	83	22	228	2	61	7	<1	.2	.1	t
5	235	Chopped	1 c	178	22	489	4	131	15	1	.3	.2	.1
5	236	Figs, dried	10 ea	187	28	477	6	122	21	2	.4	.5	1.1
		Fruit cocktail, canned, fruit and liquid:											
5	237	Heavy syrup pack	1 c	255	80	185	1	48	3	<1	<.1	<.1	.1
5	238	Juice pack	1 c	248	87	115	1	29	3	<1	t	t	t
		Grapefruit:											
		Raw 3¾″ diam, whole fruit weighs 1 lb											
		1 oz w/refuse (peel, membrane, seeds):											
5	239	Pink/red, half fruit, edible part	1 half	123	91	37	1	9	2	<1	t	t	<.1
5	240	White, half fruit, edible part[30]	1 half	118	90	39	1	10	2	<1	t	t	<.1
5	241	Canned sections with liquid	1 c	254	84	152	1	39	3	<1	<.1	<.1	.1
		Grapefruit juice:											
5	242	Raw	1 c	247	90	96	1	23	1	<1	<.1	<.1	.1
		Canned:											
5	243	Unsweetened	1 c	247	90	93	1	22	1	<1	<.1	<.1	.1
5	244	Sweetened	1 c	250	87	115	1	28	1	<1	<.1	<.1	.1
		Frozen concentrate, unsweetened											
5	245	Undiluted, 6-fl-oz can	¾ c	207	62	300	4	72	3	1	.2	.2	.3
5	246	Diluted with 3 cans water	1 c	247	89	102	1	24	1	<1	<.1	<.1	.1
		Grapes, raw, European type (adherent skin):											
5	247	Thompson seedless	10 ea	50	81	35	<1	9	1	<1	.1	t	.1
5	248	Tokay/Emperor, seeded types	10 ea	57	81	40	<1	10	1	<1	.1	t	.1
		Grape juice:											
5	249	Bottled or canned	1 c	253	84	155	1	38	1	<1	.1	t	.1
		Frozen concentrate, sweetened:											

[26]Data here are from the newest USDA *Handbook 8–14* on beverages. These data are somewhat different from that presented in *Handbook 8–9* on fruits and fruit juices.

[27]The newest USDA *Handbook 8–14* data on beverages indicates "0" for protein.

[29]The newest USDA *Handbook 8–14* data on beverages indicates "0" for fat.

[30]Weight is for edible portion. Weight with rind is 241 g for one-half.

GRP KEY: 1 = BEV 2 = DAIRY 3 = EGGS 4 = FAT/OIL 5 = FRUIT 6 = BAKERY 7 = GRAIN 8 = FISH 9 = BEEF 10 = POULTRY
11 = SAUSAGE 12 = MIXED/FAST 13 = NUTS/SEEDS 14 = SWEETS 15 = VEG/LEG 16 = MISC 22 = SOUP/SAUCE

Chol (mg)	Calc (mg)	Iron (mg)	Magn (mg)	Phos (mg)	Pota (mg)	Sodi (mg)	Zinc (mg)	VT-A (RE)	Thia (mg)	Ribo (mg)	Niac (mg)	V-B6 (mg)	Fola (μg)	VT-C (mg)
0	33	1.6	104	119	1484	14	1.28	186	.33	.37	5.84	.85	162	24
0	25	2.3	90	95	1378	24	.97	141	.25	.28	4.42	.64	142	18
0	7	.35	32	22	451	1	.19	9	.05	.11	.62	.66	24	10
0	9	.46	43	29	593	1	.25	12	.07	.15	.81	.87	31	14
0	22	1.15	108	74	1491	3	.61	31	.18	.24	2.80	.54	40	7
0	46	.8	29	30	282	0	.39	24	.04	.06	.58	.08	49	30
0	9	.24	7	15	129	9	.16	15	.07	.07	.7	.05	9	20
0	16	1.11	7	20	169	4	.14	12	.06	.15	.72	.17	19	3
0	13	.9	6	16	138	3	.14	10	.05	.12	.58	.14	16	2
0	27	3.34	15	25	240	17	.17	184	.04	.1	.43	.11	20	5
0	10	.3	8	13	152	0	.04	15	.03	.04	.3	.02	3	5
0	8	.38	5	5	45	5	.18	1	.02	.02	.09	.05	<1	90[28]
0	18	.15	5	7	68	5	.1	<1	.01	.05	.15	.06	<1	81[28]
0	11	.61	8	17	72	80	.09	6	.04	.06	.28	.05	3	6
0	27	1	29	33	541	2	.24	4	.08	.08	1.83	.16	14	0
0	58	2.14	63	70	1161	5	.52	9	.16	.18	3.92	.34	29	0
0	269	4.18	111	128	1331	21	.94	25	.13	.17	1.3	.42	16	1
0	16	.73	14	28	224	15	.21	52	.05	.05	.95	.11	1	5
0	20	.53	17	34	235	10	.21	76	.03	.04	0	.13	2	7
0	13	.15	10	11	158	0	.09	32[31]	.04	.03	.24	.05	15	47
0	14	.07	11	9	175	0	.08	1	.04	.02	.32	.05	12	39
0	36	1.02	25	25	328	4	.21	0	.1	.05	.62	.05	22	54
0	22	.49	30	37	400	2	.13	2[32]	.1	.05	.49	.11	52	94
0	17	.49	24	27	378	2	.22	2	.1	.05	.57	.05	26	72
0	20	.9	24	28	405	5	.15	2	.1	.06	.8	.05	26	67
0	56	1.02	78	101	1002	6	.38	6	.3	.16	1.6	.32	26	248
0	20	.34	26	34	337	2	.12	2	.1	.05	.54	.11	52	83
0	5	.13	3	7	92	1	.03	4	.05	.03	.15	.06	4	5
0	6	.15	4	8	105	1	.03	4	.05	.03	.17	.06	4	6
0	22	.61	24	27	334	8	.13	2	.07	.09	.66	.16	7	<1

(28) Nutrient added.
(31) Vitamin A in Texas red grapefruit would be 74 RE.
(32) Vitamin A for white grapefruit juice; pink or red grapefruit juice = 109 RE per cup.

(For purposes of calculations, use "0" for t, <1, <.1, <.01, etc.)

Table C–1 Food Composition

Grp	Ref	Food Description	Measure	Wt (g)	H₂O (%)	Ener (kcal)	Prot (g)	Carb (g)	Dietary Fiber (g)	Fat (g)	Fat Breakdown (g)		
											Sat	Mono	Poly
		FRUITS and FRUIT JUICES—Con.											
		Grape juice—con.											
5	250	Undiluted, 6-fl-oz can	¾ c	216	54	385	1	96	4	1	.2	<.1	.2
5	251	Diluted with 3 cans water	1 c	250	87	128	<1	32	1	<1	.1	t	.1
5	252	Kiwi fruit, raw, peeled (about 5 per lb with skin)	1 ea	76	83	46	1	11	3	<1	t	.2	.2
5	253	Lemons, raw, without peel and seeds (about 4 per lb whole)	1 ea	58	89	17	1	5	1	<1	t	t	.1
		Lemon juice											
		Fresh:											
5	254	Cup	1 c	244	91	60	1	21	1	t	t	t	t
5	255	Tablespoon	1 tbsp	15	91	4	<.1	1	<1	t	t	t	t
		Canned or bottled, unsweetened:											
5	256	Cup	1 c	244	92	52	1	16	1	<1	.1	<.1	.2
5	257	Tablespoon	1 tbsp	15	92	3	<1	1	<1	<.1	t	t	t
		Frozen, single strength, unsweetened:											
5	258	Cup	1 c	244	92	54	1	16	1	<1	.1	<.1	.2
5	259	Tablespoon	1 tbsp	15	92	3	<1	1	<1	<.1	t	t	t
		Lime juice:											
		Fresh:											
5	260	Cup	1 c	246	90	65	1	22	1	<1	<.1	<.1	.1
5	261	Tablespoon	1 tbsp	15	90	4	<1	1	<1	<.1	t	t	t
5	262	Canned or bottled, unsweetened	1 c	246	92	50	1	16	1	1	.1	.1	.2
5	263	Mangos, raw, edible part (weighs 300 g with skin and seeds)	1 ea	207	82	135	1	35	7	1	.1	.2	.1
		Melons, raw, without rind and cavity contents:											
5	264	Cantaloupe, 5″ diam (2⅓ lb whole (with refuse), orange flesh	½ ea	267	90	94	2	22	3	1	.1	.1	.2
5	265	Honeydew, 6½″ diam (5¼ lb whole with refuse), slice = 1/10 melon	1 slice	129	90	45	1	12	1	<1	t	t	<.1
5	266	Nectarines, raw, without pits, 2½″ diam	1 ea	136	86	67	1	16	3	1	.1	.2	.3
		Oranges, raw:											
5	267	Whole without peel and seeds, 2⅝″ dm. (weighs 180 g with peel and seeds)	1 ea	131	87	60	1	15	3	<1	t	<.1	<.1
5	268	Sections, without membranes	1 c	180	87	85	2	21	4	<1	<.1	<.1	<.1
		Orange juice:											
5	269	Fresh, all varieties	1 c	248	88	111	2	26	1	<1	.1	.1	.1
5	270	Canned, unsweetened	1 c	249	89	105	1	25	<1	<1	<.1	.1	.1
5	271	Chilled	1 c	249	88	110	2	25	<1	1	.1	.1	.2
		Frozen concentrate:											
5	272	Undiluted (6-oz can)	¾ c	213	58	339	5	81	2	<1	.1	.1	.1
5	273	Diluted with 3 parts water by volume	1 c	249	88	110	2	27	<1	<1	t	<.1	<.1
5	1345	Orange juice, from dry crystals	1 c	248	89	114	2	27	0	<1	.1	.1	.1
5	274	Orange and grapefruit juice, canned	1 c	247	89	105	1	25	<1	<1	<.1	<.1	.1
		Papayas, raw:											
5	275	½″ slices	1 c	140	89	60	1	14	2	<1	.1	.1	<.1
5	276	Whole fruit, cubes, 3½″ diam by 5⅛″, without seeds and skin (1 lb with refuse)	1 ea	304	89	117	2	30	5	<1	.1	.1	.1
5	1031	Papaya nectar, canned	1 c	250	85	142	<1	36	2	<1	.1	.1	.1

1 = BEV 2 = DAIRY 3 = EGGS 4 = FAT/OIL 5 = FRUIT 6 = BAKERY 7 = GRAIN 8 = FISH 9 = BEEF 10 = POULTRY
11 = SAUSAGE 12 = MIXED/FAST 13 = NUTS/SEEDS 14 = SWEETS 15 = VEG/LEG 16 = MISC 22 = SOUP/SAUCE

Chol (mg)	Calc (mg)	Iron (mg)	Magn (mg)	Phos (mg)	Pota (mg)	Sodi (mg)	Zinc (mg)	VT-A (RE)	Thia (mg)	Ribo (mg)	Niac (mg)	V-B6 (mg)	Fola (µg)	VT-C (mg)
0	28	.78	32	32	160	15	.28	6	.11	.2	.93	.32	9	179[34]
0	10	.26	11	11	53	5	.10	2	.04	.07	.31	.11	4	60[34]
0	20	.3	23	30	252	4	.08[32]	13	.02	.04	.4	.05[35]	17[35]	75
0	15	.35	2	9	80	1	.06	2	.02	.01	.06	.05	7	31
0	18	.08	16	14	303	2	.12	5	.07	.02	.24	.12	32	112
0	1	<.01	1	1	19	<1	.01	<1	<.01	<.01	.02	.01	2	7
0	26	.31	22	21	248	50[36]	.15	4	.10	.02	.48	.11	25	61
0	2	.02	1	1	15	3[36]	.01	<1	.01	<.01	.03	.01	2	4
0	19	.30	20	20	218	4	.12	4	.14	.03	.33	.15	23	77
0	1	.02	1	1	14	<1	.01	<1	.01	<.01	.02	.01	1	5
0	22	.08	14	18	268	2	.15	3	.05	.03	.25	.11	21	72
0	1	<.01	1	1	17	<1	.01	<1	<.01	<.01	.02	.08	1	5
0	30	.6	16	25	185	39[36]	.15	4	.08	.01	.4	.07	20	16
0	21	2.6	18	22	323	4	.07	806	.12	.12	1.21	.28	39	57
0	29	.56	19	45	825	24	.43	861	.1	.06	1.53	.31	80	113
0	8	.09	9	13	350	13	.11	5	.1	.02	.77	.08	39	32
0	6	.21	11	22	288	0	.12	100	.02	.06	1.35	.03	5	7
0	52	.14	13	18	237	<1	.09	27	.11	.05	.37	.08	40	70
0	72	.19	18	25	326	<1	.4	37	.16	.07	.51	.11	83	96
0	27	.50	27	42	496	2	.12	50	.22	.07	.99	.1	109	124
0	20	1.1	27	35	436	5	.17	44	.15	.07	.78	.22	15	86
0	25	.42	28	27	473	2	.11	19[37]	.28	.05	.7	.13	45[37]	82[37]
0	68	.75	73	121	1436	6	.38	59	.6	.14	1.53	.33	331	294
0	22	.27	24	40	474	2	.13	19	.2	.04	.5	.11	109	97
0	40	.02	5	31	50	1	—	.50	.20	.07	1.00	0	0	80
0	20	1.1	24	35	390	7	.18	29	.14	.07	.83	.06	20	72
0	33	.3	14	12	247	9	.10	282	.04	.05	.47	.03	26	92
0	72	.3	31	16	780	8	.22	612	.08	.10	1.03	.06	48	188
0	24	.86	8	1	78	14	.38	28	.02	.01	.38	.02	5	8

[32]Vitamin A for white grapefruit juice; pink or red grapefruit juice = 109 RE per cup.
[34]With added ascorbic acid.
[35]Data are estimated from other fruit data.
[36]Sodium benzoate and sodium bisulfite added as preservatives.
[37]Values for juice from California oranges indicate the following values for 1 c: 36 RE of vitamin A, 72µg of folacin, and 106 mg of vitamin C.
(For purposes of calculations, use "0" for t, <1, <.1, <.01, etc.)

Table C–1 Food Composition

Grp	Ref	Food Description	Measure	Wt (g)	H₂O (%)	Ener (kcal)	Prot (g)	Carb (g)	Dietary Fiber (g)	Fat (g)	Fat Breakdown (g)		
											Sat	Mono	Poly
		FRUITS and FRUIT JUICES—Con.											
		Peaches:											
		Raw:											
5	277	Whole, 2½″ diam, peeled, pitted (about 4 per lb with peels and pits)	1 ea	87	88	37	1	10	2	<1	t	<.1	<.1
5	278	Sliced	1 c	170	88	73	1	19	3	<1	t	.1	.1
		Canned, fruit and liquid:											
		Heavy syrup pack											
5	279	Cup	1 c	256	79	190	1	51	3	<1	<.1	.1	.1
5	280	Half	1 ea	81	79	60	<1	16	1	<1	t	<.1	<.1
		Juice pack											
5	281	Cup	1 c	248	88	109	2	29	3	<1	t	<.1	<.1
5	282	Half	1 ea	77	88	34	<1	9	1	<1	t	t	t
		Dried:											
5	283	Uncooked	10 ea	130	32	311	5	80	11	1	.1	.4	.5
5	284	Cooked, fruit and liquid	1 c	258	78	200	3	51	4	1	.1	.2	.3
		Frozen, sliced, sweetened:											
5	285	10-oz package	1 ea	284	75	267	2	68	6	<1	<.1	.1	.2
5	286	Cup, thawed measure	1 c	250	75	235	2	60	4	<1	<.1	.1	.2
5	1032	Peach nectar, canned	1 c	249	86	134	1	35	1	<1	t	<.1	<.1
		Pears:											
		Raw, with skin, cored:											
5	287	Bartlett, 2½″ diam (about 2½ per lb)	1 ea	166	84	98	1	25	5[39]	1	<.1	.1	.2
5	288	Bosc, 2½″ diam (about 3 per lb)	1 ea	141	84	85	1	21	4[39]	1	<.1	.1	.1
5	289	D'Anjou, 3″ diam (about 2 per lb)	1 ea	200	84	120	1	30	6[39]	1	<.1	.2	.2
		Canned, fruit and liquid:											
		Heavy syrup pack:											
5	290	Cup	1 c	255	80	188	1	49	4[39]	<1	t	.1	.1
5	291	Half	1 ea	79	80	59	<1	15	1[39]	<1	t	t	t
		Juice pack:											
5	292	Cup	1 c	248	86	123	1	32	4[39]	<1	t	<.1	<.1
5	293	Half	1 ea	77	86	38	<1	10	1[39]	<1	t	t	t
5	294	Dried halves	10 ea	175	27	459	3	122	19	1	.1	.2	.3
5	1033	Pear nectar, canned	1 c	250	84	149	<1	39	2	<1	t	t	t
		Pineapple:											
5	295	Raw chunks, diced	1 c	155	86	76	1	19	2	1	<.1	<.1	.2
		Canned, fruit and liquid:											
		Heavy syrup pack:											
5	296	Crushed, chunks, tidbits	1 c	255	79	199	1	52	2	<1	t	<.1	.1
5	297	Slices	1 ea	58	79	45	<1	12	1	<.1	t	t	<.1
		Juice Pack:											
5	298	Crushed, chunks, tidbits	1 c	250	84	150	1	39	2	<1	t	<.1	.1
5	299	Slices	1 ea	58	84	35	<1	9	1	<.1	t	t	t
5	300	Pineapple juice, canned, unsweetened	1 c	250	86	140	1	34	1	<1	t	t	.1
		Plantains, without peel:											
5	301	Raw slices (one whole plantain weighs 179 g without peel)	1 c	148	65	181	2	47	7[41]	1	.2	.1	.1
5	302	Cooked, boiled, sliced	1 c	154	67	179	1	48	7	<1	.1	<.1	.1

[39]Dietary fiber data vary 2.4 to 3.4 g/100 g for fresh pears; 1.6 to 2.6 g/100 g for canned pears.
[41]Dietary fiber value partially derived from data for bananas.

GRP KEY: 1 = BEV 2 = DAIRY 3 = EGGS 4 = FAT/OIL 5 = FRUIT 6 = BAKERY 7 = GRAIN 8 = FISH 9 = BEEF 10 = POULTRY
11 = SAUSAGE 12 = MIXED/FAST 13 = NUTS/SEEDS 14 = SWEETS 15 = VEG/LEG 16 = MISC 22 = SOUP/SAUCE

Chol (mg)	Calc (mg)	Iron (mg)	Magn (mg)	Phos (mg)	Pota (mg)	Sodi (mg)	Zinc (mg)	VT-A (RE)	Thia (mg)	Ribo (mg)	Niac (mg)	V-B6 (mg)	Fola (μg)	VT-C (mg)
0	4	.1	6	10	171	0	.12	47	.02	.04	.86	.02	3	6
0	9	.19	11	20	335	1	.18	91	.03	.07	1.68	.03	6	11
0	8	.69	13	29	235	16	.22	85	.03	.06	1.57	.05	8	7
0	3	.22	4	9	75	5	.07	27	.01	.02	.5	.01	3	2
0	15	.72	18	43	317	11	.26	94	.02	.04	1.44	.05	8	9
0	5	.21	6	13	98	3	.09	29	.01	.01	.45	.02	3	3
0	37	5.28	54	155	1295	9	.74	281	<.01	.28	5.69	.09	6	6
0	23	3.37	35	99	825	6	.46	51	.01	.05	3.92	.1	<1	10
0	9	1.05	14	31	369	17	.14	81	.04	.10	1.9	.05	9	268[38]
0	8	.93	12	28	325	16	.13	71	.03	.09	1.63	.04	8	236[38]
0	13	.47	11	16	101	10	.20	64	.01	.04	.72	.03	2	13
0	19	.42	9	18	208	1	.20	3	.03	.07	.17	.03	12	7
0	16	.40	8	16	176	<1	.17	3	.03	.06	.1	.03	10	6
0	22	.50	11	22	250	<1	.24	4	.04	.08	.2	.04	14	8
0	13	.56	11	18	166	13	.21	1	.03	.06	.62	.04	3	3
0	4	.17	3	5	51	4	.06	<1	.01	.02	.19	.01	1	1
0	22	.71	17	29	238	10	.22	1	.03	.03	.5	.04	5	4
0	7	.22	5	9	74	3	.07	<1	.01	.01	.15	.01	2	1
0	59	3.68	58	103	932	10	.68	1	.01	.25	2.4	.01	21	12
0	11	.65	6	7	33	8	.16	<1	<.01	.03	.32	.03	2	3
0	11	.57	21	11	175	2	.12	4	.14	.06	.65	.14	16	24
0	36	.97	40	18	265	3	.31	4	.23	.06	.73	.19	12	19
0	8	.22	9	4	60	1	.70	1	.05	.02	.17	.04	3	4
0	35	.70	35	15	305	3	.25	10	.24	.05	.71	.19	12	24
0	8	.16	8	4	71	1	.06	2	.06	.01	.17	.04	3	6
0	43	.65	34	20	335	3	.28	1	.14	.06	.64	.24	58	27[40]
0	4	.89	55	50	739	6	.27	167[42]	.08	.08	1.02	.44	33	27
0	3	.89	49	43	716	8	.21	140	.07	.08	1.16	.37	40	17

[38] With added ascorbic acid.
[40] Without added ascorbic acid. If added, contains 96 mg per cup.
[42] Vitamin A values range from 1.5 RE for white-fleshed varieties to 178 RE for yellow-fleshed varieties.

(For purposes of calculations, use "0" for t, <1, <.1, <.01, etc.)

Table C–1   Food Composition

Grp	Ref	Food Description	Measure	Wt (g)	H₂O (%)	Ener (kcal)	Prot (g)	Carb (g)	Dietary Fiber (g)	Fat (g)	Fat Breakdown (g)		
											Sat	Mono	Poly
		FRUITS and FRUIT JUICES—Con.											
		Plums, without pits:											
		Raw											
5	303	Medium 2⅛″ diam	1 ea	66	85	36	1	9	1	<1	<.1	.3	.1
5	304	Small, 1½″ diam	1 ea	28	85	15	<1	4	1	<1	t	.1	<.1
		Canned, purple, with liquid:											
		Heavy Syrup pack:											
5	305	Cup	1 c	258	76	230	1	60	4	<1	t	.2	.1
5	306	Plums	3 ea	110	76	98	<1	25	2	<1	t	.1	t
		Juice pack:											
5	307	Cup	1 c	252	84	146	1	38	4	<.1	t	<.1	t
5	308	Plums	3 ea	95	84	55	<1	14	2	<.1	t	t	t
		Prunes, dried, pitted:											
5	309	Uncooked (10 prunes weigh 97 g with pits 84 g without pits.):	10 ea	84	32	201	2	53	8[43]	<1	<.1	.3	.1
5	310	Cooked, unsweetened, fruit and liquid (250 g with pits)	1 c	212	70	227	2	60	9	<1	<.1	.3	.1
5	311	Prune juice, bottled or canned	1 c	256	81	181	2	45	3	<.1	t	<.1	t
		Raisins, seedless:											
5	312	Cup, not pressed down	1 c	145	15	435	5	115	9	1	.2	<.1	.2
5	313	One packet, ½ oz	½ oz	14	15	41	<1	11	1	<.1	t	t	t
		Raspberries:											
5	314	Raw	1 c	123	87	60	1	14	8	1	t	.1	.4
		Frozen, sweetened											
5	315	10-oz container	10 oz	284	73	293	2	74	15	<1	t	<.1	.3
5	316	Cup, thawed measure	1 c	250	73	255	2	65	12	<1	t	<.1	.2
5	317	Rhubarb, cooked, added sugar	1 c	240	68	279	1	75	5	<1	t	t	.1
		Strawberries:											
5	318	Raw, whole, capped	1 c	149	92	45	1	11	4	1	<.1	.1	.3
		Frozen, sliced, sweetened:											
5	319	10-oz container	10 oz	284	73	273	2	74	6	<1	t	.1	.2
5	320	Cup, thawed measure	1 c	255	73	245	1	66	8	<1	t	.1	.2
		Tangerines, without peel and seeds:											
5	321	Raw (2⅜″ whole)	1 ea	84	88	37	1	9	2	<1	t	<.1	<.1
5	322	Canned, light syrup, fruit and liquid	1 c	252	83	154	1	41	4	<1	<.1	<.1	.1
5	323	Tangerine juice, canned, sweetened	1 c	249	87	125	1	30	1	<1	<.1	<.1	.1
		Watermelon, raw, without rind and seeds											
5	324	Piece, 1″ thick by 10″ diam (weighs 2 lb with refuse)	1 pce	482[44]	92	152	3	35	2	2	.3	.2	1
5	325	Diced	1 c	160	92	50	1	12	1	1	.1	.1	.4
		BAKED GOODS: BREADS, CAKES, COOKIES, CRACKERS, PIES, PANCAKES, TORTILLAS											
6	326	Bagels, plain, enriched, 3½″ diam	1 ea	68	32	180	7	35	1	1	.2	.3	.4
		Biscuits:											
6	327	From home recipe	1 ea	28	28	100	2	13	1	5	1.2	2	1.3
6	328	From mix	1 ea	28	29	94	2	14	1	3	.8	1.4	.9
6	329	From refrigerated dough	1 ea	20	30	65	1	10	<1	2	.6	.9	.6
6	330	Bread crumbs, dry grated (see 364, 365 for soft crumbs)	1 c	100	7	390	13	73	4	5	1.5	1.6	1

[43]Dietary fiber data can vary between 8 and 13 g for 10 prunes.
[44]926 g with rind and seeds.

Chol (mg)	Calc (mg)	Iron (mg)	Magn (mg)	Phos (mg)	Pota (mg)	Sodi (mg)	Zinc (mg)	VT-A (RE)	Thia (mg)	Ribo (mg)	Niac (mg)	V-B6 (mg)	Fola (µg)	VT-C (mg)
0	3	.07	4	7	114	<1	.07	21	.03	.06	.33	.05	3	6
0	1	.03	2	3	48	<1	.03	9	.01	.03	.14	.02	1	3
0	23	2.17	13	34	235	49	.18	67	.04	.1	.75	.07	7	1
0	10	.92	6	14	100	21	.08	29	.02	.04	.32	.03	3	<1
0	25	.86	20	38	388	3	.28	254	.06	.15	1.19	.1	8	7
0	10	.32	8	15	147	1	.11	96	.02	.06	.45	.04	3	3
0	43	2.08	38	66	626	3	.45	167	.07	.14	1.65	.22	3	3
0	49	2.35	43	74	708	4	.51	65	.05	.21	1.53	.46	<1	6
0	31	3.02	36	64	707	10	.54	1	.04	.18	2.01	.56	1	11
0	71	3.02	48	140	1089	17	.46	1	.23	.13	1.19	.36	5	5
0	7	.29	5	14	105	2	.05	<1	.02	.01	.12	.04	1	<1
0	27	.7	22	15	187	0	.57	16	.04	.11	1.11	.07	32	31
0	43	1.85	37	48	324	3	.51	17	.05	.13	.65	.1	74	47
0	38	1.62	32	43	285	3	.45	15	.05	.11	1.5	.09	65	41
0	348	.5	30	19	230	2	.19	17	.04	.06	.48	.05	13	8
0	21	.57	16	28	247	2	.19	4	.03	.1	.34	.09	28	85
0	31	1.7	20	37	278	9	.17	7	.05	.14	1.1	.09	47	118
0	28	1.5	18	33	250	8	.15	6	.04	.13	1.02	.08	42	106
0	12	.08	10	8	132	1	.38	77	.09	.02	.13	.06	17	26
0	18	.93	19	25	197	15	.60	212	.13	.11	1.1	.11	34	50
0	45	.5	20	35	443	2	.08	105	.15	.05	.25	.08	8	55
0	38	.82	52	41	560	10	.34	176	.39	.1	.96	.69	10	47
0	13	.27	17	14	186	3	.11	59	.13	.03	.32	.23	3	15
0	20	2.1	15	61	65	300	.61	0	.26	.20	2.4	.03	16	0
t	48	.7	6	36	32	195	.15	3	.08	.08	.8	.01	2	t
t	59	.58	7	129	57	265	.18	4	.12	.11	.85	.01	2	t
1	4	.47	4	78	18	249	.09	0	.08	.05	.67	.01	1	0
5	122	4.1	31	141	152	736	.50	0	.35	.35	4.8	.02	28	0

(For purposes of calculations, use "0" for t, <1, <.1, <.01, etc.)

Table C–1　Food Composition

Grp	Ref	Food Description	Measure	Wt (g)	H₂O (%)	Ener (kcal)	Prot (g)	Carb (g)	Dietary Fiber (g)	Fat (g)	Fat Breakdown (g)		
											Sat	Mono	Poly
		BAKED GOODS—Con.											
		Breads:											
6	331	Boston brown bread, canned, 3¼" slice	1 pce	45	45	95	2	21	2	1	.26	.13	.14
		Cracked wheat bread (¼ cracked-wheat flour, ¾ enr wheat flour):											
6	332	1-lb loaf	1 ea	454	35	1190	42	227	23	16	3.1	4.3	5.7
6	333	Slice (18 per loaf)	1 pce	25	35	65	2	13	1	1	.2	.2	.3
6	334	Slice, toasted	1 pce	21	26	65	2	13	1	1	.2	.2	.3
		French/Vienna bread, enriched:											
6	335	1-lb loaf	1 ea	454	34	1270	43	230	8	18	4	6	6
6	336	French, slice, 5 × 2½ × 1"	1 pce	35	34	100	3	18	1	1	.3	.4	.5
6	337	Vienna, slice 4¾ × 4 × ½"	1 pce	25	34	70	2	13	1	1	.2	.3	.3
		French toast: see Mixed Dishes, and Fast Foods, 691											
		Italian bread, enriched:											
6	338	1-lb loaf	1 ea	454	32	1255	41	256	5	4	.6	.3	1.6
6	339	Slice, 4½ × 3¼ × ¾"	1 pce	30	32	83	3	17	<1	<1	<.1	t	.1
		Mixed grain bread, enriched:											
6	340	1-lb loaf	1 ea	454	37	1165	45	212	18	17	3	4	7
6	341	Slice (18 per loaf)	1 pce	25	37	65	2	12	2	1	.2	.2	.4
6	342	Slice, toasted	1 pce	23	27	65	2	12	2	1	.2	.2	.4
		Oatmeal bread, enriched:											
6	343	1-lb loaf	1 ea	454	37	1145	38	212	16	20	4	7	8
6	344	Slice (18 per loaf)	1 pce	25	37	65	2	12	1	1	.2	.4	.5
6	345	Slice, toasted	1 pce	23	30	65	2	12	1	1	.2	.4	.5
6	346	Pita pocket bread, enr, 6½" round	1 ea	60	31	165	6	33	1	1	.1	.1	.4
		Pumpernickel bread (⅔ rye flour, ⅓ enr. wheat flour):											
6	347	1-lb loaf	1 ea	454	37	1160	42	218	19	16	3	4	6
6	348	Slice, 5 × 4 × ⅜"	1 pce	32	37	80	3	15	2	1	.2	.3	.5
6	349	Slice, toasted	1 pce	29	28	80	3	15	1	1	.2	.3	.5
		Raisin bread, enriched:											
6	350	1-lb loaf	1 ea	454	33	1260	37	239	12	18	4	7	7
6	351	Slice (18 per loaf)	1 pce	25	33	68	2	13	1	1	.2	.4	.4
6	352	Slice, toasted	1 pce	21	24	68	2	13	1	1	.2	.4	.4
		Rye bread, light (⅓ rye flour, ⅔ enr. wheat flour):											
6	353	1-lb loaf	1 ea	454	37	1190	38	218	30	17	3.3	5.2	5.5
6	354	Slice, 4¾ × 3¾ × 7/16"	1 pce	25	37	65	2	12	2	1	.2	.3	.3
6	355	Slice, toasted	1 pce	22	28	65	2	12	2	1	.2	.3	.3
		Wheat bread (blend of enr. wheat flour and whole-wheat flour):[45]											
6	356	1-lb loaf	1 ea	454	37	1160	43	213	25	19	3.9	7.3	4.5
6	357	Slice (18 per loaf)	1 pce	25	37	65	2	12	1	1	.2	.4	.3
6	358	Slice, toasted	1 pce	23	28	65	2	12	1	1	.2	.4	.3
		White bread, enriched:											
6	359	1-lb loaf	1 ea	454	37	1210	38	222	12	18	5.6	6.5	4.2
6	360	Slice (18 per loaf)	1 pce	25	37	65	2	12	<1	1	.3	.4	.2
6	361	Slice, toasted	1 pce	22	28	65	2	12	<1	1	.3	.4	.2
6	362	Slice (22 per loaf)	1 pce	20	37	55	2	10	<1	1	.2	.3	.2
6	363	Slice, toasted	1 pce	17	28	55	2	10	<1	1	.2	.3	.2

[45]A blend of white and whole-wheat flour—no official ratio specified.

Chol (mg)	Calc (mg)	Iron (mg)	Magn (mg)	Phos (mg)	Pota (mg)	Sodi (mg)	Zinc (mg)	VT-A (RE)	Thia (mg)	Ribo (mg)	Niac (mg)	V-B6 (mg)	Fola (μg)	VT-C (mg)
3	41	.90	40	72	131	113	.35	0	.06	.04	.7	.06	8	0
0	295	12.1	218	581	608	1966	6.36	0	1.73	1.73	15.3	.42	218	t
0	16	.67	12	32	34	106	.35	0	.1	.1	.84	.02	12	t
0	16	.67	12	32	34	106	.35	0	.07	.1	.84	.02	9	t
0	499	14	91	386	409	2633	2.9	0	2.09	1.59	18.2	.24	168	t
0	39	1.08	7	30	32	203	.22	0	.16	.12	1.4	.02	13	t
0	28	.77	5	21	23	145	.16	0	.12	.09	1	.01	9	t
0	77	12.7	106	350	336	2656	3.1	0	1.86	1.06	15.1	.24	160	0
0	5	.8	7	23	22	176	.21	0	.12	.07	1	.02	11	0
0	472	14.8	222	962	990	1870	5.45	t	1.77	1.73	18.9	.47	295	
0	27	.8	12	55	56	106	.3	t	.1	.1	1.1	.03	16	t
0	27	.8	12	55	56	106	.3	t	.08	.1	1.1	.02	12	t
0	267	12	154	563	707	2231	4.45	0	2.09	1.2	15.4	.07	15	0
0	15	.7	9	31	39	124	.25	0	.12	.07	.85	<.01	1	0
0	15	.7	9	31	39	124	.25	0	.09	.07	.85	<.01	1	0
0	49	1.45	16	60	71	339	.50	0	.27	.13	2.32	.01	12	0
0	322	12.4	309	990	1966	2461	5.18	0	1.54	2.36	15	.72	222	0
0	23	.88	22	71	141	177	.4	0	.11	.17	1.06	.05	16	0
0	23	.88	22	71	141	177	.4	0	.09	.17	1.06	.05	12	0
0	463	14.1	114	395	1058	1657	2.81	1	1.5	2.81	18.6	.15	159	t
0	25	.78	6	22	59	92	.16	t	.08	.16	1.02	.01	9	t
0	25	.80	6	22	59	92	.16	t	.06	.16	1.02	.01	8	t
0	363	12.3	109	658	926	3164	5.77	0	1.86	1.45	15	.43	177	0
0	20	.68	8	36	51	175	.38	0	.1	.08	.83	.02	10	0
0	20	.68	6	36	51	175	.38	0	.08	.08	.83	.02	8	0
0	572	15.8	209	835	627	2447	4.77	t	2.09	1.45	20.5	.50	204	t
0	32	.87	12	47	35	135	.26	t	.12	.08	1.13	.03	11	t
0	32	.87	12	47	35	135	.26	t	.10	.08	1.20	.02	8	t
0	572	12.9	95	490	508	2334	2.81	t	2.13	1.41	17.0	.15	159	t
0	32	.71	5	27	28	129	.16	t	.12	.08	.94	.01	9	t
0	32	.71	5	27	28	129	.16	t	.09	.08	.94	.01	9	t
0	25	.57	4	22	22	103	.12	t	.09	.06	.75	.01	7	t
0	25	.6	4	21	22	103	.12	t	.07	.06	.75	.01	7	t

(For purposes of calculations, use "0" for t, <1, <.1, <.01, etc.)

Table C–1 Food Composition

Grp	Ref	Food Description	Measure	Wt (g)	H₂O (%)	Ener (kcal)	Prot (g)	Carb (g)	Dietary Fiber (g)	Fat (g)	Fat Breakdown (g)		
											Sat	Mono	Poly
		BAKED GOODS—Con.											
		Bread—con.											
		White bread cubes, crumbs:											
6	364	Cubes, soft	1 c	30	37	80	2	15	1	1	.4	.4	.3
6	365	Crumbs, soft	1 c	45	37	120	4	22	1	2	.6	.6	.4
		Whole-wheat bread:											
6	366	1-lb loaf	1 ea	454	38	1110	44	206	51	20	6	7	5
6	367	Slice (16 per loaf)	1 pce	28	38	70	3	13	2	1	.4	.4	.3
6	368	Slice, toasted	1 pce	25	29	70	3	13	2	1	.4	.4	.3
		Bread stuffing, prepared from mix:											
6	369	Dry type	1 c	140	33	500	9	50	4	31	6	13	10
6	370	Moist type, with egg	1 c	203	61	420	9	40	4	26	5	11	8
		Cakes, prepared from mixes:[46]											
		Angel food cake:											
6	371	Whole cake, 9 ¾″ diam tube	1 ea	635	38	1510	38	342	3	2	.4	.2	1
6	372	Piece, ¹⁄₁₂ of cake	1 pce	53	38	125	3	29	<1	<1	t	t	.1
6	373	Boston cream pie, ⅛ of cake	1 pce	120	35	260	3	44	1	8	2.8	3.1	1.5
		Coffee cake:											
6	374	Whole cake, 7 ¾ × 5 ⅛ × 1 ¼″	1 ea	430	30	1385	27	225	3	41	12	17	10
6	375	Piece, ⅙ of cake	1 pce	72	30	230	5	38	2	7	2.0	2.8	1.6
		Devil's food with chocolate frosting:											
6	376	Whole cake, 2 layer, 8 or 9″ diam	1 ea	1107	24	3755	49	645	5	136	56	51	20
6	377	Piece, ¹⁄₁₆ of cake	1 pce	69	24	235	3	40	1	8	3.5	3.2	1.2
6	378	Cupcakes, 2 ½″ diam	1 ea	42	24	143	2	25	<1	5	2.1	2.0	.7
		Gingerbread:											
6	379	Whole cake, 8″ square	1 ea	570	37	1575	18	291	3	39	10	16	11
6	380	Piece, ⅑ of cake	1 pce	63	37	174	2	32	2	4	1.1	1.8	1.2
		Yellow, with chocolate frosting, 2 layer:											
6	381	Whole cake, 8 or 9″ diam	1 ea	1108	26	3735	45	638	5	125	48	49	22
6	382	Piece, ¹⁄₁₆ of cake	1 pce	69	26	235	3	40	<1	8	3	3.1	1.4
		Cakes from home recipes with enriched flour:											
		Carrot cake, cream cheese frosting:[47]											
6	383	Whole, 9 × 13″ cake	1 ea	1536	23	6175	63	775	11	328	66	135	108
6	384	Piece, ¹⁄₁₆ of 9 × 13″ sheet cake 2¼ × 3¼″	1 pce	96	23	385	4	48	1	21	4	8	7
		Fruitcake, dark, 7½″ diam tube, 2¼″ high:[47]											
6	385	Whole cake	1 ea	1361	18	5185	74	783	38	228	48	113	52
6	386	Piece, ¹⁄₃₂ of cake, ⅔″ arc	1 pce	43	18	165	2	25	2	7	1.5	3.6	1.6
		Sheet cake, plain, no frosting:[48]											
6	387	Whole cake, 9″ square	1 ea	777	25	2830	35	434	3	108	30	45	26
6	388	Piece, ⅑ of cake	1 pce	86	25	315	4	48	<1	12	3.3	5	2.8
		Sheet cake, plain, unckd white frosting:[48]											
6	389	Whole cake, 9″ square	1 ea	1096	21	4020	37	694	3	129	42	50	26
6	390	Piece, ⅑ of cake	1 pce	121	21	445	4	77	<1	14	5	6	3
		Pound cake:[49]											
6	391	Loaf, 8½ × 3½ × 3¼″	1 ea	514	22	2025	33	265	4	94	21	41	27
6	392	Piece, ¹⁄₁₇ of loaf, ½″ slice	1 pce	30	22	120	2	15	<1	5	1.2	2.4	1.6

[46] Excepting angel food cake, cakes were made from mixes containing vegetable shortening, and frostings were made with margarine. All mixes use enriched flour.

[47] Made with vegetable oil.

[48] Cakes made with vegetable shortening; frosting with margarine.

[49] Made with margarine.

Chol (mg)	Calc (mg)	Iron (mg)	Magn (mg)	Phos (mg)	Pota (mg)	Sodi (mg)	Zinc (mg)	VT-A (RE)	Thia (mg)	Ribo (mg)	Niac (mg)	V-B6 (mg)	Fola (μg)	VT-C (mg)
0	38	.85	6	32	34	154	.19	t	.14	.09	1.13	.01	11	t
0	57	1.28	9	49	50	231	.28	t	.21	.14	1.69	.02	16	t
0	327	15.5	422	1180	799	2887	7.63	t	1.59	.95	17.4	.85	250	t
0	20	.97	26	74	50	180	.50	t	.10	.06	1.09	.05	16	t
0	20	.97	26	74	50	180	.50	t	.08	.06	1.08	.05	12	t
0	92	2.2	30	136	126	1254	.55	273	.17	.20	2.50	.02	14	0
67	81	2.03	45	134	118	1023	.78	256	.10	.18	1.62	.04	20	t
0	527	2.73	51	1086	845	3226	.82	0	.32	1.27	1.6	.08	51	0
0	44	.23	4	91	71	269	.07	0	.03	.11	.13	.01	4	0
20	26	.6	11	70	40	225	.23	70	.01	.18	.7	.05	7	0
279	262	7.30	27	748	469	1853	3.70	194	.82	.90	7.70	.12	30	1
47	44	1.22	5	125	78	310	.62	32	.14	.15	1.29	.02	5	t
598	653	22.1	200	1162	1439	2900	7.95	498	1.11	1.66	10	.32	82	1
37	41	1.40	12	72	90	181	.53	31	.07	.1	.6	.02	1	t
23	25	.85	7	44	55	110	.40	19	.04	.06	.37	.01	3	t
6	513	10.8	41	570	1562	1733	5.52	0	.86	1.03	7.4	.07	36	1
1	57	1.20	5	63	173	192	.61	0	.10	.11	.82	.01	4	t
576	1008	15.5	72	2017	1208	2515	3.31	465	1.22	1.66	11.1	.45	80	1
36	63	.97	5	126	75	157	.21	29	.08	.10	.69	.03	5	t
1183	707	21	197	998	1720	4470	8.15	246	1.83	1.97	14.7	1.38	243	23
74	44	1.3	12	62	108	279	.51	15	.11	.12	.9	.86	15	1
640	1293	37.6	340	1592	6138	2123	6.8	422	2.41	2.55	17	1.72	54	504
20	41	1.2	11	50	194	67	.22	13	.08	.08	.5	.05	2	16
552	497	11.7	108	793	614	2331	2.75	373	1.24	1.40	10.1	.26	54	2
61	55	1.3	12	88	68	258	.31	41	.14	.15	1.1	.03	15	t
636	548	11	108	822	669	2488	2.90	647	1.21	1.42	9.9	.27	110	2
70	61	1.2	12	91	74	275	.32	71	.13	.16	1.1	.03	12	t
555	339	9.3	48	473	483	1645	2.69	1033	.93	1.08	7.8	.39	55	1
32	20	.5	3	28	28	98	.16	60	.05	.06	.5	.02	3	t

(For purposes of calculations, use "0" for t, <1, <.1, <.01, etc.)

Table C–1 Food Composition

Grp	Ref	Food Description	Measure	Wt (g)	H₂O (%)	Ener (kcal)	Prot (g)	Carb (g)	Dietary Fiber (g)	Fat (g)	Fat Breakdown (g)		
											Sat	Mono	Poly
		BAKED GOODS—Con.											
		Cakes, commercial:											
		Pound cake:											
6	393	Loaf, 8½ × 3½ × 3″	1 ea	500	24	1935	26	257	4	94	52	30	4
6	394	Slice, ¹⁄₁₇ of loaf, ½″ slice	1 pce	29	24	110	2	15	<1	5	3.0	1.7	.2
		Snack cakes:											
6	395	Chocolate w/creme filling, 2 small cakes per package	1 ea	28	20	105	1	17	<1	4	1.7	1.5	.6
6	396	Sponge cake w/creme filling, 2 small cakes per package	1 ea	42	19	155	1	27	<1	5	2.3	2.1	.5
		White cake with white frosting, 2-layer cake:											
6	397	Whole cake, 8 or 9″ diam	1 ea	1140	24	4170	43	670	5	148	33	62	42
6	398	Piece, ¹⁄₁₆ of cake	1 pce	71	24	260	3	42	<1	9	2.1	3.8	2.6
		Yellow cake with chocolate frosting, 2-layer:											
6	399	Whole cake, 8 or 9″ diam	1 ea	1108	23	3895	40	620	5	175	92	59	10
6	400	Piece, ¹⁄₁₆ of cake	1 pce	69	23	245	3	39	<1	11	5.7	3.7	.6
		Cheesecake:											
6	401	Whole cake, 9″ diam	1 ea	1110	46	3350	60	317	5	213	120	66	15
6	402	Piece, ¹⁄₁₂ of cake	1 pce	92	46	278	5	26	1	18	9.9	5.4	1.2
6	1035	Cheese puffs/Cheetos®	1 oz	28.4	1	158	2	14	<1	10	4.8	3.4	.6
		Cookies made with enriched flour:											
		Brownies with nuts:											
6	403	Commercial with frosting, 1 ½ × 1 ¾ × ⅞	1 ea	25	13	100	1	16	<1	4	1.6	2	.8
6	404	Home recipe, 1¾ × 1¾ × ⅞″[47]	1 ea	20	10	95	1	11	<1	6	1.4	2.8	1.2
		Chocolate chip cookies:											
6	405	Commercial, 2¼″ diam	4 ea	42	4	180	2	28	<1	9	2.9	3.1	2.6
6	406	Home recipe, 2⅓″ diam[50]	4 ea	40	3	185	2	26	1	11	3.9	4.3	2
6	407	From refrigerated dough, 2¼″ diam	4 ea	48	5	225	2	32	1	11	4	4.4	2
6	408	Fig bars	4 ea	56	12	210	2	42	3	4	1	1.5	1
6	409	Oatmeal raisin cookies, 2⅝″ diam	4 ea	52	4	245	3	36	1	10	2.5	4.5	2.8
6	410	Peanut butter cookies, home recipe, 2⅝″ diam[50]	4 ea	48	3	245	4	28	1	14	4	5.8	2.8
6	411	Sandwich-type cookies, all	4 ea	40	2	195	2	29	<1	8	2	3.6	2.2
		Shortbread cookies:											
6	412	Commercial, small	4 ea	32	6	155	2	20	1	8	2.9	3	1.1
6	413	From home recipe, large[49]	2 ea	28	3	145	2	17	1	8	1.3	2.7	3.4
6	414	Sugar cookies from refrigerated dough, 2½″ diam	4 ea	48	4	235	2	31	<1	12	2.3	5	3.6
6	415	Vanilla wafers	10 ea	40	4	185	2	29	<1	7	1.8	3	1.8
6	416	Corn chips	1 oz	28	1	155	2	16	1	9	1.8	3.4	3.7
		Crackers:[53]											
6	1034	Armenian cracker bread	4 pce	28.4	4	117	5	19	4	2	.4	.7	1.1
6	417	Cheese crackers	10 ea	10	4	50	1	5	<1	3	.9	1.2	.3
6	418	Cheese crackers with peanut butter	4 ea	30	3	150	4	19	<1	8	1.6	3.2	1.2
6	419	Graham crackers	2 ea	14	4	60	1	11	<1	1	.4	.6	.4
6	420	Melba toast, plain	1 pce	5	4	20	1	4	<1	<1	.1	.1	.1

[47]Made with vegetable oil.
[49]Made with margarine.
[50]Made with vegetable shortening.
[53]Crackers made with enriched flour except for rye wafers and whole-wheat wafers.

Chol (mg)	Calc (mg)	Iron (mg)	Magn (mg)	Phos (mg)	Pota (mg)	Sodi (mg)	Zinc (mg)	VT-A (RE)	Thia (mg)	Ribo (mg)	Niac (mg)	V-B6 (mg)	Fola (µg)	VT-C (mg)
1100	146	9.3	48	517	443	1857	1.95	715	.96	1.12	8.1	.38	55	1
64	8	.5	3	30	26	108	.11	41	.06	.06	.5	.02	3	t
15	21	1.0	3	26	34	105	.17	4	.06	.09	.7	.01	3	0
7	14	.6	3	44	37	155	.21	9	.07	.06	.6	.02	4	0
46	536	15.5	60	1585	832	2827	1.77	194	3.19	2.05	27.6	.16	64	0
3	33	1	4	99	52	176	.11	12	.2	.13	1.7	.01	4	0
609	366	19.9	72	1884	1972	3080	3.3	488	.78	2.22	10	.45	80	0
38	23	1.24	5	117	123	192	.21	30	.05	.14	.62	.03	5	0
2053	622	5.33	111	977	1088	2464	4.66	833	.33	1.44	5.11	.71	200	56
170	52	.44	9	81	90	204	.39	69	.03	.12	.42	.06	17	5
5	18	.20	7	29	23	344	—	26	.01	.03	.20	—	—	0
14	13	.61	14	26	50	59	.36	18	.08	.07	.33	.04	5	t
18	9	.40	11	26	35	51	.31	6	.05	.05	.3	.04	4	t
5	16	.8	10	41	56	140	.3	15	.1	.23	.9	.02	4	t
18	13	1	14	34	82	82	.22	5	.06	.06	.58	.03	4	0
22	13	1.04	10	34	62	173	.24	8	.06	.10	.89	.01	4	0
27	40	1.36	15	34	162	180	.36	6	.08	.07	.73	.07	4	t
2	18	1.1	26	58	90	148	.53	12	.09	.08	1	.03	6	0
22	21	1.1	19	60	110	142	.36	5	.07	.07	1.9	.04	12	0
0	12	1.4	15	40	66	189	.21	0	.09	.07	.8	.01	1	0
27	13	.8	4	39	38	123	.15	8	.10	.09	.9	.01	3	0
0	6	.55	4	31	18	125	.13	89	.08	.06	.71	.01	2	t
29	50	.9	8	91	33	261	.24	11	.09	.06	1.1	.02	4	0
25	16	.8	6	36	50	150	.12	14	.07	.1	1	.01	4	0
0	35	.5	21	52	52	233	.44	11	.04	.05	.4	.04[51]	3[52]	1
0	21	.45	41	1	77	—	.90	1	.06	.04	1.05	.03	12	2
6	11	.35	3	17	17	112	.07	5	.05	.04	.4	.01	—	0
4	26	1.2	2	94	64	338	.06	3	.16	.12	2.4	.03	—	0
0	6	.37	6	20	36	86	.11	0	.02	.03	.6	.01	2	0
0	6	.1	—	10	11	44	—	0	.01	.01	.1	.01	—	0

[51] B6 values vary from 0 to .04 g between various brands—check label.
[52] Folacin values estimated and derived from values for cornmeal and corn tortillas.

(For purposes of calculations, use "0" for t, <1, <.1, <.01, etc.)

Table C–1   Food Composition

Grp	Ref	Food Description	Measure	Wt (g)	H₂O (%)	Ener (kcal)	Prot (g)	Carb (g)	Dietary Fiber (g)	Fat (g)	Fat Breakdown (g) Sat	Mono	Poly

BAKED GOODS—Con.

Crackers—con.

Grp	Ref	Food Description	Measure	Wt (g)	H₂O (%)	Ener (kcal)	Prot (g)	Carb (g)	Fiber (g)	Fat (g)	Sat	Mono	Poly
6	421	Rye wafers, whole grain	2 ea	14	5	55	1	10	2	1	.3	.4	.3
6	422	Saltine® crackers[54]	4 ea	12	4	50	1	9	<1	1	.5	.4	.2
6	423	Snack-type crackers, round	3 ea	9	3	45	1	6	<1	3	.6	1.2	.3
6	424	Wheat crackers, thin	4 ea	8	3	35	1	5	1	1	.5	.5	.4
6	425	Whole-wheat wafers	2 ea	8	4	35	1	5	1	2	.5	.6	.4
6	426	Croissants, 4½ × 4 × 1¾"	1 ea	57	22	235	5	27	1	12	3.5	6.7	1.4
		Danish pastry:											
6	427	Packaged ring, plain, 12 oz	1 ea	340	27	1305	21	152	3	71	22	29	16
6	428	Round piece, plain, 4¼" diam 1" high	1 ea	57	27	220	4	26	1	12	3.6	4.8	2.6
6	429	Ounce, plain	1 oz	28	28	110	2	13	<1	6	1.8	2.4	1.3
6	430	Round piece with fruit	1 pce	65	30	235	4	28	1	13	3.9	5.2	2.9
		Desserts, 3 × 3 inch piece:											
6	1348	Apple crisp	1 pce	78	58	146	1	25	1	5	1.0	2.3	1.7
6	1353	Apple cobbler	1 pce	104	56	201	2	35	2	6	1.4	2.7	1.9
6	1349	Cherry crisp	1 pce	138	73	157	2	27	2	5	1.0	2.3	1.7
6	1352	Cherry cobbler	1 pce	129	65	199	2	34	1	6	1.4	2.7	1.9
6	1350	Peach crisp	1 pce	139	72	166	2	30	2	5	1.0	2.3	1.7
6	1351	Peach cobbler	1 pce	130	64	130	2	37	2	6	1.4	2.7	1.9
		Doughnuts:											
6	431	Cake type, plain, 3¼" diam	1 ea	50	21	210	2	25	1	12	3.4	5.8	2
6	432	Yeast-leavened, glazed, 3¾" diam	1 ea	60	27	235	4	26	1	13	5.2	5.5	.9
		English muffins:											
6	433	Plain, enriched	1 ea	57	42	140	5	26	2	1	.3	.2	.3
6	434	Toasted	1 ea	50	29	140	5	26	2	1	.3	.2	.3
		Muffins, 2½" diam, 1½" high											
		From home recipe:											
6	435	Blueberry[50]	1 ea	45	37	135	3	20	2	5	1.5	2.1	1.2
6	436	Bran[47]	1 ea	45	35	125	3	19	3	6	1.4	1.6	2.3
6	437	Cornmeal	1 ea	45	33	145	3	21	2	5	1.5	2.2	1.4
		From commercial mix:											
6	438	Blueberry	1 ea	45	33	140	3	22	2	5	1.4	2	1.2
6	439	Bran	1 ea	45	28	140	3	24	3	4	1.3	1.6	1
6	440	Cornmeal	1 ea	45	30	145	3	22	2	6	1.7	2.3	1.4
		Pancakes, 4" diam:											
6	441	Buckwheat, from mix; egg and milk added	1 ea	27	58	55	2	6	1	2	.9	.9	.5
6	442	Plain, from home recipe	1 ea	27	50	60	2	9	1	2	.5	.8	.5
6	443	Plain, from mix; egg, milk, oil added	1 ea	27	54	60	2	8	1	2	.5	.9	.5
		Piecrust, with enriched flour, baked:[50]											
6	444	Home recipe, 9" shell	1 ea	180	15	900	11	79	4	60	15	26	16
		From mix:											
6	445	Piecrust for 2-crust pie	1 ea	320	19	1485	21	141	6	93	23	41	25
6	446	1 pie shell	1 ea	180	19	835	12	79	4	52	13	23	14
		Pies, 9" diam; pie crust made with veg shortening, enriched flour:											
		Apple pie:[56]											
6	447	Whole pie	1 ea	945	48	2420	22	360	19	105	25	46	29
6	448	Piece, ⅙ of pie	1 pce	158	48	405	4	60	3	18	4.1	7.6	4.9

[47]Made with vegetable oil.
[50]Made with vegetable shortening.
[54]Made with lard.
[56]Recipes updated for latest USDA values for fruits/nuts/fruit juice.

GRP KEY:1 = BEV 2 = DAIRY 3 = EGGS 4 = FAT/OIL 5 = FRUIT 6 = BAKERY 7 = GRAIN 8 = FISH 9 = BEEF 10 = POULTRY
11 = SAUSAGE 12 = MIXED/FAST 13 = NUTS/SEEDS 14 = SWEETS 15 = VEG/LEG 16 = MISC 22 = SOUP/SAUCE

Chol (mg)	Calc (mg)	Iron (mg)	Magn (mg)	Phos (mg)	Pota (mg)	Sodi (mg)	Zinc (mg)	VT-A (RE)	Thia (mg)	Ribo (mg)	Niac (mg)	V-B6 (mg)	Fola (µg)	VT-C (mg)
0	7	.5	16	44	65	115	1.60	0	.06	.03	.5	.03	10	0
4	3	.5	3	12	17	165	.09	0	.06	.05	.6	<.01	2	0
0	9	.3	2	18	12	90	.05	t	.03	.03	.3	<.01	1	0
0	3	.3	7[55]	15	17	69	.24[55]	t	.04	.03	.4	.01	3[55]	0
0	3	.24	8[55]	22	31	59	.23	0	.02	.03	.4	.01	3[55]	0
13	20	2.1	9	64	68	452	.32	13	.17	.13	1.3	.03	18	0
292	360	6.5	68	347	316	1302	2.86	99	.95	1.02	8.5	.12	84	t
49	60	1.1	11	58	53	218	.48	17	.16	.17	1.4	.02	14	t
24	30	.55	6	29	27	109	.24	9	.08	.09	.7	.01	7	t
56	17	1.3	13	80	57	233	.55	11	.16	.14	1.4	.02	16	t
0	20	.77	12	15	112	66	.09	65	.05	.04	.41	.03	3	4
1	32	.76	7	42	86	305	.17	76	.08	.07	.70	.04	3	<1
0	29	2.16	16	22	163	73	.14	144	.06	.08	.56	.05	10	3
1	39	1.78	10	46	113	311	.21	135	.09	.10	.81	.05	9	2
0	24	.00	18	30	197	71	.19	104	.05	.05	1.01	.03	5	5
1	35	.90	11	52	139	309	.24	105	.08	.08	1.15	.03	5	3
20	23	.8	12	111	58	192	.25	5	.12	.12	1.1	.02	4	t
21	17	1.4	13	55	64	222	.30	<1	.28	.12	1.8	.28	13	0
0	96	1.7	11	67	331	378	.41	0	.26	.18	2.14	.02	18	0
0	96	1.7	11	67	331	378	.41	0	.23	.18	2.14	.02	15	0
19	54	.9	11	46	47	198	.29	9	.10	.11	.9	<.01	12	1
24	60	1.4	34	125	99	189	.37	30	.11	.13	1.3	.01	9	3
23	66	.9	11	59	57	169	.31	15	.11	.11	.9	.04	5	t
45	15	.9	7	90	54	225	.21	11	.11	.13	1.17	<.01	14	<1
28	27	1.7	28	182	50	385	.95	14	.08	.12	1.9	.12	19	0
42	30	1.3	11	128	31	291	.34	16	.09	.09	.8	.04	5	t
20	59	.4	18	91	66	125	.5	17	.04	.05	.2	.06	6	t
16	27	.5	7	38	33	115	.23	10	.06	.07	.5	.02	4	t
16	36	.7	7	71	43	160	.23	7	.09	.12	.8	.01	3	t
0	25	4.5	31	90	90	1100	1.50	0	.54	.40	5.0	.17	32	0
0	131	9.3	44	272	179	2600	1.19	0	1.07	.79	9.89	.27	57	0
0	74	5.23	25	153	101	1462	.79	0	.60	.44	5.57	.15	32	0
0	170	10	69	300	600	2844	1.6	28	1.04	.76	9.5	.5	48	2
0	28	1.67	12	50	100	476	.27	5	.18	.13	1.6	.08	8	<1

[55]Values derived from whole-wheat recipes and retention values.

(For purposes of calculations, use "0" for t, <1, <.1, <.01, etc.)

Table C–1 Food Composition

Grp	Ref	Food Description	Measure	Wt (g)	H₂O (%)	Ener (kcal)	Prot (g)	Carb (g)	Dietary Fiber (g)	Fat (g)	Fat Breakdown (g)		
											Sat	Mono	Poly
BAKED GOODS—Con.													
		Pies—con.											
		Banana cream pie:[57]											
6	449	Whole pie	1 ea	1190	66	1915	38	282	10	77	27	29	15
6	450	⅙ of pie	1 pce	198	66	319	6	47	2	13	4.5	4.9	2.5
		Blueberry pie:[56]											
6	451	Whole pie	1 ea	945	51	2285	23	330	22	102	24	45	28
6	452	Piece, ⅙ of pie	1 pce	158	51	380	4	55	4	17	4.0	7.5	4.7
		Cherry pie:[56]											
6	453	Whole pie	1 ea	945	47	2465	26	363	15	107	25	47	30
6	454	Piece, ⅙ of pie	1 pce	158	47	410	4	61	2	18	4.2	7.8	4.9
		Chocolate cream pie:[58]											
6	455	Whole pie	1 ea	1051	63	1863	45	255	4	76	27	30	15
6	456	Piece, ⅙ of pie	1 pce	175	63	311	7	42	1	13	4.5	5.0	2.5
		Custard pie:											
6	457	Whole pie	1 ea	910	58	1760	46	204	4	85	28	35	17
6	458	Piece, ⅙ of pie	1 pce	152	58	293	8	34	1	14	.9	5.8	2.8
		Lemon meringue pie:[56]											
6	459	Whole Pie	1 ea	840	47	2140	31	317	5	86	21	37	22
6	460	Piece, ⅙ of pie	1 pce	140	47	355	5	53	1	14	3.5	6.2	3.7
		Peach pie:[56]											
6	461	Whole pie	1 ea	945	48	2410	24	361	17	105	25	46	29
6	462	Piece, ⅙ of pie	1 pce	158	48	405	4	61	3	17	4.1	7.7	4.8
		Pecan pie:[56]											
6	463	Whole pie	1 ea	825	20	3500	38	551	10	142	24	75	34
6	464	Piece, ⅙ of pie	1 pce	138	20	583	6	92	5	24	3.9	13	5.7
		Pumpkin pie:[56]											
6	465	Whole Pie	1 ea	910	59	2200	54	308	15	94	34	37	17
6	466	Piece, ⅙ of pie	1 pce	152	59	367	9	51	5	16	5.7	6.1	2.8
		Pies, fried, commercial:											
6	467	Apple	1 ea	85	43	255	2	32	2	14	5.8	6.6	.6
6	468	Cherry	1 ea	85	43	250	2	32	1	14	5.8	6.7	.6
		Pretzels, made with enriched flour:											
6	469	Thin sticks, 2¼″ long	10 ea	3	2	10	<1	2	<1	<1	t	<.1	<.1
6	470	Dutch twists, 2¾ × 2⅝″	1 ea	16	2	65	2	13	<1	1	.1	.2	.2
6	471	Thin twists, 3¼ × 2¼ × ¼″	10 ea	60	3	240	6	48	2	2	.4	.8	.6
		Rolls and buns, enriched:											
		Commercial:											
6	472	Cloverleaf rolls, 2½″ diam, 2″ high	1 ea	28	32	85	2	14	1	2	.5	.8	.6
6	473	Hotdog buns	1 ea	40	34	115	3	20	1	2	.5	.8	.6
6	474	Hamburger buns	1 ea	45	34	129	4	23	1	2	.6	.9	.7
6	475	Hard rolls, white, 3¾″ diam, 2″ high	1 ea	50	25	155	5	30	1	2	.4	.5	.6
6	476	Submarine rolls or hoagies, 11½ × 3 × 2½	1 ea	135	31	400	11	72	2	8	1.8	3	2.2
		From home recipe:											
6	477	Dinner rolls 2½″ diam, 2″ high	1 ea	35	26	120	3	20	1	3	.8	1.2	.9
6	478	Toaster pastries, fortified	1 ea	54	13	210	2	38	1	6	1.7	3.6	.4

[56] Recipes updated for latest USDA values for fruits/nuts/fruit juice.

[57] Recipe based on pie crust, cooked vanilla pudding, 2 bananas.

[58] Based on value for pie crust, cooked chocolate pudding with meringue.

Chol (mg)	Calc (mg)	Iron (mg)	Magn (mg)	Phos (mg)	Pota (mg)	Sodi (mg)	Zinc (mg)	VT-A (RE)	Thia (mg)	Ribo (mg)	Niac (mg)	V-B6 (mg)	Fola (µg)	VT-C (mg)
90	880	6.54	186	809	2000	2532	4.17	222	.94	1.75	7.40	1.77	116	26
15	147	1.09	31	135	333	422	.69	37	.16	.29	1.23	.30	19	4
0	155	12.3	60	274	756	2533	1.68	85	1.04	.85	10.4	.43	84	36
0	26	2.1	10	46	126	423	.28	14	.17	.14	1.73	.07	14	6
0	220	19	91	350	920	2873	1.87	416	1.13	.85	9.50	.50	93	5
0	37	3.17	15	58	153	480	.31	70	.19	.14	1.58	.08	16	1
90	958	6.46	176	881	1332	2565	4.46	204	.91	1.80	6.38	.54	66	3
15	160	1.08	29	147	222	427	.74	34	.15	.30	1.06	.09	11	<1
888	742	8.64	110	880	1040	2000	4.75	573	.82	1.60	5.50	.51	91	1
148	124	1.44	18	147	173	333	.79	96	.14	.27	.92	.08	15	4
822	150	8.4	54	412	420	2369	3.06	395	.59	.84	.50	.30	78	25
137	25	1.4	9	69	70	395	.51	66	.10	.14	.83	.05	13	4
0	160	11.3	98	332	1408	2533	2.11	690	1.04	.93	13.9	.39	72	28
0	27	1.90	16	55	235	423	.35	115	.18	.16	2.30	.07	12	5
822	210	12.0	192	777	781	1823	8.8	248	1.63	.99	6.6	.51	110	0
137	35	1.85	32	130	130	304	1.47	41	.22	.17	1.1	.08	18	0
655	1273	15.8	240	1269	2400	2029	5.96	11170[59]	.82	1.76	7.3	.64	120	6
109	212	2.63	40	211	400	338	.99	1861[59]	.14	.29	1.22	.11	20	1
14	12	.94	6	34	42	326	.14	3	.09	.06	1.0	.03	4	1
13	11	.70	7	41	61	371	.15	19	.06	.06	.60	.04	8	1
0	1	.06	1	3	3	48	.03	0	.01	.01	.13	<.01	<1	0
0	4	.32	4	15	16	258	.17	0	.05	.04	.70	<.01	3	0
0	16	1.2	15	55	61	966	.42	0	.19	.15	2.6	.01	10	0
t	33	.81	6	44	36	155	.22	t	.14	.09	1.10	.01	11	<1
0	54	1.19	8	44	56	241	.36	t	.20	.13	1.58	.01	15	<1
0	61	1.34	9	50	63	271	.41	t	.22	.15	1.78	.02	17	<1
0	24	1.40	14	46	49	313	.44	0	.20	.12	1.70	.02	17	0
0	100	3.80	31	115	128	683	1.17	0	.54	.33	4.50	.09	49	0
12	16	1.10	10	36	41	98	.32	8	.12	.12	1.20	.01	12	0
0	104	2.16	10	104	91	248	.31	150[60]	.17	.18	2.27	.2	43	4

[59]Latest USDA values of Vitamin A for canned pumpkin are almost 3.5 times greater than previously published values. Canned pumpkin is usually a blend of pumpkin and winter squash.

[60]Vitamin A values from label declaration varies from 100 to 150 RE for major brands.

(For purposes of calculations, use "0" for t, <1, <.1, <.01, etc.)

Table C–1 Food Composition

Grp	Ref	Food Description	Measure	Wt (g)	H₂O (%)	Ener (kcal)	Prot (g)	Carb (g)	Dietary Fiber (g)	Fat (g)	Fat Breakdown (g)		
											Sat	Mono	Poly
BAKED GOODS—Con.													
		Tortilla Chips:											
6	1271	Plain	1 oz	28	4	139	2	17	1	8	1.1	3.1	3.1
6	1036	Nacho flavor	1 oz	28	1	139	2	18	1	7	1.4	2.5	2.8
6	1037	Taco flavor	1 oz	28	1	140	3	18	1	7	1.4	2.5	2.7
		Tortillas:											
6	479	Corn, enriched, 6″ diam	1 ea	30	45	65	2	13	2	1	.1	.3	.6
6	480	Flour, 8″ diam	1 ea	35	27	105	3	19	1	3	.4	1.2	1.0
6	1301	Flour tortilla 10.5 in	1 ea	57	27	168	4	31	2	4	.6	1.9	1.6
6	481	Taco shells	1 ea	14	4	59	1	9	1	2	.2	.6	1.2
		Waffles, 7″ diam:											
6	482	From home recipe	1 ea	75	37	245	7	26	1	13	4	4.9	2.6
6	483	From mix, egg/milk added	1 ea	75	42	205	7	27	1	8	2.7	2.9	1.5
GRAIN PRODUCTS: CEREAL, FLOUR, GRAIN, PASTA and NOODLES, POPCORN													
		Barley, pearled:											
7	484	Dry, uncooked	1 c	200	11	700	16	158	31	2	.4	.3	1.1
7	485	Cooked	1 c	200	72	196	5	44	4	1	.1	.1	.3
		Breakfast cereals, hot, cooked:											
		Corn grits (hominy) cooked:											
7	486	Yellow, enriched, regular and quick prepared	1 c	242	85	146	4	31	5	<1	t	.1	.3
7	487	White, instant, prepared from packet	1 ea	137	85	80	2	18	3	<1	t	.1	.1
		Cream of Wheat®, cooked:											
7	488	Regular, quick, instant	1 c	244	86	140	4	29	3	1	.1	.1	.2
7	489	Mix and eat, plain, packet	1 ea	142	82	100	3	21	2	<1	<.1	<.1	.1
7	490	Malt-O-Meal® cereal, cooked	1 c	240	88	122	4	26	3	<1	<.1	<.1	.1
		Oatmeal or rolled oats, cooked:											
7	491	Regular, quick, instant, nonfortified	1 c	234	85	145	6	25	4	2	.4	.8	1
		Instant, fortified:											
7	492	Plain, from packet	¾ c	177	86	104	4	18	3	2	.3	.6	.7
7	493	Flavored, from packet	¾ c	164	76	160	5	31	3	2	.3	.7	.8
7	494	Whole-wheat cereal, cooked	1 c	242	84	150	5	33	4	1	.1	.1	.3
		Breakfast cereals, ready to eat:											
7	495	All-Bran®	⅓ c	28	3	70	4	21	9	<1	.1	.1	.3
7	1306	Alpha Bits®	1 c	28	1	111	2	25	1	1	.1	.2	.3
7	1307	Apple Jacks®	1 c	28	2	110	2	26	<1	<1	<.1	<.1	<.1
7	1308	Bran Buds®	1 c	84	3	217	12	64	23	2	.4	.3	1.1
7	1305	Bran Chex®	1 c	49	2	156	5	39	9	1	.2	.2	.8
7	1309	Buc Wheats®	.75 c	28	3	110	2	24	2	1	.1	.1	.5
7	1310	C.W. Post® plain	1 c	97	2	432	9	69	2	15	11.3	1.7	1.4
7	1311	C.W. Post® with raisins	1 c	103	4	446	9	74	2	15	11.0	1.7	1.4
7	496	Cap'n Crunch®	1 c	37	2	156	2	30	1	3	2.2	.4	.5
7	1312	Cap'n Crunchberries®	1 c	35	3	146	2	29	<1	3	1.9	.4	.5
7	1313	Cap'n Crunch®, peanut butter	1 c	35	2	154	3	27	<1	5	1.9	1.4	1.0
7	497	Cheerios®	1 c	23	5	89	3	16	2	1	.3	.5	.6
7	1314	Cocoa Krispies®	1 c	36	3	139	2	32	<1	<1	.2	.2	.2

GRP KEY: 1 = BEV 2 = DAIRY 3 = EGGS 4 = FAT/OIL 5 = FRUIT 6 = BAKERY 7 = GRAIN 8 = FISH 9 = BEEF 10 = POULTRY 11 = SAUSAGE
12 = MIXED/FAST 13 = NUTS/SEEDS 14 = SWEETS 15 = VEG/LEG 16 = MISC 22 = SOUP/SAUCE

Chol (mg)	Calc (mg)	Iron (mg)	Magn (mg)	Phos (mg)	Pota (mg)	Sodi (mg)	Zinc (mg)	VT-A (RE)	Thia (mg)	Ribo (mg)	Niac (mg)	V-B6 (mg)	Fola (µg)	VT-C (mg)
0	82	1.00	22	74	30	140	.42	1	.01	.02	.20	.08	<1	<1
0	17	.40	13	98	109	107	.42	13	.04	.03	.40	.10	—	0
0	45	.70	27	91	72	191	.42	15	.08	.09	.80	.10	—	0
0	42	.60	19	55	43	1	.36	8	.05	.03	.40	.09	6	0
0	21	.55	12	59	35	134	.27	0	.13	.08	1.20	.01	16	0
0	34	.88	19	94	56	215	.43	0	.21	.13	1.93	.02	25	0
0	26	.26	9	33	25	62	.22	1	<.01	.01	.25	.02	2	0
102	154	1.50	17	135	129	445	.65	39	.18	.24	1.50	.03	13	t
59	179	1.20	14	257	146	515	.52	49	.14	.23	.90	.03	4	t
0	32	4.2	51	378	320	6	4.47	0	.24	.1	7.9	.45	40	0
0	6	1.17	12	112	72	2	1.15	0	.05	.02	1.7	.09	10	0
0	1	1.55[61]	11	29	54	0[62]	.18	15[63]	.24[61]	.15[61]	1.96[61]	.06	2	0
0	7	1[61]	5	16	29	343	.08	0	.18[61]	.08[61]	1.3[61]	.03	1	0
0	54[64]	10.9[64]	12	43[65]	46	5[65 66]	.35	0	.24[64]	.07[64]	1.5[64]	.02	9	0
0	20[64]	8.10[64]	7	20[64]	38	241	.20	376[64]	.43[64]	.28[64]	5[64]	.01	5	0
0	5	9.6[64]	14	24[64]	31	2[66]	.17	0	.48[64]	.24[64]	5.8[64]	.02	5	0
0	20	1.59	56	178	132	1[66]	1.15	4	.26	.05	.3	.05	10	0
0	163[61]	6.32[61]	51	133	99	285[61]	1	453[61]	.53[61]	.29[61]	5.49[61]	.74	150	0
0	168[61]	6.7[61]	51	148	137	254[61]	1	460[61]	.53[61]	.38[61]	5.9[61]	.77	150	<1
0	17	1.5	53	168	171	3	1.16	0	.17	.12	2.13	.07	25	0
0	23	4.5[61]	106	264	350	320	3.7	375[61]	.37[61]	.43[61]	5[61]	.5	100	15[61]
0	8	1.80	17	51	100	219	1.50	375	.40	.40	5.00	.50	100	—
0	3	4.50	6	30	23	125	3.70	375	.40	.40	5.00	.50	100	15
0	56	13.4	267	729	1404	516	11.1	1112	1.10	1.30	14.8	1.50	297	45
0	29	7.80	126	327	394	455	2.14	11	.60	.26	8.60	.90	173	26
0	60	8.10	24	60	—	235	.30	682	.68	.77	9.00	.90	—	27
0	47	15.4	67	224	198	167	1.64	1284	1.30	1.50	17.1	1.70	342	—
0	51	16.4	74	232	260	160	1.64	1364	1.30	1.50	18.1	1.90	364	—
0	6	9.83[64]	15	47	48	278	4.01	5[61]	.66[64]	.71[64]	8.64[64]	1	238	0
0	11	9.04	14	47	49	243	3.56	0	.59	.67	8.14	.93	128	—
0	7	9.10	19	49	57	268	3.79	0	.60	.70	8.97	1.04	244	—
0	38	3.6[61]	31	109	82	246	.63	304[61]	.32[61]	.32[61]	4[61]	.4	5	12[61]
0	6	2.30	12	47	53	275	1.90	477	.50	.50	6.30	.60	127	19

[61]Nutrient added.

[62]Cooked without salt. If salt is added according to label recommendation, sodium content is 540 mg.

[63]Value for yellow corn grits; cooked white corn grits contain 0 RE of Vitamin A.

[64]Nutrient added–value based on label declaration.

[65]For regular and instant cereal. For quick cereal, phosphorus is 102 mg, and sodium is 142 mg.

[66]Cooked without salt. If added according to label recommendations, sodium content is 390 mg for Cream of Wheat; 324 mg for Malt-O-Meal; 374 mg for oatmeal.

(For purposes of calculations, use "0" for t, <1, <.1, <.01, etc.)

Table C–1 Food Composition

Grp	Ref	Food Description	Measure	Wt (g)	H₂O (%)	Ener (kcal)	Prot (g)	Carb (g)	Dietary Fiber (g)	Fat (g)	Sat	Mono	Poly
											Fat Breakdown (g)		

Grp	Ref	Food Description	Measure	Wt (g)	H₂O (%)	Ener (kcal)	Prot (g)	Carb (g)	Dietary Fiber (g)	Fat (g)	Sat	Mono	Poly
		GRAIN PRODUCTS—Con.											
		Breakfast cereals—con.											
7	1316	Cocoa Pebbles®	.67 c	21	2	87	1	18	<1	1	<.1	<.1	<.1
7	1315	Corn Bran®	1 c	36	3	124	3	30	7	1	.2	.3	.7
7	1317	Corn Chex®	1 c	28	2	111	2	25	<1	<1	.1	.3	.6
7	498	Corn Flakes, Kellogg's®	1¼ c	28	3	110	2	24	1	<1	t	t	.1
7	499	Corn Flakes, Post Toasties®	1¼ c	28	3	110	2	24	1	<1	t	t	.1
7	1318	Cracklin' Oat Bran®	1 c	60	4	229	6	41	9	9	2.1	2.3	3.5
7	1038	Crispy Wheat 'N Raisins®	1 c	43	7	150	3	35	2	1	.1	.1	.4
7	1319	Fortified Oat flakes	1 c	48	3	177	9	35	1	1	.1	.3	.3
7	500	40% Bran Flakes, Kellogg's®	1 c	39	3	125	5	31	5	1	.14	.14	.4
7	501	40% Bran Flakes, Post®	1 c	47	3	152	5	37	6	1	.2	.2	.3
7	502	Froot Loops®	1 c	28	2	111	2	25	<1	1	.2	.1	.1
7	1320	Frosted Mini-Wheats®	4 ea	31	5	111	3	26	2	<1	.1	<.1	.2
7	1321	Frosted Rice Krispies®	1 c	28	3	109	1	26	1	<1	<.1	<.1	<.1
7	1323	Fruit & Fiber® w/apples	.5 c	28	2	90	3	22	4	1	.2	.2	.6
7	1324	Fruit & Fiber® w/dates	.5 c	28	2	90	3	21	4	1	.2	.2	.6
7	1325	Fruitful Bran cereal	.75 c	34	3	110	3	27	5	0	0	0	0
7	1322	Fruity Pebbles® cereal	.875 c	28	3	115	1	24	<1	2	.5	.4	.6
7	503	Golden Grahams®	1 c	39	2	150	2	33	2	2	1.0	.1	.2
7	504	Granola, homemade	1 c	122	3	595	15	67	13	33	5.8	9.4	17
7	505	Grape Nuts®	½ c	57	3	202	7	47	4	<1	t	t	.2
7	1326	Grape Nuts® flakes	.875 c	28	3	102	3	23	2	<1	<.1	<.1	.1
7	1327	Honey & Nut Corn flakes	.75 c	28	4	113	2	23	<1	2	.2	.5	.7
7	506	Honey Nut Cheerios®	1 c	33	3	125	4	27	1	1	.1	.3	.3
7	1328	Honey Bran	1 c	35	3	119	3	29	4	1	.1	.1	.4
7	1329	Honeycomb®	1 c	22	1	86	1	20	<1	<1	.1	.1	.2
7	1330	King Vitamin® cereal	1 c	21	2	85	1	18	<1	1	.7	.2	.2
7	1039	Kix®	1 c	19	3	73	2	16	<1	<1	.1	.1	.2
7	1331	Life®	1 c	44	5	162	8	32	1	1	.1	.2	.4
7	507	Lucky Charms®	1 c	32	3	125	3	26	1	1	.2	.4	.5
7	508	Nature Valley® Granola	1 c	113	4	503	12	76	12	20	13	2.8	2.8
7	1332	Nutri-Grain™—Barley	1 c	41	3	153	5	34	2	<1	<.1	<.1	.1
7	1333	Nutri-Grain—Corn	1 c	42	3	160	3	36	3	1	.1	.3	.6
7	1334	Nutri-Grain—Rye	1 c	40	3	144	4	34	3	<1	.1	.1	.1
7	1335	Nutri-Grain—Wheat	1 c	44	3	158	4	37	3	<1	.1	.1	.3
7	1336	100% Bran	1 c	66	3	178	8	48	20	3	.6	.6	1.9
7	509	100% Natural® cereal, plain	¼ c	28	2	135	3	18	3	6	4.1	1.2	.5
7	1337	100% Natural with apples	1 c	104	2	478	11	70	5	20	15.5	1.8	1.3
7	1338	100% Natural with raisins & dates	1 c	100	4	496	11	72	4	20	13.7	3.7	1.7
7	510	Product 19®	1 c	33	3	126	3	27	<1	<1	t	t	.1
7	1339	Quisp®	1 c	30	2	124	2	25	<1	2	1.5	.3	.3
7	511	Raisin Bran, Kellogg's®	1 c	49	8	160	4	40	6	1	.2	.1	.4
7	512	Raisin Bran, Post®	1 c	56	9	174	5	43	6	1	.2	.2	.4
7	1040	Raisins, Rice & Rye™	1 c	46	9	155	3	39	<1	<1	<.1	<.1	<.1
7	1041	Rice Chex®	.75 c	19	3	75	1	17	1	1	.2	.2	.3
7	513	Rice Krispies, Kellogg's®	1 c	29	2	112	2	25	<1	<1	t	t	.1
7	514	Rice, Puffed	1 c	14	3	55	1	13	<1	<1	t	t	<.1
7	515	Shredded Wheat®	¾ c	32	5	115	3	25	4	1	.1	.1	.3

Chol (mg)	Calc (mg)	Iron (mg)	Magn (mg)	Phos (mg)	Pota (mg)	Sodi (mg)	Zinc (mg)	VT-A (RE)	Thia (mg)	Ribo (mg)	Niac (mg)	V-B6 (mg)	Fola (μg)	VT-C (mg)
0	4	1.30	9	16	35	102	1.10	282	.30	.30	3.70	.40	75	—
0	41	12.2	18	52	70	310	4.00	—	.38	.70	10.9	.86	232	—
0	3	1.80	4	11	23	271	.10	14	.40	.07	5.00	.50	100	15
0	1	1.8[61]	3	18	26	351	.06	375[61]	.37[61]	.43[61]	5[61]	.51	100	15[61]
0	1	.7[61]	3	12	33	297	.06	375[61]	.37[61]	.43[61]	5[61]	.51	100	0
0	40	3.80	116	241	355	402	3.20	794	.80	.90	10.6	1.10	212	32
0	71	6.80	35	117	174	204	.51	569	.60	.60	7.60	.80	40	—
0	68	13.7	58	176	343	429	1.50	636	.60	.70	.39	.90	169	—
0	19	11.2[61]	71	192	248	363	5.15	522[61]	.51[61]	.59[61]	6.86[61]	.7	138	0
0	21	7.47[61]	102	296	251	431	2.5	629[61]	.62[61]	.72[61]	8.3[61]	.85	166	0
0	3	4.5[61]	7	24	26	145	3.7	375[61]	.4[61]	.4[61]	5[61]	.5	100	15[61]
0	10	2.00	26	81	106	9	1.60	410	.40	.50	5.50	.60	109	16
0	1	1.80	5	27	21	240	.31	375	.40	.40	5.00	.50	100	15
0	10	4.50	60	150	—	195	1.50	375	.38	.43	5.00	.50	100	—
0	10	4.50	60	100	—	170	1.50	378	.38	.43	5.00	.50	100	—
0	10	8.10	60	150	150	240	3.75	378	.38	.43	5.00	.50	100	—
0	3	1.80	8	17	21	157	1.50	375	.40	.40	5.00	.50	100	—
0	24	6.2[61]	16	56	86	476	.34	516[61]	.5[61]	.6[61]	6.9[61]	.7	—	21[61]
0	76	4.84	141	494	612	12	4.47	4	.73	.31	2.14	.43	99	1
0	22	2.46	38	142	190	394	1.24	753[61]	.8[61]	.8[61]	10[61]	1	200	0
0	11	4.50	31	84	99	218	.57	375	.40	.40	5.00	.50	100	—
0	3	1.80	6	13	36	225	.11	375	.40	.40	5.00	.50	100	15
0	23	5.2[61]	39	122	115	299	.87	437[61]	.4[61]	.5[61]	5.8[61]	.6	4	17[61]
0	16	5.60	46	132	151	202	.90	463	.50	.50	6.20	.60	23	19
0	4	1.40	8	22	70	166	1.20	291	.30	.30	3.90	.40	78	—
0	—	12.7	7	—	26	161	.16	717	.09	1.06	12.9	1.18	286	33
0	23	5.40	8	26	29	226	.17	250	.27	.27	3.33	.33	2	10
0	154	11.6	55	238	197	229	1.55	0	.95	1.00	11.6	.05	37	—
0	36	5.1[61]	27	88	66	227	.56	424[61]	.4[61]	.5[61]	5.6[61]	.6	—	17[61]
0	71	3.78	116	354	389	232	2.19	8	.39	.19	.83	.32	85	0
0	11	1.45	32	126	108	277	5.40	540	.50	.60	7.20	.70	145	22
0	1	.89	27	120	98	276	5.50	556	.50	.60	7.40	.75	148	22
0	8	1.13	31	104	72	272	5.30	530	.50	.60	7.00	.70	141	21
0	12	1.24	34	164	120	299	5.80	583	.60	.70	7.70	.80	155	23
0	46	8.12	312	801	824	457	5.74	0	1.60	1.80	20.9	2.10	200	63
0	49	.83	34	104	138	12	.63	2	.09	.15	.6	.64	8	0
0	157	2.89	71	350	513	52	2.00	8	.33	.58	1.88	.11	17	—
0	160	3.12	124	347	538	47	2.11	8	.30	.64	2.08	.17	45	—
0	4	21[61]	12	47	51	378	.5	1769[61]	1.7[61]	2[61]	23.3[61]	2.3	466	70[61]
0	9	6.31	12	25	45	241	.18	—	.54	.76	5.80	.91	8	—
0	25	24[61]	73	200	307	293	5.0	500[61]	.51[61]	.57[61]	6.67[61]	.67	133	0
0	27	9.01[61]	96	237	349	370	3.01	750[61]	.74[61]	.85[61]	10[61]	1.02	200	0
0	10	5.60	20	50	144	350	4.70	467	.50	.60	6.30	.60	125	0
0	3	1.20	5	19	22	158	.26	1	.27	.20	3.34	.33	67	10
0	4	1.8[61]	10	34	30	340	.48	388[61]	.4[61]	.4[61]	5[61]	.5	100	15[61]
0	1	.15[61]	4	14	16	<1	.14	0	.02[61]	.01[61]	.42[61]	.01	3	0
0	12	1.35	42	112	115	3	1.05	0	.08	.09	1.67	.08	16	0

[61] Nutrient added.

(For purposes of calculations, use "0" for t, <1, <.1, <.01, etc.)

Table C–1   Food Composition

Grp	Ref	Food Description	Measure	Wt (g)	H₂O (%)	Ener (kcal)	Prot (g)	Carb (g)	Dietary Fiber (g)	Fat (g)	Fat Breakdown (g)		
											Sat	Mono	Poly
GRAIN PRODUCTS—Con.													
		Breakfast cereals—con.											
7	516	Special K®	1½ c	32	2	125	6	24	<1	<1	t	t	t
7	1340	Sugar Corn Pops	1 c	28	3	108	1	26	<1	<1	t	<.1	.1
7	518	Sugar Frosted Flakes®	1 c	35	3	133	2	32	1	<1	t	t	t
7	517	Super Sugar Crisp®	1 c	33	2	123	2	30	<1	<1	t	t	.1
7	519	Sugar Smacks®	¾ c	28	3	106	2	25	<1	<1	.1	.1	.2
7	1341	Tasteeos®	1 c	24	2	94	3	19	1	1	.2	.2	.3
7	1342	Team®	1 c	42	4	164	3	36	<1	1	.2	.2	.3
7	520	Total®, wheat, with added calcium	1 c	33	4	122	3	26	2	1	.1	.1	.4
7	521	Trix®	1 c	28	2	108	2	25	<1	<1	.2	.1	.1
7	1042	Wheat & Raisin Chex®	1 c	54	7	185	5	43	4	<1	.1	.1	.2
7	1344	Wheat Chex®	1 c	46	3	169	5	38	3	1	.2	.2	.6
7	1043	Wheat, Puffed	1 c	12	3	44	2	10	2	<1	t	t	.1
7	522	Wheaties®	1 c	29	5	101	3	23	3	1	.1	.1	.2
		Buckwheat:											
		Flour:											
7	523	Dark	1 c	98	12	338	12	71	8	3	.5	.8	.9
7	524	Light	1 c	98	12	340	6	78	6	1	.2	.4	.4
7	525	Whole grain, dry	1 c	175	11	586	23	128	16	4	.8	1.4	1.5
		Bulgar:											
7	526	Dry, uncooked	1 c	170	10	600	19	129	16	3	1.2	.3	1.2
7	527	Cooked	1 c	135	56	246	10	44	11	1	.4	.1	.4
		Cornmeal:											
7	528	Whole-ground, unbolted, dry	1 c	122	12	435	11	90	13	5	.5	1.1	2.5
7	529	Bolted, nearly whole, dry	1 c	122	12	440	11	91	12	4	.5	1.1	2.5
7	530	Degermed, enriched, dry	1 c	138	12	502	11	108	10	2	.2	.4	.9
7	531	Degermed, enriched, cooked	1 c	240	88	120	3	26	3	<1	.1	.1	.3
		Macaroni, cooked:											
7	532	Firm stage, hot	1 c	130	64	190	7	39	2	1	.1	.1	.3
7	533	Tender stage, cold	1 c	105	72	115	4	24	1	<1	.1	.1	.2
7	534	Tender stage, hot	1 c	140	72	155	5	32	2	1	.1	.1	.2
7	535	Millet, cooked	½ c	95	86	54	1	11	1	<1	.1	.1	.2
		Noodles:											
7	536	Egg noodles, cooked	1 c	160	70	200	7	37	4	2	.5	.6	.6
7	537	Chow mein, dry	1 c	45	11	220	6	26	2	11	2.1	7.3	.4
7	538	Spinach noodles, dry	3½ oz	100	10	380	14	71	7	4	1.0	1.1	1.1
7	1343	Oat bran	¼ c	25	6	58	5	17	4	1	.2	.4	.4
		Popcorn:											
7	539	Air popped, plain	1 c	8	4	30	1	6	1	<1	t	.1	.2
7	540	Popped in veg oil/salted	1 c	11	3	55	1	6	1	3	.5	1.4	1.2
7	541	Sugar-syrup coated	1 c	35	4	135	2	30	1	1	.1	.3	.6
		Rice:											
7	542	Brown rice, cooked	1 c	195	70	232	5	50	3	1	.3	.4	.4
		White, enriched, all types:											
7	543	Raw, dry	1 c	185	12	670	12	149	2	1	.2	.2	.3
7	544	Cooked without salt	1 c	205	73	223	4	50	1	<1	.1	.1	.1
7	545	Instant, prepared without salt	1 c	165	73	180	4	40	1	<1	.1	.1	.1

Chol (mg)	Calc (mg)	Iron (mg)	Magn (mg)	Phos (mg)	Pota (mg)	Sodi (mg)	Zinc (mg)	VT-A (RE)	Thia (mg)	Ribo (mg)	Niac (mg)	V-B6 (mg)	Fola (µg)	VT-C (mg)
0	9	5.06[61]	18	62	55	298	4.16	429[61]	.45[61]	.45[61]	5.63[61]	.56	112	17[61]
0	1	1.80	2	28	17	103	1.50	375	.40	.40	5.00	.50	100	15
0	1	2.2[61]	3	26	22	284	.05	463[61]	.5[61]	.5[61]	6.2[61]	.6	124	19[61]
0	7	2.1[61]	20	60	123	29	1.7	437[61]	.4[61]	.5[61]	5.8[61]	.6	116	0
0	3	1.8[61]	13	31	42	75	.28	375[61]	.37[61]	.43[61]	5[61]	.5	100	15[61]
0	11	3.80	26	96	71	183	.69	318	.30	.40	4.20	.40	9	13
0	6	2.57	19	65	71	259	.58	556	.55	.63	7.40	.80	—	22
0	200	21[61]	34	137	123	330	.15	1769[61]	1.7[61]	2[61]	23.3[61]	2.3	466	70[61]
0	6	4.5[61]	6	19	26	179	.13	375[61]	.4[61]	.4[61]	4.9[61]	.5	—	15[61]
0	—	7.70	53	163	174	306	1.19	<1	.50	.60	7.10	.70	143	2
0	18	7.30	58	182	174	308	1.23	0	.60	.17	8.10	.80	162	24
0	3	.57	17	43	42	0	.30	0	.02	.03	1.30	.02	4	0
0	44	4.6[61]	32	100	108	363	.65	388[61]	.4[61]	.4[61]	5.1[61]	.5	9	15[61]
0	32	2.5	135	298	490	1	2.65	0	.58	.16	2.75	.41	125	0
0	11	1	47	86	314	1	2.56	0	.09	.05	.47	.09	100	0
0	200	6.7	335	560	740	3	4.4	0	1.05	.26	7.7	.37	53	0
0	49	9.5	130	575	389	7	3.2	0	.48	.24	7.7	.38	80	0
0	27	2.87	57	263	151	3	2.81	0	.08	.05	4.1	.07	18	0
0	24	2.2	130	312	346	1	2.15	62	.46	.13	2.4	.57	33	0
0	21	2.2	129	272	303	1	2.15	62	.37	.1	2.3	.56	29	0
0	8	5.93	65	137	166	1	1.15	61	.61	.36	4.8	.35	29	0
0	2	1.48	17	34	38	1	.23	14	.14	.1	1.2	.06	6	0
0	14	1.69	40	85	74	1	.85	0	.23	.13	1.82	.1	4	0
0	11	1.36	32	53	60	1	.68	0	.15	.08	1.13	.07	3	0
0	15	1.82	43	90	80	2	.91	0	.2	.11	1.5	.09	4	0
0	3	1.1	38	47	64	1	.42	0	.1	.06	.4	.03	10	0
50	18	2.26	30	94	60	4	1.02	34	.22	.13	1.9	.01	7	0
5	14	.4	—	41	33	450	.1	0	.05	.03	.6	.03	10	0
0	41	4.54	38	154	460	35	2.2	18	.98	.47	6.89	.27	73	0
0	13	1.23	58	94	137	6	.66	0	.15	.03	.23	.05	10	—
0	1	.2	23	22	20	<1	.22	1	.03	.01	.2	.02	3	0
0	3	.27	25	31	19	86	.28	2	.01	.02	.1	.02	3	0
0	2	.5	29	47	90	<1	.29	3	.13	.02	.4	.03	3	0
0	23	1.17	72	142	137	0	1.05	0	.18	.04	2.73	.29	10	0
0	44	5.4	63	174	170	9	2.41	0	.81	.06	6.48	.3	19	0
0	21	2.87	23	57	57	0	.84	0	.22	.02	2.05	.1	4	0
0	5	1.32	17	31	0	0[67]	.64	0	.22	.02	1.65	.02	7	0

[61] Nutrient added.

[67] If prepared with salt according to label recommendation, sodium would be 608 mg.

(For purposes of calculations, use "0" for t, <1, <.1, <.01, etc.)

Table C–1   Food Composition

Grp	Ref	Food Description	Measure	Wt (g)	H$_2$O (%)	Ener (kcal)	Prot (g)	Carb (g)	Dietary Fiber (g)	Fat (g)	Fat Breakdown (g) Sat	Mono	Poly
GRAIN PRODUCTS—Con.													
		Rice—con.											
		White, parboiled/converted rice:											
7	546	Raw, dry	1 c	185	10	683	14	150	4	1	.2	.2	.4
7	547	Cooked, hot	1 c	175	73	186	4	41	1	<1	t	t	<.1
7	548	Wild rice, cooked	½ c	100	76	92	4	19	3	<1	.1	<.1	.1
7	549	Rye flour, medium	1 c	115	11	392	13	85	17	2	.4	.5	.9
7	1044	Soy flour, low fat	1 c	88	3	370	51	34	12	6	.9	1.3	3.3
		Spaghetti, cooked:											
7	550	Firm stage, hot	1 c	130	64	190	7	39	2	1	.1	.1	.3
7	551	Tender stage, hot	1 c	140	72	155	5	32	2	1	.1	.1	.2
7	552	Whole-wheat spaghetti, cooked	1 c	123	67	151	7	33	5	<1	.1	.1	.2
7	1302	Tapioca, dry	1 c	152	13	535	1	131	2	<1	.1	.1	.1
7	553	Wheat bran	½ c	18	12	38	3	11	8	1	.1	.1	.4
		Wheat germ:											
7	554	Raw	1 c	75	12	272	20	35	12	8	1.4	1.2	4.9
7	555	Toasted	1 c	113	4	431	33	56	16	12	2.1	1.8	7.3
7	556	Rolled wheat, cooked	1 c	240	80	142	4	32	5	1	.1	.1	.3
7	557	Whole-grain wheat, cooked	⅓ c	50	86	28	1	6	1	<1	<.1	<.1	.1
		Wheat flour (unbleached):											
		All-purpose white flour, enriched:											
7	558	Sifted	1 c	115	12	419	12	88	3	1	.2	.1	.5
7	559	Unsifted	1 c	125	12	455	13	95	3	1	.2	.1	.6
7	560	Cake or pastry flour, enriched, sifted	1 c	96	12	349	7	76	3	1	.2	.1	.4
7	561	Self-rising, enriched, unsifted	1 c	125	12	440	12	93	3	1	.2	.1	.6
7	562	Whole wheat, from hard wheats	1 c	120	12	400	16	85	15	2	.3	.3	1.1
MEATS: FISH and SHELLFISH													
8	1045	Bass, baked or broiled	3.5 oz.	100	70	125	24	0	0	4	.9	1.6	1.2
		Bluefish:											
8	1046	Baked or broiled	3.5 oz.	100	68	159	26	0	0	5	1.1	2.1	1.3
8	1047	Fried in bread crumbs	3.5 oz.	100	61	205	23	5	0	10	2.1	4.3	2.5
		Clams:											
8	563	Raw meat only	3 oz	85	82	63	11	2	<1	1	.1	.1	.2
8	564	Canned, drained	3 oz	85	64	126	22	4	t	2	.2	.2	.5
8	1290	Steamed, meat only	20 ea	90	64	133	23	5	<1	2	.2	.2	.5
		Cod:											
8	565	Baked with butter	3½ oz	100	75	132	23	0	0	3	.4	.3	.5
8	566	Batter fried	3½ oz	100	61	199	20	8	0	10	3.9	5.5	.9
8	567	Poached, no added fat	3½ oz	100	76	102	22	0	0	1	.2	.1	.3
		Crab, meat only:											
8	1048	Blue crab, cooked	1 c	135	77	138	27	0	0	2	.3	.4	.9
8	1049	Dungeness Crab, cooked	.75 c	101	74	85	18	<1	0	2	.3	.6	1.1
8	568	Canned	1 c	135	76	133	28	0	0	2	.3	.3	.6
8	569	Fish sticks, breaded pollock	2 ea	57	46	155	9	14	<1	7	1.8	2.9	1.8
		Flounder/sole, baked with lemon juice:											
8	570	With butter	3 oz	85	73	120	16	<1	0	6	3.2	1.5	.5
8	571	With margarine	3 oz	85	73	120	16	<1	0	6	1.2	2.3	1.9
8	572	Without added fat	3 oz	85	78	99	21	0	0	1	.3	.3	.4
		Haddock:											
8	573	Breaded/fried[68]	3 oz	85	61	175	17	7	<1	9	2.4	3.9	2.4
8	1050	Smoked	3.5 oz	100	72	116	25	0	0	1	.2	.2	.3

[68]Dipped in egg, milk and bread crumbs; fried in vegetable shortening.

GRP KEY: 1 = BEV 2 = DAIRY 3 = EGGS 4 = FAT/OIL 5 = FRUIT 6 = BAKERY 7 = GRAIN 8 = FISH 9 = BEEF 10 = POULTRY
11 = SAUSAGE 12 = MIXED/FAST 13 = NUTS/SEEDS 14 = SWEETS 15 = VEG/LEG 16 = MISC 22 = SOUP/SAUCE

Chol (mg)	Calc (mg)	Iron (mg)	Magn (mg)	Phos (mg)	Pota (mg)	Sodi (mg)	Zinc (mg)	VT-A (RE)	Thia (mg)	Ribo (mg)	Niac (mg)	V-B6 (mg)	Fola (μg)	VT-C (mg)
0	111	5.4	34	370	278	17	2.03	0	.81	.07	6.5	.49	23	0
0	33	1.4	11	100	75	9	.56	0	.19	.02	2.1	.18	7	0
0	5	1.1	33	85	55	2	1.17	0	.11	.16	1.6	1.31	35	0
0	36	2.72	90	340	304	1	1.67	0	.36	.16	2.45	.25	91	0
0	165	5.27	202	522	2262	16	1.04	4	.33	.25	1.90	.46	361	0
0	14	2.08	39	70	89	1	1.03	0	.23	.13	1.82	.1	9	0
0	15	2	41	74	83	1	1.07	0	.2	.11	1.5	.09	8	0
0	19	1.06	68	106	200	16	1.44	0	.21	.09	1.54	.87	25	0
0	16	1.06	5	22	28	5	—	0	0	.15	0	0	13	0
0	21	1.95	91	223	205	3	2.34	0	.14	.06	4.86	.25	46	0
0	54	4.5	252	838	620	2	11	0	1.51	.51	3.15	.69	246	0
0	50	8.71	362	1294	1070	4	18.9	0	1.89	.93	6.32	1.13	474	0
0	19	1.7	58	182	202	2	1.96	0	.17	.07	2.2	.08	27	0
0	3	.3	12	30	29	1	.44	0	.04	.01	.4	.03	6	0
0	18	5.06	24	100	109	2	.76	0	.74	.46	6.08	.05	18	0
0	20	5.5	26	109	119	3	.83	0	.8	.5	6.61	.05	20	0
0	15	4.23	20	70	91	2	.63	0	.61	.38	5.08	.04	19	0
0	331	5.5	26	583	113	1349	.83	0	.8	.5	6.61	.05	20	0
0	49	5.16	168	446	444	4	2.96	0	.66	.14	5.16	.38	58	0
80	86	1.61	32	216	385	75	.70	35	.10	.03	2.40	.35	9	0
63	9	.62	42	290	477	77	1.04	127	.08	.11	7.78	.53	2	<1
60	8	.53	37	285	413	67	.90	120	.06	.08	5.50	.37	2	<1
29	39	11.9	8	144	267	47	1.16	77	.09	.18	1.5	.07	13	9
57	78	23.8	16	287	534	95	2.32	145	.01	.36	2.85	.07	4	3
60	83	25.2	17	304	565	100	2.46	154	.01	.38	3.02	.08	4	4
60	20	.49	42	140	245	224	.58	30	.09	.08	2.51	.28	10	<1
55	80	.5	36	200	370	100	.5	26	.04	.04	2.2	.24	9	<1
55	14	.49	42	138	244	78	.58	14	.09	.08	2.51	.28	11	<1
135	140	1.22	45	278	437	376	5.70	20	.14	.12	3.00	.33	20	2
64	46	.37	46	184	359	299	4.33	14	.04	.16	2.92	.33	20	2
120	137	1.13	52	351	505	450	5.42	14	.11	.11	1.85	.41	22	0
64	11	.42	14	103	149	332	.38	18	.07	.1	1.21	.03	10	0
68	16	.28	50	187	272	145	.53	54	.07	.1	1.85	.20	10	1
55	16	.28	50	187	273	151	.53	69	.07	.1	1.85	.20	10	1
58	16	.28	50	246	292	89	.53	10	.07	.1	1.85	.20	10	1
55	34	1.15	26	183	270	123	.85	20	.06	.1	2.9	.13	14	0
77	49	1.40	54	251	415	763	.50	22	.05	.05	5.07	.40	3	<1

(For purposes of calculations, use "0" for t, <1, <.1, <.01, etc.)

Table C–1 Food Composition

Grp	Ref	Food Description	Measure	Wt (g)	H₂O (%)	Ener (kcal)	Prot (g)	Carb (g)	Dietary Fiber (g)	Fat (g)	Fat Breakdown (g)		
											Sat	Mono	Poly
MEATS: FISH and SHELLFISH—Con.													
		Halibut:											
8	574	Broiled with butter and lemon juice	3 oz	85	72	140	23	0	0	6	3.3	1.6	.7
8	1051	Smoked	3.5 oz	100	49	224	21	0	0	15	2.5	4.8	6.9
8	1054	Raw	3.5 oz	100	78	110	21	0	0	2	.3	.7	.8
8	575	Herring, pickled	3 oz	85	55	223	12	8	0	15	2.0	10	1.4
8	1052	Lobster meat, cooked w/ moist heat	1 c	145	77	142	30	2	0	1	.2	.2	1
8	576	Ocean perch, breaded/fried	3 oz	85	59	185	16	7	<1	11	3	5	3
8	1056	Octopus, raw	3.5 oz.	100	80	82	15	2	0	1	.2	.2	.2
		Oysters:											
		Raw:											
8	577	Eastern	1 c	248	85	170	18	10	0	6	1.6	.6	1.8
8	578	Pacific	1 c	248	82	200	23	12	0	6	1.3	.9	2.2
		Cooked:											
8	579	Eastern, breaded, fried, medium	6 ea	88	65	173	8	10	<1	11	2.8	4.1	2.9
8	580	Western, simmered	3½ oz	100	71	135	19	7	0	2	.5	.4	.9
		Pollock, cooked:											
8	581	Baked or broiled	3 oz	85	74	96	20	0	0	1	.2	.1	.6
8	1055	Moist heat, poached	3.5 oz	100	72	128	23	0	0	1	.2	.1	.6
		Salmon:											
8	582	Canned pink, solids and liquid	3 oz	85	69	118	17	0	0	5	1.3	1.5	1.7
8	583	Broiled or baked	3 oz	85	62	183	23	0	0	9	1.6	4.5	2.1
8	584	Smoked	3 oz	85	72	99	16	0	0	4	.8	1.7	.8
8	585	Atlantic sardines, canned, drained, 2 = 24 g	3 oz	85	60	177	21	0	0	11	1.4	3.6	4.7
8	586	Scallops, breaded, cooked from frozen	6 ea	93	59	200	17	9	<1	10	2.5	4.2	2.7
		Shrimp:											
8	587	Cooked, boiled, 18 large shrimp	3½ oz	100	77	99	21	0	0	1	.3	.2	.4
8	588	Canned, drained	⅔ c	85	73	102	20	1	0	2	.3	.3	.6
8	589	Fried, 4 large = 30 g[71]	12 ea	90	53	206	19	10	<1	11	1.9	3.4	4.6
8	1057	Raw, large, about 7 g each	14 ea	100	76	106	20	1	0	2	.3	.3	.7
8	1053	Snapper, baked or broiled	3.5 oz	100	70	128	26	0	0	2	.4	.3	.6
8	1060	Squid, fried in flour[70a]	3 oz	85	65	149	15	7	<1	6	1.6	2.3	1.8
		Swordfish:											
8	1058	Baked or broiled	3.5 oz	100	76	121	20	0	0	4	1.1	1.6	.9
8	1059	Raw	3.5 oz	100	69	155	25	0	0	5	1.4	2.0	1.2
8	590	Trout, baked or broiled	3 oz	85	63	129	22	<1	0	4	.7	1.1	1.3
		Tuna, light, canned, drained solids:											
8	591	Oil pack	3 oz	85	60	169	25	0	0	7	1.3	2.5	2.5
8	592	Water pack	3 oz	85	71	111	25	0	0	<1	.1	.1	.1
8	1061	Raw	3.5 oz	100	80	108	23	0	0	1	.2	.2	.3
MEATS: BEEF, LAMB, PORK and others													
		BEEF, cooked[72]											
		Braised, simmered, pot roasted:											
		Relatively fat, like chuck blade:											
9	593	Lean and fat, piece 2½ × 2½ × ¾"	3 oz	85	43	325	22	0	0	26	11	12	1
9	594	Lean only	3 oz	85	53	230	26	0	0	13	5.3	5.8	.4

[71]Dipped in egg, bread crumbs, and flour; fried in vegetable shortening.

[70a]Recipe is 94.6% squid, 4.9% flour, and 0.6% salt.

[72]Outer layer of fat removed to about 1/2" of the lean. Deposits of fat within the cut remain.

Chol (mg)	Calc (mg)	Iron (mg)	Magn (mg)	Phos (mg)	Pota (mg)	Sodi (mg)	Zinc (mg)	VT-A (RE)	Thia (mg)	Ribo (mg)	Niac (mg)	V-B6 (mg)	Fola (µg)	VT-C (mg)
45	51	.91	91	242	490	100	.43	174	.06	.08	6.06	.34	6	<1
100	48	.84	83	222	450	480	.42	45	.05	.07	5.80	.33	5	<1
32	47	.84	83	222	450	54	.42	47	.06	.08	5.85	.34	12	<1
11	65	1.04	8	76	59	740	.45	219	.03	.12	2.8	.11	2	0
104	88	.57	51	268	510	551	4.23	38	<1	1	1.55	.112	16	t
46	92	1.2	26	191	241	138	.41	20	.10	.11	2	.22	6	0
48	53	5.30	—	186	—	—	1.68	<1	.03	.04	2.10	.36	—	<1
136	111	16.6	135	344	568	277	226[69]	223	.34	.41	3.3	.12	25	24
136	20	12.7	55	402	417	262	41.2[69]	223	.17	.58	5	.12	25	72
72	54	6.12	51	140	215	367	76.7[69]	86	.13	.18	1.45	.06	12	7
48	16	10.2	44	322	334	210	33[69]	81	.14	.46	3.82	.10	17	7
82	5	.24	31	250	329	98	.51	19	.06	.07	1.4	.06	4	t
70	60	.53	1	252	400	98	.54	9	.04	.18	3.14	.27	12	0
37	181[70]	.72	29	279	277	471	.78	14	.02	.16	5.6	.10	13	0
74	6	.47	26	234	319	56	.43	53	.18	.14	5.67	.19	14	0
20	9	.72	15	139	149	666	.26	22	.02	.09	4.01	.24	2	0
121	325[70]	2.5	33	417	337	429	1.11	57	.07	.19	4.5	.14	10	0
57	39	.76	55	219	310	431	.99	21	.04	.10	1.4	.18	11	0
195	39	3.09	34	137	182	224	1.56	18	.03	.03	2.59	.13	4	<1
147	50	2.32	35	198	179	143	1.07	15	.02	.03	2.34	.09	2	0
159	60	1.13	36	196	213	310	1.24	24	.12	.12	2.76	.09	7	0
152	52	2.41	37	205	185	148	1.11	3	.03	.03	2.55	.10	3	2
47	40	.24	37	201	522	57	.44	12	.05	.08	3.46	.27	9	<1
221	33	.86	33	213	237	260	1.5	0	.05	.39	2.21	.05	—	4
39	4	.81	27	263	288	90	1.15	36	.04	.10	9.68	.33	14	1
50	6	1.04	34	337	369	115	1.47	41	.04	.12	11.8	.38	16	1
62	73	2.07	33	272	539	29	1.18	19	.07	.19	2.3	.42	6	3
15	11	1.2	26	265	176	301	.77	20	.03	.09	10.1	.32	5	0
15	10	2.7	26	158	267	303	.77	20	.03	.10	13.2	.32	5	0
45	16	.73	38	191	329	37	.52	18	.43	.05	9.80	.90	30	—
87	11	2.52	15	162	190	53	6.66	<1	.06	.20	2.0	.21	5	0
90	11	3.13	19	200	223	60	8.73	<1	.07	.24	2.27	.25	5	0

[69] Value varies widely.

[70] If bones are discarded, calcium value is greatly reduced.

(For purposes of calculations, use "0" for t, <1, <.1, <.01, etc.)

Table C-1   Food Composition

Grp	Ref	Food Description	Measure	Wt (g)	H₂O (%)	Ener (kcal)	Prot (g)	Carb (g)	Fiber (g)	Fat (g)	Fat Breakdown (g) Sat	Mono	Poly
		MEATS: BEEF, LAMB, PORK and others—Con.											
		BEEF—Con.											
		Relatively lean, like round:											
9	595	Lean and fat, piece 4⅛ × 2¼ × ¾″	3 oz	85	54	222	25	0	0	13	5	6	1
9	596	Lean only	3 oz	85	57	189	27	0	0	8	2.9	3.8	.3
		Ground beef, broiled, patty 3 × ⅝″:											
9	597	Lean	3 oz	85	56	231	21	0	0	16	6	7	1
9	598	Regular	3 oz	85	54	246	21	0	0	18	7	8	1
		Roasts, oven cooked, no added liquid:											
		Relatively fat, rib:											
9	601	Lean and fat, piece 4⅛ × 2¼ × ½″	3 oz	85	46	324	19	0	0	27	11	12	1
9	602	Lean only	3 oz	61	58	204	23	0	0	12	5	5	.4
		Relatively lean, round:											
9	603	Lean and fat, piece 2½ × 2½ × ¾″	3 oz	85	57	213	23	0	0	13	5	6	.5
9	604	Lean only	3 oz	75	63	162	24	0	0	6	2.3	2.6	.3
		Steak, broiled, relatively lean, sirloin,											
9	605	Lean and fat, piece 2 ½ × 2½ × ¾″	3 oz	85	54	238	22	0	0	16	6.6	7.0	.6
9	606	Lean only	3 oz	72	60	172	24	0	0	8	3.0	3.2	.3
		Steak, broiled, relatively fat, T-bone:											
9	1063	Lean and fat	3 oz	85	50	276	20	0	0	21	8.7	9.1	.8
9	1064	Lean only	3 oz	85	60	182	24	0	0	9	3.5	3.5	.3
		Variety meats:											
9	1086	Brains, pan fried	3 oz	85	71	167	11	0	0	14	3.2	3.4	2.0
9	599	Heart, simmered	3 oz	85	64	140	25	<1	0	5	1.4	1.1	1.2
9	600	Liver, fried	3 oz	85	56	184	23	7	0	7	2.4	1.5	1.5
9	1062	Tongue, cooked	3 oz	85	56	241	19	<1	0	18	7.6	8.1	.7
9	607	Beef, canned, corned	3 oz	85	58	213	23	0	0	13	5	5	.5
9	608	Beef, dried, cured	1 oz	28	57	47	8	<1	0	1	.4	.5	.1
		LAMB, cooked:											
		Chops (3 per lb with bone):											
		Arm chops, braised:											
9	609	Lean and fat	2.2 oz	63	44	220	20	0	0	15	7	6	1
9	610	Lean part of #609	1.7 oz	48	49	135	17	0	0	7	3	3	.4
		Loin chops, broiled:											
9	611	Lean and fat	2.8 oz	80	54	235	22	0	0	16	7	6	1
9	612	Lean part of #611	2.3 oz	64	61	140	19	0	0	6	2.6	2.4	.4
9	1067	Cutlet, grilled	3 oz	85	64	189	24	0	0	9	5.1	4.6	.7
		Leg, roasted											
9	613	Lean and fat, piece 4⅛ × 2¼ × ½″	3 oz	85	59	205	22	0	0	13	6	5	.8
9	614	Lean only	3 oz	85	64	163	23	0	0	7	2.8	2.6	.5
		Rib, roasted:											
9	615	Lean and fat, piece 2½ × 2½ × ¾″	3 oz	85	47	315	18	0	0	26	12	11	1.5
9	616	Lean only from #615	2 oz	57	60	130	15	0	0	7	3.2	3	5
		Shoulder roast:											
9	1066	Lean only	3 oz	85	49	239	30	0	0	12	5.1	4.6	.7
9	1065	Lean and fat	3 oz	85	49	297	27	0	0	20	9.3	8.1	1.2
		Variety meats:											
9	1069	Brains, cooked	3.5 oz	100	77	126	12	0	0	9	3.6	3.1	.9
9	1068	Heart, cooked	1 c	145	65	360	40	2	0	21	10.3	7.9	2.6
9	1070	Sweetbreads, cooked	3.5 oz	100	60	230	19	6	0	15	7.4	6.0	.8
9	1071	Tongue, cooked	3.5 oz	100	57	289	18	0	0	24	9.8	12.1	1.8

Chol (mg)	Calc (mg)	Iron (mg)	Magn (mg)	Phos (mg)	Pota (mg)	Sodi (mg)	Zinc (mg)	VT-A (RE)	Thia (mg)	Ribo (mg)	Niac (mg)	V-B6 (mg)	Fola (µg)	VT-C (mg)
81	5	2.76	20	217	248	43	4.36	<1	.06	.21	3.29	.29	9	0
81	4	2.94	21	231	262	44	4.66	<1	.06	.22	3.47	.31	10	0
74	9	1.79	18	134	256	65	4.56	<1	.04	.18	4.39	.22	8	0
76	9	2.07	17	144	248	70	4.40	<1	.03	.16	4.91	.23	8	0
72	10	1.8	16	144	250	54	4.40	<1	.06	.15	2.8	.21	6	0
68	10	2.2	21	181	320	63	5.90	<1	.07	.18	3.5	.26	7	0
70	6	2.3	21	188	300	53	5.41	<1	.08	.21	2.95	.31	6	0
69	5	2.5	23	205	328	55	6.01	<1	.08	.23	3.18	.34	7	0
67	7	1.91	20	166	299	54	3.91	<1	.07	.15	4.02	.32	6	0
65	7	2.1	25	185	336	57	4.44	<1	.08	.17	4.54	.36	7	0
71	8	2.16	20	150	288	51	3.79	<1	.08	.18	3.32	.28	6	0
68	6	2.55	25	177	346	56	4.59	<1	.09	.21	3.94	.33	7	0
1696	8	1.89	12	328	301	134	1.15	0	.11	.22	3.21	.33	5	3
164	5	6.38	22	213	198	54	2.66	0	.12	1.31	3.46	.18	2	1
410	9	5.34	20	392	309	90	4.63	9119[69]	.18	3.52	12.3	1.22	187	19
91	6	2.88	14	121	153	51	4.08	0	.03	.30	1.83	.14	4	<1
73	17	1.77	12	94	116	855	3.03	0	.02	.13	2.07	.11	5	1
18	2	1.28	9	49	126	984	1.49	0	.02	.09	1.06	.06	2	0
77	16	1.5	11	132	195	46	2.9	2	.04	.16	4.4	.11	2	0
59	12	1.3	11	111	162	36	2.26	1	.03	.13	3	.11	2	0
78	16	1.4	21	162	272	62	3.11	2	.09	.21	5.5	.12	18	0
60	12	1.3	18	145	241	54	2.69	1	.08	.18	4.4	.1	16	0
89	8	1.87	24	204	323	64	3.57	<1	.13	.26	5.07	.19	3	0
78	8	1.73	20	162	273	57	3.79	2	.09	.25	5.5	.17	3	0
76	7	1.75	20	175	288	58	3.89	1	.09	.23	5.36	.19	3	0
77	19	1.4	15	139	224	60	2.9	2	.08	.18	5.5	.14	3	0
50	12	1.2	15	111	179	46	2.33	<1	.05	.13	3.50	.13	2	0
104	21	2.30	19	197	287	64	4.20	<1	.05	.23	5.31	.19	3	0
104	21	2.02	15	178	263	62	3.91	<1	.05	.22	5.94	.14	3	0
1804	11	1.40	15	320	190	210	1.40	<1	.10	.24	2.10	.08	6	17
395	20	11.7	51	450	536	217	2.63	45	.45	1.83	9.30	.55	6	—
408	34	1.80	23	420	260	210	2.10	<1	.03	.24	2.10	.02	14	18
270	11	3.40	13	200	110	80	2.83	0	.13	.45	7.60	.10	4	6

[69]Value varies widely.

(For purposes of calculations, use "0" for t, <1, <.1, <.01, etc.)

Table C–1 Food Composition

Grp	Ref	Food Description	Measure	Wt (g)	H₂O (%)	Ener (kcal)	Prot (g)	Carb (g)	Dietary Fiber (g)	Fat (g)	Fat Breakdown (g)		
											Sat	Mono	Poly
		MEATS: BEEF, LAMB, PORK and other—Con.											
		PORK, cured, cooked (see also #669–672):											
9	617	Bacon, medium slices	3 pce	19	13	109	6	<1	0	9	3.3	4.5	1.1
9	1087	Breakfast strips, cooked	3 pce	34	27	156	10	<1	0	13	4.3	5.6	1.9
9	618	Canadian-style bacon	2 pce	47	62	86	11	1	0	4	1.3	1.9	.4
		Ham, roasted											
9	619	Lean and fat, 2 pieces 4⅛ × 2¼ × ¼″	3 oz	85	58	207	18	0	0	14	5.1	7	2
9	620	Lean only	3 oz	85	66	133	21	0	0	5	1.6	2.2	.5
9	621	Ham, canned, roasted	3 oz	85	66	140	18	<1	0	7	2.4	3.5	.8
		PORK, fresh, cooked:											
		Chops, loin (cut 3 per lb with bone):											
		Braised:											
9	1291	Lean and fat	1 ea	71	44	261	19	0	0	20	7.2	9.1	2.2
9	1292	Lean only	1 ea	55	51	150	18	0	0	8	2.8	3.6	.0
		Broiled:											
9	622	Lean and fat	3.1 oz	87	50	275	24	0	0	19	7	9	2
9	623	Lean only from #622	2.5 oz	72	57	166	23	0	0	8	2.6	3.4	.9
		Pan fried:											
9	624	Lean and fat	3.1 oz	89	45	334	21	0	0	27	10	13	3
9	625	Lean only for #624	2.4 oz	67	54	178	19	0	0	11	3.7	4.8	1.3
		Leg, roasted:											
9	626	Lean and fat, piece 2½ × 2½ × ¾″	3 oz	85	53	250	21	0	0	18	6	8	2
9	627	Lean only from #626	3 oz	85	60	187	24	0	0	9	3.2	4.2	1.1
		Rib, roasted:											
9	628	Lean and fat, piece 2½ × 2½ × ¾″	3 oz	85	51	270	21	0	0	20	7	9	2
9	629	Lean only	3 oz	85	57	210	24	0	0	12	4.1	5.3	1.4
		Shoulder, braised:											
9	630	Lean and fat, 3 pieces 2½ × 2½ × ¼″	3 oz	85	47	293	23	0	0	22	8	10	2
9	631	Lean only	3 oz	85	54	208	27	0	0	10	4	5	1.3
9	1088	Spareribs, cooked	6.25 oz	177	40	703	51	0	0	54	20.8	25.1	6.2
9	1095	Rabbit, cooked	1 c	140	64	276	40	0	0	10	4.3	2.1	3.4
		VEAL, medium fat, cooked:											
9	632	Veal cutlet, braised or broiled, 4⅛ × 2¼ × ½″	3 oz	85	61	154	28	0	0	3	1.4	1.6	.7
9	633	Veal rib roasted, 2 pieces 4⅛ × 2¼ × ¼″	3 oz	85	67	136	22	0	0	5	1.7	2.3	.5
9	634	Veal liver, simmered	3 oz	85	53	222	25	3	0	11	5	3	4
9	1096	Venison, roasted	3.5 oz	100	66	146	30	0	0	2	1.4	.6	.2
		MEATS: POULTRY and POULTRY PRODUCTS											
		CHICKEN, cooked:											
		Fried, batter dipped:[74]											
10	635	Breast (5.6 oz with bones)	1 ea	140	52	364	35	13	<1	19	5	8	4
10	636	Drumstick (3.4 oz with bones)	1 ea	72	53	193	16	6	<1	11	3	5	3
10	637	Thigh	1 ea	86	52	238	19	8	<1	14	4	6	3
10	638	Wing	1 ea	49	46	159	10	5	<1	11	3	4	3
		Fried, flour coated:[74]											
10	639	Breast (4.2 oz with bones)	1 ea	98	57	218	31	2	<1	9	2.4	3.4	1.9
10	1212	Breast, without skin	1 ea	86	60	161	29	<1	0	4	1.1	1.5	.9

[74] Fried in vegetable shortening.

GRP KEY: 1 = BEV 2 = DAIRY 3 = EGGS 4 = FAT/OIL 5 = FRUIT 6 = BAKERY 7 = GRAIN 8 = FISH 9 = BEEF 10 = POULTRY
11 = SAUSAGE 12 = MIXED/FAST 13 = NUTS/SEEDS 14 = SWEETS 15 = VEG/LEG 16 = MISC 22 = SOUP/SAUCE

Chol (mg)	Calc (mg)	Iron (mg)	Magn (mg)	Phos (mg)	Pota (mg)	Sodi (mg)	Zinc (mg)	VT-A (RE)	Thia (mg)	Ribo (mg)	Niac (mg)	V-B6 (mg)	Fola (μg)	VT-C (mg)
16	2	.32	5	64	92	303	.62	0	.13	.05	1.39	.05	1	6[73]
36	5	.67	9	90	158	714	1.25	0	.25	.13	2.58	.12	1	15
27	5	.38	10	138	181	719	.79	0	.38	.09	3.22	.21	2	10[73]
53	6	.74	16	182	243	1009	1.97	0	.51	.19	3.8	.32	3	0
47	6	.8	19	193	269	1128	2.19	0	.58	.22	4.27	.4	3	0
35	6	.91	16	188	298	908	1.97	0	.82	.21	4.27	.33	4	19[73]
73	6	.82	14	141	245	46	2.15	2	.43	.21	4.24	.26	3	<1
58	5	.77	13	131	230	41	2.05	2	.38	.20	3.82	.25	3	<1
84	4	.71	22	184	312	61	1.68	3	.87	.24	4.35	.35	4	<1
71	4	.66	22	176	302	56	1.61	2	.83	.22	3.99	.34	4	<1
92	4	.75	23	190	323	64	1.74	3	.91	.25	4.58	.35	4	<1
71	3	.67	21	178	305	57	1.61	2	.84	.22	4.03	.34	4	<1
79	5	.85	18	210	280	50	2.43	2	.54	.27	3.89	.33	9	<1
80	6	.95	21	239	317	54	2.77	2	.59	.3	4.2	.38	10	<1
69	9	.76	16	190	313	37	1.67	3	.5	.24	4.17	.3	7	<1
67	10	.85	18	218	360	40	1.9	3	.54	.26	4.6	.34	7	<1
93	6	1.4	16	162	286	74	3.43	3	.46	.26	4.43	.23	3	<1
95	6	1.64	19	189	339	85	4.16	3	.5	.3	5	.35	4	<1
214	83	3.27	43	462	566	165	8.14	5	.72	.68	9.69	.62	7	0
127	22	2.38	31	321	404	51	2.00	3	.08	.25	15.8	.70	6	0
116	8	.92	28	251	373	72	3.00	t	.08	.35	11.4	.37	14	0
115	17	.9	20	182	264	92	3.97	t	.06	.27	6.9	.21	13	0
280	11	12.1	22	456	385	100	5.23	6464[69]	.21	3.56	14	.62	272	31
65	20	3.50	29	264	336	70	—	0	.37	.28	7.40	—	—	0
119	28	1.75	34	258	282	385	1.33	28	.16	.2	14.7	.6	8	0
62	12	.97	14	106	134	194	1.67	19	.08	.16	3.67	.2	6	0
80	16	1.24	18	134	165	248	1.75	25	.1	.2	4.92	.23	8	0
39	10	.63	8	59	68	157	.67	17	.05	.07	2.58	.15	3	0
88	16	1.17	29	228	253	74	1.07	15	.08	.13	13.5	.57	4	0
78	14	.98	27	212	237	68	.93	6	.07	.11	12.7	.55	4	0

[69] Value varies widely.

[73] Values based on products containing added ascorbic acid or sodium ascorbate. If none added, ascorbic acid content would be negligible.

(For purposes of calculations, use "0" for t, <1, <.1, <.01, etc.)

Grp	Ref	Food Description	Measure	Wt (g)	H₂O (%)	Ener (kcal)	Prot (g)	Carb (g)	Dietary Fiber (g)	Fat (g)	Sat	Mono	Poly

MEATS: POULTRY and POULTRY PRODUCTS—Con.
CHICKEN—con.

Grp	Ref	Food Description	Measure	Wt (g)	H₂O (%)	Ener (kcal)	Prot (g)	Carb (g)	Dietary Fiber (g)	Fat (g)	Sat	Mono	Poly
10	640	Drumstick (2.6 oz with bones)	1 ea	49	57	120	13	1	<1	7	1.8	2.7	1.6
10	641	Thigh	1 ea	62	54	162	17	2	<1	9	2.5	3.6	2.1
10	1099	Thigh, without skin	1 ea	52	59	113	15	1	<1	5	1.5	2.0	1.3
10	642	Wing	1 ea	32	49	103	8	1	<1	7	1.9	2.8	1.6

Roasted:

Grp	Ref	Food Description	Measure	Wt (g)	H₂O (%)	Ener (kcal)	Prot (g)	Carb (g)	Dietary Fiber (g)	Fat (g)	Sat	Mono	Poly
10	643	All types of meat	1 c	140	64	266	41	0	0	10	2.9	3.7	2.4
10	644	Dark meat	1 c	140	63	286	38	0	0	14	3.7	5.0	3.2
10	645	Light meat	1 c	140	65	242	43	0	0	6	1.8	2.2	1.4
10	646	Breast, without skin	½ ea	86	65	142	27	0	0	3	.9	1.1	.7
10	647	Drumstick	1 ea	44	67	76	13	0	0	2	.7	.8	.6
10	648	Thigh	1 ea	62	59	153	16	0	0	10	2.9	3.8	2.1
10	1100	Thigh, without skin	1 ea	52	63	109	14	0	0	6	1.6	2.2	1.3
10	649	Stewed, all types	1 c	140	67	248	38	0	0	9	2.6	3.3	2.2
10	1102	Chicken gizzards, simmered	1 ea	22	67	34	6	<1	0	1	.2	.2	.2
10	1101	Chicken hearts, simmered	1 ea	3.3	65	6	1	<1	0	<1	.1	.1	.1
10	650	Chicken liver, simmered	1 ea	20	68	30	5	2	0	1	.4	.3	.2

DUCK, roasted:

Grp	Ref	Food Description	Measure	Wt (g)	H₂O (%)	Ener (kcal)	Prot (g)	Carb (g)	Dietary Fiber (g)	Fat (g)	Sat	Mono	Poly
10	1293	Meat with skin, about 2.7 cups	½ duck	382	52	1287	73	0	0	108	37	49	14
10	651	Meat only, about 1.5 cups	½ duck	221	64	445	52	0	0	25	9.2	8.2	3.2

GOOSE, domesticated, roasted:

Grp	Ref	Food Description	Measure	Wt (g)	H₂O (%)	Ener (kcal)	Prot (g)	Carb (g)	Dietary Fiber (g)	Fat (g)	Sat	Mono	Poly
10	1294	Meat only, 4.2 cups	½ goose	591	57	1406	171	0	0	75	27	26	9
10	1295	Meat w/skin, about 5.5 cups	½ goose	774	52	2362	195	0	0	170	53	79	20

TURKEY, roasted, meat only:

Grp	Ref	Food Description	Measure	Wt (g)	H₂O (%)	Ener (kcal)	Prot (g)	Carb (g)	Dietary Fiber (g)	Fat (g)	Sat	Mono	Poly
10	652	Dark meat	3 oz	85	63	159	24	0	0	6	2.1	1.4	1.8
10	653	Light meat	3 oz	85	66	133	25	0	0	3	.9	.5	.7
10	654	All types, chopped or diced	1 c	140	65	238	41	0	0	7	2.3	1.5	2.0
10	655	All types, sliced	3 oz	85	65	145	25	0	0	4	1.4	.9	1.2
10	1103	Ground turkey, cooked	3.5 oz	100	60	225	26	0	0	13	4.5	5.4	3.2

Turkey breast:

Grp	Ref	Food Description	Measure	Wt (g)	H₂O (%)	Ener (kcal)	Prot (g)	Carb (g)	Dietary Fiber (g)	Fat (g)	Sat	Mono	Poly
10	1104	Barbecued	1 oz	28	70	40	6	0	0	1	.4	.5	.3
10	1105	Hickory smoked	1 oz	28	70	35	6	1	0	1	.3	.3	.3
10	1106	Gizzard, cooked	1 ea	67	65	109	20	<1	0	3	.7	.5	.7
10	1107	Heart, cooked	1 ea	16	64	28	4	<1	0	1	.3	.2	.3
10	1108	Liver, cooked	1 ea	75	66	127	18	3	0	4	1.4	1.1	1.1

Poultry food products (see also #664, 668, 673, 676, 1076, 1080):

Grp	Ref	Food Description	Measure	Wt (g)	H₂O (%)	Ener (kcal)	Prot (g)	Carb (g)	Dietary Fiber (g)	Fat (g)	Sat	Mono	Poly
10	656	Canned, boneless chicken	5 oz	142	69	235	31	0	0	11	3.1	4.5	2.5
10	657	Chicken frankfurter, 10/pkg.	1 ea	45	58	115	6	3	0	9	2.5	3.8	1.8
10	658	Chicken roll, light meat	2 pce	57	69	90	11	1	0	4	1.2	1.7	.9
10	659	Gravy and turkey, frozen package	5 oz	142	85	95	8	7	<1	4	1.2	1.4	.7
10	1296	Poultry sandwich spread	1 tbsp	13	60	25	2	1	0	2	.5	.4	.8
10	660	Turkey loaf, breast meat	2 pce	42	72	46	10	0	0	1	.2	.2	.1
10	661	Turkey patties, breaded, fried	1 ea	64	50	181	9	10	<1	12	3	4.8	3
10	662	Turkey, frozen, roasted, seasoned	3 oz	85	68	130	18	3	0	5	1.6	1	1.4

MEATS: SAUSAGES and LUNCHMEATS
Beerwurst/beer salami:

Grp	Ref	Food Description	Measure	Wt (g)	H₂O (%)	Ener (kcal)	Prot (g)	Carb (g)	Dietary Fiber (g)	Fat (g)	Sat	Mono	Poly
11	1072	Beef	1 pce	23	54	75	3	<1	0	7	2.8	3.3	.2
11	1074	Pork	1 pce	23	62	55	3	<1	0	4	1.4	2.1	.5
11	1075	Berliner	1 pce	23	61	53	4	1	0	4	1.4	1.8	.4

(76)Cooked weight is half the weight of raw sausage.

GRP KEY: 1 = BEV 2 = DAIRY 3 = EGGS 4 = FAT/OIL 5 = FRUIT 6 = BAKERY 7 = GRAIN 8 = FISH 9 = BEEF 10 = POULTRY 11 = SAUSAGE 12 = MIXED/FAST 13 = NUTS/SEEDS 14 = SWEETS 15 = VEG/LEG 16 = MISC 22 = SOUP/SAUCE

Chol (mg)	Calc (mg)	Iron (mg)	Magn (mg)	Phos (mg)	Pota (mg)	Sodi (mg)	Zinc (mg)	VT-A (RE)	Thia (mg)	Ribo (mg)	Niac (mg)	V-B6 (mg)	Fola (µg)	VT-C (mg)
44	6	.66	11	86	112	44	1.42	12	.04	.11	2.96	.17	4	0
60	8	.93	15	116	147	55	1.56	18	.06	.15	4.31	.21	5	0
53	7	.76	14	103	134	49	1.45	11	.05	.13	3.70	.20	4	0
26	5	.4	6	48	57	25	.56	12	.02	.04	2.14	.13	1	0
125	21	1.69	35	273	340	120	2.94	22	.1	.25	12.8	.65	8	0
130	21	1.86	33	250	336	130	3.92	30	.1	.32	9.17	.5	11	0
118	21	1.49	38	302	345	108	1.73	12	.09	.16	17.4	.84	5	0
73	13	.89	25	196	220	64	.86	5	.06	.1	11.8	.52	3	0
41	5	.57	11	81	108	42	1.4	8	.03	.1	2.67	.17	4	0
58	8	.83	14	108	137	52	1.46	30	.04	.13	3.95	.19	4	0
49	6	.68	12	95	124	46	1.34	10	.04	.12	3.39	.18	4	0
116	20	1.63	29	210	252	98	2.79	21	.07	.23	8.56	.37	8	0
43	2	.91	4	34	39	15	.96	12	.01	.05	.87	.03	12	<1
8	1	.30	1	7	4	2	.24	<1	<.01	.02	.09	.01	3	<1
126	3	1.7	2	62	28	10	.87	983	.03	.35	.89	.12	154	3
320	43	10.3	62	595	780	227	7.12	241	.67	1.03	18.4	.70	25	0
198	26	5.97	44	449	557	143	5.75	51	.57	1.04	11.3	.55	22	0
569	84	17.0	148	1828	2291	447	16.0	71	.54	2.31	24.1	2.75	13	0
708	104	21.9	169	2091	2546	543	16.0	162	.60	2.50	32.3	2.89	17	0
72	27	1.99	21	174	247	67	3.8	0	.05	.21	3.1	.3	8	0
59	16	1.14	24	186	259	54	1.73	0	.05	.12	5.81	.46	5	0
107	35	2.49	37	298	418	99	4.34	0	.09	.26	7.62	.64	10	0
64	21	1.51	23	181	254	60	2.64	0	.05	.16	4.63	.39	6	0
84	29	1.66	20	193	236	115	3.45	0	.08	.27	6.01	.26	3	<1
16	2	.12	7	74	57	156	.35	0	.01	.03	2.73	.11	1	<1
13	1	.20	7	79	59	208	.30	0	.01	.03	2.75	.11	1	<1
155	10	3.64	13	86	141	37	2.79	37	.02	.22	2.06	.08	36	1
36	2	1.10	4	33	29	9	.84	1	.01	.14	.52	.05	13	<1
469	8	5.85	11	204	146	48	2.32	2806	.04	1.07	4.46	.39	499	1
88	20	2.2	17	158	196	714	2.13	48	.02	.18	8.99	.5	4	3
45	43	.9	8	48	38	616	1	17	.03	.05	1.39	.09	2	0
28	24	.55	10	89	129	331	.41	14	.04	.07	3	.31	2	0
26	20	1.32	11	115	87	787	.99	18	.03	.18	2.55	.14	2	0
4	1	.08	3	4	24	49	.25	6	<.01	.01	.22	.01	1	<1
17	3	.17	9	97	118	608	.48	0	.02	.05	3.54	.15	2	0[75]
40	9	1.41	12	173	176	512	1.5	7	.06	.12	1.47	.13	3	0
45	4	1.4	20	207	253	578	2.37	0	.04	.14	5.3	.24	5	0
13	2	.31	3	24	42	214	.61	0	.03	.03	.66	.05	1	3
13	2	.17	3	24	58	285	.40	0	.13	.04	.75	.08	1	7
11	3	.27	3	30	65	298	.57	0	.09	.05	.72	.05	1	2

[75]If sodium ascorbate is added, product contains 11 mg ascorbic acid.

(For purposes of calculations, use "0" for t, <1, <.1, <.01, etc.)

Table C–1 Food Composition

Grp	Ref	Food Description	Measure	Wt (g)	H₂O (%)	Ener (kcal)	Prot (g)	Carb (g)	Dietary Fiber (g)	Fat (g)	Fat Breakdown (g)		
											Sat	Mono	Poly
MEATS: SAUSAGES and LUNCHMEATS—Con.													
		Bologna:											
11	1297	Beef	1 pce	23	55	72	3	<1	0	7	2.7	3.1	.2
11	663	Beef and pork	1 pce	28	54	89	3	1	0	8	3.0	3.8	.7
65	1298	Pork	1 pce	23	61	57	4	<1	0	5	1.6	2.3	.5
11	664	Turkey	1 pce	28	66	56	4	<1	0	4	1.5	1.9	1.2
11	665	Braunschweiger sausage	2 pce	57	48	205	8	2	0	18	6.2	8.5	2.1
11	1073	Brotwurst, link	1 ea	70	51	226	10	2	0	20	7.0	9.3	2.0
11	666	Brown-and-serve sausage links, cooked	1 ea	13	45	50	2	<1	0	5	1.7	2.2	.5
11	1089	Cheesefurter/cheese smoki	1 ea	43	53	141	6	1	0	13	4.5	5.9	1.3
11	1090	Corned beef loaf, jellied	1 pce	28	67	46	7	0	0	2	.8	.9	.1
		Frankfurters (see also #657)											
11	1077	Beef, large link, 8/pkg.	1 ea	57	54	184	6	1	0	17	6.8	8.2	.7
11	1078	Beef and Pork, large link, 8/pkg.	1 ea	57	54	183	6	1	0	17	6.1	7.8	1.6
11	667	Beef and pork, smaller link, 10/pkg.	1 ea	45	54	145	5	1	0	13	4.8	6.2	1.2
11	668	Turkey, smaller link, 10/pkg.	1 ea	45	63	102	6	1	0	8	2.7	3.3	2.1
		Ham:											
11	669	Ham lunchmeat, canned, 3 x 2 x ½″	1 pce	21	52	70	3	<1	0	6	2.3	3.0	.8
11	670	Chopped ham, packaged	2 pce	22	61	98	7	<1	0	8	2.6	3.9	.9
11	671	Ham lunchmeat, regular	2 pce	57	65	103	10	2	0	6	1.9	2.8	.7
11	672	Ham lunchmeat, extra lean	2 pce	57	70	75	11	1	0	3	.9	1.3	.3
11	673	Turkey ham	2 pce	57	72	73	11	1	0	3	1.0	.8	.8
11	1091	Keilbasa sausage	1 pce	26	54	81	3	1	0	7	2.6	3.4	.8
11	1092	Knockwurst sausage-link	1 ea	68	56	209	8	1	0	19	6.9	8.7	2.0
11	1093	Mortadella lunchmeat	1 pce	15	52	47	2	<1	0	4	1.4	1.7	.5
11	1097	Olive loaf lunchmeat	2 pce	57	58	133	7	5	<1	9	3.3	4.5	1.1
11	1080	Pastrami, turkey	2 pce	57	72	74	11	1	0	4	1.0	1.2	.9
11	1081	Pepperoni sausage, small slices	4 pce	22	27	109	5	1	0	10	3.6	4.6	1
11	1094	Pickle & pimento loaf	2 pce	57	57	149	7	3	<1	12	4.5	5.4	1.5
11	1082	Polish sausage	1 oz.	28	53	92	4	<1	0	8	2.9	3.8	.9
		Pork sausage, cooked:											
11	674	Link, small	1 ea	13	45	48	3	<1	0	4	1.4	1.8	.5
11	1079	Patty	1 pce	27	45	100	5	<1	0	8	2.9	3.8	1.0
		Salami:											
11	675	Pork and beef	2 pce	57	60	143	8	1	0	11	4.6	5.2	1.1
11	676	Turkey	2 pce	57	66	111	9	<1	0	8	2.3	2.6	2.0
11	677	Dry, beef and pork	2 pce	20	35	85	5	1	0	7	2.4	3.4	.6
		Sandwich spreads (see also #1296):											
11	1300	Ham salad	1 c	240	63	518	21	26	<1	37	12.1	17.3	6.5
11	678	Pork and beef	1 tbsp	15	60	35	1	2	0	3	.9	1.1	.4
		Smoked Link Sausage:											
11	1083	Beef and pork	1 ea	68	39	265	15	1	0	22	7.7	10.0	2.6
11	1084	Pork	1 ea	68	52	229	9	1	0	21	7.2	9.7	2.2
11	1085	Summer sausage	1 pce	23	48	80	4	1	0	7	2.8	3.2	.4
11	1076	Turkey breakfast sausage	1 pce	28	60	65	6	0	0	4	1.6	1.8	1.2
11	679	Vienna sausage, canned	1 ea	16	60	45	2	<1	0	4	1.5	2.0	.3

Chol (mg)	Calc (mg)	Iron (mg)	Magn (mg)	Phos (mg)	Pota (mg)	Sodi (mg)	Zinc (mg)	VT-A (RE)	Thia (mg)	Ribo (mg)	Niac (mg)	V-B6 (mg)	Fola (μg)	VT-C (mg)
13	3	.32	2	19	36	230	.46	0	.01	.03	.61	.04	1	4
16	3	.43	3	26	51	289	.55	0	.05	.04	.73	.05	1	6[73]
14	3	.18	3	33	65	272	.47	0	.12	.04	.90	.06	1	8
28	23	.43	4	37	56	248	.49	0	.02	.05	1.04	.05	1	<1
89	6	5.32	6	96	113	652	1.62	2406	.14	.87	4.78	.19	57	5[73]
44	34	.72	11	94	197	778	1.47	0	.18	.16	2.31	.09	2	20
9	1	.1	2	14	25	105	.15	0	.05	.02	.40	.03	1	0
29	25	.46	5	76	89	465	.97	3	.11	.07	1.25	.05	1	8
12	3	.58	3	18	25	294	1.08	0	<.01	.03	.46	.04	1	2
27	7	.76	7	47	90	584	1.21	0	.03	.06	1.44	.06	2	14
29	6	.66	7	49	95	639	1.05	0	.11	.07	1.50	.08	2	15
23	5	.52	6	39	75	504	.83	0	.09	.05	1.18	.06	2	12[73]
39	58	.77	8	83	88	454	1	17	.04	.08	1.7	.10	2	<1
13	1	.15	2	17	45	271	.31	0	.08	.04	.66	.04	1	<1
21	3	.4	5	58	119	573	.77	0	.23	.07	1.4	.13	2	1[73]
32	4	.56	11	140	188	746	1.21	0	.49	.14	2.98	.19	2	16[73]
27	4	.43	10	124	198	810	1.09	0	.53	.13	2.74	.26	2	15[73]
32	5	1.56	12	138	163	548	1.58	0	.04	.15	2.72	.16	4	0
17	11	.38	4	38	70	280	.52	0	.06	.06	.75	.05	1	6
39	7	.62	8	67	136	687	1.13	0	.23	.10	1.86	.11	2	18
8	3	.21	2	15	24	187	.32	0	.02	.02	.40	.02	<1	4
22	62	.31	11	72	169	842	.78	0	.17	.15	1.04	.13	1	5
30	5	.81	10	142	155	569	1.46	0	.05	.15	2.48	.16	4	<1
8	2	.31	4	26	76	449	.55	0	.07	.06	1.09	.06	—	<1
21	54	.58	10	79	193	787	.79	<1	.17	.14	1.16	.11	1	8
20	3	.41	4	39	67	248	.55	0	.14	.04	.98	.05	1	0
11	4	.16	2	24	47	168	.33	0	.1	.03	.59	.04	1	<1
22	9	.34	5	50	97	349	.68	0	.20	.07	1.22	.09	2	<1
37	7	1.51	9	65	112	604	1.21	0	.14	.21	2.02	.12	1	7[73]
46	11	.93	9	73	125	535	1.25	0	.06	.15	2.23	.14	5	<1
16	2	.3	4	28	76	372	.64	0	.12	.06	.97	.1	0	6[73]
88	19	1.42	23	286	359	2187	2.64	42	1.04	.29	5.02	.36	3	14
6	2	.12	1	9	16	152	.15	1	.03	.02	.26	.02	<1	0
46	20	.79	13	110	228	1020	1.92	0	.48	.18	3.08	.24	2	1
48	7	.99	8	73	129	642	1.44	0	.18	.12	2.19	.12	2	13
16	2	.47	3	23	53	334	.47	0	.04	.07	.94	.07	1	5
23	5	.52	6	52	76	191	.97	0	.03	.08	1.42	.08	1	—
8	2	.14	1	8	16	152	.26	0	.01	.02	.26	.02	<1	0

[73]Values based on products containing added ascorbic acid or sodium ascorbate. If none added, ascorbic acid content would be negligible.

(For purposes of calculations, use "0" for t, <1, <.1, <.01, etc.)

Table C-1 Food Composition

Grp	Ref	Food Description	Measure	Wt (g)	H₂O (%)	Ener (kcal)	Prot (g)	Carb (g)	Dietary Fiber (g)	Fat (g)	Fat Breakdown (g)		
											Sat	Mono	Poly
MIXED DISHES and FAST FOODS													
		MIXED DISHES:											
		Beef stew with vegetables:											
12	680	Homemade	1 c	245	82	220	16	15	3	11	4.4	4.5	.5
12	1109	Canned	1 c	245	83	194	14	18	1	8	3.1	3.1	.4
12	1116	Beef, macaroni & tomato sauce casserole	1 c	226	80	189	10	25	2	6	2.1	2.3	.4
12	681	Beef pot pie, homemade[77]	1 pce	210	55	515	21	39	1	30	8	13	7
12	682	Chicken à la king, home recipe	1 c	245	68	470	27	12	1	34	13	13	6
12	683	Chicken and noodles, home recipe	1 c	240	71	365	22	26	1	18	5	7	4
12	684	Chicken chow mein, canned	1 c	250	89	95	7	18	5	1	.1	.1	.8
12	685	Chicken chow mein, home recipe	1 c	250	78	255	23	10	4	11	4	4	3
12	686	Chicken pot pie, home recipe[77]	1 pce	232	57	545	23	42	2	31	10	16	7
12	1112	Chicken salad w/celery	.5 c	78	53	266	11	1	<1	25	4.1	7.2	12.0
12	687	Chili with beans, canned	1 c	255	76	286	15	30	8	14	6	6	1
12	688	Chop suey with beef and pork	1 c	250	75	300	26	13	2	17	4	7	4
12	689	Corn pudding[78]	1 c	250	76	271	11	32	9	13	6.3	4.3	1.7
12	690	Cole slaw[79]	1 c	120	82	84	2	15	2	3	.5	.9	1.6
12	1110	Corned beef hash-canned	1 c	220	67	382	18	22	1	10	4.2	4.9	.5
12	1113	Egg salad	1 c	183	66	438	19	3	<1	39	8.4	13.2	13.5
12	691	French toast, home recipe[81]	1 pce	65	53	123	5	15	1	4	1.1	1.4	1.1
12	1355	Green pepper, stuffed	1 ea	172	76	217	10	16	1	13	5.3	5.2	.6
		Lasagna:											
12	1346	With meat	1 pce	245	64	398	26	30	2	20	9.2	7.2	1.5
12	1111	Without meat	1 pce	218	64	316	20	30	2	14	6.9	4.7	1.3
12	1117	Frozen entree	1 pce	205	73	275	17	19	1	12	6.3	4.2	1.2
		Macaroni and cheese:											
12	692	Canned[82]	1 c	240	80	230	9	26	1	10	5	3	1
12	693	Home recipe[49]	1 c	200	58	430	17	40	1	22	10	7	4
12	1115	Macaroni salad-no cheese	1 c	141	61	371	3	18	1	33	5.1	9.5	17.2
		Meat Loaf:											
12	1120	Beef	1 pce	87	62	193	16	4	<1	12	4.8	5.2	.6
12	1119	Beef and pork (1/3)	1 pce	87	59	212	15	5	<1	15	5.5	6.3	1.2
12	1303	Moussaka (lamb and eggplant)	1 c	250	79	250	21	16	6	11	3.6	4.3	1.9
12	715	Potato salad with mayonnaise and egg[85]	1 c	250	76	358	7	28	4	21	4	6	9
12	694	Quiche lorraine, 1/8 of 8″ quiche[77]	1 pce	176	47	600	13	29	1	48	23	18	4
		Spaghetti (enriched) in tomato sauce:											
		With cheese:											
12	695	Canned	1 c	250	80	190	6	39	3	2	.4	.4	.5
12	696	Home recipe	1 c	250	77	260	9	37	3	9	3	3.6	1.2
		With meatballs:											
12	697	Canned	1 c	250	78	260	12	39	3	10	2	4	3
12	698	Home recipe	1 c	248	70	330	19	39	3	12	4	4	2

[49]Made with margarine.

[77]Crust made with vegetable shortening and enriched flour.

[78]Recipe: 55% yellow corn, 23% whole milk, 14% egg, 4% sugar, 3% salt, and 1% pepper.

[79]Recipe: 41% cabbage; 12% celery; 12% table cream; 12% sugar; 7% green pepper; 6% lemon juice; 4% onion; 3% pimento; 3% vinegar; 2% each for salt, dry mustard, and white pepper.

[81]Recipe: 35% whole milk, 32% white bread, 29% egg, and cooked in 4% margarine.

[82]Made with corn oil.

[85]Recipe: 62% potatoes; 12% egg; 8% mayonnaise; 7% celery; 6% sweet pickle relish; 2% onion; 1% each for green pepper, pimiento, salt, and dry mustard.

Chol (mg)	Calc (mg)	Iron (mg)	Magn (mg)	Phos (mg)	Pota (mg)	Sodi (mg)	Zinc (mg)	VT-A (RE)	Thia (mg)	Ribo (mg)	Niac (mg)	V-B6 (mg)	Fola (µg)	VT-C (mg)
71	29	2.9	40	184	613	292	5.3	569	.15	.17	4.7	.28	37	17
15	23	3.18	39	56	417	992	4.23	262	.07	.12	2.43	.20	31	7
22	30	2.39	37	118	562	974	2.07	111	.19	.17	3.51	.30	23	16
42	29	3.8	6	149	334	596	3.17	517	.29	.29	4.8	.24	29	6
221	127	2.5	20	358	404	760	1.8	272	.1	.42	5.4	.23	11	12
103	26	2.4	37	247	211	600	2.14	130	.05	.17	4.3	.16	9	1
8	45	1.3	14	85	418	725	1.3	28	.05	.1	1	.09	12	13
75	58	2.50	28	293	473	718	2.12	50	.08	.23	4.3	.41	19	10
56	70	3.0	25	232	343	594	2.0	735	.32	.32	4.9	.46	29	5
48	16	.66	11	80	137	199	.80	31	.03	.08	3.25	.17	4	1
43	119	8.75	115	393	932	1330	5.10	86	.12	.27	.91	.34	41	4
68	60	4.80	32	248	425	1053	3.58	60	.28	.38	5.0	.32	22	33
230	100	1.40	38	143	402	138	1.26	89	1.03	.32	2.47	.30	63	7
10[80]	54	.70	12	38	218	28	.24	98	.08	.07	.33	.18	32	39
132	29	4.40	3	147	440	1354	4.38	0	.12	.40	4.60	.41	15	8
629	94	3.39	21	282	211	428	2.24	257	.12	.45	.16	.18	74	0
73	79	1.08	12	82	96	189	.47	57	.15	.17	1.09	.04	18	<1
38	15	2.32	23	91	227	210	2.58	29	.11	.10	2.96	.22	14	83
56	460	3.08	41	393	507	783	3.23	168	.22	.33	3.64	.35	16	7
30	457	2.38	35	345	424	760	1.93	168	.21	.28	2.01	.22	14	7
90	246	2.48	52	253	437	967	1.25	97	.19	.33	2.70	.29	25	6
24	199	1.0	31	182	139	730	1.20	72	.12	.24	1.0	.02	8	<1
24	27	1.14	23	50	162	315	.34	40	.10	.07	.67	.07	7	3
98	29	1.90	19	123	227	340	3.50	26	.06	.18	3.19	.18	8	1
97	33	1.39	18	128	238	392	2.86	26	.19	.19	3.07	.19	8	1
143	129	2.75	44	245	695	485	3.29	125	.25	.32	4.78	.35	44	7
170	48	1.63	39	130	635	1323	.78	83	.19	.15	2.23	.35	17	25
44	362	1.8	37	322	240	1086	1.20	232	.20	.40	1.8	.05	10	1
285	211	1.4	23	276	283	653	1.95	454	.11	.32	1.2	.15	17	<1
3	40	2.8	21	88	303	955	1.12	120	.35	.28	4.5	.13	6	10
8	80	2.3	26	135	408	955	1.3	140	.25	.18	2.3	.20	8	13
23	53	3.3	20	113	245	1220	2.39	100	.15	.18	2.3	.12	5	5
89	124	3.7	40	236	665	1009	2.45	159	.25	.30	.4	.20	10	22

[80]From dairy cream in recipe.

(For purposes of calculations, use "0" for t, <1, <.1, <.01, etc.)

Table C–1   Food Composition

Grp	Ref	Food Description	Measure	Wt (g)	H₂O (%)	Ener (kcal)	Prot (g)	Carb (g)	Dietary Fiber (g)	Fat (g)	Fat Breakdown (g)		
											Sat	Mono	Poly
MIXED DISHES and FAST FOOD—Con.													
12	716	Spinach soufflé[86]	1 c	136	74	218	11	3	4	18	7	7	3
12	717	Tuna salad[87]	1 c	205	63	383	33	19	2	19	3	6	9
12	1121	Tuna noodle casserole, recipe	1 c	202	73	251	21	24	<1	7	2.0	1.5	3.2
12	1270	Waldorf salad	1 c	142	58	424	4	13	4	42	5.6	11.2	23.1
		FAST FOODS and SANDWICHES: see end of this appendix for additional Fast Foods.											
		Burrito:[83]											
12	699	Beef and bean	1 ea	175	54	390	21	40	5	18	7	7	2
12	700	Bean	1 ea	174	55	322	13	47	8	10	4	3	2
		Cheeseburger:											
12	701	Regular	1 ea	112	46	300	15	28	1	15	7	6	1
12	702	4-oz patty	1 ea	194	46	524	30	40	2	31	15	12	1
12	703	Chicken patty sandwich	1 ea	157	52	436	25	34	1	22	6	10	5
12	704	Corn dog	1 ea	111	45	330	10	27	<1	20	8	10	1
12	705	Enchilada[84]	1 ea	230	72	235	20	24	2	16	8	7	.6
12	706	English muffin with egg, cheese, bacon	1 ea	138	49	360	18	31	2	18	8	8	.7
		Fish sandwich:											
12	707	Regular, with cheese	1 ea	140	43	420	16	39	1	23	6	7	8
12	708	Large, without cheese	1 ea	170	48	470	18	41	1	27	6	9	10
		Hamburger with bun:											
12	709	Regular	1 ea	98	46	245	12	28	1	11	4	5	1
12	710	4-oz patty	1 ea	174	50	445	25	38	1	21	7	12	1
12	711	Hotdog/frankfurter and bun	1 ea	85	53	260	8	21	1	15	5	7	2
12	712	Cheese pizza, ⅛ of 15″ round[77]	1 pce	120	46	290	15	39	2	9	4	3	1
		SANDWICHES:											
		Avocado, cheese, tomato & lettuce:											
12	1276	On white bread, firm	1 ea	205	59	464	15	39	7	29	9.1	11.8	6.0
12	1278	On part-whole wheat	1 ea	195	60	432	14	33	8	29	8.7	11.8	6.0
12	1277	On whole wheat	1 ea	209	58	459	16	39	13	29	9.1	11.9	6.2
		Bacon, lettuce & tomato sandwich:											
12	1137	On white bread, soft	1 ea	135	54	333	11	30	2	19	5.2	7.4	5.5
12	1139	On part-whole wheat	1 ea	135	54	327	12	28	3	19	4.9	7.5	5.5
12	1138	On whole-wheat	1 ea	149	53	355	13	34	8	20	5.4	7.7	5.7
		Cheese sandwich, grilled:											
12	1140	On white bread, soft	1 ea	117	37	399	17	28	1	24	12.7	7.6	2.3
12	1142	On part-whole wheat	1 ea	117	37	393	18	27	3	24	12.5	7.7	2.3
12	1141	On whole wheat	1 ea	131	38	420	20	33	7	25	12.9	7.9	2.6
		Chicken salad sandwich:											
12	1143	On white bread, soft	1 ea	99.7	44	300	10	28	1	16	3.0	4.9	7.5
12	1145	On part-whole wheat	1 ea	99.7	44	294	11	27	3	16	2.8	5.0	7.5
12	1144	On whole wheat	1 ea	114	44	321	12	33	8	17	3.2	5.2	7.8
12	1146	Corned beef & swiss cheese on rye	1 ea	147	45	429	27	25	5	24	9.4	8.2	5.0
		Egg salad sandwich:											
12	1147	On white bread, soft	1 ea	111	47	325	9	28	1	19	3.9	6.2	7.7
12	1149	On part whole-wheat	1 ea	111	47	319	10	27	3	19	3.7	6.3	7.7
12	1148	On whole wheat	1 ea	125	47	346	12	33	7	20	4.1	6.4	8.0

[77] Crust made with vegetable shortening and enriched flour.
[83] Made with a 10½″-diameter flour tortilla.
[84] USDA data were unspecified for type of enchilada.
[86] Recipe: 29% whole milk, 26% spinach, 13% egg white, 13% cheddar cheese, 7% egg yolk, 7% butter, 4% flour, 1% salt and pepper.
[87] Made with drained chunk light tuna, celery, onion, pickle relish, and mayonnaise-type salad dressing.

Chol (mg)	Calc (mg)	Iron (mg)	Magn (mg)	Phos (mg)	Pota (mg)	Sodi (mg)	Zinc (mg)	VT-A (RE)	Thia (mg)	Ribo (mg)	Niac (mg)	V-B6 (mg)	Fola (µg)	VT-C (mg)
184	230	1.34	37	231	202	763	1.29	675	.09	.31	.48	.12	62	3
27	35	2.0	40	365	365	824	1.15	55	.06	.14	13.3	.17	15	5
52	37	1.94	31	182	224	869	.97	34	.14	.17	8.59	.24	13	1
22	44	.98	41	88	279	246	.69	41	.10	.06	.37	.16	19	6
52	165	2.7	61	274	388	516	3.30	58	.26	.29	4.36	.73	48	5
15	181	2.53	76	243	427	1030	2.37	58	.26	.23	2.40	1.01	55	5
44	135	2.30	22	174	219	672	2.53	65	.26	.24	3.70	.11	20	1
104	236	4.45	43	320	407	1224	5.27	128	.33	.49	7.37	.23	23	3
68	44	1.87	30	173	194	2732	1.00	16	.29	.26	9.21	.37	18	4
37	34	1.94	22	303	164	1252	1.44	<1	.28	.17	3.27	.11	2	3
19	322	3.29	76	198	653	1332	1.20	352	.18	.26	.40	.25	19	<1
213	197	3.10	28	290	201	832	1.86	160	.46	.50	3.71	.15	35	1
56	132	1.85	29	223	274	667	.95	25	.32	.27	3.30	.10	24	3
90	61	2.23	34	246	375	621	.88	15	.35	.24	3.52	.12	43	1
32	56	2.20	19	107	202	463	2.0	14	.23	.24	3.80	.12	16	1
71	75	4.84	38	225	404	763	5.01	28	.38	.38	7.85	.28	24	2
23	59	1.71	13	83	113	745	1.19	<1	.29	.19	2.48	.07	17	12
56	220	1.60	36	216	230	699	1.81	106	.34	.29	4.20	.04	40	2
32	312	3.02	54	242	557	556	1.69	160	.41	.43	3.98	.25	74	11
32	299	3.09	66	274	562	518	1.87	160	.36	.40	4.02	.29	76	11
32	279	3.52	105	353	608	660	2.46	160	.35	.37	4.18	.36	91	11
21	81	2.22	22	138	253	647	1.06	50	.42	.25	3.71	.10	35	13
21	80	2.57	36	181	269	661	1.30	50	.42	.26	4.13	.15	41	13
21	60	3.00	76	260	315	803	1.89	50	.41	.23	4.29	.21	55	13
55	424	1.82	25	489	158	1155	2.24	214	.28	.38	2.14	.06	25	<1
55	424	2.17	39	531	174	1169	2.49	214	.28	.38	2.56	.10	30	<1
55	404	2.61	78	610	219	1311	3.07	214	.26	.35	2.72	.17	45	<1
25	80	1.94	18	102	136	401	.76	18	.28	.21	3.73	.11	22	1
25	79	2.30	32	144	152	415	.00	18	.28	.22	4.15	.15	28	1
25	59	2.73	71	223	197	557	1.59	18	.27	.19	4.31	.22	43	1
85	331	3.98	32	310	174	1045	4.37	85	.23	.41	3.65	.14	25	0
163	96	2.49	17	133	119	447	.92	73	.29	.29	2.14	.07	38	<1
163	95	2.85	31	176	135	461	1.16	73	.29	.29	2.56	.11	44	<1
163	75	3.28	71	255	180	603	1.75	73	.28	.26	2.72	.18	59	<1

(For purposes of calculations, use "0" for t, <1, <.1, <.01, etc.)

Table C–1 Food Composition

Grp	Ref	Food Description	Measure	Wt (g)	H₂O (%)	Ener (kcal)	Prot (g)	Carb (g)	Dietary Fiber (g)	Fat (g)	Fat Breakdown (g)		
											Sat	Mono	Poly
		MIXED DISHES and FAST FOODS—Con.											
		SANDWICHES—con.											
		Ham sandwich:											
12	1279	On rye bread	1 ea	116	55	242	16	25	5	9	1.9	3.2	2.8
12	1151	On white bread, soft	1 ea	122	54	262	16	28	1	9	2.2	3.4	2.7
12	1153	On part whole wheat	1 ea	122	54	256	17	27	3	9	2.0	3.5	2.7
12	1152	On whole wheat	1 ea	136	53	283	18	33	7	10	2.4	3.7	3.0
		Ham & cheese sandwich:											
12	1280	On soft white bread	1 ea	151	51	369	22	29	1	18	7.8	6.0	3.0
12	1282	On part whole wheat bread	1 ea	151	51	363	23	28	3	18	7.6	6.1	3.0
12	1281	On whole wheat	1 ea	165	50	390	25	33	7	19	8.0	6.2	3.3
12	1150	Ham & swiss on rye	1 ea	145	51	350	24	26	5	17	7.0	5.3	3.1
		Ham salad sandwich:											
12	1154	On white bread, soft	1 ea	125	48	345	10	34	1	19	4.8	7.2	5.9
12	1156	On part whole wheat	1 ea	125	48	339	11	33	3	19	4.6	7.3	6.0
12	1155	On whole wheat	1 ea	139	47	366	12	38	7	20	5.0	7.5	6.2
12	1157	Patty melt sandwich: ground beef & cheese on rye	1 ea	177	45	567	32	25	5	38	14.1	13.9	6.5
		Peanut butter & jam sandwich:											
12	1158	On soft white bread	1 ea	100	27	347	12	45	3	15	2.8	6.8	4.3
12	1160	On part whole wheat	1 ea	100	27	341	12	44	5	15	2.5	6.9	4.3
12	1159	On whole wheat	1 ea	114	29	368	14	50	9	16	3.0	7.1	4.6
12	1161	Reuben sandwich, grilled: corned beef, swiss cheese, sauerkraut on rye	1 ea	233	61	480	28	29	7	28	10.2	10.0	6.2
		Roast beef sandwich:											
12	713	On a bun	1 ea	150	52	345	22	34	1	13	4	7	2
12	1162	On soft white bread	1 ea	122	51	286	17	28	1	11	2.5	3.7	4.4
12	1164	On part whole-wheat bread	1 ea	122	51	280	18	27	3	11	2.3	3.8	4.4
12	1163	On whole wheat bread	1 ea	136	50	307	19	32	7	12	2.7	3.9	4.7
		Tuna salad sandwich:											
12	1165	On soft white	1 ea	116	47	309	13	32	2	14	2.6	4.1	6.6
12	1167	On part whole-wheat bread	1 ea	116	47	303	14	31	3	14	2.4	4.2	6.7
12	1166	On whole-wheat bread	1 ea	130	47	331	15	37	8	15	2.8	4.4	6.9
		Turkey sandwich:											
12	1168	On soft white bread	1 ea	122	52	277	18	28	1	10	2.1	3.2	4.5
12	1170	On part whole wheat	1 ea	122	52	271	18	26	3	11	1.9	3.3	4.5
12	1169	On whole wheat	1 ea	136	51	298	20	32	7	11	2.3	3.4	4.8
		Turkey ham sandwich:											
12	1272	On rye bread	1 ea	116	55	239	15	25	5	9	1.9	2.6	3.3
12	1273	On soft white bread	1 ea	122	55	259	16	29	1	9	2.2	2.8	3.2
12	1275	On part whole wheat	1 ea	122	54	253	16	28	3	9	2.0	2.9	3.2
12	1274	On whole wheat	1 ea	136	53	281	18	33	7	10	2.4	3.1	3.5
12	714	Taco, corn tortilla, beef filling	1 ea	78	52	207	14	10	1	13	5	5	2
		Tostada:											
12	1114	With refried beans	1 ea	157	69	212	10	26	7	9	3.6	2.5	2.3
12	1118	With beans & beef	1 ea	192	67	332	18	20	4	21	9.4	7.2	2.6
12	1354	With beans & chicken	1 ea	157	67	249	19	19	4	11	4.4	3.5	2.9
		Vegetarian Foods:											
12	1175	Nuteena	1 ea	34	52	89	7	3	1	6	—	—	—
12	1171	Proteena	1 pce	67	58	160	8	5	1	12	—	—	—
12	1172	Redi-burger	1 pce	71	56	140	17	5	2	6	—	—	—
12	1173	Vege-Burger	1 pce	68	57	130	14	5	1	6	—	—	—
12	1174	Breakfast links	.5 c	108	73	110	22	4	1	1	—	—	—

GRP KEY: 1 = BEV   2 = DAIRY   3 = EGGS   4 = FAT/OIL   5 = FRUIT   6 = BAKERY   7 = GRAIN   8 = FISH   9 = BEEF   10 = POULTRY
11 = SAUSAGE   12 = MIXED/FAST   13 = NUTS/SEEDS   14 = SWEETS   15 = VEG/LEG   16 = MISC   22 = SOUP/SAUCE

Chol (mg)	Calc (mg)	Iron (mg)	Magn (mg)	Phos (mg)	Pota (mg)	Sodi (mg)	Zinc (mg)	VT-A (RE)	Thia (mg)	Ribo (mg)	Niac (mg)	V-B6 (mg)	Fola (µg)	VT-C (mg)
29	49	1.94	25	203	311	1261	1.91	4	.74	.30	4.50	.32	23	14
29	80	2.17	25	191	271	1199	1.50	4	.80	.31	4.94	.29	23	14
29	79	2.52	39	234	287	1213	1.74	4	.80	.32	5.36	.33	29	14
29	59	2.96	78	313	333	1355	2.33	4	.79	.29	5.52	.40	44	14
56	256	2.28	31	405	318	1610	2.44	88	.81	.42	4.96	.31	26	14
56	256	2.64	45	447	334	1624	2.69	88	.81	.42	5.38	.35	31	14
56	236	3.07	84	526	379	1766	3.27	88	.79	.39	5.54	.42	46	14
55	325	1.99	35	376	342	1336	3.03	77	.75	.40	4.52	.34	25	14
27	77	2.00	18	134	156	887	1.02	19	.52	.25	3.36	.11	21	4
27	77	2.36	32	177	172	901	1.26	19	.52	.25	3.78	.15	26	4
27	57	2.79	71	256	217	1043	1.85	19	.51	.22	3.94	.22	41	4
107	228	3.33	40	423	410	923	6.63	139	.25	.45	6.08	.31	26	<1
0	83	2.23	55	153	246	403	1.06	1	.30	.21	5.39	.12	42	<1
0	82	2.59	69	195	262	417	1.30	1	.30	.21	5.81	.16	47	<1
0	62	3.02	108	274	308	559	1.89	1	.28	.18	5.97	.23	62	<1
85	358	5.20	44	328	313	1642	4.55	133	.25	.43	3.80	.24	27	12
55	60	4.04	38	222	338	757	3.66	32	.39	.33	6.02	.28	42	2
30	80	2.86	23	157	298	757	2.63	8	.31	.29	5.10	.21	23	<1
30	79	3.22	37	200	314	771	2.87	8	.31	.29	5.52	.25	29	<1
30	59	3.65	76	279	359	912	3.46	8	.29	.26	5.68	.32	44	<1
25	80	2.27	23	133	199	559	.65	22	.28	.21	5.43	.14	30	2
25	80	2.63	37	176	215	573	.89	22	.28	.22	5.85	.19	36	2
25	60	3.06	76	255	260	715	1.48	22	.26	.19	6.01	.25	51	2
29	76	1.87	23	192	223	1151	1.00	8	.29	.24	6.82	.23	23	<1
29	76	2.23	37	235	239	1165	1.24	8	.28	.24	7.24	.27	28	<1
29	56	2.66	77	314	285	1307	1.83	8	.27	.21	7.40	.34	43	<1
35	50	3.04	27	214	273	986	2.37	4	.25	.32	4.46	.21	24	0
35	81	3.28	26	203	233	924	1.96	5	.31	.34	4.90	.18	24	<1
35	80	3.63	40	245	249	938	2.20	5	.30	.34	5.32	.23	29	<1
35	60	4.06	80	324	295	1080	2.79	5	.29	.31	5.48	.29	44	<1
45	85	1.29	23	141	183	141	2.89	27	.03	.13	2.49	.16	13	1
15	177	1.93	62	195	422	618	1.55	74	.06	.14	.85	1.01	47	6
62	186	2.16	52	247	442	483	3.57	132	.08	.24	2.94	.67	37	6
53	162	1.69	48	242	358	474	1.94	81	.07	.19	4.53	.73	34	3
<1	11	1.96	—	—	43	203	—	<1	1.65	.17	3.77	.20	—	<1
0	21	1.20	40	111	200	120	.87	10	.47	.58	.14	.45	60	—
0	22	1.60	31	99	280	460	1.20	26	.64	.50	7.80	.50	23	—
0	19	1.40	13	56	120	370	1.20	10	.60	.40	6.70	.80	17	—
0	32	2.70	24	105	110	190	1.10	10	.53	.68	5.00	.56	27	—

(For purposes of calculations, use "0" for t, <1, <.1, <.01, etc.)

607

Table C–1   Food Composition

Grp	Ref	Food Description	Measure	Wt (g)	H₂O (%)	Ener (kcal)	Prot (g)	Carb (g)	Dietary Fiber (g)	Fat (g)	Fat Breakdown (g)		
											Sat	Mono	Poly
NUTS, SEEDS and PRODUCTS													
		Almonds:											
13	1365	Dry roasted, salted	1 c	138	3	810	23	33	18	71	6.8	46.2	15.0
13	718	Slivered, packed, unsalted	1 c	135	4	795	27	28	15[88]	70	7	46	15
		Whole, dried, unsalted:											
13	719	Cup	1 c	142	4	837	28	29	17[88]	74	7	48	16
13	720	Ounce	1 oz	28	4	167	6	6	3[88]	15	1	10	3
13	721	Almond butter	1 tbsp	16	1	101	2	3	1	9	1	6	2
13	722	Brazil nuts, dry (about 7)	1 oz	28	3	186	4	4	3	19	5	7	7
		Cashew nuts:											
		Dry roasted, salted:											
13	723	Cup	1 c	137	2	787	21	45	8	63	13	37	11
13	724	Ounce	1 oz	28	2	163	4	9	2	13	3	8	2
		Oil roasted, salted:											
13	725	Cup	1 c	130	4	748	21	37	8	63	12	37	11
13	726	Ounce	1 oz	28	4	163	5	8	2	14	3	8	2
		Dry roasted, unsalted											
13	1366	Dry roasted	1 c	137	2	787	21	45	8	64	12.6	37.4	10.7
13	1367	Oil roasted	1 c	130	4	748	21	37	8	63	12.4	36.9	10.6
13	727	Cashew butter	1 tbsp	16	3	94	3	4	1	8	2	5	1
13	728	European chestnuts, roasted, 1 c = approx 17 kernels	1 c	143	40	350	5	76	19	3	.6	1.1	1.2
		Coconut:											
		Raw											
13	729	Piece 2 × 2 × ½″	1 pce	45	47	159	2	7	5	15	13	.6	.2
13	730	Shredded/grated[94]	1 c	80	47	283	3	12	9	27	24	1	.3
		Dried, shredded/grated:											
13	731	Unsweetened	1 c	78	3	515	5	19	12	50	45	2	.6
13	732	Sweetened	1 c	93	16	466	3	44	9	33	29	1	.4
		Filberts (hazelnuts), chopped:											
13	733	Cup	1 c	115	5	727	15	18	7	72	5	57	7
13	734	Ounce	1 oz	28	5	179	4	4	2	18	1	14	2
		Macadamia nuts, oil roasted:											
		Salted:											
13	735	Cup	1 c	134	2	962	10	17	7	103	15	81	2
13	736	Ounce	1 oz	28	2	204	2	4	1	22	3	17	.4
13	1368	Unsalted	1 c	134	2	962	10	17	7	103	15.4	80.9	1.8
		Mixed nuts:											
13	737	Dry roasted, salted	1 c	137	2	814	24	35	12	70	10	43	15
13	738	Oil roasted, salted	1 c	142	2	876	24	30	13	80	12	45	19
13	1369	Oil roasted, unsalted	1 c	142	2	876	24	30	13	80	12.4	45.0	18.9

[88]Values reported for dietary fiber in almonds vary from 7.0 to 14.3g/100 g
[94]1 c packed = 130 g.

GRP KEY: 1 = BEV 2 = DAIRY 3 = EGGS 4 = FAT/OIL 5 = FRUIT 6 = BAKERY 7 = GRAIN 8 = FISH 9 = BEEF 10 = POULTRY
11 = SAUSAGE 12 = MIXED/FAST 13 = NUTS/SEEDS 14 = SWEETS 15 = VEG/LEG 16 = MISC 22 = SOUP/SAUCE

Chol (mg)	Calc (mg)	Iron (mg)	Magn (mg)	Phos (mg)	Pota (mg)	Sodi (mg)	Zinc (mg)	VT-A (RE)	Thia (mg)	Ribo (mg)	Niac (mg)	V-B6 (mg)	Fola (µg)	VT-C (mg)
0	389	5.25	419	756	1063	1076	6.76	0	.18	.83	3.89	.10	88	1
0	359	4.94	400	702	988	15	3.94	0	.28	1.05	4.54	.15	79	1
0	378	5.20	420	738	1034	15[89]	4.15	0	.30	1.11	4.77	.16	83	1
0	75	1.04	84	147	208	3[89]	.83	0	.06	.22	.96	.03	17	<1
0	43	.59	49	84	121	2[90]	.49	0	.02	.1	.46	.01	0	<1
0	50	.97	64	170	170	<1	1.30	t	.28	.04	.46	.07	1	<1
0	62	8.22	356	671	774	877[91]	7.67	0	.27	.27	1.92	.35	95	0
0	13	1.70	74	139	160	181[91]	1.59	0	.06	.06	.4	.07	20	0
0	53	5.33	332	554	689	814[92]	6.18	0	.55	.23	2.34	.33	88	0
0	12	1.16	72	121	151	177[92]	1.35	0	.12	.05	.51	.07	19	0
0	62	8.22	356	671	774	21	7.67	0	.27	.27	1.92	.35	95	0
0	53	5.33	332	554	689	22	6.18	0	.55	.23	2.34	.33	88	0
0	7	.09	41	73	87	2[93]	.83	0	.05	.03	.26	.04	11	0
0	42	1.30	47	153	846	3	.82	4	.35	.25	1.92	.71	100	37
0	6	1.09	14	51	160	9	.50	0	.03	.01	.24	.02	12	2
0	12	1.94	26	90	285	16	.88	0	.05	.02	.43	.04	21	3
0	20	2.59	70	161	423	29	1.57	0	.05	.08	.47	2.34	7	1
0	14	1.79	47	100	313	244	1.69	0	.03	.02	.44	.29	9	1
0	216	3.76	328	359	512	3	2.76	8	.57	.13	1.31	.7	83	1
0	53	.93	81	89	126	1	.68	2	.14	.03	.32	.17	20	<1
0	60	2.41	157	268	441	348[95]	1.47	1	.28	.15	2.71	.33	79	0
0	13	.51	33	57	94	74[95]	.31	<1	.06	.03	.57	.07	17	0
0	60	2.41	157	268	441	9	1.47	1	.28	.15	2.71	.33	79	0
0	96	5.07	308	596	817	917[96]	5.21	2	.27	.27	6.44	.41	69	1
0	153	4.56	334	659	825	926[96]	7.22	3	.71	.32	7.19	.34	118	1
0	153	4.56	334	659	825	16	7.22	3	.71	.32	7.19	.34	118	1

[89] Salted almonds contain 1108 mg sodium per cup, 221 mg/oz.
[90] Salted almond butter contains 72 mg sodium per tablespoon.
[91] Dry-roasted cashews without salt contain 21 mg sodium per cup, or 4 mg/oz.
[92] Oil-roasted cashews without salt contain 22 mg sodium per cup, or 5 mg/oz.
[93] Salted cashew butter contains 98 mg sodium per tablespoon.
[95] Macadamia nuts without salt contain 9 mg sodium per cup, or 2 mg/oz.
[96] Mixed nuts without salt contain about 15 mg sodium per cup.

(For purposes of calculations, use "0" for t, <1, <.1, <.01, etc.)

Table C–1 Food Composition

Grp	Ref	Food Description	Measure	Wt (g)	H$_2$O (%)	Ener (kcal)	Prot (g)	Carb (g)	Dietary Fiber (g)	Fat (g)	Fat Breakdown (g) Sat	Mono	Poly
NUTS, SEEDS and PRODUCTS—Con.													
		Peanuts:											
		Oil roasted, salted:											
13	739	Cup	1 c	145	2	841	39	27	13	71	10	36	23
13	740	Ounce	1 oz	28	2	165	8	5	2	14	2	7	4
13	1370	Oil roasted, unsalted	1 c	145	2	841	39	27	13	71	9.9	35.5	22.6
		Dried, unsalted:											
13	741	Cup	1 c	146	7	827	38	24	13	72	10	36	23
13	742	Ounce	1 oz	28	7	161	7	5	3	14	2	7	4
13	743	Peanut butter	1 tbsp	16	2	95	5	3	1	8	1.4	4.0	2.3
		Pecans, halves:											
		Dried, unsalted:											
13	744	Cup	1 c	108	5	720	8	20	7[99]	73	6	46	18
13	745	Ounce	1 oz	28	5	190	2	5	2[99]	19	1.5	12	5
13	1372	Dry roasted, salted	¼ c	28.4	1	187	2	6	2	18	1.5	11.5	4.6
13	746	Pine nuts/piñons, dried	1 oz	28	6	161	3	5	2	17	3	7	7
		Pistachio nuts:											
13	747	Dried, shelled	1 oz	28	4	164	6	7	1	14	2	9	2
13	1373	Dry roasted, salted, shelled	1 c	128	2	776	19	35	14	68	8.6	45.7	10.3
		Pumpkin kernals											
13	748	Dried, unsalted	1 oz	28	7	154	7	5	2	13	2.5	4	6
13	1374	Roasted, salted	1 c	227	7	1185	75	31	9	96	18.1	29.7	43.6
13	749	Sesame seeds, hulled, dried	¼ c	38	5	221	10	4	6	21	3	8	9
		Sunflower seed kernels:											
13	750	Dry	¼ c	36	5	205	8	7	2	18	2	3	12
13	751	Oil roasted	¼ c	34	3	208	7	5	2	19	2	4	13
13	752	Tahini (sesame butter)	1 tbsp	15	3	91	3	3	2	8	1	3	4
		Black walnuts, chopped:											
13	753	Cup	1 c	125	4	759	30	15	7	71	5	16	47
13	754	Ounce	1 oz	28	4	172	7	3	2	16	1	4	11
		English walnuts, chopped:											
13	755	Cup	1 c	120	4	770	17	22	7	74	7	17	47
13	756	Ounce	1 oz	28	4	182	4	5	2	18	2	4	11
SWEETENERS and SWEETS: see also Dairy (milk desserts) and Baked Goods													
14	757	Apple butter	2 tbsp	35	52	66	<1	17	<1	<1	.1	<.1	.1
14	1124	Butterscotch topping	3 tbsp	50	31	156	1	40	0	<1	—	—	—
		Cake frosting:											
14	1127	Canned, average of all types	2.5 tbsp	39	15	160	0	24	0	7	1.7	2.9	1.7
14	1123	Prepared from mix	2.5 tbsp	39	15	167	0	28	0	6	—	—	—
		Candy:											
14	1128	Almond Joy® candy bar	1 oz	28.4	7	151	2	19	<1	8	6.7	.6	.1
14	758	Caramel, plain or chocolate	1 oz	28	8	115	1	22	<1	3	2.2	.3	.1

[99] Dietary fiber data calculated/derived from data on other nuts.

GRP KEY: 1 = BEV 2 = DAIRY 3 = EGGS 4 = FAT/OIL 5 = FRUIT 6 = BAKERY 7 = GRAIN 8 = FISH 9 = BEEF 10 = POULTRY 11 = SAUSAGE 12 = MIXED/FAST 13 = NUTS/SEEDS 14 = SWEETS 15 = VEG/LEG 16 = MISC 22 = SOUP/SAUCE

Chol (mg)	Calc (mg)	Iron (mg)	Magn (mg)	Phos (mg)	Pota (mg)	Sodi (mg)	Zinc (mg)	VT-A (RE)	Thia (mg)	Ribo (mg)	Niac (mg)	V-B6 (mg)	Fola (μg)	VT-C (mg)
0	125	2.78	273	734	1020	626[97]	9.6	0	.43	.15	21.5	.58	153	0
0	24	.54	53	144	200	123[97]	1.88	0	.08	.03	4.20	.11	30	0
0	125	2.78	2.73	734	1020	22	9.60	0	.43	1.46	21.5	.58	153	0
0	85	4.72	263	559	1047	23	4.78	0	.97	.19	20.7	.43	153	0
0	17	.92	51	109	204	5	.93	0	.19	.04	4.02	.08	30	0
0	5	.29	28	60	110	75[98]	.47	0	.02	.02	2.15	.06	13	2
0	39	2.30	138	314	423	1[100]	5.91	14	.92	.14	.96	.20	42	1
0	10	.61	36	83	111	<1	1.55	4	.24	.04	.25	.05	11	1
0	10	.62	38	86	105	221	1.61	4	.09	.04	.26	.05	12	1
0	2	.87	67	10	178	20	1.22	1	.35	.06	1.24	.08	19	<1
0	38	1.93	45	143	310	2[101]	.38	7	.22	.05	.31	.06	17	<1
0	90	4.06	166	609	1242	998	1.74	30	.54	.32	1.80	.27	74	0
0	12	4.25	152	333	229	5[102]	2.12	11	.06	.09	.50	.03	26	<1
0	98	33.9	1212	2600	1830	1305	16.9	88	.25	.66	3.60	.20	115	0
0	49	2.93	130	291	153	15	2.23	<1	.27	.03	1.76	.30	38	0
0	42	2.44	128	254	248	1	1.82	2	.83	.10	1.62	.46	85	<1
0	19	2.26	43	385	163	205[103]	1.76	2	.11	.10	1.40	.40	79	<1
0	21	.83	53	119	69	5	1.57	1	.24	.02	.85	.06	15	1
0	73	3.84	253	580	655	1	4.28	37	.27	.14	.86	.70	83	1
0	16	.87	57	132	149	0	.97	8	.06	.03	.20	.16	19	<1
0	113	2.93	203	380	602	12	3.28	15	.46	.18	1.25	.67	79	4
0	27	.69	48	90	142	3	.78	4	.11	.04	.30	.16	19	1
0	5	.25	2	13	89	1	.01	0	<.01	.01	.08	.01	<1	1
0	24	.10	3	23	34	111	—	<1	0	.04	0	—	—	0
0	—	—	—	—	—	91	—	0	—	—	—	—	—	—
0	—	—	—	—	—	84	—	0	—	—	—	—	—	—
0	2	.78	—	—	—	—	—	0	—	—	—	—	—	—
1	42	.4	6	35	54	64	.15	<1	.01	.05	.1	<.01	0	t

[97] Peanuts without salt contain 22 mg sodium per cup, or 4 mg/oz.
[98] Peanut butter without added salt contains 3 mg sodium per tablespoon.
[100] Salted pecans contain 816 mg sodium per cup, or 214 mg/oz.
[101] Salted pistachios contain approx 221 mg sodium per ounce.
[102] Salted pumpkin/squash kernels contain approximately 163 mg sodium per ounce.
[103] Unsalted sunflower seeds contain 1 mg sodium per ¼ cup.

(For purposes of calculations, use "0" for t, <1, <.1, <.01, etc.)

Table C–1 Food Composition

Grp	Ref	Food Description	Measure	Wt (g)	H₂O (%)	Ener (kcal)	Prot (g)	Carb (g)	Dietary Fiber (g)	Fat (g)	Fat Breakdown (g)		
											Sat	Mono	Poly
		SWEETENERS and SWEETS—Con.											
		Candy—con.											
		Chocolate (see also, #784, 785, 971):											
		Milk chocolate:											
14	759	Plain	1 oz	28	1	145	2	16	1	9	5.4	3	.3
14	760	With almonds	1 oz	28	2	150	3	15	1	10	4.4	4.7	1.0
14	761	With peanuts	1 oz	28	1	155	5	10	2	12	3.5	5.2	2.7
14	762	With rice cereal	1 oz	28	2	140	2	18	1	7	4.4	2.5	.2
14	763	Semisweet chocolate chips	1 c	170	1	860	7	97	5	61	36	20	2
14	764	Sweet dark chocolate	1 oz	28	1	150	1	16	1	10	5.9	3.3	.3
14	1133	English toffee candy bar	1 ea	32	2	220	1	11	<1	19	—	—	—
14	765	Fondant candy, uncoated(mints, candy corn, other)	1 oz	28	3	105	0	27	0	0	0	0	0
14	766	Fudge, chocolate	1 oz	28	8	115	1	21	2	3	2.1	1	.1
14	767	Gum drops	1 oz	28	12	98	0	25	0	<1	t	t	.1
14	768	Hard candy, all flavors	1 oz	28	1	109	0	28	0	0	0	0	0
14	769	Jelly beans	1 oz	28	6	104	t	26	0	<.1	t	t	.1
14	1134	M&M's Plain choc. candies®	48 grm	48	1	237	3	33	<1	10	—	—	—
14	1135	M&M's Peanut choc candies®	47 grm	47.3	2	240	5	28	1	12	—	—	—
14	1130	MARS® bar	1 ea	50	7	240	4	30	1	11	4.8	4.4	.8
14	1129	MILKY WAY® candy bar	1 ea	60	7	260	3	43	<1	9	5.4	3.0	.3
14	1132	REESE's® peanut butter cup	2 ea	45	4	240	6	22	2	14	—	—	—
14	1131	SNICKERS® candy bar, 2.2oz size	1 ea	61.2	7	290	7	37	2	14	—	—	—
14	1125	Caramel topping	3 tbsp	50	31	155	1	39	<1	—	—	—	—
14	771	Gelatin salad/dessert	½ c	120	84	70	2	17	<1	0	0	0	0
		Honey:											
14	772	Cup	1 c	339	17	1030	1	279	0	0	0	0	0
14	773	Tablespoon	1 tbsp	21	17	65	<.1	17	0	0	0	0	0
		Jams or preserves:											
14	774	Tablespoon	1 tbsp	20	29	54	<1	14	<1	<.1	0	t	t
14	775	Packet	1 ea	14	29	38	<.1	10	<1	<.1	0	t	t
		Jellies:											
14	776	Tablespoon	1 tbsp	18	28	49	<.1	13	<1	<.1	t	t	t
14	777	Packet	1 ea	14	28	39	<.1	10	<1	<.1	t	t	t
14	1136	Marmalade	1 tbsp	20	29	52	<1	14	<1	0	0	0	0
14	770	Marshmallows	4 ea	28	17	90	t	23	0	0	0	0	0
14	1126	Marshmallow creme topping	3 tbsp	50	20	158	<1	40	0	0	0	0	0
14	778	Popsicles, 3 oz when fluid	1 ea	95	80	70	0	18	0	0	0	0	0
		Sugars:											
14	779	Brown sugar	1 c	220	2	820	0	212	0	0	0	0	0
		White sugar, granulated:											
14	780	Cup	1 c	200	1	770	0	199	0	0	0	0	0
14	781	Tablespoon	1 tbsp	12	1	45	0	12	0	0	0	0	0
14	782	Packet	1 ea	6	1	25	0	6	0	0	0	0	0
14	783	White sugar, powdered, sifted	1 c	100	<1	385	0	99	0	0	0	0	0
		Syrups:											
		Chocolate:											
14	784	Thin type	2 tbsp	38	37	85	1	22	1	<1	.2	.1	.1
14	785	Fudge type	2 tbsp	38	25	125	2	21	1	5	3	2	.2
14	786	Molasses, blackstrap [104]	2 tbsp	40	24	85	0	22	0	0	0	0	0
14	787	Pancake table syrup (corn and maple)	¼ c	84	25	244	0	64	0	0	0	0	0

[104] Light molasses would contain about 66 mg calcium, 2.1 mg iron, 18 mg magnesium, and 366 mg potassium for 2 tbsp.

Chol (mg)	Calc (mg)	Iron (mg)	Magn (mg)	Phos (mg)	Pota (mg)	Sodi (mg)	Zinc (mg)	VT-A (RE)	Thia (mg)	Ribo (mg)	Niac (mg)	V-B6 (mg)	Fola (μg)	VT-C (mg)
6	50	.4	16	61	96	23	.37	10	.02	.1	.1	.02	<1	t
5	61	.56	33	77	125	23	.48	8	.03	.13	.31	.02	4	t
3	32	.68	35	87	155	19	.68	8	.11	.07	2.2	.05	16	t
6	48	.2	13	57	100	46	.29	8	.01	.08	.1	.01	<1	t
0	51	5.8	230	178	593	24	2.39	3	.1	.14	.9	.04	22	t
0	7	.6	32	41	86	5	.42	1	.01	.04	.1	.01	5	t
0	0	.20	—	0	50	90	—	5	.53	.05	.10	.04	—	0
0	2	.1	—	2	1	57	.1	0	<.01	<.01	.01	.01	0	0
1	22	.3	14	24	42	54	.16	16	.01	.03	.1	.01	2	t
0	2	.1	—	—	1	10	0	5	0	<.01	.01	0	0	0
0	6	.1	<1	2	1	7	0	0	0	0	0	0	0	0
0	1	.30	—	1	11	7	0	0	0	<.01	.01	—	0	0
0	79	.76	30	65	171	41	.57	13	.03	.12	.27	.01	5	—
0	59	.67	38	64	162	29	.66	<1	.03	.09	1.48	.03	5	—
0	85	.55	37	63	176	85	.59	<1	.02	.16	.48	.01	5	—
14	86	.49	22	80	167	140	.45	25	.03	.15	.20	.01	7	1
3	35	.68	47	87	168	92	.69	8	.03	.05	2.12	.06	17	—
0	70	.49	39	75	209	170	.69	5	.03	.11	1.84	.02	6	—
0	28	.10	3	23	33	152	—	<1	0	.05	0	—	—	0
0	2	.10	<1	23	91	55	.03	0	.01	.01	.20	<.01	0	0
0	17	1.70	7	20	173	17	.40	0	.02	.14	1.0	.06	32	3
0	1	.11	<1	1	11	1	.02	0	<.01	.01	.06	<.01	2	<1
0	4	.20	1	2	18	2	.01	t	<.01	.01	.04	<.01	2	<1
0	3	.14	<1	1	13	1	<.01	t	<.01	.01	.03	<.01	1	<1
0	2	.12	<1	1	16	4	0	t	<.01	<.01	.04	<.01	2	1
0	1	.09	<1	1	12	3	0	t	<.01	<.01	.03	<.01	2	1
0	7	.12	1	3	123	4	—	1	—	—	—	<.01	1	2
0	1	.45	1	2	2	25	<.01	0	0	<.01	.01	<.01	0	0
0	16	—	—	6	16	29	—	0	—	—	—	—	—	5
0	0	.01	—	0	4	11	0	0	0	0	0	0	0	0
0	187	4.80	135	56	757	97	.08	0	.02	.07	.20	0	0	0
0	3	.10	<1	.1	7	5	.04	0	0	0	0	0	0	0
0	<1	.01	<1	t	t	t	<.01	0	0	0	0	0	0	0
0	<1	<.01	<1	t	t	t	<.01	0	0	0	0	0	0	0
0	0	.08	<1	0	4	2	<.01	0	0	0	0	0	0	0
0	6	.75	26	49	85	36	.39	1	.02	.02	.11	<.01	3	0
0	38	.50	18	60	82	42	.39	13	.08	.08	.08	<.01	3	0
0	274[104]	10.1[104]	103[104]	34	1171[104]	38	0	0	.08	.08	.80	.11	6	0
0	2	.06	2	8	14	38	.08	0	0	0	0	t	<1	0

[104] Light molasses would contain about 66 mg calcium, 2.1 mg iron, 18 mg magnesium, and 366 mg potassium for 2 tbsp.

(For purposes of calculations, use "0" for t, <1, <.1, <.01, etc.)

Table C–1   Food Composition

Grp	Ref	Food Description	Measure	Wt (g)	H₂O (%)	Ener (kcal)	Prot (g)	Carb (g)	Dietary Fiber (g)	Fat (g)	Fat Breakdown (g)		
											Sat	Mono	Poly
VEGETABLES AND LEGUMES													
15	788	Alfalfa seeds, sprouted	1 c	33	91	10	1	1	1	<1	t	t	.1
15	789	Artichokes, cooked globe (300 g with refuse)	1 ea	120	87	53	3	12	10	<1	<.1	t	.1
		Artichoke hearts:											
15	1177	Cooked from frozen	9 oz	240	87	108	7	22	18	1	.3	<.1	.5
15	1176	Marinated	6 oz	170	59	168	4	13	11	14	2.0	3.0	7.7
		Asparagus, green, cooked:											
		From raw:											
15	790	Cuts and tips	½ c	90	92	23	2	4	2	<1	.1	t	.1
15	791	Spears, ½″ diam at base	4 spears	60	92	15	2	3	1	<1	<.1	t	.1
		From frozen:											
15	792	Cuts and tips	1 c	180	91	50	5	9	3	1	.2	t	.3
15	793	Spears, ½″ diam at base	4 spears	60	91	17	2	3	1	<1	.1	t	.1
15	794	Canned, spears, ½″ diam at base	4 spears	80	95	11	2	2	1	1	.1	t	.2
15	795	Bamboo shoots, canned, drained slices	1 c	131	94	25	2	4	3	1	.1	t	.2
		Beans (see also Great northern, #855; Kidney beans, #860; Navy beans, #876; Pinto beans, #898; Refried beans, #921; Soybeans, #925):											
15	796	Black beans, cooked	1 c	172	66	227	15	41	15	1	.2	.1	.4
		Lima beans:											
15	797	Thick seeded (Fordhooks), cooked from frozen	½ c	85	74	85	5	16	5	<1	.1	t	.1
15	798	Thin seeded (baby), cooked from frozen	½ c	90	72	94	6	18	8	<1	.1	t	.1
15	799	Cooked from dry, drained	1 c	188	70	217	15	39	18	1	.2	.1	.3
		Snap beans/green beans, cuts and french style:											
15	800	Cooked from raw	1 c	125	89	44	2	10	3	<1	.1	t	.2
15	801	Cooked from frozen	1 c	135	92	36	2	8	4	<1	<.1	t	.1
15	802	Canned, drained	1 c	136	93	26	2	6	2	<1	<.1	t	.1
		Navy beans, canned:											
15	803	Beans w/pork and tomato sauce	1 c	253	73	247	13	49	14	3	1.0	1.1	.3
15	804	Beans w/pork and sweet sauce	1 c	253	71	282	13	53	14	4	1.4	1.6	.5
15	805	Beans with frankfurters	1 c	257	70	366	17	40	18	17	6	7	2
		Bean sprouts (mung):											
15	806	Raw	1 c	104	90	31	3	6	3	<1	<.1	t	.1
15	807	Cooked, stir fried	1 c	124	84	62	5	13	3	<1	<.1	.1	.1
15	808	Cooked, boiled, drained	1 c	124	93	26	3	5	3	<1	<.1	t	<.1
		Beets:											
		Cooked from fresh:											
15	809	Sliced or diced	½ c	85	91	26	1	6	2	<.1	t	t	t
15	810	Whole beets, 2″ diam	2 beets	100	91	31	1	7	2	<.1	t	t	t

614

Chol (mg)	Calc (mg)	Iron (mg)	Magn (mg)	Phos (mg)	Pota (mg)	Sodi (mg)	Zinc (mg)	VT-A (RE)	Thia (mg)	Ribo (mg)	Niac (mg)	V-B6 (mg)	Fola (μg)	VT-C (mg)
0	11	.32	9	23	26	2	.30	5	.03	.04	.16	.01	12	3
0	47	1.62	47	72	316	79	.43	17	.07	.06	.71	.1	53	9
0	50	1.34	74	146	634	127	.86	39	.15	.38	2.20	.21	285	12
0	39	1.62	48	102	438	900	.54	28	.06	.17	1.38	.15	149	52
0	22	.59	17	55	279	4	.43	75	.09	.11	.95	.13	88	25
0	14	.4	11	37	186	2	.29	50	.06	.07	.63	.09	59	16
0	41	1.15	23	99	392	7	1.01	147	.12	.19	1.87	.16	176	44
0	14	.38	8	33	131	2	.34	49	.04	.06	.62	.06	59	15
0	11	.5	8	30	122	278[105]	.32	38	.05	.07	.7	.04	69	13
0	10	.42	6	33	105	9	.30	1	.03	.03	.18	—	40	1
0	47	3.60	121	241	611	1	1.92	1	.42	.10	.87	.12	256	0
0	19	1.16	29	54	347	45	.37	16	.06	.05	.91	.10	55	11
0	25	1.76	50	101	370	26	.50	15	.06	.05	.69	.10	58	5
0	32	4.50	82	208	955	4	1.79	0	.30	.10	.79	.30	156	0
0	58	1.60	32	48	373	4	.45	83[106]	.09	.12	.77	.07	42	12
0	61	1.11	29	33	151	17	.84	71[107]	.07	.10	.56	.08	42	11
0	36	1.22	18	26	147	339[108]	.39	47[109]	.02	.08	.27	.05	43	6
17	141	8.30	88	297	759	1113	2.60	31	.13	.12	1.26	.18	57	8
17	155	4.20	87	266	673	849	3.80	29	.12	.15	.89	.22	95	8
15	123	4.45	71	267	604	1105	4.79	40	.15	.14	2.32	.12	77	6
0	14	.95	22	56	154	6	.43	2	.09	.13	.78	.09	63	14
0	16	2.40	38	70	200	14	1.12	3	.17	.22	1.49	.10	72	20
0	15	.81	18	34	125	12	.58	2	.06	.13	1.01	.05	35	14
0	9	.53	31	26	266	42	.21	1	.03	.01	.23	.03	49	5
0	11	.62	37	31	312	49	.25	1	.03	.01	.27	.03	86	6

[105] Special dietary pack contains 3 mg sodium
[106] For green varieties; yellow beans contain 10 RE/cup.
[107] For green varieties; yellow beans contain 15 RE.
[108] Dietary pack contains 3 mg sodium.
[109] For green varieties; yellow beans contain 14 RE.

(For purposes of calculations, use "0" for t, <1, <.1, <.01, etc.)

615

Table C–1 Food Composition

Grp	Ref	Food Description	Measure	Wt (g)	H₂O (%)	Ener (kcal)	Prot (g)	Carb (g)	Dietary Fiber (g)	Fat (g)	Fat Breakdown (g)		
											Sat	Mono	Poly
		VEGETABLES and LEGUMES—Con.											
		Beets—con.											
		Canned:											
15	811	Sliced or diced	½ c	85	91	27	1	6	2	<1	t	t	<.1
15	812	Pickled slices	½ c	114	82	74	1	19	2	<1	t	t	<.1
15	813	Beet greens, cooked, drained	1 c	144	89	40	4	8	3	<1	<.1	.1	.1
		Black-eyed peas, cooked:											
15	814	From dry, drained	1 c	171	70	198	13	36	21	1	.2	.1	.4
15	815	From fresh, drained	1 c	165	72	179	13	30	12	1	.3	.1	.6
15	816	From frozen, drained	1 c	170	66	224	14	40	14	1	.3	.1	.5
		Broccoli:											
		Raw:											
15	817	Chopped	1 c	88	91	24	3	5	3	<1	.1	t	.1
15	818	Spears	1 spear	151	91	42	5	8	6	1	.1	<.1	.3
		Broccoli—con.											
		Cooked from raw:											
15	819	Spears	1 spear	180	90	53	5	10	7	<1	.1	<.1	.2
15	820	Chopped	1 c	156	90	46	5	9	6	<1	.1	<.1	.2
		Cooked from frozen:											
15	821	Spear, small piece	1 spear	30	91	8	1	2	1	<.1	t	t	t
15	822	Chopped	1 c	184	91	51	6	10	6	<1	<.1	t	.1
		Brussels sprouts:											
15	823	Cooked from raw	1 c	156	87	60	6	14	6	1	.2	.1	.4
15	824	Cooked from frozen	1 c	155	87	65	6	13	5	1	.1	.1	.3
		Cabbage, common varieties:											
15	825	Raw, shredded or chopped	1 c	70	92	16	1	4	2	<1	t	t	.1
15	826	Cooked, drained	1 c	150	94	32	1	7	4	<1	.1	<.1	.2
		Chinese cabbage:											
15	1178	Bok-choy or Pak-choi, raw, shredded	1 c	70	95	9	1	2	1	<1	t	t	.1
15	827	Bok choy or Pak-choi, cooked, drained	1 c	170	96	20	3	3	3	<1	<.1	t	.1
15	828	Pe-Tsai, raw, chopped	1 c	76	94	11	1	2	2	<1	<.1	t	.1
		Cabbage, red, coarsely chopped:											
15	829	Raw	1 c	70	92	19	1	4	2	<1	t	t	.1
15	830	Cooked	½ c	75	94	16	1	3	4	<1	t	t	.1
15	831	Savoy cabbage, coarsely chopped, raw	1 c	70	91	20	1	4	2	<.1	t	t	<.1
		Carrots:											
		Raw:											
15	832	Whole, 7½ × 1⅛"	1 carrot	72	88	31	1	7	2	<1	t	t	.1
15	833	Grated	½ c	55	88	24	1	6	2	<1	t	t	<.1
		Cooked, sliced, drained:											
15	834	Cooked from raw	½ c	78	87	35	1	8	3	<1	<.1	t	.1
15	835	Cooked from frozen	½ c	73	90	26	1	6	3	<.1	t	t	<.1
15	836	Canned, sliced, drained	½ c	73	93	17	<1	4	1	<1	<.1	t	.1
15	837	Carrot juice	½ c	123	89	49	1	11	2	<1	<.1	t	.1
		Cauliflower:											
15	838	Raw, flowerets	½ c	50	92	12	1	2	1	<.1	t	t	<.1
		Cooked, drained, flowerets:											
15	839	From raw	½ c	62	92	15	1	3	1	<1	t	t	.1
15	840	From frozen	1 c	180	94	34	3	7	3	<1	.1	<.1	.2

Chol (mg)	Calc (mg)	Iron (mg)	Magn (mg)	Phos (mg)	Pota (mg)	Sodi (mg)	Zinc (mg)	VT-A (RE)	Thia (mg)	Ribo (mg)	Niac (mg)	V-B6 (mg)	Fola (μg)	VT-C (mg)
0	13	1.55	13	15	126	233[110]	.18	1	.01	.04	.15	.05	22	4
0	13	.47	17	19	169	301	.30	1	.03	.06	.29	.03	35	3
0	165	2.74	97	58	1308	346	.72	734	.17	.42	.72	.19	47	36
0	42	4.30	91	266	476	6	2.20	3	.35	.1	.85	.17	356	1
0	46	2.36	83	197	693	7	1.30	105	.11	.18	1.8	.08	173	3
0	40	3.60	85	208	638	9	2.42	13	.42	.11	1.24	.16	240	5
0	42	.78	22	58	286	24	.36	136[111]	.06	.10	.56	.14	62	82
0	72	1.33	38	99	490	41	.60	233[111]	.10	.18	.96	.24	107	141
0	205	2.06	108	86	293	20	.55	254[111]	.15	.37	1.36	.36	123	113
0	178	1.78	94	74	254	16	.48	220[111]	.13	.32	1.18	.31	107	98
0	15	.18	6	16	54	7	.09	44[111]	.02	.02	.14	.04	26	12
0	94	1.13	37	101	331	44	.56	272[111]	.10	.15	.84	.24	104	74
0	56	1.88	32	87	491	17	.50	112	.17	.12	.95	.31	94	97
0	38	1.15	37	84	504	36	.55	91	.16	.18	.83	.27	157	71
0	32	.40	10	16	172	12	.12	9	.04	.02	.21	.07	40	33
0	50	.59	23	38	308	29	.24	13	.09	.08	.34	.10	31	36
0	74	.56	13	26	176	<1	.29	210	.03	.05	.35	.07	57	32
0	158	1.77	18	49	630	57	.43	437	.05	.11	.73	.30	32	44
0	59	.23	10	22	181	7	.17	91	.03	.04	.30	.18	60	21
0	36	.35	11	29	144	8	.15	3	.05	.02	.21	.15	19	40
0	28	.27	8	21	105	6	.11	2	.03	.01	.15	.11	9	26
0	25	.28	20	29	161	20	.26	70	.05	.02	.21	.13	32	22
0	19	.36	11	32	233	25	.14	2025	.07	.04	.67	.11	10	7
0	15	.28	8	24	178	19	.11	1547	.05	.03	.51	.08	8	5
0	24	.48	10	24	177	52	.23	1915	.03	.04	.40	.19	11	2
0	21	.35	7	19	115	43	.18	1292	.02	.03	.32	.09	8	2
0	19	.47	6	17	131	176[112]	.19	1006	.01	.02	.40	.08	7	2
0	29	.56	17	51	358	36	.22	3159	.11	.07	.47	.27	5	11
0	14	.29	7	23	178	7	.09	1	.04	.03	.32	.12	33	36
0	17	.26	7	22	200	4	.15	1	.04	.04	.34	.13	32	34
0	31	.74	16	43	250	33	.23	4	.07	.10	.56	.16	74	56

[110]Dietary pack contains 39 mg sodium.

[111]Vitamin A for whole plant: leaves are 1600 RE/100 g raw; flower clusters are 300/100 g raw; stalks are 40 RE/100 g raw.

[112]Dietary pack contains 31 mg sodium.

(For purposes of calculations, use "0" for t, <1, <.1, <.01, etc.)

Table C–1 Food Composition

Grp	Ref	Food Description	Measure	Wt (g)	H₂O (%)	Ener (kcal)	Prot (g)	Carb (g)	Dietary Fiber (g)	Fat (g)	Fat Breakdown (g)		
											Sat	Mono	Poly
		VEGETABLES and LEGUMES—Con.											
		Celery, pascal type, raw:											
15	841	Large outer stalk, 8 × 1½″ (at root end)	1 stalk	40	95	6	<1	1	1	<.1	t	t	t
15	842	Diced	½ c	60	95	10	<1	2	1	<.1	t	t	<.1
		Chard, swiss:											
15	1179	Raw, chopped	1 c	36	93	7	1	1	1	<1	t	t	<.1
15	1180	Cooked	1 c	175	93	35	3	7	4	<1	<.1	t	.1
		Chick-peas (see Garbanzo, #854)											
		Collards, cooked, drained:											
15	843	From raw	1 c	145	96	20	2	4	4	<1	.1	<.1	.1
15	844	From frozen	1 c	170	88	61	5	12	5	1	.1	.1	.4
		Corn:											
		Cooked, drained:											
15	845	From raw, on cob, 5″ long	1 ear	77	70	83	3	19	3	1	.2	.3	.5
15	846	From frozen, on cob, 3½″ long	1 ear	63	73	59	2	14	3	<1	.1	.1	.2
15	847	Kernels, cooked from frozen	½ c	82	76	67	2	17	3	<.1	t	t	<.1
		Canned:											
15	848	Cream style	½ c	128	79	93	2	23	2	<1	.1	.2	.3
15	849	Whole kernel, vacuum pack	1 c	210	77	166	5	41	3	1	.2	.3	.5
		Cowpeas; (see Black-eyed peas, #814–816)											
15	850	Cucumbers with peel, ⅛″ thick, 2⅛″ diam	6 slices	28	96	4	<1	1	<1	<.1	t	t	t
		Dandelion greens:											
15	851	Raw	1 c	55	86	25	1	5	1	<1	<.1	<.1	.2
15	852	Chopped, cooked, drained	1 c	105	90	35	2	7	1	1	.2	<.1	.4
15	853	Eggplant, cooked	1 c	160	92	45	1	11	6	<1	.1	<.1	.2
15	854	Garbanzo beans (chick-peas), cooked	1 c	164	60	269	15	45	11	4	.4	1.0	2.0
15	855	Great northern beans, cooked	1 c	177	69	210	15	37	11	1	.3	<.1	.3
15	856	Escarole/curly endive, chopped	1 c	50	94	9	1	2	1	<1	t	t	<.1
15	857	Jerusalem artichokes, raw slices	1 c	150	78	114	3	26	2	<.1	—	t	t
		Kale, cooked, drained:											
15	858	From raw	1 c	130	91	42	3	7	4	1	.1	<.1	.3
15	859	From frozen	1 c	130	90	39	4	7	3	1	.1	<.1	.3
15	860	Kidney beans, canned	1 c	256	78	208	13	38	19	<1	.1	.1	.4
		Kohlrabi:											
15	1181	Raw slices	1 c	140	91	38	2	9	2	<1	t	t	.1
15	861	Cooked	1 c	165	90	48	3	11	2	<1	t	t	.1
		Leeks:											
15	1183	Raw, chopped	1 c	104	83	63	2	15	2	<1	.1	<.1	.4
15	1182	Cooked, chopped	.5 c	52	91	16	<1	4	2	<1	t	t	.1
15	862	Lentils, cooked from dry	1 c	198	70	231	18	40	10	1	.1	.1	.4
		Lentils, sprouted:											
15	1288	Stir fried	3.5 oz	100	69	101	9	21	4	<1	.1	.1	.2
15	1289	Raw	1 c	77	67	81	7	17	3	<1	<.1	.1	.2
		Lettuce:											
		Butterhead/Boston types:											
15	863	Head, 5″ diam	1 head	163	96	21	2	4	3	<1	<.1	t	.2
15	864	Leaves, 2 inner or outer	2 leaves	15	96	2	<1	<1	<1	<.1	t	t	t

Chol (mg)	Calc (mg)	Iron (mg)	Magn (mg)	Phos (mg)	Pota (mg)	Sodi (mg)	Zinc (mg)	VT-A (RE)	Thia (mg)	Ribo (mg)	Niac (mg)	V-B6 (mg)	Fola (µg)	VT-C (mg)
0	14	.19	5	10	114	35	.07	5	.01	.01	.12	.01	4	3
0	22	.29	7	16	170	53	.10	8	.02	.02	.18	.02	5	4
0	18	.65	29	17	136	77	.16	259	.01	.03	.14	.03	20	11
0	102	3.96	150	58	961	313	.59	1198	.06	.15	.63	.12	57	32
0	113	.60	16	15	135	27	.93	322	.03	.06	.34	.06	55	14
0	357	1.90	52	46	427	85	.46	1017	.08	.20	1.08	.19	129	45
0	2	.47	25	79	192	13	.37	17[113]	.17	.06	1.24	.18	36	5
0	2	.38	18	47	158	3	.40	13[113]	.11	.04	.96	.14	19	3
0	2	.25	15	39	114	4	.29	20[113]	.06	.06	1.05	.18	19	2
0	4	.49	22	65	172	365[114]	.68	12[113]	.03	.07	1.23	.08	57	6
0	11	.88	48	134	390	572[115]	.97	51[113]	.09	.15	2.46	.12	104	17
0	4	.08	3	5	42	1	.07	1	.01	.01	.09	.02	4	1
0	103	1.71	20	36	218	42	.62	770	.11	.14	.39	.02	64	19
0	147	1.89	26	44	244	46	.80	1229	.14	.18	.50	.04	82	19
0	10	.56	21	35	397	5	.24	10	.12	.03	.96	.14	23	2
0	80	4.74	78	275	477	11	2.51	4	.19	.10	.86	.23	282	2
0	121	3.77	88	293	692	4	1.55	<1	.28	.10	1.21	.21	181	2
0	26	.42	8	14	157	11	.40	103	.04	.04	.20	.01	71	3
0	21	5.10	26	117	644	6	.11	3	.30	.09	1.95	.11	15	6
0	94	1.17	23	36	296	30	.31	962	.07	.09	.70	.18	30	53
0	179	1.22	23	36	417	20	.23	826	.06	.15	.87	.11	31	33
0	69	3.14	79	269	658	889	1.41	0	.28	.18	1.29	.11	126	3
0	34	.56	27	64	490	28	.32	5	.07	.03	.56	.21	14	87
0	41	.66	31	74	561	34	.32	6	.07	.03	.64	.18	13	89
0	61	2.18	29	36	187	21	.17	10	.06	.03	.42	.24	67	13
0	16	.57	7	9	45	5	.12	2	.01	.01	.10	.08	16	2
0	37	6.59	71	356	731	4	2.50	2	.34	.14	2.10	.35	358	3
0	14	3.10	35	153	284	9	1.60	4	.22	.09	1.20	.16	84	13
0	19	2.47	28	133	248	8	1.16	4	.18	.10	.87	.15	77	13
0	52	.49	18	38	419	8	.42	158	.10	.10	.49	.11	119	13
0	5	.05	2	3	39	1	.04	15	.01	.01	.05	.01	11	1

[113]For yellow varieties; white varieties contain only a trace of vitamin A.

[114]Dietary pack contains 4 mg sodium per ½ cup.

[115]Dietary pack contains 6 mg sodium per cup.

(For purposes of calculations, use "0" for t, <1, <.1, <.01, etc.)

Table C–1   Food Composition

Grp	Ref	Food Description	Measure	Wt (g)	H₂O (%)	Ener (kcal)	Prot (g)	Carb (g)	Dietary Fiber (g)	Fat (g)	Fat Breakdown (g)		
											Sat	Mono	Poly
		VEGETABLES and LEGUMES—Con.											
		Lettuce—con.											
		Iceberg/crisphead:											
15	865	Head, 6″ diam	1 head	539	96	70	5	11	9	1	.1	<.1	.5
15	866	Wedge, ¼ of head	1 wedge	135	96	18	1	3	2	<1	<.1	t	.1
15	867	Chopped or shredded	1 c	56	96	7	1	1	1	<1	t	t	.1
15	868	Loose leaf, chopped	1 c	56	94	10	1	2	1	<1	t	t	.1
		Romaine:											
15	869	Chopped	1 c	56	95	9	1	1	1	<1	t	t	.1
15	870	Inner leaf	1 leaf	10	95	2	<1	<1	<1	<.1	t	t	t
		Mushrooms:											
15	871	Raw, sliced	½ c	35	92	9	1	2	1	<1	t	t	.1
15	872	Cooked from raw, pieces	½ c	78	91	21	2	4	2	<1	<.1	t	.1
15	873	Canned, drained	½ c	78	91	19	1	4	2	<1	<.1	t	.1
		Mustard greens:											
15	874	Cooked from raw	1 c	140	94	21	3	3	3	<1	t	.2	.1
15	875	Cooked from frozen	1 c	150	94	29	3	5	3	<1	t	.2	.1
15	876	Navy beans, cooked from dry	1 c	182	63	259	16	50	16	1	.3	.1	.4
		Okra, cooked:											
15	877	From fresh pods	8 pods	85	90	27	2	6	2	<1	<.1	t	<.1
15	878	From frozen slices	½ c	92	91	34	2	8	2	<1	.1	.1	.1
		Onions:											
		Raw:											
15	879	Chopped	1 c	160	91	54	1	12	3	<1	.1	.1	.2
15	880	Sliced	1 c	115	91	39	1	8	2	<1	.1	<.1	.1
15	881	Cooked, drained, chopped	½ c	105	92	29	1	7	2	<1	<.1	t	.1
15	882	Dehydrated flakes	¼ c	14	4	45	1	12	1	<.1	t	t	<.1
		Spring onions:											
15	883	Chopped, bulb and top	½ c	50	91	13	1	3	1	<.1	t	t	<.1
15	1185	Green tops only, chopped,	1 c	100	92	34	2	6	3	<1	.1	.1	.2
15	1184	White part only, chopped	1 c	100	92	50	1	10	3	<1	<.1	t	.1
15	884	Onion rings, breaded, prepared f/frozen	2 rings	20	29	81	1	8	<1	5	1.7	2.2	1
		Parsley:											
		Raw:											
15	885	Chopped	½ c	30	88	10	1	2	2	<.1	t	t	<.1
15	886	Sprigs	10 sprigs	10	88	3	<1	1	1	<.1	t	t	t
15	887	Freeze dried	¼ c	1	2	4	<1	1	1	<.1	t	t	<.1
15	888	Parsnips, sliced, cooked	1 c	156	78	125	2	30	5	1	.1	.2	.1
		Peas:											
		Black-eyed (see Black-eyed peas, #814–816)											
15	889	Edible pods, cooked	1 c	160	89	67	5	11	4	<1	.1	<.1	.2
		Green:											
15	890	Canned, drained	½ c	85	82	59	4	11	4	<1	.1	<.1	.1
15	891	Cooked from frozen	½ c	80	80	63	4	11	4	<1	<.1	t	.1
15	892	Split, green, cooked from dry	1 c	196	69	231	16	41	10	1	.1	.2	.3
		Peas and carrots:											
15	1187	Cooked from frozen	.5 c	80	86	38	2	8	3	<1	.1	<.1	.2
15	1186	Canned, with liquid	.5 c	128	88	48	3	11	4	<1	.1	<.1	.2

Chol (mg)	Calc (mg)	Iron (mg)	Magn (mg)	Phos (mg)	Pota (mg)	Sodi (mg)	Zinc (mg)	VT-A (RE)	Thia (mg)	Ribo (mg)	Niac (mg)	V-B6 (mg)	Fola (µg)	VT-C (mg)
0	102	2.70	49	108	852	48	1.19	178	.25	.16	1.01	.22	302	21
0	26	.68	12	27	213	12	.30	45	.06	.04	.25	.05	76	5
0	11	.28	5	11	89	5	.12	19	.03	.02	.11	.02	31	2
0	38	.78	6	14	148	5	.19	106	.03	.04	.22	.03	60	10
0	20	.62	3	25	162	4	.19	146	.06	.06	.28	.03	76	13
0	4	.11	1	5	29	1	.03	26	.01	.01	.05	.06	14	2
0	2	.43	4	36	130	1	.30	0	.04	.16	1.44	.03	7	1
0	5	1.36	9	68	278	2	.68	0	.06	.23	3.48	.07	14	3
0	9	.62	6	52	101	332	.56	0	.05	.17	1.25	.06	10	0
0	104	1.56	21	57	283	22	.30	424	.06	.09	.61	.18	20	35
0	152	1.68	20	36	209	38	.30	671	.06	.08	.39	.16	20	21
0	128	4.5	107	285	669	2	1.93	<1	.37	.11	.97	.30	255	1
0	54	.38	48	48	274	4	.47	49	.11	.05	.74	.16	39	14
0	88	.62	47	42	215	3	.57	47	.09	.11	.72	.04	134	11
0	40	.59	16	46	248	3	.29	0	.1	.02	.16	.25	32	13
0	29	.43	12	33	178	2	.21	0	.07	.01	.12	.18	23	10
0	29	.21	11	24	159	8	.19	0	.04	.01	.08	.19	13	6
0	36	.22	13	42	227	3	.26	0	.01	.01	.03	.22	23	11
0	30	.94	10	16	128	2	.22	250	.04	.07	.10	.03	8	23
0	56	2.20	21	39	260	7	.22	400	.07	.10	.60	0	80	51
0	40	.89	16	40	230	7	.25	<1	.07	.03	.33	.10	36	27
0	6	.34	4	16	26	75	.08	5	.06	.03	.72	.02	3	<1
0	39	1.86	13	12	161	12	.22	156	.02	.03	.21	.05	55	27
0	13	.62	4	4	54	4	.07	52	.01	.01	.07	.02	18	9
0	2	.75	5	8	88	5	.09	89	.02	.03	.15	.02	22	2
0	58	.90	46	108	573	16	.40	0	.13	.08	1.10	.15	91	20[116]
0	67	3.15	42	89	383	6	.60	30	.21	.12	.86	.23	48	77
0	17	.81	15	57	147	186[117]	.60	65	.10	.07	.62	.05	38	8
0	19	1.25	23	72	134	70	.75	77	.23	.14	1.18	.09	47	8
0	26	2.52	71	195	710	4	1.96	1	.37	.11	1.74	.09	127	1
0	18	.75	13	39	127	55	.36	621	.18	.06	.92	.07	21	7
0	29	.97	<1	58	128	332	.74	739	.10	.07	.74	.11	24	8

[116] Value for Vitamin C is highest right after harvest and drops after that.
[117] Dietary pack contains 1.7 mg sodium.

(For purposes of calculations, use "0" for t, <1, <.1, <.01, etc.)

Table C–1 Food Composition

Grp	Ref	Food Description	Measure	Wt (g)	H₂O (%)	Ener (kcal)	Prot (g)	Carb (g)	Dietary Fiber (g)	Fat (g)	Fat Breakdown (g) Sat	Mono	Poly
		VEGETABLES and LEGUMES—Con.											
		Peppers, hot:											
		Hot green chili:											
15	893	Canned	½ c	68	92	17	1	4	1	<.1	t	t	<.1
15	894	Raw	1 pepper	45	88	18	1	4	1	<.1	t	t	<.1
15	895	Jalapenos, chopped, canned	½ c	68	90	17	1	3	2	<1	.4	t	.2
		Peppers, sweet, green:											
15	896	Whole pod (90 g with refuse), raw	1 pod	74	93	18	1	4	1	<1	.1	t	.2
15	897	Cooked, chopped (1 pod cooked = 73 g)	½ c	68	95	12	<1	3	1	<1	<.1	t	.1
		Sweet red pepper											
15	1286	Raw, chopped	.5 c	50	93	12	<1	3	1	<1	<.1	t	.1
15	1287	Cooked, chopped	.5 c	68	95	12	<1	3	1	<1	<.1	t	.1
15	898	Pinto beans, cooked from dry	1 c	171	64	235	14	44	20	1	.2	.2	.3
15	1191	Poi - two finger	1 c	240	72	269	1	65	6	<1	.1	<.1	.1
		Potatoes:[122]											
		Baked in oven, 4¾ × 2⅓″ diam:											
15	899	With skin	1 potato	202	71	220	5	51	5	<1	.1	t	.1
15	900	Flesh only	1 potato	156	75	145	3	34	2	<1	<.1	t	.1
15	901	Skin only	1 ea	58	47	115	2	27	2	<.1	t	t	<.1
		Baked in microwave, 4¾ × 2⅓″ diam:											
15	902	With skin	1 potato	202	72	212	5	49	5	<1	.1	t	.1
15	903	Flesh only	1 potato	156	74	156	3	36	2	<1	<.1	t	.1
15	904	Skin only	1 ea	58	64	77	3	17	2	<.1	t	t	<.1
		Boiled, about 2½″ diam:											
15	905	Peeled after boiling	1 potato	136	77	119	3	27	2	<1	<.1	t	.1
15	906	Peeled before boiling	1 potato	135	78	116	2	27	2	<1	<.1	t	.1
		French fried, strips 2-3½″ long, frozen											
15	907	Oven heated	10 strips	50	53	111	2	17	1	4	2.1	1.8	.3
15	908	Fried in veg oil	10 strips	50	38	158	2	20	1	8	2.5	1.6	3.8
15	1188	Fried in veg. and animal oil	10 strips	50	38	158	2	20	1	8	3.4	4.0	.5
15	909	Hashed brown, from frozen	1 c	156	56	340	5	44	3	18	7	8	2
		Mashed:											
15	910	Home recipe with milk[123]	1 c	210	78	162	4	37	3	1	.7	.3	.1
15	911	Home recipe with milk and margarine	1 c	210	76	222	4	35	3	9	2.2	3.7	2.5
15	912	Prepared from flakes; water, milk, butter, salt added	1 c	210	76	237	4	32	3	12	7.2	3.3	.5
		Potato products, prepared:											
		Au gratin:											
15	913	From dry mix	1 c	245	79	228	6	32	4	10	6.3	3	.3
15	914	From home recipe[125]	1 c	245	74	322	12	28	4	19	12	5	1
		Potato salad (see Mixed Dishes #715)											
		Scalloped:											
15	915	From dry mix	1 c	245	79	228	5	31	3	11	6.5	3.0	.5
15	916	Home recipe[127]	1 c	245	81	210	7	26	3	9	5.5	2.6	.4
15	1192	Potato puffs, cooked from frozen	.5 c	62	53	138	2	19	1	7	3.2	2.7	.5
15	917	Potato chips (14 chips = about 1 oz)	14 chips	28	2	148	2	15	1	10	2.6	1.8	5.2

[122]Vitamin C varies with length of storage. After 3 months of storage approximately two-thirds of the ascorbic acid remains; after 6 to 7 months, about one-third remains.

[123]Recipe: 84% potatoes, 15% whole milk, 1% salt.

[125]Recipe: 55% potatoes, 30% whole milk, 9% cheddar cheese, 3% butter, 2% flour, 1% salt.

[127]Recipe: 59% potatoes, 36% whole milk, 2% butter, 2% flour, 1% salt.

GRP KEY: 1 = BEV 2 = DAIRY 3 = EGGS 4 = FAT/OIL 5 = FRUIT 6 = BAKERY 7 = GRAIN 8 = FISH 9 = BEEF 10 = POULTRY
11 = SAUSAGE 12 = MIXED/FAST 13 = NUTS/SEEDS 14 = SWEETS 15 = VEG/LEG 16 = MISC 22 = SOUP/SAUCE

Chol (mg)	Calc (mg)	Iron (mg)	Magn (mg)	Phos (mg)	Pota (mg)	Sodi (mg)	Zinc (mg)	VT-A (RE)	Thia (mg)	Ribo (mg)	Niac (mg)	V-B6 (mg)	Fola (μg)	VT-C (mg)
0	5	.34	8	12	143	10	.02	42[118]	.01	.03	.54	.08	35	46
0	8	.54	11	21	153	3	.14	35[119]	.04	.04	.43	.13	11	109
0	18	1.90	8	12	92	995	.13	116	.02	.03	.34	.08	35	9
0	4	.94	10	16	144	2	.13	39[120]	.06	.04	.41	.12	13	95[120]
0	3	.60	7	10	88	1	.08	26[121]	.04	.02	.25	.07	10	76[121]
0	3	.63	7	11	98	2	.09	285	.04	.03	.28	.08	9	95
0	3	.60	7	10	88	1	.08	256	.04	.02	.25	.07	10	113
0	82	4.47	95	273	800	3	1.85	<1	.32	.16	.68	.27	294	4
0	37	2.11	58	94	439	28	2.04	5	.31	.10	2.64	—	—	10
0	20	2.75	55	115	844	16	.65	0	.22	.07	3.32	.70	22	26
0	8	.55	39	78	610	8	.45	0	.16	.03	2.18	.47	14	20
0	20	2.20	25	59	332	12	.28	0	.07	.07	1.78	.35	13	8
0	22	2.50	54	212	903	16	.73	0	.24	.07	3.46	.70	24	31
0	8	.64	39	170	641	11	.51	0	.20	.04	2.54	.50	19	24
0	27	3.44	22	48	377	9	.30	0	.04	.04	1.29	.28	10	9
0	7	.42	30	60	515	6	.41	0	.14	.03	1.96	.41	14	18
0	10	.42	26	54	443	7	.37	0	.13	.03	.18	.36	12	10
0	4	.67	11	43	229	15	.21	0	.06	.02	1.15	.12	8	6
0	10	.38	17	47	366	108	.19	0	.09	.01	1.63	.12	15	5
0	10	.38	17	47	366	108	.19	0	.09	.01	1.63	.12	15	5
0	24	2.36	27	112	680	53	.50	0	.17	.03	3.78	.20	26	10
4	55	.57	39	100	628	636	.60	12	.19	.08	2.35	.49	17	14
4[124]	54	.55	37	97	607	619	.58	41	.18	.11	2.27	.47	17	13
4[124]	103	.46	37	118	490	697	.37	44	.23	.08	1.41	.02	9	20
12	203	.78	37	233	537	1076	.59	76	.05	.20	2.30	.10	3	8
56[126]	292	1.56	48	277	970	1064	1.69	93	.16	.28	2.43	.43	20	24
27	88	.93	34	137	497	835	.61	51	.05	.14	2.52	.10	3	8
29[128]	140	1.41	46	154	926	821	.98	46	.17	.23	2.58	.44	21	26
0	19	.97	12	30	236	462	.19	1	.12	.05	1.34	.14	.10	4
0	7	.34	17	43	369	133[129]	.30	0	.04	.01	1.19	.14	13	12

[118] For green chili peppers; red varieties contain 809 RE vitamin A.
[119] For green chili peppers; red varieties contain 484 RE vitamin A.
[120] For green sweet peppers; red varieties contain 570 RE vitamin A and 141 mg ascorbic acid.
[121] For green sweet peppers; red varieties contain 256 RE vitamin A and 113 mg ascorbic acid.
[124] For margarine; if butter is used, cholesterol = 25 mg for 29 total mg.
[126] For butter; if margarine is used, cholesterol = 37 mg.
[128] For butter; if margarine is used cholesterol = 15 mg.
[129] If no salt is added, sodium = 2 mg.

(For purposes of calculations, use "0" for t, <1, <.1, <.01, etc.)

Table C–1 Food Composition

Grp	Ref	Food Description	Measure	Wt (g)	H₂O (%)	Ener (kcal)	Prot (g)	Carb (g)	Dietary Fiber (g)	Fat (g)	Fat Breakdown (g)		
											Sat	Mono	Poly
		VEGETABLES and LEGUMES—Con.											
		Pumpkin:											
15	918	Cooked from raw, mashed	1 c	245	94	50	2	12	4	<1	.1	t	t
15	919	Canned	1 c	245	90	83	3	20	5	1	.4	.1	<.1
15	920	Red radishes	10 radishes	45	95	7	<1	2	1	<1	t	t	t
15	921	Refried beans, canned	1 c	253	72	270	16	47	22	3	1	1.2	.4
15	1375	Rutabaga, cooked cubes	.5 c	85	90	29	1	7	1	<1	<.1	<.1	.1
15	922	Sauerkraut, canned with liquid	1 c	236	92	44	2	10	4	<1	.1	<.1	.1
		Seaweed:											
15	923	Kelp, raw	1 oz	28	82	12	1	3	1	<1	.1	<.1	t
15	924	Spirulina, dried	1 oz	28	5	82	16	7	1	2	.8	.2	.6
15	925	Soybeans, cooked from dry	1 c	172	63	298	29	17	5	15	2.2	3.4	8.7
		Soybean products:											
15	926	Miso	½ c	138	46	283	16	39	7	8	1.2	1.9	4.7
15	927	Tofu	½ c	124	85	94	10	2	2	6	.9	1.3	3.4
		Spinach:											
15	928	Raw, chopped	1 c	56	92	12	2	2	2	<1	<.1	t	.1
		Cooked, drained:											
15	929	From raw	1 c	180	91	41	5	7	4	<1	.1	t	.2
15	930	From frozen (leaf)	1 c	190	90	53	6	10	5	<1	.1	t	.2
15	931	Canned, drained solids	1 c	214	92	50	6	7	6	1	.2	<.1	.5
		Spinach soufflé (see #716 Mixed Dishes)											
		Squash, summer varieties, cooked slices:											
15	932	Varieties averaged	1 c	180	94	36	2	8	3	1	.1	<.1	.2
15	933	Crookneck	1 c	180	94	36	2	8	3	1	.1	<.1	.2
15	934	Zucchini	1 c	180	95	29	1	7	4	<.1	t	t	<.1
		Squash, winter varieties, cooked:											
		Average of all varieties, baked:											
15	935	Mashed	1 c	245	89	96	2	21	7	2	.3	.1	.7
15	936	Baked cubes	1 c	205	89	79	2	18	6	1	.3	.1	.5
		Acorn squash:											
15	937	Baked, mashed	1 c	245	83	137	3	36	7	<1	<.1	t	.1
15	1218	Boiled, mashed	1c	245	90	83	2	22	6	<1	<.1	t	.1
15	938	Butternut, baked cubes	1 c	205	88	83	2	22	6	<1	<.1	t	.1
		Butternut squash:											
15	1219	Baked, mashed	1 c	245	88	99	2	26	7	<1	<.1	t	.1
15	1193	Cooked from frozen	1 c	240	88	94	3	24	7	<1	<.1	t	.1
		Hubbard squash:											
15	1194	Baked, mashed	1 c	240	85	120	6	26	6	1	.3	.1	.6
15	1195	Boiled, mashed	1 c	236	91	70	4	15	7	1	.2	.1	.4
15	1196	Spaghetti squash, baked or boiled	1 c	155	92	45	1	10	4	<1	.1	<.1	.2
15	1189	Succotash, cooked from frozen	1 c	170	74	158	7	34	9	2	.3	.3	.7
		Sweet potatoes:											
		Cooked, 5 × 2″ diam:											
15	939	Baked in skin, peeled	1 potato	114	73	118	2	28	3	<1	<.1	t	.1
15	940	Boiled without skin	1 potato	151	73	160	2	37	5	<1	.1	t	.2

Chol (mg)	Calc (mg)	Iron (mg)	Magn (mg)	Phos (mg)	Pota (mg)	Sodi (mg)	Zinc (mg)	VT-A (RE)	Thia (mg)	Ribo (mg)	Niac (mg)	V-B6 (mg)	Fola (μg)	VT-C (mg)
0	37	1.40	22	74	564	3	.45	265	.08	.19	1.01	.16	33	12
0	64	3.41	56	85	504	12	.42	5404	.06	.13	.9	.14	30	10
0	9	.13	4	8	104	11	.13	t	<.01	.02	.14	.03	12	10
0	118	4.5	99	214	994	1071	3.45	0	.12	.14	1.23	.28	150	15
0	36	.40	18	42	244	15	.26	0	.06	.03	.54	.08	13	19
0	72	3.47	31	46	401	1561	.44	4	.05	.05	.34	.31	4	35
0	48	.81	34	12	25	66	.35	3	.01	.04	.13	—	51	—
0	34	8.08	55	33	386	297	—	16	.68	1.04	3.63	.10	—	3
0	175	8.84	148	421	886	1	1.98	2	.27	.49	.69	.40	93	3
0	92	3.78	58	211	226	5032	4.58	12	.13	.35	1.19	.3	46	0
0	130	6.65	127	120	150	9	1.00	11	.10	.06	.24	.06	19	<1
0	55	1.52	44	27	312	44	.30	448	.04	.11	.41	.11	109	16
0	244	6.42	157	100	838	126	1.37	1750	.17	.43	.88	.44	262	40
0	277	2.89	131	91	566	163	1.33	1756	.11	.32	.80	.28	204	23
0	271	4.92	162	94	740	683[131]	.99	1878	.03	.30	.83	.21	209	31
0	48	.64	44	69	346	2	.71	52[132]	.08	.07	.92	.12	36	9
0	48	.64	44	69	346	2	.71	52[132]	.09	.09	.92	.17	36	10
0	23	.63	40	72	455	5	.32	43[132]	.07	.07	.77	.14	30	8
0	34	.81	20	49	1071	2	.64	872	.21	.06	1.72	.18	69	24
0	28	.67	16	41	895	3	.54	730	.17	.05	1.43	.15	57	20
0	108	2.28	104	111	1071	11	.42	105	.41	.03	2.16	.48	46	26
0	65	1.37	63	67	645	6	.27	63	.25	.02	1.30	.29	28	16
0	84	1.23	59	55	582	7	.27	1435	.15	.04	1.99	.25	39	31
0	100	1.47	71	66	697	8	.32	1715	.18	.04	2.38	.30	47	37
0	46	1.40	22	34	319	4	.29	801	.12	.09	1.11	.17	29	8
0	41	1.13	53	55	859	19	.36	1450	.18	.11	1.34	.41	39	23
0	23	.67	32	33	504	12	.22	945	.10	.07	.79	.24	23	15
0	33	.52	17	21	182	28	.31	17	.06	.03	1.26	.15	12	6
0	25	1.51	39	119	451	77	.76	39	.13	.12	2.22	.16	57	10
0	32	.52	23	63	397	12	.33	2488	.08	.14	.7	.28	26	28
0	32	.8	15	41	278	20	.4	2575	.08	.21	1	.36	22	26

[131]Dietary pack contains 58 mg sodium.
[132]Applies to squash including skin; flesh has no appreciable vitamin A value.

(For purposes of calculations, use "0" for t, <1, <.1, <.01, etc.)

Table C–1 Food Composition

Grp	Ref	Food Description	Measure	Wt (g)	H₂O (%)	Ener (kcal)	Prot (g)	Carb (g)	Dietary Fiber (g)	Fat (g)	Fat Breakdown (g)		
											Sat	Mono	Poly
		VEGETABLES and LEGUMES—Con.											
		Sweet potatoes—con.											
15	941	Candied, 2½ × 2″	1 pce	105	67	144	1	29	2	3	1.4	.7	.2
		Canned:											
15	942	Solid pack, mashed	1 c	265	74	258	5	59	6	<1	.1	t	.2
15	943	Vacuum pack, mashed	1 c	255	76	233	4	54	5	1	.1	t	.2
15	944	Vacuum pack, 2¾ × 1″	1 pce	40	76	36	1	8	1	<1	t	t	<.1
		Tomatoes:											
		Raw:											
15	945	Whole, 2⅗″ diam	1 tomato	123	94	24	1	5	2	<1	<.1	<.1	.1
15	946	Chopped	1 c	180	94	35	2	8	3	<1	.1	.1	.2
15	947	Cooked from raw	1 c	240	92	60	3	14	4	1	.1	.1	.3
15	948	Canned, solids and liquid	1 c	240	94	47	2	10	3	1	.1	.1	.2
15	949	Tomato juice, canned	1 c	244	94	42	2	10	2	<1	t	t	.1
		Tomato products, canned:											
15	950	Paste	1 c	262	74	220	10	49	11	2	.3	.4	.9
15	951	Puree	1 c	250	87	102	4	25	6	<1	<.1	<.1	.1
15	952	Sauce	1 c	245	89	74	3	18	4	<1	.1	.1	.2
15	953	Turnips, cubes, cooked from raw	½ c	78	94	14	1	4	2	<1	t	t	<.1
		Turnip greens, cooked:											
15	954	From raw (leaves and stems)	1 c	144	94	29	2	6	4	<1	.1	t	.1
15	955	From frozen (chopped)	½ c	82	90	24	3	4	4	<1	.1	t	.1
15	956	Vegetable juice cocktail, canned	1 c	242	94	46	2	11	2	<1	<.1	<.1	.1
		Vegetables, mixed:											
15	957	Canned, drained	1 c	163	87	77	4	15	6	<1	.1	<.1	.2
15	958	Frozen, cooked, drained	1 c	182	83	107	5	24	7	<1	.1	t	.1
		Water chestnuts, canned:											
15	959	Slices	½ c	70	86	35	1	9	2	<.1	t	t	t
15	960	Whole	4 ea	28	86	14	<1	4	1	<1	t	t	t
15	1190	Watercress, fresh, chopped	.5 c	17	95	2	<1	<1	<1	<1	t	t	t
		MISCELLANEOUS											
		Baking powders for home use:											
		Sodium aluminum sulfate:											
16	962	With monocalcium phosphate monohydrate	1 tsp	3	2	5	t	1	0	0	0	0	0
16	963	With monocalcium phosphate monohydrate, calcium sulfate	1 tsp	3	1	5	t	1	0	0	0	0	0
16	964	Straight phosphate	1 tsp	4	2	5	t	1	0	0	0	0	0
16	965	Low sodium	1 tsp	4	1	5	t	1	0	0	0	0	0
16	1204	Baking soda	1 tsp	3	1	0	0	0	0	0	0	0	0
16	966	Basil, ground	1 tbsp	5	6	11	1	3	1	<1	—	—	—
16	961	Carob flour	1 c	103	3	185	5	92	34	1	.1	.2	.2

Chol (mg)	Calc (mg)	Iron (mg)	Magn (mg)	Phos (mg)	Pota (mg)	Sodi (mg)	Zinc (mg)	VT-A (RE)	Thia (mg)	Ribo (mg)	Niac (mg)	V-B6 (mg)	Fola (μg)	VT-C (mg)
0[133]	27	1.2	12	27	198	73	.16	440	.02	.04	.41	.17	12	7
0	77	3.4	61	133	536	191	.54	3857	.07	.23	2.4	.48	42	13
0	56	2.27	57	125	796	136	.46	2036	.09	.14	1.89	.49	42	67
0	9	.36	9	20	125	21	.07	319	.02	.02	.3	.08	7	11
0	9	.59	14	28	255	10	.13	139	.07	.06	.74	.09	12	22[134]
0	12	.86	20	42	372	15	.19	204	.11	.09	1.08	.14	17	32[134]
0	20	1.44	33	70	624	25	.32	325	.17	.14	1.72	.15	23	50
0	63[135]	1.45	29	46	529	390[136]	.38	145	.11	.07	1.76	.22	35	36
0	22	1.41	27	46	537	881[137]	.34	136	.12	.08	1.64	.27	9	45
0	92	7.84	134	207	2442	170[138]	2.1	647	.41	.5	8.44	1	4	111
0	37	2.32	60	99	1051	49[139]	.54	340	.18	.14	4.29	.38	39	88
0	34	1.88	46	78	908	1481[140]	.6	240	.16	.14	2.82	.33	39	32
0	18	.17	6	15	106	39	.08	0	.02	.02	.23	.05	7	9
0	198	1.15	32	41	293	41	.29	792	.07	.1	.59	.26	171	40
0	125	1.59	21	27	184	12	.34	654	.04	.06	.38	.06	32	18
0	27	1.02	27	41	467	883	.48	283	.1	.07	1.76	.34	38	67
0	44	1.71	26	68	474	243	.67	1899	.07	.08	.94	.13	39	8
0	46	1.49	40	93	308	64	.89	779	.13	.22	1.55	.14	35	6
0	3	.61	3	14	82	6	.27	t	.01	.02	.25	—	8	1
0	1	.25	1	5	33	2	.11	t	<.01	.01	.1	—	3	<1
0	20	.03	4	10	56	7	.03	80	.02	.02	.03	.02	34	7
0	58	0	t	87	5	329	0	0	0	0	0	0	0	0
0	183	0	—	45	4	290	0	0	0	0	0	0	0	0
0	239	0	—	359	6	312	0	0	0	0	0	0	0	0
0	207	0	—	314	891	t	0	0	0	0	0	0	0	0
0	0	—	—	—	—	821	—	0	0	0	0	0	0	0
0	95	1.89	18	22	154	2	.26	42	.01	.01	.31	—	—	3
0	359	3.03	56	81	852	36	.94	2	.06	.48	1.95	.38	30	<1

[133] For recipe using margarine; if butter is used, cholesterol = 8 mg.

[134] Year-round average. From June through October, ascorbic acid is approximately 32 mg and 47 mg, respectively, for one tomato and 1 c chopped tomato. From November through May, market samples average around 12 and 18 mg, respectively.

[135] Calcium is added as a firming agent.

[136] Dietary pack contains 31 mg sodium.

[137] If no salt is added, sodium content is 24 mg.

[138] If salt is added, sodium content is 2070 mg.

[139] If salt is added, sodium content is 998 mg.

[140] With salt added.

(For purposes of calculations, use "0" for t, <1, <.1, <.01, etc.)

Table C–1   Food Composition

Grp	Ref	Food Description	Measure	Wt (g)	H₂O (%)	Ener (kcal)	Prot (g)	Carb (g)	Dietary Fiber (g)	Fat (g)	Fat Breakdown (g) Sat	Mono	Poly
		MISCELLANEOUS—Con.											
		Catsup:											
16	967	Cup	1 c	273	69	290	5	69	4	1	.2	.2	.4
16	968	Tablespoon	1 tbsp	17	69	18	<1	4	<1	<.1	t	t	<.1
16	1200	Cayenne (red pepper)	1 tbsp	5.3	8	17	1	3	2	1	.2	.2	.4
16	969	Celery seed	1 tsp	2	6	9	<1	1	<1	1	<.1	.3	.1
16	970	Chili powder	1 tsp	3	8	8	<1	1	1	<1	.1	.1	.2
		Chocolate:											
16	971	Baking, unsweetened	1 oz	28	2	145	4	7	4	15	9	5	.5
		For other chocolate items, see Sweeteners and Sweets, #759, 763, 764											
16	972	Coriander, fresh	¼ c	4	93	<1	<1	<1	<1	<.1	—	—	—
16	1197	Cornstarch	1 tbsp	8	12	29	<1	7	<1	<1	t	t	<.1
16	973	Cinnamon	1 tsp	2	10	6	<1	2	1	<.1	t	t	t
16	974	Curry powder	1 tsp	2	10	6	<1	1	<1	<1	t	.2	<.1
16	1202	Dill weed, dried	1 tbsp	3.1	7	8	1	2	<1	<1	—	—	—
		Garlic:											
16	975	Cloves	4 cloves	12	59	18	1	4	<1	<.1	t	t	<.1
16	976	Powder	1 tsp	3	6	9	<1	2	<1	<.1	t	t	t
16	977	Gelatin, dry, plain	1 envelope	7	13	25	6	0	1	0	0	0	0
16	978	Ginger root, raw, sliced	5 slices	11	87	8	<1	2	<1	<.1	t	t	t
16	1198	Horseradish, prepared	1 tbsp	15	87	6	<1	1	<1	<1	t	t	t
16	1199	Hummous/Humous	1 c	246	65	420	12	50	4	21	3.1	8.8	7.8
16	979	Mustard, prepared, (1 packet =1 tsp)	1 tsp	5	80	4	<1	<1	<1	<1	t	.2	t
		Miso (see #926 under Vegetables and Legumes, Soybean products):											
		Olives:											
16	980	Green	10 olives	39	78	45	<1	<1	1	6	.6	3.6	.3
16	981	Ripe, pitted[141]	10 olives	47	73	78	<1	1	1.5	10	1.6	6.8	1.0
16	982	Onion powder	1 tsp	2.1	5	5	<1	2	<1	<.1	t	t	t
16	983	Oregano, ground	1 tsp	2	7	5	<1	1	<1	<1	t	t	.1
16	984	Paprika	1 tsp	2	10	6	<1	1	<1	<1	t	t	.2
16	985	Pepper, black	1 tsp	2	11	5	<1	1	<1	<.1	<.1	<.1	<.1
		Pickles:											
16	986	Dill, medium, 3¾ × 1¼″ diam	1 pickle	65	93	5	<1	1	1	<1	<.1	t	<.1
16	987	Fresh pack, slices, 1½″ diam × ¼″ thick	4 slices	30	79	20	<1	5	<1	<.1	t	t	t
16	988	Sweet, small, about 2½ × ¾″ diam	1 pickle	15	61	20	<.1	6	<1	<.1	t	t	t
16	989	Pickle relish, sweet	1 tbsp	15	63	20	<.1	5	<1	<.1	t	t	<.1
16	1201	Sage-ground	1 tbsp	2	8	6	<1	1	<1	<1	.1	<.1	<.1
		Popcorn (see Grain Products, #539–541)											
22	1347	Salsa, from recipe	.85 c	184	91	79	2	9	3	5	.7	3.4	.5
16	990	Salt	1 tsp	6	0	0	0	0	0	0	0	0	0
		Salt substitute:											
16	1205	Morton Salt substitute	1 tbsp	6	0	0	0	<1	0	0	0	0	0
16	1206	No Salt, packet, Norcliff Thayer	1 ea	.75	0	0	0	0	0	0	0	0	0
16	1207	Light Salt, Morton	1 tsp	6	0	0	0	0	0	0	0	0	0
16	991	Vinegar, cider	1 tbsp	15	94	2	0	1	0	0	0	0	0

[141]This is the most recent tested data from the California Olive Industry, October 1986.

Chol (mg)	Calc (mg)	Iron (mg)	Magn (mg)	Phos (mg)	Pota (mg)	Sodi (mg)	Zinc (mg)	VT-A (RE)	Thia (mg)	Ribo (mg)	Niac (mg)	V-B6 (mg)	Fola (µg)	VT-C (mg)
0	60	2.2	57	137	991	2845	.59	382	.25	.19	4.4	.29	14	41
0	4	.14	4	9	62	177	.04	24	.02	.01	.27	.02	1	3
0	8	.41	8	16	107	7	.13	221	.02	.05	.46	—	—	4
0	38	.90	10	11	30	4	.14	<1	.01	.01	.1	—	—	<1
0	7	.37	4	8	50	26	.07	91	.01	.02	.21	—	1	2
0	22	1.9	82	109	235	1	1.01	1	.02	.1	.38	.01	18	0
0	4	.08	1	1	22	1	—	11	<.01	<.01	.03	—	—	<1
0	—	.04	<1	2	0	0	<.01	0	0	.01	0	—	—	0
0	28	.86	1	1	11	1	.05	1	<.01	<.01	.03	.02	—	1
0	10	.59	5	7	31	1	.08	2	<.01	<.01	.07	—	—	<1
0	50	1.50	13	16	110	6	.10	—	.01	.01	.09	.05	—	—
0	22	.2	3	18	48	2	1.06	0	.02	.01	.08	.40	<1	4
0	2	.08	2	12	31	1	.07	0	.01	<.01	.02	.57	2	<1
0	1	0	2	0	2	6	0	0	0	0	0	<.01	0	0
0	2	.05	5	3	46	1	.22	0	<.01	<.01	.08	.02	2	1
0	9	.10	4	5	44	14	.18	0	.01	<.01	.06	.01	2	1
0	124	3.87	71	275	427	599	2.70	6	.23	.13	1.01	.98	146	19
0	4	.1	3	4	7	63	.03	0	<.01	.01	.07	<.01	0	<1
0	24	.6	9	6	21	936	.03	12	<.01	<.01	.01	.01	<1	<1
0	52	1.04	10	10	10	355	.14	5	<.01	<.01	.01	.01	<1	<1
0	8	.06	3	7	20	1	.05	0	01	<.01	.01	.03	3	<1
0	24	.66	4	3	25	<1	.07	10	<.01	t	.09	—	—	1
0	4	.50	4	7	49	1	.09	127	.01	.04	.32	—	—	2
0	9	.61	4	4	26	1	.03	<1	<.01	<.01	.02	0	—	0
0	17	.7	6	14	130	741	.18	7	<.01	.01	.01	<.01	1	4
0	10	.55	2	8	60	201	0	4	t	.01	<.01	<.01	0	2
0	2	.25	2	2	30	107	<.01	1	<.01	<.01	<.01	<.01	0	1
0	3	.13	1	2	30	107	.01	2	t	t	<.01	0	0	1
0	33	.56	9	2	21	0	.09	12	.02	.01	.11	—	—	1
0	18	.86	19	41	347	191	.20	150	.09	.07	.93	.16	28	39
0	14	<.01	2	3	.3	2132	t	0	0	0	0	0	0	0
0	30	0	t	28	2800	t	0	0	0	0	0	0	0	0
0	—	—	—	—	385	0	—	0	0	0	0	0	0	0
0	3	0	4	0	1500	1100	0	0	0	0	0	0	0	0
0	1	.09	<1	1	15	t	02	0	0	0	0	0	0	0

(For purposes of calculations, use "0" for t, <1, <.1, <.01, etc.)

Table C–1 Food Composition

Grp	Ref	Food Description	Measure	Wt (g)	H₂O (%)	Ener (kcal)	Prot (g)	Carb (g)	Dietary Fiber (g)	Fat (g)	Fat Breakdown (g)		
											Sat	Mono	Poly
		MISCELLANEOUS—Con.											
		Yeast:											
16	992	Baker's, dry, active, package	1 package	7	5	20	3	3	2	<1	t	.1	t
16	993	Brewer's, dry	1 tbsp	8	5	25	3	3	3	<.1	t	t	0
		SOUPS, SAUCES, AND GRAVIES											
		SOUPS, canned, condensed:											
		Unprepared, condensed:											
22	1210	Cream of celery	1 c	251	85	180	3	18	1	11	2.8	2.6	5.0
22	1215	Cream of chicken	1 c	251	82	233	7	19	<1	15	4.2	.8	3.0
22	1216	Cream of mushroom	1 c	251	81	257	4	19	<1	19	5.2	3.6	8.9
22	1220	Onion	1 c	246	86	114	8	16	1	3	.5	1.5	1.3
		Prepared with equal volume of whole milk:											
22	994	Clam chowder, New England	1 c	248	85	163	9	17	1	7	3.0	2.3	1.1
22	1209	Cream of celery	1 c	248	87	165	6	15	<1	10	4.0	2.5	2.7
22	995	Cream of chicken	1 c	248	85	191	7	15	<1	12	5	4	2
22	996	Cream of mushroom	1 c	248	85	205	6	15	<1	14	5	3	5
22	1214	Cream of potato	1 c	248	87	148	6	17	<1	6	3.8	1.7	.6
22	1213	Oyster stew	1 c	245	89	134	6	10	0	8	5.1	2.1	.3
22	997	Tomato	1 c	248	85	160	6	22	<1	6	2.9	1.6	1.1
		Prepared with equal volume of water:											
22	998	Bean with bacon	1 c	253	84	173	8	23	3	6	1.5	2.2	1.8
22	999	Beef broth, bouillon, consommé	1 c	240	98	16	3	<1	0	1	.3	.2	t
22	1000	Beef noodle	1 c	244	92	84	5	9	<1	3	1.2	1.2	.5
22	1001	Chicken noodle	1 c	241	92	75	4	9	1	2	.7	1.1	.6
22	1002	Chicken rice	1 c	241	94	60	4	7	1	2	.5	.9	.4
22	1208	Chili beef soup	1 c	250	85	169	7	22	1	7	3.3	2.8	.3
22	1003	Clam chowder, Manhatten	1 c	244	90	78	4	12	1	2	.4	.4	1.3
22	1004	Cream of chicken	1 c	244	91	115	3	9	1	7	2.1	3.3	1.5
22	1005	Cream of mushroom	1 c	244	90	130	2	9	1	9	2.4	1.7	4.2
22	1006	Minestrone	1 c	241	91	80	4	11	1	3	.5	.7	1.1
22	1211	Onion soup-canned	1 c	241	93	57	4	8	<1	2	.3	.8	.7
22	1007	Split pea with ham	1 c	253	82	189	10	28	1	4	1.8	1.8	.6
22	1008	Tomato	1 c	244	90	86	2	17	<1	2	.4	.4	1.0
22	1009	Vegetable beef	1 c	244	92	79	6	10	1	2	.9	.8	.1
22	1010	Vegetarian vegetable	1 c	241	92	70	2	12	2	2	.3	.8	.7
		SOUPS, dehydrated:											
		Unprepared, dry products:											
22	1011	Bouillon	1 packet	6	3	14	1	1	<1	1	.3	.2	t
22	1012	Onion	1 packet	7	4	20	1	4	<1	<1	.1	.2	.1
		Prepared with water:											
22	1299	Beef broth	1 c	244	97	19	1	2	<1	1	.3	.3	<.1
22	1376	Chicken broth	1 c	244	97	21	1	1	<1	1	.3	.4	.4
22	1013	Chicken noodle	¾ c	188	94	40	2	6	<1	1	.2	.4	.3
22	1122	Cream of chicken	1 c	261	91	107	2	13	1	5	3.4	1.2	.4
22	1014	Onion	¾ c	184	96	20	1	4	<1	<1	.1	.3	.1
22	1217	Split pea	1 c	255	87	133	8	23	1	2	.4	.7	.3
22	1015	Tomato vegetable	¾ c	189	94	41	1	8	<1	1	.3	.3	.1

Chol (mg)	Calc (mg)	Iron (mg)	Magn (mg)	Phos (mg)	Pota (mg)	Sodi (mg)	Zinc (mg)	VT-A (RE)	Thia (mg)	Ribo (mg)	Niac (mg)	V-B6 (mg)	Fola (µg)	VT-C (mg)
0	4	1.1	16	90	140	4	.43	t	.17	.38	2.7	.14	266	t
0	17[142]	1.39	18	140	152	10	.63	t	1.25	.34	3.16	.4	313	t
28	80	1.25	13	75	246	1899	.30	61	.06	.10	.67	.03	5	<1
20	68	1.21	5	75	174	1973	1.26	112	.06	.12	1.64	.03	3	<1
3	64	1.05	9	84	167	2032	1.19	0	.06	.17	1.62	.03	7	2
0	53	1.35	5	22	138	2116	1.23	0	.07	.05	1.21	.10	31	3
22	187	1.48	23	157	300	992	1.3	40	.07	.24	1.03	.13	12	4
32	186	.69	22	151	309	1010	.20	68	.07	.25	.44	.06	9	1
27	180	.67	18	152	273	1046	.68	94	.07	.26	.92	.07	8	1
20	178	.59	20	156	270	1076	.64	38	.08	.28	.81	.06	15	2
22	166	.54	17	160	323	1060	.68	67	.08	.24	.64	.09	9	1
32	167	1.04	21	162	235	1040	10.3	45	.07	.23	.34	.06	7	4
17	159	1.82	23	148	450	932	.29	109	.13	.25	1.52	.16	21	68
3	81	2.05	44	132	403	952	1.03	89	.09	.03	.57	.04	32	2
1	15	.41	9	31	130	782	.6	0	<.01	.05	1.87	.07	2	0
5	15	1.1	6	46	100	952	1.54	63	.07	.06	1.07	.04	4	<1
7	17	.78	7	36	55	900	.55	71	.05	.06	1.39	.01	2	<1
7	17	.75	1	22	101	815	.26	66	.02	.02	1.13	.02	1	<1
12	43	2.40	30	148	525	1035	1.40	503	.06	.08	1.07	.16	10	4
2	34	1.89	10	58	261	1808	.93	92	.06	.05	1.34	.08	10	3
10	34	.61	3	37	88	986	.63	56	.03	.06	.82	.02	2	<1
2	46	.5	5	49	100	1032	.59	0	.05	.09	.7	.02	3	1
2	34	.92	7	56	312	911	.74	234	.05	.04	.94	.10	16	1
0	26	.67	2	11	69	1053	.61	0	.03	.02	.60	.05	15	1
8	22	2.28	48	213	399	1008	1.32	44	.15	.08	1.48	.07	3	1
0	13	1.76	8	34	263	872	.24	69	.09	.05	1.42	.11	15	67
5	17	1.11	6	41	173	956	2	189	.04	.05	1.03	.08	11	2
0	21	1.08	7	35	209	823	.46	301	.05	.05	.92	.06	11	1
1	4	.1	3	19	27	1019	.01	<1	<.01	.02	.27	.01	—	0
<1	10	.14	3	23	47	627	.06	<1	.02	.04	.4	.01	2	<1
1	5	.08	4	26	36	1358	.01	<1	<.01	.02	.36	.02	0	<1
1	15	.08	4	13	25	1484	.01	4	.01	.03	.20	.02	—	<1
2	24	.37	5	24	23	957	.15	5	.05	.04	.66	.01	1	<1
3	76	—	—	96	215	1184	—	—	—	.20	—	.05	—	—
0	9	.14	6	22	48	635	.06	<1	.02	.04	.36	<.01	2	<1
3	22	1.01	46	134	238	1220	.59	5	.22	.15	1.34	.05	15	—
0	6	.47	15	23	78	856	.13	15	.04	.03	.59	.04	2	5

[142]Value varies from 6 to 60 mg.

(For purposes of calculations, use "0" for t, <1, <.1, <.01, etc.)

631

Table C–1   Food Composition

Grp	Ref	Food Description	Measure	Wt (g)	H₂O (%)	Ener (kcal)	Prot (g)	Carb (g)	Dietary Fiber (g)	Fat (g)	Fat Breakdown (g)		
											Sat	Mono	Poly
		SOUPS, SAUCES, AND GRAVIES—Con.											
		SAUCES—con.											
		From dry mixes, prepared with milk:											
22	1016	Cheese sauce	1 c	279	77	305	16	23	<1	17	9	5	2
22	1017	Hollandaise	1 c	259	84	240	5	14	–	20	12	6	1
22	1018	White sauce	1 c	264	81	240	10	21	<1	13	6	5	2
		From home recipe:											
22	1019	White sauce, medium[143]	1 c	250	73	395	10	24	<1	30	9	12	7
		Ready to serve:											
22	1020	Barbeque sauce	1 tbsp	16	81	10	<1	2	<1	<1	<.1	.1	.1
22	1021	Soy sauce	1 tbsp	18	71	9	1	2	0	t	0	0	0
		Spaghetti sauce: canned:											
22	1377	Plain	1 c	249	75	272	5	40	3	12	1.7	6.1	3.3
22	1378	With meat	.8 c	206	75	220	8	27	1	10	2.5	4.5	1.5
22	1379	With mushrooms	.75 c	185	75	162	2	9	2	5	.6	2.3	1.2
22	1380	Teriyaki sauce	1 tbsp	18	84	15	1	3	0	<1	t	t	<.1
		GRAVIES:											
		Canned:											
22	1022	Beef	1 c	233	88	124	9	11	<1	5	2.8	2.3	.2
22	1023	Chicken	1 c	238	85	189	5	13	<1	14	3.4	6.1	3.6
22	1024	Mushroom	1 c	238	89	120	3	13	<1	6	1	3	2.4
		From dry mix:											
22	1025	Brown	1 c	261	91	80	3	14	<1	2	.9	.8	.1
22	1026	Chicken	1 c	260	91	85	3	14	<1	2	.5	.9	.4

[143]Made with enriched flour, margarine, and whole milk.

Chol (mg)	Calc (mg)	Iron (mg)	Magn (mg)	Phos (mg)	Pota (mg)	Sodi (mg)	Zinc (mg)	VT-A (RE)	Thia (mg)	Ribo (mg)	Niac (mg)	V-B6 (mg)	Fola (μg)	VT-C (mg)
53	569	.3	32	438	552	1565	.95	117	.15	.56	.3	.1	12	2
52	124	.9	—	127	124	1564	—	220	.05	.18	.1	.5	—	t
34	425	.3	30	256	444	797	1.15	92	.08	.45	.5	.08	14	3
32	292	.9	35	238	381	888	1.05	340	.15	.43	.8	.1	12	2
0	3	.13	1	3	27	128	.03	14	<.01	<.01	.06	.02	1	1
0	3	.36	6	20	32	1029	.07	0	.01	.02	.61	.03	3	0
0	70	1.62	60	90	957	1236	.53	306	.14	.15	3.75	.40	39	28
17	36	2.80	15	106	444	1045	1.05	189	.20	.16	3.40	.27	13	2
0	22	1.50	22	45	500	744	.51	362	.12	.12	1.40	.24	19	14
0	4	.31	11	28	41	690	.02	0	<.01	.01	.23	.02	4	0
7	14	1.63	3	70	189	117	2.33	0	.07	.08	1.54	.02	7	0
5	48	1.1	5	69	260	1375	1.91	264	.04	.1	1.06	.02	3	0
0	17	1.6	—	36	252	1357	1.66	0	.08	.15	1.6	.05	0	0
2	66	.2	10	47	61	1147	.01	0	.04	.09	.9	<.01	—	0
3	39	.3	—	47	62	1134	.32	0	.05	.15	.8	.03	—	3

(For purposes of calculations, use "0" for t, <1, <.1, <.01, etc.)

Grp	Ref	Food Description	Measure	Wt (g)	H_2O (%)	Ener (kcal)	Prot (g)	Carb (g)	Dietary Fiber (g)	Fat (g)	Fat Breakdown (g) Sat	Mono	Poly
ARBY'S													
12	1402	Bac'n Cheddar, deluxe	1 ea	226	56	526	27	33	<1	37	10	16	11
		Roast beef sandwiches:											
12	1403	Regular	1 ea	147	51	353	22	32	<1	15	7	5	2
12	1404	Junior	1 ea	86	48	218	12	22	<1	9	4	3	2
12	1405	Super	1 ea	234	58	501	25	50	<1	22	9	8	5
12	1406	Deluxe	1 ea	247	62	486	26	43	<1	23	9	8	5
12	1407	Beef 'n Cheddar	1 ea	197	57	455	26	28	<1	27	8	12	7
		Chicken Sandwiches:											
12	1408	Chicken breast sandwich	1 ea	195	52	509	26	36	<1	29	6	11	12
12	1409	Chicken salad sandwich	1 ea	156	53	386	18	33	<1	20	—	—	—
12	1410	Chicken salad & croissant	1 ea	150	50	472	22	16	<1	36	—	—	—
12	1411	Chicken club sandwich	1 ea	210	44	621	26	57	<1	32	—	—	—
12	1412	Hot ham and cheese sandwich	1 ea	156	62	292	23	19	<1	14	5	6	3
12	1413	Turkey deluxe sandwich	1 ea	197	61	375	24	33	<1	17	4	5	8
		Baked Potatoes											
12	1414	Plain	1 ea	312	75	290	8	66	6	<1	t	t	t
12	1415	Deluxe, w/butter & sour cream	1 ea	340	74	648	18	59	6	38	22	10	2
12	1416	W/broccoli & cheese	1 ea	340	70	541	13	72	6	22	10	7	3
12	1417	W/mushrooms & cheese	1 ea	321	70	506	16	61	6	22	10	7	3
12	1418	Taco	1 ea	425	70	619	23	73	6	27	11	9	3
		Milkshakes											
12	1419	Chocolate	1 ea	340	74	451	10	77	<1	12	3	7	2
12	1420	Jamocha	1 ea	326	75	368	9	59	0	11	3	6	2
12	1421	Vanilla	1 ea	312	75	330	11	46	0	12	4	5	2

Source: Arby's Inc, Atlanta Georgia for the basic nutrients. Values for dietary fiber, magnesium, phosphorus, potassium, zinc, vitamin A (in RE's), B6, folacin, some of the fatty acids, and percent water, are estimates calculated from known values for major ingredients.

Grp	Ref	Food Description	Measure	Wt (g)	H_2O (%)	Ener (kcal)	Prot (g)	Carb (g)	Dietary Fiber (g)	Fat (g)	Sat	Mono	Poly
BURGER KING													
		Croissant Sandwiches											
12	1422	With egg, bacon & cheese	1 ea	119	49	335	15	20	<1	24	13	8	2
12	1423	With egg, sausage & cheese	1 ea	163	49	538	19	20	<1	41	20	12	3
12	1424	With egg, ham & cheese	1 ea	145	58	335	18	20	<1	20	12	7	1
		Whopper Sandwiches											
12	1425	Whopper	1 ea	265	57	640	27	42	<1	41	16	19	4
12	1426	Whopper w/ cheese	1 ea	289	57	723	31	43	<1	48	20	20	3
12	1427	Double beef	1 ea	351	56	850	46	52	<1	52	20	24	5
12	1428	Double w/cheese	1 ea	374	55	950	51	54	<1	60	24	28	4
12	1429	Whopper, Junior	1 ea	136	52	370	15	31	<1	17	6	8	1
12	1430	Whopper, Junior w/cheese	1 ea	158	55	420	17	32	<1	20	9	8	1
12	1431	Hamburger	1 ea	109	46	275	15	29	<1	12	5	6	<1
12	1432	Cheeseburger	1 ea	120	45	317	17	30	<1	15	7	6	1
12	1433	Bacon double cheeseburger	1 ea	159	41	510	33	27	<1	31	14	15	2
12	1434	Chicken sandwich	1 ea	230	46	688	26	56	<1	40	11	17	10
12	1435	Chicken tenders	1 ea	95	50	204	20	10	0	10	3	4	2
12	1436	Ham & cheese sandwich	1 ea	230	59	471	24	44	<1	23	10	8	4
12	1437	Whaler fish sandwich	1 ea	189	45	488	19	45	<1	27	6	9	10
12	1438	Whaler sandwich w/cheese	1 ea	201	45	530	21	46	<1	30	7	9	10
12	1439	French fries, regular	1 svg	74	37	227	3	24	<1	13	5	4	1
12	1440	Onion rings, regular	1 svg	79	37	274	4	28	<1	16	5	7	4
		Milkshakes											
12	1441	Chocolate, medium	1 ea	273	76	320	8	46	<1	12	—	—	—
12	1442	Vanilla, medium	1 ea	273	74	321	9	49	<1	10	—	—	—

Chol (mg)	Calc (mg)	Iron (mg)	Magn (mg)	Phos (mg)	Pota (mg)	Sodi (mg)	Zinc (mg)	VT-A (RE)	Thia (mg)	Ribo (mg)	Niac (mg)	V-B6 (mg)	Fola (µg)	VT-C (mg)
83	100	2.70	—	—	422	1672	—	85	.15	.26	6	—	—	4
39	80	3.60	16	120	200	588	2.4	t	.23	.43	7.6	.20	14	<1
20	40	1.80	8	60	197	345	1.2	t	.15	.26	4	.10	7	t
40	100	4.50	25	190	500	798	3.8	225	.38	.60	9	.30	21	36
59	100	6.30	25	190	500	1288	3.8	10	.30	.34	5	.30	22	t
63	80	5.40	24	260	335	955	3.3	86	.12	.34	5	.22	19	<1
83	100	3.60	30	180	390	1082	1.0	17	.23	.26	10	.38	18	<1
30	—	—	—	—	—	630	—	—	—	—	—	—	—	—
12	—	—	—	—	—	725	—	—	—	—	—	—	—	—
108	—	—	—	—	—	1300	—	—	—	—	—	—	—	—
45	200	1.80	31	405	312	1350	2.4	60	.98	.51	6	.31	26	24
39	80	2.70	30	250	346	1047	2.3	30	.23	.43	12	.52	20	5
0	20	1.80	80	175	1300	12	1.0	0	.30	.14	5	1.08	30	63
72	300	2.70	83	200	1340	475	1.1	300	.23	.43	6	1.10	33	63
24	150	2.70	97	400	1400	475	2.0	200	.30	.34	6	1.15	60	63
21	300	2.70	91	440	1345	635	2.1	250	.23	.43	7	1.25	36	63
145	450	3.60	105	530	1425	1065	4.7	860	.38	.26	8	1.40	38	63
36	300	1.10	48	350	410	341	1.2	85	.12	.60	.4	.14	14	2
35	300	1.10	36	350	525	262	1.1	85	.09	.51	3	.14	14	t
32	300	.70	36	350	686	281	1.1	85	.12	.60	t	.14	37	2
249	136	2.00	20	249	182	762	1.5	150	.32	.30	2	.06	24	t
293	145	2.90	19	292	284	1042	2.4	150	.36	.32	4	.06	24	t
262	136	2.20	24	317	256	987	1.9	150	.49	.32	3	.06	24	t
94	80	4.90	43	237	547	842	4.5	60	.33	.41	7	.40	35	14
117	210	4.90	47	360	570	1126	5.1	85	.34	.48	7	.40	35	14
188	91	7.30	60	387	760	1080	8.5	60	.34	.56	10	.50	45	14
211	222	7.30	65	510	730	1535	9.1	85	.35	.63	10	.50	45	14
41	40	2.80	24	127	275	486	2.3	30	.23	.25	4	.20	17	6
52	105	2.80	27	189	287	628	2.6	85	.23	.29	4	.20	17	6
37	37	2.70	23	124	235	509	2.4	15	.23	.25	4	.12	18	3
48	102	3.80	26	186	247	651	2.6	70	.23	.29	4	.13	24	3
104	168	3.80	37	328	363	728	5.1	85	.31	.42	6	.30	30	t
82	79	3.30	54	274	375	1423	1.2	13	.45	.31	10	.40	18	t
47	18	.70	24	236	200	636	.6	5	.08	.08	7	.34	10	t
70	195	3.20	42	384	419	1534	2.4	85	.87	.42	6	.31	25	7
84	t	2.20	40	249	366	592	.1	20	.28	.21	4	.13	3	t
95	112	2.20	43	311	378	734	1.1	40	.27	.24	4	.13	3	t
14	t	.50	21	114	360	160	.3	0	.10	.30	7.5	.23	20	t
0	124	.80	18	195	173	665	.4	—	t	t	t	.07	8	t
—	260	1.60	46	262	567	202	1.0	—	.13	.55	t	—	—	t
—	295	t	32	284	505	205	1.0	—	.11	.57	t	—	—	t

Table C–1   Food Composition

Grp	Ref	Food Description	Measure	Wt (g)	H$_2$O (%)	Ener (kcal)	Prot (g)	Carb (g)	Dietary Fiber (g)	Fat (g)	Fat Breakdown (g)		
											Sat	Mono	Poly
		BURGER KING—Con.											
		Pies											
12	1443	Apple pie	1 ea	125	51	305	3	44	<1	12	—	—	—
12	1444	Cherry pie	1 ea	128	42	357	4	55	<1	13	—	—	—
12	1445	Pecan pie	1 ea	113	20	459	5	64	1	20	3	11	5

Source: Burger King Corporation for basic nutrients. Values for fatty acids, dietary fiber, vitamin A (RE's), folacin and percent water, calculated from known values for major ingredients.

Grp	Ref	Food Description	Measure	Wt (g)	H$_2$O (%)	Ener (kcal)	Prot (g)	Carb (g)	Dietary Fiber (g)	Fat (g)	Sat	Mono	Poly
		DAIRY QUEEN											
		Ice cream cones											
12	1446	Small	1 ea	85	65	140	3	22	0	4	2	1	<1
12	1447	Regular	1 ea	142	65	240	6	38	0	7	—	—	—
12	1448	Large	1 ea	213	65	340	9	57	0	10	—	—	—
		Dipped ice cream cones											
12	1449	Small	1 ea	92	58	190	3	25	<1	9	—	—	—
12	1450	Regular	1 ea	156	58	340	6	42	<1	16	—	—	—
12	1451	Large	1 ea	234	58	510	9	64	<1	24	—	—	—
		Sundaes											
12	1452	Small	1 ea	106	60	190	3	33	<1	4	—	—	—
12	1453	Regular	1 ea	177	60	310	5	56	<1	8	—	—	—
12	1454	Large	1 ea	248	60	440	8	78	<1	10	—	—	—
12	1455	Banana Split	1 ea	383	67	540	9	103	<1	11	—	—	—
12	1456	Peanut buster parfait	1 ea	305	52	740	16	94	<1	34	—	—	—
12	1457	Hot fudge brownie delight	1 ea	266	55	600	9	85	<1	25	—	—	—
12	1458	Strawberry shortcake	1 ea	312	61	540	10	100	<1	11	—	—	—
12	1459	Buster bar	1 ea	149	45	460	10	41	<1	29	—	—	—
12	1460	Dilly bar	1 ea	85	55	210	3	21	<1	13	—	—	—
12	1461	DQ ice cream sandwich	1 ea	60	47	140	3	24	<1	4	—	—	—
		Milkshakes:											
12	1462	Small	1 ea	291	63	490	10	82	<1	13	—	—	—
12	1463	Regular	1 ea	418	63	710	14	120	<1	19	—	—	—
12	1464	Large	1 ea	588	63	990	19	168	<1	26	—	—	—
		Malted milkshakes:											
12	1465	Small	1 ea	291	60	520	10	91	<1	13	—	—	—
12	1466	Regular	1 ea	418	60	760	14	134	<1	18	—	—	—
12	1467	Large	1 ea	588	60	1060	20	187	<1	25	—	—	—
12	1468	Float	1 ea	397	76	410	5	82	0	7	—	—	—
12	1469	Freeze	1 ea	397	72	500	9	89	0	12	—	—	—
		Mr. Misty											
12	1470	Regular	1 ea	330	81	250	0	63	0	0	0	0	0
12	1471	Kiss	1 ea	89	81	70	0	17	0	0	0	0	0
12	1472	Freeze	1 ea	411	72	500	9	91	0	12	—	—	—
12	1473	Float	1 ea	411	78	390	5	74	0	7	—	—	—
12	1474	Chicken sandwich	1 ea	220	46	670	29	46	<1	41	8	15	17
12	1475	Fish filet sandwich	1 ea	170	52	400	20	41	<1	16	4	6	6
12	1476	Fish filet sandwich w/cheese	1 ea	177	51	440	24	39	<1	21	7	7	6
		Hamburgers											
12	1477	Single	1 ea	148	51	360	21	33	<1	16	6	7	1
12	1478	Double	1 ea	210	52	530	36	33	<1	28	10	13	2
12	1479	Triple	1 ea	272	52	710	51	33	<1	45	17	21	4
		Cheeseburgers											
12	1480	Single	1 ea	162	51	410	24	33	<1	20	8	8	1
12	1481	Double	1 ea	239	51	650	43	34	<1	37	15	14	2
12	1482	Triple	1 ea	301	52	820	58	34	<1	50	20	20	3

Chol (mg)	Calc (mg)	Iron (mg)	Magn (mg)	Phos (mg)	Pota (mg)	Sodi (mg)	Zinc (mg)	VT-A (RE)	Thia (mg)	Ribo (mg)	Niac (mg)	V-B6 (mg)	Fola (µg)	VT-C (mg)
4	t	1.20	t	31	122	412	.2	4	.27	.16	.6	.03	7	5
6	t	1.10	12	37	166	204	.2	15	.24	.16	.5	.03	4	8
4	24	1.10	16	84	204	374	<1	16	.28	.18	.6	.06	15	t
10	100	.40	13	100	134	45	.47	30	.03	.17	t	.04	2	t
15	150	.70	20	200	220	80	.70	60	.06	.34	t	.06	3	t
25	250	1.40	30	300	330	115	1.0	90	.12	.51	t	.09	4	t
10	100	.40	13	100	134	55	.47	30	.03	.17	t	.04	2	t
20	150	.70	20	200	220	100	.70	60	.06	.34	t	.06	3	t
30	250	1.40	30	300	330	145	1.0	90	.12	.51	t	.09	4	t
10	100	.40	13	150	145	75	.45	30	.03	.17	.17	.03	2	t
20	200	1.10	26	200	290	120	.90	60	.06	.34	.3	.06	4	t
30	250	1.40	40	300	435	165	1.35	120	.12	.43	.4	.09	6	t
30	250	1.80	60	350	670	150	2.1	225	.15	.51	.4	.80	9	15
30	250	1.80	50	450	500	250	1.5	90	.15	.43	2	.10	7	t
20	200	1.80	30	300	300	225	.90	90	.12	.34	.3	.06	4	t
25	250	1.80	—	300	—	215	—	—	.23	.51	t	—	—	12
10	100	1.10	—	250	—	175	—	—	.12	.17	2	—	—	t
10	100	.40	—	100	—	50	—	—	.03	.17	t	—	—	t
5	60	.04	—	60	—	40	—	—	.03	.07	.4	—	—	t
35	350	1.80	30	400	480	180	.10	75	.15	.60	.3	.14	3	t
50	450	2.70	43	500	690	260	.14	105	.23	.77	.4	.20	4	t
70	700	3.60	60	800	960	360	.20	150	.30	1.2	.8	.28	6	t
35	350	2.70	30	400	480	180	.10	75	.15	.60	.4	.14	3	t
50	450	4.50	43	600	690	260	.14	105	.30	.85	.8	.20	4	t
70	700	5.40	60	800	960	360	.20	150	.38	1.2	1.20	.28	6	t
20	200	1.10	—	200	—	85	—	60	.06	.26	t	—	—	t
30	300	1.80	—	350	—	180	—	120	.15	.51	t	—	—	t
0	t	t	—	t	—	10	—	0	t	t	t	—	—	t
0	t	t	—	t	—	10	—	—	t	t	t	—	—	t
30	300	1.40	—	200	—	140	—	—	.12	.51	t	—	—	t
20	200	.70	—	200	—	95	—	—	.06	.26	t	—	—	t
75	t	.40	15	60	200	870	.5	8	.06	t	.1	.16	9	9
50	60	.70	20	200	370	875	.3	<1	.15	.26	3	.16	40	<1
60	150	.40	22	250	370	1035	.3	30	.15	.26	3	.16	20	<1
45	100	3.60	33	150	290	630	4.5	10	.30	.17	5	.18	16	t
85	100	6.30	45	300	410	660	6.4	20	.45	.34	9	.28	23	t
135	100	9.00	60	450	532	690	8.2	28	.60	.51	14	.33	29	t
50	200	3.60	35	250	300	790	5.0	110	.30	.17	5	.20	20	t
95	350	6.30	50	500	443	980	7.3	160	.45	.43	9	.30	30	t
145	350	9.00	65	700	550	1010	9.2	200	.60	.60	14	.55	37	t

Table C–1 Food Composition

Grp	Ref	Food Description	Measure	Wt (g)	H₂O (%)	Ener (kcal)	Prot (g)	Carb (g)	Dietary Fiber (g)	Fat (g)	Fat Breakdown (g)		
											Sat	Mono	Poly
		DAIRY QUEEN-Con.											
		Hotdogs											
12	1483	Regular	1 ea	100	50	280	11	21	<1	16	6	7	2
12	1484	With cheese	1 ea	114	49	330	15	21	<1	21	8	8	2
12	1485	With chili	1 ea	128	55	320	13	23	2	20	8	8	2
		Super Hotdogs											
12	1486	Regular	1 ea	175	48	520	17	44	<1	27	9	12	3
12	1487	With cheese	1 ea	196	48	580	22	45	<1	34	11	13	3
12	1488	With chili	1 ea	218	53	570	21	47	2	32	11	13	3
12	1489	French fries, small	1 svg	71	47	200	2	25	<1	10	4	3	<1
12	1490	French fries, large	1 svg	113	47	320	3	40	<1	16	7	5	1
12	1491	Onion Rings	1 svg	85	28	280	4	31	<1	16	5	7	4

Source: International Dairy Queen Inc., Minneapolis, MN for basic nutrients. Values for dietary fiber, magnesium, potassium, zinc, fatty acids, vitamin A (RE's), B6, folacin and percent water, calculated from known values for the major ingredients.

Grp	Ref	Food Description	Measure	Wt (g)	H₂O (%)	Ener (kcal)	Prot (g)	Carb (g)	Dietary Fiber (g)	Fat (g)	Sat	Mono	Poly
		JACK IN THE BOX											
12	1492	Breakfast Jack sandwich	1 ea	126	49	307	18	30	<1	13	—	—	—
12	1493	Canadian crescent	1 ea	134	42	472	19	25	<1	31	—	—	—
12	1494	Sausage crescent	1 ea	156	38	584	22	28	<1	43	—	—	—
12	1495	Supreme crescent	1 ea	146	38	547	20	27	<1	40	—	—	—
12	1496	Pancakes breakfast	1 ea	232	45	626	16	79	<1	27	—	—	—
12	1497	Scrambled egg breakfast	1 ea	267	51	719	26	55	<1	44	—	—	—
12	1498	Hamburger	1 ea	98	44	276	13	30	<1	12	—	—	—
12	1499	Cheeseburger	1 ea	113	44	323	16	32	<1	15	—	—	—
12	1500	Jumbo Jack	1 ea	205	57	485	26	38	<1	26	—	—	—
12	1501	Jumbo Jack w/cheese	1 ea	246	56	630	32	45	<1	35	—	—	—
12	1502	Bacon cheeseburger supreme	1 ea	231	45	724	34	44	<1	46	—	—	—
12	1503	Swiss & baconburger	1 ea	231	52	643	33	31	<1	43	—	—	—
12	1504	Ham & swiss burger	1 ea	203	44	638	36	37	<1	39	—	—	—
12	1505	Chicken supreme	1 ea	228	52	601	31	39	<1	36	—	—	—
12	1506	Moby Jack sandwich	1 ea	137	40	444	16	39	<1	25	—	—	—
12	1507	Club Pita	1 ea	177	64	284	22	30	<1	8	—	—	—
		Tacos											
12	1508	Regular	1 ea	81	57	191	8	16	<1	11	—	—	—
12	1509	Super	1 ea	135	63	288	12	21	<1	17	—	—	—
12	1510	Chicken strips dinner	1 ea	180	23	689	40	65	—	30	—	—	—
12	1511	Shrimp dinner	1 ea	165	16	731	22	77	<1	37	—	—	—
12	1512	Pasta seafood salad	1 ea	150	52	394	15	32	2	22	—	—	—
12	1513	Taco salad	1 ea	358	81	377	31	10	1	24	—	—	—
		Nachos											
12	1514	Cheese	1 svg	155	36	571	15	49	—	35	—	—	—
12	1515	Supreme	1 svg	340	70	718	23	66	—	40	—	—	—
12	1516	French fries	1 svg	68	40	221	2	27	<1	12	—	—	—
12	1517	Hash brown potatoes	1 svg	90	60	68	2	15	<1	12	—	—	—
12	1518	Onion rings	1 svg	108	28	382	5	39	<1	23	—	—	—
		Milkshakes											
12	1519	Chocolate	1 ea	322	77	330	11	55	0	7	—	—	—
12	1520	Strawberry	1 ea	328	77	320	10	55	0	7	—	—	—
12	1521	Vanilla	1 ea	317	76	320	10	57	0	6	—	—	—
12	1522	Apple turnover	1 ea	119	38	410	4	45	<1	24	—	—	—

Source: Jack in the Box Restaurants, Foodmaker, Inc., San Diego, CA for basic nutrients. Some values for dietary fiber, magnesium, phosphorus, potassium, zinc, vitamin A (RE's), B6, folacin, and fatty acids, calculated from known values for major ingredients.

Chol (mg)	Calc (mg)	Iron (mg)	Magn (mg)	Phos (mg)	Pota (mg)	Sodi (mg)	Zinc (mg)	VT-A (RE)	Thia (mg)	Ribo (mg)	Niac (mg)	V-B6 (mg)	Fola (μg)	VT-C (mg)
45	80	1.40	21	100	130	830	1.4	t	.12	.14	3	.08	20	<1
55	150	1.40	24	200	140	990	1.9	85	.12	.17	3	.08	24	<1
55	80	1.80	38	150	170	985	1.8	60	.15	.26	4	.17	30	<1
80	150	2.70	24	150	210	1365	2.8	t	.23	.26	5	.14	35	<1
100	250	1.40	38	300	220	1605	2.5	100	.23	.26	5	.16	39	<1
100	150	2.70	48	250	250	1595	2.5	60	.23	.43	6	.25	45	<1
10	t	.34	16	60	450	115	t	0	.06	t	.8	.16	15	9
15	t	1.08	24	100	700	185	.3	0	.09	.03	1.2	.30	25	15
15	20	.72	16	60	110	140	.3	15	.09	t	.4	.08	10	2
203	170	3.10	24	310	190	871	1.8	—	.47	.41	3	.11	—	<1
226	125	3.40	—	—	—	851	—	—	.50	.40	3.6	—	—	3
187	170	2.90	—	—	—	1012	—	—	.60	.51	4.6	—	—	t
178	150	2.70	—	—	—	1053	—	—	.64	.54	4.2	—	—	t
85	100	2.70	36	633	237	1670	1.9	—	.60	.43	5	.19	3	27
260	250	2.40	55	483	635	1110	3.0	—	.68	.59	5	.34	1	12
29	70	2.70	20	115	165	521	1.8	9	.36	.24	3.2	.10	—	1
42	160	2.70	22	194	177	749	2.3	57	.36	.27	3.3	.10	—	1
64	97	6.90	35	208	390	905	3.7	—	.51	.21	7	.25	—	5
110	250	4.50	49	411	499	1665	4.8	—	.53	.34	12	.31	—	5
70	310	4.90	—	—	—	1307	—	—	.56	.51	8.8	—	—	3
99	230	4.70	—	—	—	1354	—	—	.45	.41	6.8	—	—	3
117	268	6.10	—	—	—	1330	—	—	.76	.48	7.6	—	—	10
60	240	3.00	—	—	—	1582	—	—	.52	.37	10.6	—	—	4
47	160	2.20	30	263	246	820	1.1	—	.40	.25	2.8	.08	—	<1
43	80	—	—	—	—	953	—	—	.78	.29	5.9	—	—	4
21	100	1.10	35	146	257	460	1.2	—	.07	.17	1.0	.13	—	<1
37	150	1.60	45	198	347	765	1.8	—	.12	.08	1.4	.18	—	2
100	110	4.00	—	—	—	1213	—	—	.45	.29	18.6	—	—	12
157	370	4.90	—	—	—	1510	—	—	.39	.17	7	—	—	12
48	208	5.90	—	—	—	1570	—	—	.38	.23	1.8	—	—	21
102	280	4.30	—	—	—	1436	—	—	.18	.53	6	—	—	7
37	370	1.40	—	—	—	1154	—	—	.11	.19	1	—	—	3
65	410	3.20	—	—	—	1782	—	—	.15	.26	3.2	—	—	8
8	10	.50	23	75	360	164	.26	<1	.07	.03	1.20	.18	—	3
0	t	.70	—	—	—	15	—	<1	.03	t	.08	—	—	4
27	30	1.40	16	69	109	407	.40	<1	.21	.12	1.80	.06	—	3
25	350	.70	55	330	650	270	1.20	—	.15	.59	.60	.18	—	3
25	350	.40	40	328	613	240	1.10	—	.15	.43	.40	.16	—	3
25	350	.30	38	312	599	230	1.00	<1	.15	.34	.40	.20	—	<1
15	11	1.40	10	33	69	350	.20	—	.23	.12	2.50	.03	—	<1

Table C–1 Food Composition

Grp	Ref	Food Description	Measure	Wt (g)	H₂O (%)	Ener (kcal)	Prot (g)	Carb (g)	Dietary Fiber (g)	Fat (g)	Fat Breakdown (g)		
											Sat	Mono	Poly
KENTUCKY FRIED CHICKEN													
		Original Recipe:											
12	1253	Center breast	1 ea	95	52	236	24	7	<1	14	4	7	2
12	1251	Side breast	1 ea	69	39	199	16	7	<1	12	3	5	3
12	1250	Drumstick	1 ea	47	53	117	12	3	<1	7	2	3	2
12	1252	Thigh	1 ea	88	49	257	18	7	<1	18	4	7	4
12	1249	Wing	1 ea	42	44	136	10	4	<1	9	2	4	2
		Dinners:											
12	1254	2 pce dinner, white	1 ea	322	64	604	30	48	1	32	7	12	10
12	1255	2 pce dinner, dark	1 ea	346	65	643	35	46	1	35	8	13	11
12	1256	2 pce dinner, combination	1 ea	341	63	661	33	48	1	38	8	14	11
		Extra crispy recipe:											
12	1261	Center breast	1 ea	104	39	297	24	14	<1	16	4	7	4
12	1259	Side breast	1 ea	84	39	286	17	14	<1	18	5	7	4
12	1258	Drumstick	1 ea	58	51	155	13	5	<1	9	2	4	2
12	1260	Thigh	1 ea	107	45	343	20	13	<1	23	6	10	6
12	1257	Wing	1 ea	53	36	201	11	9	<1	14	4	6	3
		Dinners:											
12	1262	2 pce dinner, white	1 ea	348	60	755	33	60	1	43	10	16	12
12	1263	2 pce dinner, dark	1 ea	375	62	765	38	55	1	54	11	16	13
12	1264	2 pce dinner, combination	1 ea	371	60	902	36	58	1	48	12	18	14
12	1265	Mashed potatoes	⅓ c	80	81	60	2	12	<1	1	<1	<1	<1
12	1266	Chicken gravy	⅓ c	78	76	59	2	4	<1	4	1	2	<1
12	1267	Dinner roll	1 ea	21	31	61	2	11	<1	1	<1	<1	<1
12	1268	Corn on the cob	1 ea	143	70	176	5	32	2	3	<1	1	1
12	1269	Coleslaw	⅓ c	79	76	103	1	12	<1	6	1	2	3
12	1381	Kentucky nuggets	1 ea	16	44	46	3	2	<1	3	1	2	<1
		Kentucky nugget sauces											
12	1382	Barbeque	2 tbsp	30	51	35	<1	7	—	1	<1	<1	<1
12	1383	Sweet & sour	2 tbsp	30	50	58	<1	13	—	1	<1	<1	<1
12	1384	Honey sauce	1 tbsp	15	50	49	0	12	—	<1	—	—	—
12	1385	Mustard sauce	2 tbsp	30	52	36	1	6	—	1	—	—	—
12	1386	Kentucky fries	1 svg	119	45	268	5	33	<1	13	3	8	1
12	1387	Mashed potatoes & gravy	⅓ c	86	80	62	2	10	<1	1	<1	<1	<1
12	1388	Buttermilk biscuit	1 ea	75	27	269	5	32	<1	14	4	8	1
12	1389	Potato salad	⅓ c	90	76	141	2	13	1	9	1	3	5
12	1390	Baked beans	⅓ c	89	71	105	5	18	6	1	<1	<1	<1
12	1391	Chicken Little sandwich	1 ea	57	52	177	6	17	1	9	2	3	3

Source: Kentucky Fried Chicken Corporation

Grp	Ref	Food Description	Measure	Wt (g)	H₂O (%)	Ener (kcal)	Prot (g)	Carb (g)	Dietary Fiber (g)	Fat (g)	Sat	Mono	Poly
LONG JOHN SILVER'S													
		Fish, batter fried											
12	1523	Fish & fryes, 3 pce	1 ea	350	55	853	43	64	<1	48	—	—	—
12	1524	Fish & fryes, 2 pce	1 ea	260	53	651	30	53	<1	36	—	—	—
12	1525	Fish dinner, 3 pce	1 ea	540	60	1180	47	93	<1	70	—	—	—
		Fish, breaded & fried											
12	1526	Fish dinner, 3 pce	1 ea	450	60	940	35	84	<1	52	—	—	—
12	1527	Fish dinner, 2 pce	1 ea	400	60	818	26	76	<1	46	—	—	—
		Chicken											
12	1528	Chicken plank dinner, 3 pce	1 ea	370	60	885	32	72	<1	51	—	—	—
12	1529	Chicken plank dinner, 4 pce	1 ea	440	60	1037	41	82	<1	59	—	—	—
12	1530	Chicken nugget dinner, 6 pce	1 ea	300	60	699	23	54	<1	45	—	—	—
12	1531	Clam chowder	1 svg	185	85	128	7	15	<1	5	—	—	—

GRP KEY: 1 = BEV 2 = DAIRY 3 = EGGS 4 = FAT/OIL 5 = FRUIT 6 = BAKERY 7 = GRAIN 8 = FISH 9 = BEEF 10 = POULTRY
11 = SAUSAGE 12 = MIXED/FAST 13 = NUTS/SEEDS 14 = SWEETS 15 = VEG/LEG 16 = MISC 22 = SOUP/SAUCE

Chol (mg)	Calc (mg)	Iron (mg)	Magn (mg)	Phos (mg)	Pota (mg)	Sodi (mg)	Zinc (mg)	VT-A (RE)	Thia (mg)	Ribo (mg)	Niac (mg)	V-B6 (mg)	Fola (µg)	VT-C (mg)
87	30	1.17	28	205	267	631	.72	6	.08	.11	7.57	.31	8	2
70	50	.98	19	151	176	558	.77	4	.06	.08	5.66	.20	6	1
63	12	.80	13	95	122	207	1.29	3	.04	.09	2.38	.09	4	1
109	34	1.45	22	169	217	566	1.65	5	.08	.16	4.03	.17	9	2
55	22	.68	10	76	86	302	.58	3	.03	.04	2.28	.10	4	1
133	142	3.31	61	326	643	1528	1.88	77	.22	.19	10.0	.50	39	37
180	116	3.90	66	363	720	1441	3.47	77	.25	.32	8.46	.46	42	37
172	126	3.78	64	344	684	1536	2.76	77	.24	.27	8.36	.47	41	37
79	62	1.29	29	218	244	584	.77	6	.11	.11	7.89	.30	11	2
65	57	1.12	21	157	188	564	.88	5	.12	.13	5.37	.24	9	2
66	11	.95	14	100	147	263	1.32	4	.07	.11	3.07	.16	6	1
109	49	1.49	24	185	228	549	1.73	7	.12	.19	5.35	.17	11	2
59	16	.65	12	77	100	312	.67	3	.06	.09	2.94	.11	5	1
132	143	6.03	65	333	689	1544	2.08	77	.31	.29	10.4	.56	43	37
183	130	4.09	70	383	776	1480	3.58	77	.32	.38	10.4	.54	46	37
176	135	6.40	68	361	729	1529	2.93	77	.31	.35	10.3	.49	45	37
<1	21	.28	14	41	218	228	.16	5	.01	.04	.96	.11	7	5
2	9	.48	2	10	21	398	.04	1	.01	.03	.47	<.01	2	<1
1	21	.53	6	28	29	118	.20	1	.10	.04	.98	.01	7	<1
<1	7	.79	53	134	323	12	.99	27	.14	.11	1.80	.22	71	2
4	29	.19	9	20	115	171	.13	28	.03	.03	.20	.07	10	19
12	2	.13	4	29	33	140	.22	30	.02	.03	1.00	.04	1	2
1	6	.24	5	10	75	450	.05	37	.01	.01	.19	.02	3	<1
1	5	.16	2	5	39	148	.02	6	.01	.02	.04	.01	1	<1
t	1	.11	<1	<1	6	10	<.01	0	.01	<.01	.04	t	1	3
1	10	.26	6	15	23	346	.09	1	.02	.01	.16	.02	3	1
1	24	.94	28	78	606	81	.31	0	.17	.06	2.70	.18	20	3
1	19	.35	9	28	137	297	.11	5	.01	.04	1.00	.08	8	1
1	77	1.22	9	264	95	521	.29	30	.28	.13	1.80	.03	8	<1
11	10	.32	15	32	256	396	.29	27	.07	.02	.60	.19	7	3
1	54	1.43	29	90	229	387	1.29	10	.06	.04	.50	.07	32	2
20	39	1.40	10	105	114	398	.93	6	.15	.14	1.65	.07	11	<1
17	—	—	—	—	—	611	—	—	—	—	—	—	—	—
27	—	—	—	—	—	1543	—	—	—	—	—	—	—	—
56	—	—	—	—	—	2076	—	—	—	—	—	—	—	—
55	—	—	—	—	—	763	—	—	—	—	—	—	—	—
37	—	—	—	—	—	1579	—	—	—	—	—	—	—	—
95	—	—	—	—	—	2161	—	—	—	—	—	—	—	—
127	—	—	—	—	—	1297	—	—	—	—	—	—	—	—
75	—	—	—	—	—	1402	—	—	—	—	—	—	—	—
64	—	—	—	—	—	986	—	—	—	—	—	—	—	—

Table C–1 Food Composition

Grp	Ref	Food Description	Measure	Wt (g)	H₂O (%)	Ener (kcal)	Prot (g)	Carb (g)	Dietary Fiber (g)	Fat (g)	Fat Breakdown (g)		
											Sat	Mono	Poly
LONG JOHN SILVER'S—Con.													
12	1532	Clam dinner	1 ea	460	60	955	22	100	<1	58	—	—	—
12	1533	Fish & chicken dinner	1 ea	460	60	935	36	73	<1	55	—	—	—
12	1534	Oyster dinner	1 ea	360	60	789	17	78	<1	45	—	—	—
12	1535	Scallop dinner	1 ea	320	60	747	17	66	<1	45	—	—	—
12	1536	Seafood platter	1 ea	410	60	976	29	85	<1	58	—	—	—
12	1537	Batter fried shrimp dinner	1 ea	300	60	711	17	60	<1	45	—	—	—
12	1538	Fish sandwich platter	1 ea	400	60	835	30	84	<1	42	—	—	—
		Salads											
12	1539	Ocean chef	1 ea	320	85	229	27	13	2	8	—	—	—
12	1540	Seafood	1 ea	480	85	426	19	22	2	30	—	—	—
12	1541	Cole slaw	1 svg	98	70	182	1	11	<1	15	—	—	—
12	1542	Fries	1 svg	85	42	247	4	31	<1	12	—	—	—
12	1543	Hush puppies	1 ea	47	37	145	3	18	<1	7	—	—	—

Source: Long John Silver's Inc., Lexington, KY.

Grp	Ref	Food Description	Measure	Wt (g)	H₂O (%)	Ener (kcal)	Prot (g)	Carb (g)	Dietary Fiber (g)	Fat (g)	Sat	Mono	Poly
McDONALD'S													
		Sandwiches											
12	1221	Big Mac	1 ea	200	48	570	25	39	1	35	12	13	8
12	1222	Quarter Pounder	1 ea	160	49	427	25	29	1	24	9	11	2
12	1223	Quarter Pounder w/cheese	1 ea	186	48	525	30	31	1	32	13	12	2
12	1224	Filet-O-Fish sandwich	1 ea	143	44	435	15	36	<1	26	6	9	9
12	1225	Hamburger	1 ea	100	46	263	12	28	<1	11	4	5	1
12	1226	Cheeseburger	1 ea	114	45	318	15	29	<1	16	7	6	1
12	1227	French fries	1 svg	68	37	220	3	26	<1	12	5	4	1
12	1228	Chicken McNuggets	6 ea	109	49	323	19	15	<1	20	5	11	2
		Sauces											
12	1229	Mustard Sauce	1 ea	30	53	63	1	11	<1	2	<1	1	1
12	1230	Barbecue	1 ea	32	51	60	<1	14	<1	<1	<1	<1	<1
12	1231	Sweet & sour	1 ea	32	50	64	<1	15	<1	<1	<1	<1	<1
		Milkshakes											
12	1232	Chocolate	10 fl oz	291	70	383	10	66	<1	9	4	2	<1
12	1233	Strawberry	10 fl oz	290	72	362	9	62	<1	9	4	3	<1
12	1234	Vanilla	10 fl oz	291	73	352	10	60	<1	8	4	3	<1
		Sundaes											
12	1235	Hot fudge	1 ea	164	60	357	7	58	<1	11	5	3	1
12	1236	Strawberry	1 ea	164	62	320	6	54	<1	9	3	3	1
12	1237	Caramel	1 ea	165	57	361	7	61	<1	10	3	3	1
12	1238	Soft ice cream cone	1 ea	115	65	189	4	31	<1	5	2	1	<1
		Pies											
12	1239	Fried Apple	1 ea	85	45	253	2	29	<1	14	5	7	1
12	1240	Fried Cherry	1 ea	88	44	260	2	32	<1	14	5	7	1
		Cookies, package											
12	1241	McDonaldland cookies	1 pkg	67	3	308	4	49	<1	10	4	5	1
12	1242	Chocolate chip cookies	1 pkg	69	3	342	4	45	<1	16	8	6	1
		Breakfast items:											
12	1243	English muffin, w/butter	1 ea	63	42	186	5	30	<1	5	2	2	1
12	1244	Egg McMuffin	1 ea	138	51	340	19	31	<1	16	6	5	2
12	1245	Hot Cakes w/butter & syrup	1 ea	214	46	500	8	94	<1	10	4	4	1
12	1246	Scrambled eggs	1 ea	98	70	180	13	3	<1	13	5	5	2
12	1247	Sausage	1 svg.	53	43	210	10	1	<1	19	7	9	2
12	1248	Hash brown potato patty	1 ea	55	56	144	1	15	<1	9	3	5	1
12	1392	Sausage McMuffin	1 ea	115	38	427	18	30	<1	26	10	11	3

Chol (mg)	Calc (mg)	Iron (mg)	Magn (mg)	Phos (mg)	Pota (mg)	Sodi (mg)	Zinc (mg)	VT-A (RE)	Thia (mg)	Ribo (mg)	Niac (mg)	V-B6 (mg)	Fola (µg)	VT-C (mg)
113	—	—	—	—	—	1086	—	—	—	—	—	—	—	—
12	—	—	—	—	—	367	—	—	—	—	—	—	—	—
13	—	—	—	—	—	1	—	—	—	—	—	—	—	—
1	—	—	—	—	—	405	—	—	—	—	—	—	—	—
106	—	—	—	—	—	2025	—	—	—	—	—	—	—	—
75	—	—	—	—	—	1352	—	—	—	—	—	—	—	—
119	—	—	—	—	—	2797	—	—	—	—	—	—	—	—
101	—	—	—	—	—	1900	—	—	—	—	—	—	—	—
76	—	—	—	—	—	1526	—	—	—	—	—	—	—	—
25	—	—	—	—	—	1918	—	—	—	—	—	—	—	—
25	—	—	—	—	—	2433	—	—	—	—	—	—	—	—
25	—	—	—	—	—	853	—	—	—	—	—	—	—	—
83	203	4.90	38	314	249	979	4.69	38	.48	.38	7.20	.27	21	3
80	98	4.30	37	249	322	718	5.11	23	.35	.32	7.20	.27	23	3
107	255	4.84	41	382	341	1195	5.70	128	.37	.41	7.07	.23	23	3
47	133	2.47	27	229	150	800	.89	28	.36	.23	3.00	.10	20	2
29	84	2.85	19	126	142	506	2.09	14	.31	.22	4.08	.12	17	2
40	169	2.84	23	205	157	730	2.60	67	.30	.24	4.33	.12	21	2
9	9	.61	27	101	564	109	.32	5	.12	.02	2.26	.22	19	13
63	11	1.25	26	283	302	512	.89	27	.16	.14	7.52	.38	11	2
3	8	.17	6	15	23	259	.09	1	.01	<.01	.08	.01	3	<1
<1	4	.12	5	10	75	309	.05	5	.01	.01	.08	.02	3	1
<1	2	.08	2	5	39	186	.02	20	.01	.01	.07	.01	1	<1
30	320	.84	45	306	533	300	1.16	72	.13	.44	.50	.14	14	3
32	322	.17	34	289	487	207	1.02	86	.12	.44	.35	.14	11	4
31	329	.18	34	326	500	200	1.05	79	.12	.70	.35	.14	35	3
27	215	.61	35	236	410	170	.98	58	.07	.31	1.12	.13	11	2
25	174	.38	28	180	290	90	.80	58	.07	.30	1.03	.05	20	3
31	200	.23	30	230	338	145	.87	70	.07	.31	1.01	.05	13	4
24	183	.12	17	160	182	109	.64	55	.06	.36	.44	.06	3	1
7	14	.62	6	27	39	398	.16	3	.02	.02	.19	.02	5	1
8	12	.59	7	27	39	427	.15	11	.03	.02	.25	.02	3	1
10	12	1.47	11	74	52	358	.34	8	.23	.23	2.85	.03	6	1
18	29	1.56	29	108	170	313	.50	23	.12	.21	1.70	.03	6	1
15	117	1.51	13	74	71	310	.50	42	.28	.49	2.61	.04	17	1
259	226	2.93	26	322	168	885	1.92	145	.47	.44	3.77	.21	30	1
47	3	2.23	28	501	187	1070	.69	64	.26	.36	2.27	.12	9	5
514	61	2.53	13	264	135	205	1.66	187	.08	.47	.20	.20	65	1
39	16	.82	9	95	127	423	1.47	9	.27	.11	2.07	.18	1	1
4	5	.40	13	67	247	325	.17	1	.06	.01	.82	.13	6	4
59	168	2.25	24	186	215	942	1.68	114	.70	.25	4.14	.15	23	1

Table C–1   Food Composition

Grp	Ref	Food Description	Measure	Wt (g)	H₂O (%)	Ener (kcal)	Prot (g)	Carb (g)	Dietary Fiber (g)	Fat (g)	Fat Breakdown (g)		
											Sat	Mono	Poly
McDONALD'S—Con.													
12	1393	Sausage McMuffin w/egg	1 ea	165	47	517	23	32	<1	33	13	14	4
12	1394	Biscuit, plain	1 ea	85	27	330	5	37	<1	18	8	7	2
12	1395	Biscuit w/sausage	1 ea	121	32	467	12	35	<1	31	12	14	4
12	1396	Biscuit w/sausage & egg	1 ea	175	43	585	20	36	<1	40	15	17	5
12	1397	Biscuit w/bacon, egg & cheese	1 ea	145	41	483	17	33	<1	32	10	14	3
		Salads											
12	1398	Chef salad	1 ea	273	84	226	21	6	2	13	6	4	1
12	1399	Shrimp salad	1 ea	264	88	99	14	5	2	3	1	1	<1
12	1400	Garden salad	1 ea	204	91	91	6	4	2	6	3	2	<1
12	1401	Chicken salad oriental	1 ea	280	88	146	23	5	2	4	1	1	1

Source: McDonald's Corporation, Oak Brook, Illinois. Some values for Salads estimated from known values for major ingredients.

Grp	Ref	Food Description	Measure	Wt (g)	H₂O (%)	Ener (kcal)	Prot (g)	Carb (g)	Dietary Fiber (g)	Fat (g)	Sat	Mono	Poly
TACO BELL													
		Burritos:											
12	1544	Bean	1 ea	191	58	360	13	54	8	11	5	5	1
12	1545	Beef	1 ea	191	58	402	22	38	2	17	8	7	1
12	1546	Bean & beef	1 ea	191	58	381	17	46	5	14	7	6	1
12	1547	Burrito supreme	1 ea	248	66	422	17	46	5	19	9	8	1
12	1548	Double beef supreme	1 ea	262	66	465	23	41	2	23	11	10	1
12	1549	Enchirito	1 ea	213	66	382	20	30	5	20	10	8	1
12	1550	Fajita (steak taco)	1 ea	142	65	235	15	20	2	11	5	4	1
		Tacos:											
12	1551	Regular	1 ea	78	55	184	10	11	1	11	6	3	1
12	1552	Taco bellgrande	1 ea	170	63	351	18	20	2	22	13	6	1
12	1553	Taco light	1 ea	170	59	411	19	18	2	29	18	8	1
12	1554	Soft taco	1 ea	92	52	228	12	18	2	12	5	4	1
		Tostadas:											
12	1555	Regular	1 ea	156	67	243	10	28	7	11	5	4	1
12	1556	Beefy tostada	1 ea	198	69	322	15	22	4	20	10	8	1
12	1557	Bellbeefer	1 ea	177	63	312	17	32	<1	13	6	4	2
12	1558	Mexican pizza	1 ea	269	55	714	28	43	5	48	31	14	2
12	1559	Taco salad with salsa	1 ea	601	73	949	36	63	5	62	40	18	3
		Nachos:											
12	1560	Regular	1 ea	106	40	356	7	38	<1	19	12	5	1
12	1561	Bellgrande	1 ea	333	58	719	23	65	6	49	23	20	2
12	1562	Pintos & cheese	1 ea	128	69	194	9	19	7	10	5	4	<1
12	1563	Taco sauce	1 ea	3.7	96	2	<1	<1	<1	<1	<1	<1	<1
12	1564	Salsa	1 ea	90.7	95	18	1	4	1	<1	<1	<1	<1
12	1565	Cinnamon Crispas	1 ea	47.3	1	266	3	27	<1	16	13	2	1

Source: Taco Bell Corporation, California for most nutrient values. Values for Dietary fiber, mono-unsaturated fat, magnesium, phosphorus, zinc, folacin, Vitamin B6, Vitamin A in REs, and percentage water are estimates calculated from known values of major ingredients.

Grp	Ref	Food Description	Measure	Wt (g)	H₂O (%)	Ener (kcal)	Prot (g)	Carb (g)	Dietary Fiber (g)	Fat (g)	Sat	Mono	Poly
WENDY's													
		Hamburgers:											
12	1566	Single, on white bun, no toppings	1 ea	117	41	350	21	27	<1	18	7	9	1
12	1567	Single, on multigrain bun, no toppings	1 ea	211	45	527	30	28	2	33	12	13	2
12	1568	Double, on white bun, no toppings	1 ea	197	44	560	41	32	<1	34	7	13	8
12	1569	Big classic	1 ea	241	63	470	26	36	2	25	7	10	5

Chol (mg)	Calc (mg)	Iron (mg)	Magn (mg)	Phos (mg)	Pota (mg)	Sodi (mg)	Zinc (mg)	VT-A (RE)	Thia (mg)	Ribo (mg)	Niac (mg)	V-B6 (mg)	Fola (µg)	VT-C (mg)
287	196	3.47	30	288	294	1044	2.36	198	.84	.50	4.46	.20	33	<1
9	74	1.30	10	299	108	786	.33	54	.21	.15	1.70	.03	9	<1
48	82	2.05	17	353	231	1147	1.31	18	.56	.22	3.39	.12	12	1
285	119	3.43	24	476	312	1301	2.10	126	.53	.49	3.85	.19	35	1
263	2	2.57	20	461	232	1269	1.55	196	.30	.43	2.32	.10	44	2
125	222	1.30	25	200	400	850	1.40	125	.35	.33	5.20	.04	60	20
187	64	.87	60	180	420	570	1.90	71	.13	.13	1.70	.06	60	10
110	104	.63	18	80	280	100	.40	65	.08	.16	.94	.06	60	10
92	47	1.40	20	140	350	270	.66	120	.14	.17	7.60	.34	61	22
14	120	2.19	65	210	427	921	2.05	65	.66	.39	2.74	1.00	55	2
59	103	2.11	35	225	313	994	4.00	100	.31	.44	3.44	.23	27	2
36	111	2.15	50	220	370	958	2.67	80	.49	.42	3.09	.59	38	2
35	142	2.21	50	227	437	952	3.00	185	.45	.45	3.14	.52	40	9
59	140	2.45	52	230	434	1054	4.00	200	.34	.49	3.68	.30	30	9
56	260	2.10	61	263	423	1260	3.51	157	.39	.41	2.12	.61	29	3
14	119	3.03	24	150	207	507	3.18	133	.41	.34	2.74	.17	15	3
32	78	1.10	16	100	159	274	2.12	42	.07	.14	1.07	.12	10	1
55	165	1.91	18	100	334	470	2.12	132	.13	.28	1.91	.12	13	5
57	156	2.07	18	100	316	575	2.12	128	.10	.28	1.78	.12	13	5
32	116	2.27	18	100	178	516	2.12	42	.39	.22	2.74	.12	10	1
18	161	1.81	62	195	401	670	1.55	84	.40	.22	1.15	1.01	47	3
40	185	1.96	43	206	408	764	2.97	152	.24	.29	1.61	.56	31	6
39	174	2.36	22	125	299	855	2.10	121	.16	.30	1.73	.12	<1	5
81	453	3.08	80	400	449	1364	5.40	355	.36	.39	2.00	1.11	60	7
85	393	5.92	130	460	1222	1763	5.59	450	.69	.78	4.00	1.30	140	25
9	178	.99	40	200	158	423	.80	27	.03	.16	.09	.14	4	2
43	323	4.19	100	400	763	1312	4.30	280	.52	.47	2.36	.98	33	12
19	139	1.75	110	156	384	733	2.17	87	.43	.21	1.15	.21	68	1
0	2	.07	—	—	13	126	—	19	<.01	<.01	.06	—	—	<1
0	36	.60	—	—	163	376	—	112	.02	.14	—	—	—	2
2	25	.71	—	—	36	122	—	<1	.03	.02	.18	—	—	<1
65	32	4.50	20	118	220	410	2.10	—	.22	.25	5.00	.12	<1	<1
86	167	4.01	46	368	464	814	4.65	—	.35	.31	5.55	.28	36	6
125	48	6.30	42	339	431	575	8.35	—	.22	.43	9.00	.47	29	<1
81	43	4.55	34	200	468	901	5.11	31	.26	.24	4.80	.25	30	12

Table C–1 Food Composition

Grp	Ref	Food Description	Measure	Wt (g)	H₂O (%)	Ener (kcal)	Prot (g)	Carb (g)	Dietary Fiber (g)	Fat (g)	Fat Breakdown (g)		
											Sat	Mono	Poly
		WENDY'S—Con.											
		Cheeseburgers:											
12	1570	Bacon cheeseburger	1 ea	147	46	460	29	23	<1	28	13	13	2
12	1571	Single, w/all toppings	1 ea	215	50	548	30	32	2	33	13	12	5
12	1572	Double, w/all toppings	1 ea	291	50	735	48	27	2	48	18	18	6
		Baked Potatoes:											
12	1573	Plain	1 ea	250	75	249	6	52	5	<1	<1	<1	<1
12	1574	W/bacon & cheese	1 ea	372	71	610	16	55	5	31	17	11	3
12	1575	W/broccoli & cheese	1 ea	377	74	502	13	56	5	25	11	8	4
12	1576	W/cheese	1 ea	404	71	727	17	56	5	32	20	10	2
12	1577	W/chili & cheese	1 ea	453	72	653	21	64	8	28	14	12	1
12	1578	W/sour cream & chives	1 ea	280	71	405	7	54	5	18	11	5	1
12	1579	Chili	1 c	256	77	260	21	26	5	8	3	4	<1
12	1580	French fries	1 svg	106	43	306	4	38	<1	15	7	5	2
12	1581	Frosty dairy dessert	1 c	216	35	354	7	53	0	13	5	3	2
12	1582	Chocolate chip cookie	1 ea	64	5	320	3	40	1	17	6	6	5

Source: Wendy's International, for most nutrient values. Some of the values for Dietary fiber, the types of fatty acids, magnesium, phosphorus, zinc, folacin, Vitamin B6, Vitamin A in REs, and percentage water are estimates calculated from known values of major ingredients.

Chol (mg)	Calc (mg)	Iron (mg)	Magn (mg)	Phos (mg)	Pota (mg)	Sodi (mg)	Zinc (mg)	VT-A (RE)	Thia (mg)	Ribo (mg)	Niac (mg)	V-B6 (mg)	Fola (µg)	VT-C (mg)
65	136	3.60	33	296	332	860	5.14	82	.27	.28	5.70	.24	25	1
84	177	4.00	33	339	430	864	4.41	111	.34	.35	5.29	.25	28	6
165	180	5.40	50	470	620	883	8.80	112	.36	.53	10.0	.46	31	6
0	34	2.82	67	169	1362	58	.65	0	.28	.11	3.82	.70	68	10
36	207	3.94	79	657	1602	1560	2.81	250	.52	.39	7.68	.82	68	13
20	226	3.44	76	449	1478	435	.76	370	.31	.27	4.06	.77	95	33
27	742	3.04	67	423	1472	1371	.65	240	.28	.21	3.84	.70	68	7
18	686	4.58	85	354	1682	1538	2.07	220	.32	.23	5.07	.80	83	9
5	45	2.82	68	177	1376	171	.68	15	.28	.13	3.82	.70	69	7
30	64	4.50	60	320	594	1070	3.78	300	.15	.17	3.00	.26	40	6
15	13	1.02	45	197	689	105	.51	0	.15	.04	2.96	.27	33	12
45	257	.86	43	238	518	194	.92	143	.11	.45	.31	.12	17	<1
7	10	1.09	15	62	102	237	.46	0	.05	.08	.58	.03	6	0

647

D

Vitamin/Mineral Supplements Compared

Tables D–1, D–2, and D–3 are useful for comparing the essential vitamin and mineral contents of supplements commonly available in the United States. Note that blank columns have been provided for the addition of locally available products you may wish to compare with those shown here.*

Not all ingredients in vitamin/mineral preparations are of proven benefit. To facilitate meaningful comparison, the tables list only the nutrients known to be essential in human nutrition. Other nutrients and compounds found on the labels of these supplements are listed in the table notes.

When a supplement is needed that supplies certain nutrients, these tables will ease the task of selecting an appropriate one. Note, for example, that some preparations marketed for the elderly are composed largely of alcohol, with few vitamins or minerals. These are "tonics," not vitamin/mineral supplements. A tonic may be useful if the only need is for comfort and the benefit of the placebo effect, but if an elderly person needs a balanced assortment of vitamins and minerals and cannot easily take pills, it may be advisable to suggest a liquid preparation designated for infants.

Note the very low levels of calcium present in some of these preparations. A product that supplies 20 milligrams of calcium provides only two percent of an adult's RDA for calcium and would have no significant impact on a person's calcium nutrition.

*These tables are reprinted, with permission, from L. K. DeBruyne and S. R. Rolfes, *Selection of Supplements,* a 1986 monograph in the *Nutrition Clinics* series available from Stickley Publishing Co., 210 Washington Sq., Philadelphia, PA 19106.

TABLE D–1 Supplements for Infants and Children

Company	Lederle	Miles Laboratories	Mead-Johnson	Mead-Johnson	Radiance	Chocks
Product	Centrum Jr.	Flintstones with Iron	Poly-Vi-Sol	Poly-Vi-Sol Iron and Zinc	Chewable for Children	Bugs Bunny plus Iron
Age of Intended Users	Children over 4	Children over 2	Infants	Children and Adults	Children 2 to 12	Children over 2
Recommended Daily Dose	1 Chewable	1 Chewable	1 ml Dropper	1 Chewable	1 Chewable	1 Chewable
Vitamins						
Vitamin A (IU)	5000	2500	1500	2500	4000	2500
Vitamin D (IU)	400	400	400	400	400	400
Vitamin E (IU)	15	15	5	15	3.4	15
Vitamin C (mg)	60	60	35	60	60	60
Thiamin (B_1) (mg)	1.5	1.05	0.5	1.05	2	1.05
Riboflavin (B_2) (mg)	1.7	1.2	0.6	1.2	2.4	1.2
Vitamin B_6 (mg)	2	1.05	0.4	1.05	2	1.05
Vitamin B_{12} (μg)	6	4.5	2	4.5	10	4.5
Niacin (mg)	20	13.5	8	13.5	10	13.5
Folacin (mg)	0.4	0.3	—	0.3	—	0.3
Minerals						
Calcium (mg)	—	—	—	—	19	—
Phosphorus (mg)	—	—	—	—	—	—
Iron (mg)	18	15	—	12	12	15
Potassium (mg)	1.6	—	—	—	4	—
Mangnesium (mg)	25	—	—	—	22	—
Zinc (mg)	10	—	—	8	—	—
Copper (mg)	2	—	—	—	0.2	—
Iodine (μg)	—	—	—	—	—	—
Manganese (mg)	1	—	—	—	—	—
Cost per day[a]						

[a]Divide the total retail price for the container by the number of doses per container. For example, XYZ Vitamins are sold in bottles of 100 tablets, and the recommended dose is 2 tablets per day; there are 50 doses in the bottle. At $5.00 per bottle, XYZ Vitamins cost $.10 per day.

TABLE D–1 (continued)

	Neolife	J. B. Williams	Upjohn	Amway	Shaklee	Richardson Vicks	Ross Labs	Miles Labs	Other
	Vita Squares	Popeye with Mins/ Iron	Unicap	Nutrilite	Vita-Lea Children	Life-Stage Children	Vi-Daylin with Iron	Flintstones Complete	
	Children over 2	Children	Children	Children	Children over 4	Children 4 to 12	Children under 4	Children over 4	
	3 Chewables	1 Chewable	1 Chewable	1 Chewable	2 Chewables	2 Chewables	1 Dropper	1 Chewable	
	3000	2500	5000	2500	2000	5000	1500	5000	
	400	400	400	400	400	400	400	400	
	9	15	15	10	10	30	5	30	
	60	60	60	40	60	60	35	60	
	1.5	1.05	1.5	0.7	1.1	1.5	0.5	1.5	
	1.5	1.2	1.7	0.8	1.2	1.7	0.6	1.7	
	1.2	1.05	2	0.7	1.5	2	0.4	2	
	3	4.5	6	3	3	6	1.5	6	
	10	13.5	20	9	14	20	8	20	
	0.2	0.3	0.4	0.2	0.3	0.4	—	0.4	
	—	—	—	—	130	—	—	100	
	—	—	—	—	100	—	—	100	
	3	15	—	5	10	9	10	18	
	—	—	—	—	—	—	—	—	
	—	40	—	—	60	—	—	20	
	—	12	—	—	1.5	—	—	15	
	0.002	1.5	—	—	0.2	—	—	—	
	75	105	—	—	15	—	—	150	
	1	—	—	—	—	—	—	2.5	

Note: Radiance chewables also contain 2 mg pantothenic acid, 10 mg biotin, 2 mg inositol, and 2 mg of a choline compound.
Neolife chewables also contain 10 mg pantothenic acid, 0.075 mg inositol, 0.05 mg of a choline compound, 15 mg biotin, and 15 mg PABA.
Williams chewables also contain 2.5 mg pantothenic acid and 37.5 mg biotin.
Amway chewables also contain 5 mg pantothenic acid.
Shaklee chewables also contain 4 mg pantothenic acid and 0.1 mg biotin.
Lederle chewables also contain 1.4 mg chlorine (recommended daily dose for children 2 to 4 is ½ tablet).
Richardson Vicks chewables also contain 10 mg pantothenic acid and 0.3 mg biotin.

TABLE D–2 Supplements for Adults

Company	Lederle	Parke-Davis	Squibb	Miles Labs	Radiance	Neolife	Amway
Product	Centrum A to Zinc	Myadec	Theragran M	One-a-Day Plus Iron	Nutri-Mega	Formula IV	Nutrilite Double X
Recommended Daily Dose	*1 Tablet*	*1 Tablet*	*1 Tablet*	*1 Tablet*	*2 Tablets*	*2 Capsules*	*9 Tablets*
Vitamins							
Vitamin A (IU)	5000	10,000	10,000	5000	10,000	4000	15,000
Vitamin D (IU)	400	400	400	400	400	400	400
Vitamin E (IU)	30	30	15	30	300	10	30
Vitamin C (mg)	90	250	200	60	300	90	500
Thiamin (B_1) (mg)	2.25	10	10.3	1.5	50	10	15
Riboflavin (B_2) (mg)	2.6	10	10	1.7	50	10	15
Vitamin B_6 (mg)	3	5	4.1	2	50	10	15
Vitamin B_{12} (g)	9	6	5	6	50	10	9
Niacin (mg)	20	100	100	20	50	50	35
Folacin (mg)	0.4	0.4	—	0.4	0.4	0.4	0.4
Minerals							
Calcium (mg)	162	—	—	—	200	—	900
Phosphorus (mg)	125	—	—	—	50	—	450
Iron (mg)	27	20	12	18	18	25	18
Potassium (mg)	7.7	—	—	—	30	10	—
Magnesium (mg)	100	100	65	—	50	35	300
Zinc (mg)	22.5	20	1.5	—	15	—	15
Copper (mg)	3	2	2	—	2	2	2
Iodine (μg)	150	150	150	—	150	100	150
Manganese (mg)	7.5	1.25	1	—	30	10	5
Cost per day [a]							

[a]Divide the total retail price for the container by the number of doses per container. For example, XYZ Vitamins are sold in bottles of 100 tablets, and the recommended dose is 2 tablets per day; there are 50 doses in the bottle. At $5.00 per bottle, XYZ Vitamins cost $.10 per day.

TABLE D–2 (continued)

J. B. Williams	Origin	Miles Labs	Mineralab	Richardson Vicks	Richardson Vicks	J. B. Williams	Upjohn	Squibb	Other
Vitabank	Multi-vitamin	One-a-Day Plus Minerals	Added Protection III	Lifestage— Women	Lifestage— Men	Femiron	Unicap Plus Iron	Theragran Z	
1 Tablet	1 Tablet	1 Tablet	6 Tablets	1 Tablet	1 Tablet	1 Tablet	1 Tablet	1 Tablet	
5000	10,000	5000	10,000	5000	10,000	5000	5000	10,000	
400	400	400	200	400	400	400	400	400	
30	30	30	400	30	50	15	15	15	
90	250	60	1200	100	200	60	60	200	
2.25	20	1.5	100	3	10	1.5	1.5	10.3	
2.6	20	1.7	50	3.4	10	1.7	1.7	10	
3	5	2	100	4	5	2	2	4.1	
9	6	6	100	12	6	6	6	5	
20	150	20	40	40	100	20	20	100	
0.4	0.4	0.4	0.8	0.4	0.4	0.4	0.4	—	
170	100	129.6	500	—	—	10	—	—	
130	—	100	—	—	—	—	—	—	
18	30	18	20	27	18	20	18	12	
7.5	5	5	99	—	—	—	—	—	
100	50	100	500	100	100	—	—	—	
15	7.5	15	30	15	15	—	—	22.5	
2	1	2	2	2	2	—	—	2	
150	150	150	200	150	150	—	—	150	
2.5	1.5	2.5	20	—	1.25	—	—	1	

Note: Lederle Centrum A to Zinc also contains 10 mg pantothenic acid, 45 μg biotin, 25 μg selenium, 15 μg molybdenum, 15 μg chromium, and 7 mg chlorine.

Radiance Nutri-Mega also contains 50 mg pantothenic acid, 50 μg biotin, 50 mg inositol, 50 mg PABA, 50 mg of a choline compound, and 80 mg lecithin.

Neolife Formula IV also contains 12 mg pantothenic acid, 65 mg inositol, 30 mg PABA, 30 mg lecithin, 40 mg diastase, 45 mg lipase (pancreatin), 168 mg linoleic acid, 40 mg pancrein, and 10 mg betaine.

Origin Multivitamins also contains 20 mg pantothenic acid, 25 μg biotin, 10 mg inositol, and 20 mg of a choline compound.

Amway Nutrilite Double X also contains 10 mg panthothenic acid, 5 μg chromium, and 5 μg selenium.

J.B. Williams Vitabank also contains 18 mg pantothenic acid and 25 μg selenium.

Miles Labs One-a-Day plus Minerals also contains 10 mg pantothenic acid, 10 μg chromium, 10 μg selenium, and 10 μg molybdenum.

Miles Labs One-a-Day plus Iron also contains 30 μg biotin, 10 mg pantothenic acid, and 50 μg vitamin K.

Squibb Theragran Z and M also contain 18.4 mg pantothenic acid.

Parke-Davis Myadec also contains 20 mg pantothenic acid.

Mineral Lab Added Protection III also contains 500 mg pantothenic acid, 300 μg biotin, 150 mg of a choline compound, 100 mg inositol, 50 mg PABA, 100 mg citrus bioflavinoid complex, 200 μg chromium, 200 μg selenium, 100 μg molybdenum, 5000 IU beta-carotene, 150 mg niacinamide, and 100 μg trace elements.

Richardson Vicks Lifestage for Women and Men also contain 10 and 20 mg pantothenic acid, respectively.

Upjohn Unicap plus Iron also contains 10 mg pantothenic acid.

TABLE D–3 Supplements and Tonics for the Elderly

Company	Ross Labs	Lederle	J.B. Williams	J.B. Williams	Upjohn	Other
Product	Vi-Daylin Plus Iron	Gevrabon	Geritol	Geritol	Unicap Senior	
Recommended Daily Dose	*1 Tsp*	*1 Oz*	*1 Oz*	*1 Tablet*	*1 Tablet*	
Vitamins						
Vitamin A (IU)	2500	—	—	—	5000	
Vitamin D (IU)	400	—	—	—	—	
Vitamin E (IU)	15	—	—	—	15	
Vitamin C (mg)	60	—	—	75	60	
Thiamin (B_1) (mg)	1.05	5	5	5	1.2	
Riboflavin (B_2) (mg)	1.2	2.5	5	5	1.7	
Vitamin B_6 (mg)	1.05	1	1	0.5	2	
Vitamin B_{12} (μg)	4.5	1	1.5	3	6	
Niacin (mg)	13.5	50	100	30	14	
Folacin (mg)	—	—	—	—	0.4	
Minerals						
Calcium (mg)	—	—	—	2	—	
Phosphorus (mg)	—	—	—	—	—	
Iron (mg)	10	15	100	50	10	
Potassium (mg)	—	—	—	—	5	
Magnesium (mg)	—	2	—	—	—	
Zinc (mg)	—	2	—	—	15	
Copper (mg)	—	—	—	—	2	
Iodine (μg)	—	100	—	—	150	
Manganese (mg)	—	2	—	—	1	
Alcohol (%)	0.5	18	12	—	—	
Cost per day[a]						

[a]Divide the total retail price for the container by the number of doses per container. For example, XYZ Vitamins are sold in bottles of 100 tablets, and the recommended dose is 2 tablets per day; there are 50 doses in the bottle. At $5.00 per bottle, XYZ Vitamins cost $.10 per day.

Note: Lederle Gevrabon also contains 100 mg inositol and 100 mg of a choline compound.
J.B. Williams Geritol also contains 100 mg of a choline compound, 50 mg methionine, and 4 mg panthenol.
Upjohn Unicap Senior also contains 10 mg pantothenic acid.

E

Enteral Formulas

As you can see from this appendix, the number of commercially prepared formulas available to meet the nutrient needs of people unable to meet these needs using regular foods is staggering. By the time this appendix has gone to press, even more formulas may be on the market. The information presented here can help you see the similarities and differences among formulas so that you can select the most appropriate one for your client.

Source: Sandoz Nutrition Corporation, Clinical Products Division, Minneapolis, MN.

TABLE E–1. Enteral Formulas[†]

Product	Manufacturer	Form	Major Protein Sources	Major Fat Sources	Major Carbohydrate Sources	Protein (g/1,000 ml)	Fat (g/1,000 ml)	Carbohydrate (g/1,000 ml)	kCalories/ml	mOsm/kg
					Nutrient Sources					
Amin-Aid®[1]	Kendall McGaw	Powder	Free essential amino acids plus histidine	Partially hydrogenated soybean oil	Maltodextrin, sucrose	19.4	46.2	366	2.0	1095
Citrotein®	SandozNutrition	Powder	Egg white solids	Partially hydrogenated soybean oil	Sucrose, maltodextrin	41	1.6	122	0.66	480 Punch
Compleat® Modified Formula	SandozNutrition	Liquid	Beef, calcium caseinate	Beef, corn oil	Hydrolyzed cereal solids, fruits and vegetables	43	37	141	1.07	300
Compleat® Regular Formula	SandozNutrition	Liquid	Beef, nonfat milk	Beef, corn oil	Hydrolyzed cereal solids, fruits, vegetables, maltodextrin, lactose	43	43	128	1.07	405
Criticare HN®	Mead Johnson	Liquid	Enzymatically hydrolyzed casein, free amino acids	Safflower oil	Maltodextrin, modified corn starch	38	3	222	1.06	650
Enrich™	Ross	Liquid	Sodium and calcium caseinates, soy protein isolate	Corn oil	Hydrolyzed corn starch, sucrose, soy polysaccharide	39.7	37.2	162	1.1	480
Ensure®	Ross	Liquid	Sodium and calcium caseinates, soy protein isolate	Corn oil	Corn syrup, sucrose	37.2	37.2	145	1.06	450
Ensure® HN	Ross	Liquid	Sodium and calcium caseinates, soy protein isolate	Corn oil	Corn syrup, sucrose	44.4	35.5	141	1.06	470
Ensure Plus®	Ross	Liquid	Sodium and calcium caseinates, soy protein isolate	Corn oil	Corn syrup, sucrose	54.9	53.3	200	1.5	600
Ensure Plus® HN	Ross	Liquid	Sodium and calcium caseinates, soy protein isolate	Corn oil	Corn syrup, sucrose	62.6	49.9	200	1.5	650

[†]Based on manufacturers' available literature.
[*]Value not provided in available literature.
[+]Retinol equivalents
[++]Tocopherol equivalents
[1]Does not contain vitamins or electrolytes.
[2]One packet Sustacal Powder mixed with whole milk to prepare a 40 kcal/fl oz serving.
[3]At 1.0 kcal/ml dilution.
[4]Does not contain fat-soluble vitamins or electrolytes.

BCAA: Branched-chain amino acids
MCT: Medium-chain triglycerides

Volume to meet 100% of U.S. RDA	Vitamin A (IU)	Vitamin D (IU)	Vitamin E (IU)	Vitamin C (mg)	Folacin (μg)	Thiamin (mg)	Riboflavin (mg)	Niacin (mg)	Vitamin B6 (mg)	Vitamin B12 (μg)	Biotin (mg)	Pantothenic Acid (mg)	Calcium (g)	Phosphorus (g)	Iodine (μg)	Iron (mg)	Magnesium (mg)	Copper (mg)	Zinc (mg)	Vitamin K (μg)	Choline (g)	Potassium g (mEq)	Sodium g (mEq)	Chloride g (mEq)	Manganese (mg)	Selenium (μg)
—	—	—	—	—	—	—	—	—	—	—	—	—	—	—	—	—	—	—	—	—	—	*(<6)	*(<15)	—	—	—
1270	5250	420	31.5	236	830	3.15	3.5	42	4.3	12.6	0.63	20.9	1.06	1.06	158	37.8	420	2.1	16	—	0.35	0.71 (18.2)	0.71 (31)	0.94 (26.5)	5.1	—
1500	3330	267	20	60	270	1.5	1.7	13.3	2.0	4.0	0.20	6.7	0.67	0.93	100	12	267	1.3	10	67	0.20	1.4 (35.9)	0.67 (29.1)	0.47 (13.3)	2.7	67
1500	3330	267	20	60	270	1.5	1.7	13	2.0	4.0	0.20	6.7	0.67	1.3	100	12	267	1.3	10	67	0.20	1.4 (35.9)	1.3 (56.5)	0.87 (24.5)	2.7	67
1892	2642	211	40	159	211	2.0	2.3	26.4	2.6	8.0	0.16	13.2	0.53	0.53	80	9.5	211	1.0	10.6	131	0.26	1.32 (34)	0.63 (27)	1.06 (30)	2.6	*
1391	3593	287	32.5	215	431	1.6	1.9	21.5	2.2	6.7	0.33	10.8	0.719	0.719	108	12.9	287	1.4	16.2	51	0.43	1.564 (40.0)	0.845 (36.8)	1.437 (40.5)	3.6	*
1887	2642	211	23.8	158.5	211	1.6	1.8	21.1	2.1	6.3	0.16	5.3	0.528	0.528	79.5	9.5	211	1.1	11.9	38	0.32	1.564 (40.0)	0.845 (36.8)	1.437 (40.5)	2.6	*
1320	3775	304	34.2	226.6	456	1.7	1.9	22.7	2.28	7.2	0.34	11.3	0.757	0.757	113	13.6	302	1.5	17.0	55	0.45	1.564 (40.0)	0.930 (40.5)	1.437 (40.5)	3.8	*
1600	3525	283	31.7	211	566	2.1	2.4	28.2	2.8	8.5	0.42	14.1	0.706	0.706	106	12.7	283	1.4	15.8	51	0.42	2.113 (54.1)	1.141 (49.6)	1.987 (56)	3.5	*
947	5283	423	47.8	317	845	3.2	3.6	42	4.2	12.7	0.63	21.1	1.056	1.056	159	19.0	423	2.1	23.8	76	0.63	1.818 (46.5)	1.184 (51.5)	1.606 (45.3)	5.3	*

TABLE E–1. Enteral Formulas[†]

Product	Manufacturer	Form	Major Protein Sources	Major Fat Sources	Major Carbohydrate Sources	Protein (g/1,000 ml)	Fat (g/1,000 ml)	Carbohydrate (g/1,000 ml)	kCalories/ml	mOsm/kg
Entrition®	Biosearch	Liquid	Sodium and calcium caseinates	Corn oil	Maltodextrin	35	35	136	1.0	300
Fortison™	Chesebrough-Pond's	Liquid	Calcium and sodium caseinates	Partially hydrogenated soybean oil	Maltodextrin, sucrose	35	40	125	1.0	300
Hepatic-Aid®II[1]	Kendall McGaw	Powder	Free amino acids (46% BCAA)	Partially hydrogenated soybean oil	Maltodextrin, sucrose	44.1	36.2	169	1.1	560
Isocal®	Mead Johnson	Liquid	Calcium and sodium caseinates, soy protein isolate	Soybean oil, MCT	Maltodextrin	34	44	133	1.06	300
Isocal® HCN	Mead Johnson	Liquid	Calcium and sodium caseinates	Soybean oil, MCT	Corn syrup	75	91	225	2.0	690
Isotein HN®	SandozNutrition	Powder	Delactosed lactalbumin	Partially hydrogenated soybean oil, MCT	Maltodextrin, monosaccharides	68	34	156	1.2	300
Magnacal®	Chesebrough-Pond's	Liquid	Calcium and sodium caseinates	Partially hydrogenated soybean oil	Maltodextrin, sucrose	70	80	250	2.0	590
Meritene® Liquid	SandozNutrition	Liquid	Concentrated sweet skim milk	Corn oil	Lactose, corn syrup solids, sucrose	57.6	32	110	0.96	505 van.
Meritene® Powder (prepared w/ whole milk)	SandozNutrition	Powder	Nonfat milk	Milk fat	Lactose, sucrose, corn syrup solids	69	34	119	1.0	690
Osmolite®	Ross	Liquid	Sodium and calcium caseinates, soy protein isolate	MCT, corn oil, soybean oil	Hydrolyzed cornstarch	37.2	38.5	145	1.06	300
Osmolite® HN	Ross	Liquid	Sodium and calcium caseinates, soy protein isolate	MCT, corn oil, soybean oil	Hydrolyzed cornstarch	44.4	36.8	141	1.06	310
Precision High Nitrogen Diet®	SandozNutrition	Powder	Egg white solids	Partially hydrogenated soybean oil	Maltodextrin, sucrose	43.9	1.3	216	1.05	525
Precision Isotonic Diet®	SandozNutrition	Powder	Egg white solids	Partially hydrogenated soybean oil	Glucose, oligosaccharides, sucrose	29	30	144	1.0	300
Precision LR Diet®	SandozNutrition	Powder	Egg white solids	Partially hydrogenated soybean oil	Maltodextrin, sucrose	26	1.6	248	1.1	530 Van.

[†]Based on manufacturers' available literature.
[*]Value not provided in available literature.
[+]Retinol equivalents
[++]Tocopherol equivalents
[1]Does not contain vitamins or elecrolytes.
[2]One packet Sustacal Powder mixed with whole milk to prepare a 40 kcal/fl oz serving.
[3]At 1.0 kcal/ml dilution.
[4]Does not contain fat-soluble vitamins or electrolytes.

BCAA: Branched-chain amino acids
MCT: Medium-chain triglycerides

Volume to meet 100% of U.S. RDA	Vitamin A (IU)	Vitamin D (IU)	Vitamin E (IU)	Vitamin C (mg)	Folacin (μg)	Thiamin (mg)	Riboflavin (mg)	Niacin (mg)	Vitamin B$_6$ (mg)	Vitamin B$_{12}$ (μg)	Biotin (mg)	Pantothenic Acid (mg)	Calcium (g)	Phosphorus (g)	Iodine (μg)	Iron (mg)	Magnesium (mg)	Copper (mg)	Zinc (mg)	Vitamin K (μg)	Choline (g)	Potassium g (mEq)	Sodium g (mEq)	Chloride g (mEq)	Manganese (mg)	Selenium (μg)
2000	2500	200	30	150	400	1.5	1.7	20	2.0	6.0	0.3	10	0.50	0.50	75	9.0	200	1.0	7.5	100	0.4	1.2 (30.7)	0.70 (30.5)	1.0 (28.2)	2.0	*
2000	2500	200	30	150	200	1.5	1.7	20	2	6	0.15	5	0.5	0.5	75	9	200	1.0	15	150	0.25	1.25 (32)	0.50 (22)	0.85 (24)	2.5	*
—	—	—	—	—	—	—	—	—	—	—	—	—	—	—	—	—	—	—	—	—	—	* (<6)	* (<15)	—	—	—
1892	2638	211	40	158	211	2.0	2.3	26	2.6	8.0	0.16	3	0.634	0.528	80	9.5	211	1.1	10.6	132	0.26	1.32 (34)	0.53 (23)	1.06 (30)	2.6	*
1500	3330	270	50	200	270	2.5	2.9	33	3.3	10	0.20	16.7	0.67	0.67	100	12	270	2.0	20	165	0.33	1.4 (36)	0.80 (35)	1.2 (34)	3.3	*
1770	2820	226	17	51	230	1.27	1.47	11.3	1.7	3.4	0.17	5.7	0.56	0.56	85	10.2	226	1.13	8.5	57	0.06	1.07 (27.4)	0.62 (27)	0.96 (27.1)	2.3	85
1000	5000	400	60	300	400	3	3.4	40	4	12	0.3	10	1.0	1.0	150	18	400	2	30	300	0.50	1.250 (32.1)	1.00 (43.5)	0.950 (26.8)	5	*
1250	4000	320	24	72	320	1.8	2.1	16	2.4	4.8	0.24	8.0	1.2	1.2	120	14.4	320	1.6	12	—	0.08	1.6 (41)	0.88 (38.3)	1.6 (45.1)	3.2	—
1040	4800	385	28.8	57.7	380	1.5	2.6	19.2	1.9	6.9	0.29	9.6	2.2	1.9	146	17.3	385	1.9	14.4	77	0.21	2.8 (71.8)	1.1 (47.8)	2.2 (62.1)	3.8	—
1887	2642	211	23.8	158.5	423	1.6	1.8	21.1	2.1	6.3	0.32	10.6	0.528	0.528	79.5	9.5	211	1.1	11.9	38	0.32	1.014 (25.9)	0.634 (27.6)	0.845 (23.8)	2.62	*
1320	3804	304	34.2	139	465	1.7	1.9	22.8	2.3	7.2	0.35	11.4	0.76	0.76	114	1.39	304	1.5	17.3	55	0.59	1.564 (40)	0.930 (40.5)	1.437 (40.5)	3.8	*
2850	1760	140	10.5	31.6	140	0.79	0.91	7.0	1.1	2.1	0.11	3.5	0.35	0.35	52.6	6.3	140	0.70	5.3	35.1	0.04	0.91 (23.3)	0.98 (42.6)	1.19 (33.6)	1.4	61
1560	3210	256	19.2	57.7	260	1.44	1.67	12.8	1.92	3.85	0.19	6.41	0.64	0.64	96.2	11.5	256	1.28	9.6	64.1	0.06	0.96 (24.6)	0.77 (19.7)	1.03 (44.8)	2.7	64
1710	2920	235	17.5	52.6	240	1.3	1.5	11.7	1.8	3.5	0.18	5.9	0.58	0.58	88	10.5	234	1.2	8.8	58.5	0.06	0.88 (22.6)	0.70 (30.4)	1.1 (31)	2.4	58.5

TABLE E–1. Enternal Formulas[†]

Product	Manufacturer	Form	Nutrient Sources — Major Protein Sources	Major Fat Sources	Major Carbohydrate Sources	Protein (g/1,000 ml)	Fat (g/1,000 ml)	Carbohydrate (g/1,000 ml)	kCalories/ml	mOsm/kg
Pulmocare®	Ross	Liquid	Sodium and calcium caseinates	Corn oil	Sucrose, hydrolyzed cornstarch	62.6	92.1	106	1.5	490
Resource® Instant Crystals™	SandozNutrition	Instant Crystals	Sodium and calcium caseinates, soy protein isolate	Hydrogenated soybean oil	Maltodextrin, sucrose	37.2	37.2	145	1.06	450
Ross SLD™	Ross	Powder	Egg white solids	*	Hydrolyzed cornstarch, sucrose	37.5	0.5	137	0.82	550
Stresstein®	SandozNutrition	Powder	Free amino acids (44% BCAA)	MCT, soybean oil	Maltodextrin	70	28	170	1.2	910
Sustacal®	Mead Johnson	Liquid	Calcium and sodium caseinates, soy protein isolate	Partially hydrogenated soybean oil	Sucrose, corn syrup	61	23	140	1.0	625
Sustacal® HC	Mead Johnson	Liquid	Calcium and sodium caseinates	Partially hydrogenated soybean oil	Corn syrup solids, sugar	61	58	190	1.5	650
Sustacal® Powder[2]	Mead Johnson	Powder	Nonfat milk	Milk fat	Lactose, sugar, corn syrup solids	77	34	180	1.33	899
Sustogen®	Mead Johnson	Powder	Nonfat milk, powdered whole milk, calcium caseinate	Milk fat	Corn syrup solids, lactose, dextrose	111.5	16.5	312	1.7	*
Traumacal™ Fulfil™	Mead Johnson	Liquid	Calcium and sodium caseinates	Soybean oil, MCT	Corn syrup, sugar	82.5	68.5	142.5	1.5	550
Traum-Aid® HBC	Kendall McGaw	Powder	Free amino acids (50% BCAA)	Partially hydrogenated soybean oil, MCT	Maltodextrins	56	12.4	166	1.0	675
Travasorb®	Travenol	Liquid	Sodium and calcium caseinates, soy protein isolate	Corn oil, partially hydrogenated soybean oil	Sucrose, corn syrup solids	35	35	136	1.06	488
Travasorb® HN	Travenol	Powder	Enzymatically hydrolyzed lactalbumin	MCT, safflower oil	Glucose oligosaccharides	45	13.4	175	1.0	560
Travasorb® Hepatic	Travenol	Powder	Free amino acids (50% BCAA)	MCT, sunflower oil	Glucose oligosaccharides	28.6	14.3	209	1.1	690
Travasorb® MCT[3]	Travenol	Powder	Lactalbumin, potassium caseinates	MCT, sunflower oil	Corn syrup solids	49.3	33	123	1.0	312
Travasorb® MCT Liquid Diet	Travenol	Liquid	Casein, lactalbumin, and other whey proteins	MCT, safflower oil	Maltodextrin	74	50	185	1.5	488

[†]Based on manufacturers' available literature.
*Value not provided in available literature.
[+]Retinol equivalents
[++]Tocopherol equivalents
[1]Does not contain vitamins or elecrolytes.
[2]One packet Sustacal Powder mixed with whole milk to prepare a 40 kcal/fl oz serving.
[3]At 1.0 kcal/ml dilution.
[4]Does not contain fat-soluble vitamins or electrolytes.

BCAA: Branched-chain amino acids
MCT: Medium-chain triglycerides

Volume to meet 100% of U.S. RDA	Vitamin A (IU)	Vitamin D (IU)	Vitamin E (IU)	Vitamin C (mg)	Folacin (μg)	Thiamin (mg)	Riboflavin (mg)	Niacin (mg)	Vitamin B$_6$ (mg)	Vitamin B$_{12}$ (μg)	Biotin (mg)	Pantothenic Acid (mg)	Calcium (g)	Phosphorus (g)	Iodine (μg)	Iron (mg)	Magnesium (mg)	Copper (mg)	Zinc (mg)	Vitamin K (μg)	Choline (g)	Potassium g (mEq)	Sodium g (mEq)	Chloride g (mEq)	Manganese (mg)	Selenium (μg)
960	5283	423	47.8	317	845	3.17	3.59	42	4.2	12.7	0.63	21.1	1.056	1.056	161	19.0	423	2.11	23.7	76	0.63	1.902 (48.8)	1.310 (57.0)	1.691 (47.6)	5.28	*
1896	2642	211	24.1	161	211	1.6	1.8	21.1	2.1	6.3	0.16	5.3	0.55	0.55	80	9.5	211	1.1	15.9	38	0.55	1.56 (40)	0.85 (36.8)	1.4 (40.5)	2.1	—
1200	4167	333	37.5	75	500	1.92	2.17	25	2.5	7.5	0.38	12.5	0.83	0.83	125	15	333	1.67	19.2	30	0.38	0.833 (21)	0.833 (36)	1.00 (28.2)	4.17	*
2000	2500	200	15	30	200	0.75	0.85	10	1.1	3.0	0.15	5.0	0.5	0.5	75	9.0	200	1.0	7.5	35	0.05	1.1 (28.2)	0.65 (28.3)	1.0 (28.2)	2.0	62.5
1080	4690	376	28	56	380	1.4	1.7	20	2.0	5.6	0.28	9.8	1.0	0.93	140	17	380	2	13.7	234	0.23	2.08 (53)	0.94 (41)	1.58 (44)	2.8	*
1200	4220	338	25	76	506	1.9	2.1	25	2.5	7.6	0.38	12.7	0.85	0.85	127	15	338	1.7	12.7	210	0.21	1.48 (38)	0.84 (37)	1.27 (36)	2.5	*
800	6254	498	37.5	75	498	1.9	2.25	26	2.6	7.5	0.38	13	2.2	1.8	187	22	506	2.6	18.8	*	*	3.4 (87)	1.2 (53.5)	1.8 (51)	3.8	*
1030	5275	422	47	316	422	4.0	4.5	52.8	5.3	15.8	0.32	26.4	3.4	2.5	158	19	422	2.1	21	264	0.53	3.38 (86.5)	1.27 (55)	2.85 (80.2)	5.3	*
2000	2500	200	38	150	200	1.9	2.2	25	2.5	7.5	0.15	12.5	0.75	0.75	75	9.0	200	1.5	15	125	0.25	1.4 (36)	1.2 (52)	1.6 (45)	2.5	*
3000	1667	133	20	33	133	0.5	0.57	6.7	0.67	2.0	0.1	3.3	0.40	0.40	50	6.0	133	0.67	6.7	50	0.14	1.167 (30)	0.533 (23)	0.833 (23.4)	1.3	50
1896	2637	211	32	160	211	1.6	1.8	21.1	2.1	6.3	0.16	5.3	0.527	0.527	80	9.5	210	1.05	15.8	1013	0.53	1.266 (32.5)	0.738 (32)	1.055 (29.7)	2.1	*
2000	2500	200	15	45	200	0.75	0.85	10	1.0	3.0	0.15	5.0	0.5	0.5	75	9.0	200	1.0	7.5	75	0.14	1.17 (30)	0.92 (40)	1.37 (38.6)	1.25	*
2100	486 R.E.+	197	4.9 T.E.++	44	195	0.68	0.77	8.7	1.06	1.4	0.07	2.6	0.38	0.47	71	8.6	186	0.95	7.1	50	0.20	1.14 (29)	0.445 (19.3)	0.690 (19.4)	1.21	*
2000	2500	200	30	150	200	1.5	1.7	20	2.0	6.0	0.15	5.0	0.5	0.5	75	9.0	200	1.0	15	75	0.23	1.74 (44.6)	0.350 (15.2)	1.21 (34.1)	2.0	*
1333	3743	300	45	225	300	2.25	2.5	30.0	3.0	9.0	0.22	7.5	0.75	0.75	112	13.5	300	1.5	22.5	112	0.34	1.48 (25.6)	0.524 (22.8)	1.81 (51.1)	3.0	*

TABLE E–1. Enteral Formulas[†]

Product	Manufacturer	Form	Major Protein Sources	Major Fat Sources	Major Carbohydrate Sources	Protein (g/1,000 ml)	Fat (g/1,000 ml)	Carbohydrate (g/1,000 ml)	kCalories/ml	mOsm/kg
			Nutrient Sources							
Travasorb® Renal[4]	Travenol	Powder	Free amino acids	MCT, sunflower oil	Glucose oligosaccharides, sucrose	22.9	17.7	271	1.35	590
Travasorb® Standard	Travenol	Powder	Hydrolyzed lactalbumin	MCT, sunflower oil	Glucose oligosaccharides	30	13.4	190	1.0	560
TwoCal™ HN	Ross	Liquid	Sodium and calcium caseinates, soy protein isolate	Corn oil, MCT	Hydrolyzed corn starch, sucrose	83.4	90.5	216.4	2.0	740
Vital® HN	Ross	Powder	Protein components, (partially hydrolyzed whey, meat, and soy), free amino acids	Safflower oil, MCT	Hydrolyzed corn starch, sucrose	41.7	10.8	185	1.0	460
Vitaneed®	Chesebrough-Pond's	Liquid	Beef, sodium, and calcium caseinates	Soybean oil, beef	Maltodextrin, pureed fruit and vegetables	35	40	125	1.0	310
Vivonex® High Nitrogen	Norwich-Eaton	Powder	Free amino acids	Safflower oil	Glucose oligosaccharides	46	0.87	210	1.0	810
Vivonex® Standard	Norwich-Eaton	Powder	Free amino acids	Safflower oil	Glucose oligosaccharides	20.4	1.5	231	1.0	550
Vivonex® T.E.N.	Norwich-Eaton	Powder	Free amino acids (33.1% BCAA)	Safflower oil	Maltodextrins, modified starch	38	3.0	206	1.0	630

[†]Based on manufacturers' available literature.
[*]Value not provided in available literature.
[+]Retinol equivalents
[++]Tocopherol equivalents
[1]Does not contain vitamins or elecrolytes.
[2]One packet Sustacal Powder mixed with whole milk to prepare a 40 kcal/fl oz serving.
[3]At 1.0 kcal/ml dilution.
[4]Does not contain fat-soluble vitamins or electrolytes.

BCAA: Branched-chain amino acids
MCT: Medium-chain triglycerides

Volume to meet 100% of U.S. RDA	Vitamin A (IU)	Vitamin D (IU)	Vitamin E (IU)	Vitamin C (mg)	Folacin (μg)	Thiamin (mg)	Riboflavin (mg)	Niacin (mg)	Vitamin B$_6$ (mg)	Vitamin B$_{12}$ (μg)	Biotin (mg)	Pantothenic Acid (mg)	Calcium (g)	Phosphorus (g)	Iodine (μg)	Iron (mg)	Magnesium (mg)	Copper (mg)	Zinc (mg)	Vitamin K (μg)	Choline (g)	Potassium g (mEq)	Sodium g (mEq)	Chloride g (mEq)	Manganese (mg)	Selenium (μg)
2100	—	—	—	43	48	0.71	0.81	9.5	4.8	—	0.14	2.6	—	—	—	—	—	—	—	—	0.19	—	—	—	—	—
2000	2500	200	15	45	200	0.75	0.85	10	1.0	3.0	0.15	5.0	0.50	0.50	75	9.0	200	1.0	7.5	75	0.143	1.17 (30)	0.92 (40)	1.5 (42.3)	1.25	*
950	5263	421	48	189.5	674	2.52	2.86	33.6	3.36	10.1	0.506	16.8	1.06	1.06	160	19	422	2.10	24	75.8	0.8	2.316 (59.4)	1.052 (45.7)	1.558 (44.5)	6.32	*
1500	3333	267	30	60	267	1.0	1.1	13.3	1.5	4.0	0.20	6.7	0.667	0.667	100	12.0	267	1.3	10.0	47	0.13	1.333 (34.1)	0.467 (20.3)	0.900 (25.4)	2.5	*
2000	2500	200	30	150	200	1.5	1.7	20	2.0	6.0	0.15	5.0	0.50	0.50	75	9.0	200	1.0	15	150	0.25	1.25 (32)	0.50 (22)	0.85 (24)	2.5	*
3000	1667	133	10.0	20	133	0.5	0.6	6.7	0.7	2.0	0.10	3.3	0.333	0.333	50	6.0	133	0.7	5.0	22	0.02	1.173 (30.0)	0.529 (23.0)	0.815 (23.0)	0.9	50
1800	2778	222	16.7	33	222	0.8	0.9	11.1	1.1	3.3	0.17	5.6	0.556	0.556	83	10.0	222	1.1	8.3	37	0.04	1.172 (30.0)	0.468 (20.4)	0.722 (20.4)	1.6	84
2000	2500	200	15.0	60	400	1.5	1.7	20.0	2.0	6.0	0.30	10.0	0.50	0.50	75	9.0	200	1.0	10.0	22.3	0.07	0.782 (20.0)	0.460 (20.0)	0.819 (23.1)	0.94	50

TABLE E–2. Enteral Protein Modules[†]

Product	Manufacturer	Form	Nutrient Source — Major Protein Source	g or ml of Product/1,000 kcal	Protein (g/1,000 kcal)	Fat (g/1,000 kcal)	Carbohydrate (g/1,000 kcal)	% kCal from Protein	% kCal from Fat	% kCal from Carbohydrate	kCalories/ml or g of Product	Calcium (g)	Phosphorus (g)	Potassium g (mEq)	Sodium g (mEq)	Chloride g (mEq)
						Nutritional Profile								**Nutrient Analysis per 1,000 kCal**			
Casec®	Mead Johnson	Powder	Calcium caseinates	270 g	238	5	0	95	5	0	3.7 kcal/g	4.3	2.2	0.027 (0.7)	0.41 (18)	0.027 (0.8)
Nutrisource® Amino Acids	SandozNutrition	Powder	Free amino acids	256 g	249	0	0	100	0	0	3.9 kcal/g	0	0	0	0	0
Nutrisource® Amino Acids-High Branched Chain	Sandoz Nutrition	Powder	Free amino acids (44% BCAA)	256 g	249	0	0	100	0	0	3.8 kcal/g	0	0	0	0	0
Nutrisource® Protein	SandozNutrition	Powder	Delactosed lactalbumin, egg white solids	248 g	188	21	17	75	19	6	4.0 kcal/g	0.890	0.744	1.414 (36)	0.670 (29)	0.15 (4.3)
ProMod™	Ross	Powder	Whey protein with lecithin	236 g	179	21.4*	24*	71	19	10	4.2 kcal/g	0.82*	0.79*	2.3* (59)	0.46* (20.4)	**
Propac®	Chesebrough-Pond's	Powder	Whey protein	250 g	192	20	13	77	18	5	4.0 kcal/g	1.5	0.77	1.3 (33)	0.58 (25)	0.17 (4.8)
R.D.P.[1]	Navaco	Powder	Whey protein with lecithin	278 g	209	11	14	84	10	6	3.6 kcal/g	1.02	0.89	2.3 (58)	0.64 (28)	0.64 (18)

[†]Based on manufacturer's available literature.
**Value not provided in available literature.

[1]Also contains trace minerals.

*Does not exceed.

TABLE E–3. Enteral Carbohydrate Modules†

Product	Manufacturer	Form	Nutrient Source / Major Protein Source	g or ml of Product/1,000 kcal	Protein (g/1,000 kcal)	Fat (g/1,000 kcal)	Carbohydrate (g/1,000 kcal)	% kCal from Protein	% kCal from Fat	% kCal from Carbohydrate	kCalories/ml or g of Product	Calcium (g)	Phosphorus (g)	Potassium g (mEq)	Sodium g (mEq)	Chloride g (mEq)
												Nutrient Analysis per 1,000 kCal				
Liquid Carbohydrate Supplement	Navaco	Liquid	Glucose polymers	400 ml	0	0	250	0	0	100	2.5 kcal/ml	0.07	0.03	0.07 (2.0)	0.25 (11)	**
Moducal®	Mead Johnson	Powder	Maltodextrins	263 g	0	0	250	0	0	100	3/8 kcal/g	**	**	0.01 (0.3)	0.18 (8)	0.44 (12)
Nutrisource® Carbohydrate	SandozNutrition	Liquid	Deionized corn syrup solids	313 ml	0	0	250	0	0	100	3.2 kcal/ml	0.001	0.006	0.004 (<1)	0.006 (<1)	0.003 (<1)
Polycose® Liquid	Ross	Liquid	Hydrolyzed corn starch	500 ml	0	0	250	0	0	100	2.0 kcal/ml	0.15	0.03	0.10 (2.6)	0.29 (12)	0.54 (15)
Polycose® Powder	Ross	Powder	Hydrolyzed corn starch	263 g	0	0	250	0	0	100	3.8 kcal/g	0.15	0.03	0.10 (2.6)	0.30 (13)	0.56 (16)
Pure Carbohydrate Supplement	Navaco	Powder	Glucose polymers	250 g	0	0	250	0	0	100	4.0 kcal/g	0.02	0.03	Trace	0.04 (1.6)	**
Sumacal®	Chesebrough-Pond's	Powder	Maltodextrins	263 g	0	0	250	0	0	100	3.8 kcal/g	**	**	**	0.26 (11)	0.55 (15)

†Based on manufacturer's available literature.
**Value not provided in available literature.

TABLE E–4. Enteral Fat Modules[†]

Product	Manufacturer	Form	Nutrient Source Major Fat Source	Nutritional Profile g or ml of Product/1,000 kcal	Protein (g/1,000 kcal)	Fat (g/1,000 kcal)	Carbohydrate (g/packet)	% kCal from Protein	% kCal from Fat	% kCal from Carbohydrate	kCalories/ml or g of Product
High Fat Supplement[1]	Navaco	Powder	Partially hydrogenated coconut oil	163 g	8	77	66[2]	3	70	26	6.12 kcal/g
MCT® Oil	Mead Johnson	Liquid	Coconut oil	130 ml	0	122	0	0	100	0	7.7 kcal/ml
Microlipid®	Chesebrough-Pond's	Liquid	Safflower Oil	222 ml	0	111	0	0	100	0	4.5 kcal/ml
Nutrisource® Lipid-Long Chain Triglycerides	SandozNutrition	Liquid	Soybean oil	455 ml	0	111	0	0	100	0	2.2 kcal/ml
Nutrisource® Lipid-Medium Chain Triglycerides	SandozNutrition	Liquid	Coconut oil	490 ml	0	120	0	0	100	0	2.0 kcal/ml

[†]Based on manufacturers' available literature.
[1]Contains trace amounts of calcium, phosphorus, and sodium.
[2]Contains dried corn syrup as major carbohydrate source.

TABLE E–5. Enteral Vitamin Modules[†]

| Product | Manufacturer | Form | Nutritional Profile | | | | Nutrient Analysis per Packet[¶] | | | | | | | | | | | | | |
			Protein (g/packet)	Fat (g/packet)	Carbohydrate (g/packet)	kCalories/packet	Vitamin A (IU)	Vitamin D (IU)	Vitamin E (IU)	Vitamin C (mg)	Folacin (μg)	Thiamin (mg)	Riboflavin (mg)	Niacin (mg)	Vitamin B_6 (mg)	Vitamin B_{12} (μg)	Biotin (mg)	Pantothenic Acid (mg)	Vitamin K (μg)	Choline (g)
Nutrisource® Vitamins	SandozNutrition	Powder	0	0	9	36	5000	200	10	60	400	1.4	1.6	18	2.2	3.0	0.15	5.5	70	0.10

†Based on manufacturer's available literature.
¶One 10-g packet.

TABLE E–6. Enteral Mineral Modules[†]

Product	Manufacturer	Form	Protein (g/packet)	Fat (g/packet)	Carbohydrate (g/packet)	kCalories/packet	Calcium (g)	Phosphorus (g)	Iodine (μg)	Iron (mg)	Magnesium (mg)	Copper (mg)	Zinc (mg)	Potassium g (mEq)	Sodium g (mEq)	Chloride g (mEq)	Manganese (mg)	Selenium (μg)	Chromium (μg)	Molybdenum (μg)
			Nutritional Profile				**Nutrient Analysis per Packet[¶]**													
Nutrisource® Minterals for Amino Acid Formulas	SandozNutrition	Powder	0	0	3	12	0.80	0.80	150	18	350	2	15	2.2 (56.3)	1.3 (56.5)	2.0 (56.4)	4	125	125	325
Nutrisource® Minerals for Amino Acid Formulas-Electrolyte Restricted	SandozNutrition	Powder	0	0	12	48	0.80	0.80	150	18	350	2	15	0.005 (0.2)	0.015 (0.7)	0.025 (0.7)	4	125	125	325
Nutrisource® Minerals for Protein Formulas	SandozNutrition	Powder	0	0	6	24	0.65	0.65	150	18	350	2	15	1.75 (44.8)	1.0 (43.5)	1.8 (50.8)	4	125	125	325
Nutrisource® Minerals for Protein Formulas-Electrolyte Restricted	SandozNutrition	Powder	0	0	13	52	0.65	0.65	150	18	350	2	15	0.005 (0.2)	0.015 (0.7)	0.025 (0.7)	4	125	125	325

[†]Based on manufacturers' available literature.
[¶]One 24-g packet.

GLOSSARY

acid-base balance: the balance maintained in the body between too much and too little acid. Blood pH, for example, is regulated normally between 7.38 and 7.42.

acidosis: too much acid in the blood and body fluids.

acute: developing rapidly and lasting for only a short time. Conditions that develop slowly and are of long duration are described as *chronic*.

adequacy: the characteristic of a diet that provides all the essential nutrients and kcalories necessary to maintain health and body weight. Ideally, a diet will be more than just adequate; it will be optimal, providing an assortment and balance of nutrients and kcalories that maintain a favorable body weight and the best possible state of health.

ADH (antidiuretic hormone): a hormone released by the pituitary gland in response to high osmotic pressure of the blood. The kidney responds by reabsorbing water.

aerobic: requiring oxygen.

aerobic metabolism: that part of energy nutrient breakdown that requires oxygen for completion, such as the metabolism of fat.

albumin: the chief blood protein used to assess nutrition status.

alkalosis: too much base in the blood and body fluids.

allergy: an immune reaction to a foreign substance, such as some component of food, in which antibodies are produced.

amino (a-MEEN-oh) **acid:** a building block of protein; a compound containing an amino group and an acid group attached to

a central carbon, which also carries a distinctive side chain.
amino = containing nitrogen

amylase: a starch-digesting enzyme secreted by the pancreas.

anaerobic (AN-air-ROE-bic): refers to processes that do not involve oxygen.
an = without

anaerobic metabolism: that part of energy nutrient breakdown that can take place without oxygen—for example, the first steps in the breakdown of glucose.

angina (an-JYE-nah or ANN-juh-nuh): pain in the region of the heart caused by lack of oxygen.

anion (AN-eye-un): a negatively charged ion.

anorexia nervosa: literally, "nervous lack of appetite," a disorder (most commonly seen in teenage girls) involving self-starvation to the extreme.

anthropometric: relating to measurement of the physical characteristics of the body, such as height and weight.
anthropos = human
metric = measuring

antibody: a large protein of the blood and body fluids, produced in response to invasion of the body by unfamiliar molecules (mostly proteins); it inactivates the invaders and so protects the body. The invaders are called *antigens*.
anti = against

antigen: a molecule foreign or unfamiliar to the body.

antigen skin testing: a test of the immune system's competence in which an antigen is

injected just under the skin. A reaction means the immune system is working normally.

antioxidant: a compound that protects other compounds from oxidation by being oxidized itself.

antiscorbutic factor: the original name for vitamin C.
anti = against
scorbutic = causing scurvy

anus (AY-nus): terminal sphincter muscle of the GI tract.

appendix: a narrow blind sac extending from the beginning of the colon; a vestigial organ with no known function.

appetite: the desire to eat, which normally accompanies hunger; by itself a pleasant sensation.

areola (a-REE-uh-luh): the colored halo around the nipple. Beneath the areola lie the ducts that bring milk from the mammary glands. Pumping action on the areola promotes flow of milk from the glands through the ducts.
areola = a small space

artery: a vessel that carries blood away from the heart.

ascites (uh-SITE-eez): a type of edema characterized by the accumulation of fluid in the abdominal cavity.

ascorbic acid: one of the two active forms of vitamin C. Many people consistently and incorrectly refer to all vitamin C by this name.
a = without
scorbic = having scurvy

atrophy (AT-tro-fee): a decrease in size from disuse.

basal metabolism: the total energy output of a body at rest after a 12-hour fast; also called *basal metabolic rate* or *BMR.*

beriberi: the thiamin-deficiency disease; it pointed the way to the first discovery of a vitamin, thiamin.

beta-carotene: an orange pigment found in plants.

bicarbonate: an alkaline secretion of the pancreas contained in pancreatic juice. (Bicarbonate also occurs widely in all cell fluids.)

bifidus (BIFF-id-us or by-FEED-us) **factor:** a factor in breast milk that favors growth of the "friendly" bacteria *lactobacillus* (lack-toh-bo-SILL-us) *bifidus* in the infant's intestinal tract so that other, less desirable intestinal inhabitants will not flourish.

bile: an exocrine secretion of the liver (the liver also performs a multitude of metabolic functions). Bile flows from the liver into the gallbladder where it is stored until needed.

bilirubin: a pigment in the bile whose concentration in the blood may become elevated as a result of some disorders.

bioelectrical impedance: a clinical test of body fatness based on the electrolyte level and electrical resistance of fat versus lean body tissue. The results at this time are not as accurately reproducible as those obtained by hydrostatic weighing or fatfold measurements.

blenderized diet: a liquid diet made from a combination of table foods. Blenderized diets usually contain pureed meat, vegetables, fruits, milk, and starches with vitamins and minerals added as necessary. They can be made in a blender or purchased commercially.

blind loop syndrome: the problems of fat malabsorption and vitamin B_{12} depletion that can result from the overgrowth of bacteria in a bypassed segment of the intestine.

bolus (BOH-lus): the portion of food swallowed at one time.

bolus delivery: delivery of a 4- to 6-hour volume of feeding solution within a few minutes.

bonding: the forming of a bond between mother and infant. A critical event in bonding, thought to be mediated by chemical messengers in breast milk, occurs in the first 45 minutes after birth.

brown sugar: sugar crystals contained in molasses syrup with natural flavor and color;

91% to 96% pure sucrose. (Some refiners add syrup to refined white sugar to make brown sugar.)

buffer: a compound that can reversibly combine with hydrogen ions to help maintain a constant pH.

buffer: a substance or mixture in a solution that is capable of neutralizing both acids and bases and thereby capable of maintaining the original concentration of hydrogen ions (pH) in the solution.

bulimia, bulimarexia: binge eating (literally, eating like an ox). Known popularly as "pigging out" or "blind munchies." When followed by self-induced vomiting or the taking of laxatives, this form of eating behavior has been called the *binge-purge syndrome.*

calcium rigor: hardness or stiffness of the muscles caused by high blood calcium.

calcium tetany: intermittent spasms of the extremities due to nervous and muscular excitability, which is caused by low blood calcium.

calisthenics: exercise routines or muscular development that use the weight of the body as resistance.

calorie: a unit in which energy is measured.

cancer cachexia (ka-KEX-ee-uh): a syndrome induced by many cancers, major symptoms are anorexia with inadequate food intake, accelerated metabolism and wasting, and general ill health associated with cancer.

capillary (CAP-ill-ary): a small vessel that branches from an artery. Capillaries connect arteries to veins. Exchange of oxygen, nutrients, and waste materials takes place across capillary walls.

carbohydrate: an energy nutrient composed of monosaccharides.
carbo = carbon
hydrate = water

cardiac sphincter (CARD-ee-ack SFINK-ter): sphincter muscle at the junction between the esophagus and the stomach.
sphincter = band (binder)

cardiovascular endurance: a component of fitness, the ability of the cardiovascular system to sustain effort over a long time.

catalyst (CAT-uh-list): a compound that facilitates chemical reactions without itself being destroyed in the process.

cathartic (ca-THART-ic): a strong laxative.
cata = down

cation (CAT-eye-un): a positively charged ion.

celiac (SEE-lee-ack) **disease:** a sensitivity to gliadin that causes flattening of the intestinal villi and generalized malabsorption; also called *gluten-sensitive enteropathy* (EN-ter-OP-ah-thee) or *celiac sprue.*

cell salts: a mineral preparation sold in health-food stores that is supposed to have been prepared from living, healthy cells. It is not necessary to take such preparations, and it may be dangerous.

cellulose (CELL-you-loce): a plant polysaccharide composed of glucose, indigestible by humans; one of the fibers.

central veins: the larger-diameter veins located close to the heart.

chemotherapy: the use of drugs to arrest or destroy cancer cells.
chemo = chemical
Chemotherapeutic drugs also are called **antineoplastic agents.**

chloride: the ionic form of chlorine (Cl^-).

cholecystitis (KO-lee-sis-TIE-tis): inflammation of the gallbladder.

cholesterol: one of the sterols.

chylomicron (kye-lo-MY-cron): the lipoprotein formed in the intestinal wall cells following digestion and absorption of fat. Released from these cells, chylomicrons transport ingested fats to all cells of the body which remove the fats they need, leaving chylomicron remnants to be picked up by the liver cells. The liver cells dismantle the chylomicron remnants and construct other lipoproteins for further transport of lipids.

chyme (KIME): the semiliquid mass of partly digested food expelled by the stomach into the duodenum.
chymos = juice

cirrhosis (sih-ROW-sis): a disease of the liver characterized by scarring. *Laennec's cirrhosis* is the type associated with alcohol abuse and malnutrition.

CoA (coh-AY): nickname for a small molecule that participates in metabolism. As pyruvate breaks down to the smaller compound *acetic acid,* a molecule of CoA is attached to it, making *acetyl CoA* (ASS-uh-teel or uh-SEET-ul co-AY).

coenzyme (co-EN-zime): small molecule that works with an enzyme to promote the enzyme's activity. Many coenzymes have B vitamins as part of their structure.

co = with

cofactor: a mineral element that, like a coenzyme, works with an enzyme to facilitate a chemical reaction.

collagen: the characteristic protein of connective tissue.

kolla = glue

gennan = to produce

collaterals: small blood vessels that develop to divert blood flow away from an obstructed organ. These blood vessels are also called **shunts.**

colon (COAL-un): the large intestine. Its segments are the ascending colon, the transverse colon, the descending colon, and the sigmoid colon.

sigmoid = shaped like the letter S (*sigma* in Greek)

colostrum (co-LAHS-trum): a yellowish, milklike secretion from the breast, rich in protective factors; present for up to two weeks before milk appears.

complementary proteins: two or more proteins whose amino acid assortments complement each other in such a way that the essential amino acids missing from each are supplied by the other.

complete formula: a liquid formula that, when given in sufficient volume, supplies all the nutrients needed.

complete protein: a protein containing all the amino acids essential in human nutrition in amounts adequate for human use.

complex carbohydrates: the polysaccharides (starch, glycogen, and cellulose).

confectioners' sugar: finely powdered sucrose; 99.9% pure.

congestive heart failure: a syndrome in which the heart can no longer adequately pump blood through the circulatory system.

continuous drip administration: delivery of a feeding solution continuously over a 16- to 24-hour period.

convenience food: a food prepared or packaged in such a way that it is easy to cook and serve at home.

corn sweeteners: corn syrup and sugars derived from corn.

corn syrup: a syrup produced by the action of enzymes on cornstarch, containing mostly glucose. See also *high-fructose corn syrup*.

cornea (KOR-nee-uh): the transparent membrane covering the outside of the front of the eye.

creatinine (cree-AT-in-een or cree-AT-in-in) **excretion:** an indicator of lean body mass. Creatinine is a waste product produced by active muscle.

cretinism (CREE-tin-ism): an iodine-deficiency disease characterized by mental and physical retardation.

Crohn's disease: inflammation and ulceration along the length of the GI tract, often with granulomas.

crude fiber (CF): the residue of plant food remaining after extraction with dilute acid followed by dilute alkali in a laboratory procedure; that is, the fiber that remains in food after a harsh chemical digestive procedure.

cyanosis: a bluish or grayish color of the skin.

cystic fibrosis (CF): a hereditary disorder that affects many organs, including the pancreas, lungs, liver, heart, gallbladder, and small intestine.

desiccated liver: dehydrated liver; a powder sold in health food stores that is supposed to contain all the nutrients found in liver in concentrated form. This supplement has no particular nutritional merit, even though it may not be dangerous, and grocery store liver is considerably less expensive. *Desiccated* means "totally dried."

dextrose: a form of glucose that is very soluble in water and is therefore used in IV solutions. Dextrose contains a little water; therefore, while glucose provides 4 kcal/g, dextrose provides only 3.4 kcal/g.

diabetes mellitus (dye-uh-BEE-teez MELL-ih-tus or mell-EYE-tus): a disorder of energy metabolism caused by an absolute or a relative deficiency of insulin. When the word *diabetes* is used alone it refers to diabetes mellitus. *mellitus* = honey sweet (from sugar in the urine)

diagnosis: the disease a person has or is thought to have.

dia = through

gnosis = knowing

diet order: a physician's written statement in the medical record of what diet a client should receive.

diffusion and osmosis: the movement of water across a membrane to equalize the concentration of particles on both sides of the membrane. Water moves from the less concentrated to the more concentrated side.

dipeptide: two amino acids bonded together.

di = two

peptide = amino acid

dissociation: physical separation of the ions in an ionic compound. A salt that partly dissociates in water is an *electrolyte*.

diuretic (dye-yoo-RET-ic): a drug that promotes the excretion of water through the kidneys. Only some diuretics increase the urinary loss of potassium. Others called **potassium-sparing** diuretics are less likely to result in a potassium deficiency.

diverticulosis (DYE-ver-tic-you-LOH-sis): a condition in which pouches of intestinal lining balloon out through the muscles of the intestinal wall. The pouches are called **diverticula** (DYE-ver-TIC-you-luh; the singular is **diverticulum**); they can become inflamed, a condition called **diverticulitis** (DYE-ver-tic-you-LIGH-tus).

draught reflex (DRAFT): the reflex that moves the hindmilk toward the nipple after the infant has drawn off the foremilk.

dumping syndrome: the symptoms that result from the rapid emptying of undigested food into the jejunum; sweating, weakness, diarrhea shortly after eating, and hypoglycemia later.

duodenum (doo-oh-DEEN-um or doo-ODD-num): the top portion of the small intestine (about "12 fingers' breadth" long, in ancient terminology).

dysentery (DIS-en-terry): an infection of the gastrointestinal tract caused by an amoeba or bacterium that gives rise to severe diarrhea.

dys = bad

entery = intestine

dyspepsia: a vague term used to describe abdominal discomfort. Dyspepsia is a symptom, not a disease.

dys = bad, difficult

peptein = to digest.

edema (e-DEE-muh): an accumulation of fluid that can be seen in many disorders. In one case, PCM, protein in the blood is depleted and water cannot be held there. Instead, water seeps into the interstitial space and accumulates. Hormonal imbalances in protein deficiency also contribute to edema.

eicosanoids (eye-COSS-a-noids): derivatives of a 20-carbon fatty acid; hormonelike compounds that regulate blood pressure, clotting, and other body functions.

electrolyte solution: a solution that can conduct electricity.

electrolytes: charged minerals, such as sodium, potassium, magnesium, and chloride.

embolism: the sudden closure of a blood vessel caused by an embolus.

embolus (EM-boh-luss): a thrombus that breaks loose.

empty-kcalorie food: a popular term used to denote foods that contain no nutrients, only kcalories. Actually, since almost all foods contain some nutrients, most nutritionists prefer to say "food of low nutrient density."

end-stage renal disease (ESRD): the severe state of renal disease in which diet alone is no longer effective in maintaining normal kidney function.

engineered food: a food subjected to a complex technical process, such as extraction of certain components.

enteric hyperoxaluria (en-TER-ick HIGH-per-ox-sa-LOO-reeah): a condition of excess oxalate absorption that comes about because calcium is unable to bind oxalate in the gut. It leads to kidney stone formation.

enzyme: a protein catalyst.

epiglottis (epp-ee-GLOT-tiss): cartilage in the throat that guards the entrance to the trachea and prevents fluid or food from entering it when a person swallows.
epi = upon (over)
glottis = back of tongue

esophageal varices (ee-SOF-ah-GEE-al VAIR-ih-seez): tangles of distended blood vessels that protrude into the esophagus.

esophagus (e-SOFF-uh-gus): food pipe.

essential amino acid: an amino acid that the body cannot synthesize in amounts sufficient to meet physiological need. Nine amino acids are known to be essential for human adults.

essential fatty acids: fatty acids that cannot be synthesized in the body in amounts sufficient to meet physiological need.

ethnic diets: diets associated with particular national origins, races, cultural heritages, or geographic locations.

fabricated food: a food put together from highly processed ingredients, such as meat-substitute burgers made from textured vegetable protein.

fast food: foods prepared quickly in a fast-food restaurant, such as a hamburger stand or fried-chicken place.

fasting hypoglycemia: chronic low blood glucose, the symptom of an underlying disorder of the pancreas, liver, pituitary gland, or other body organ or system; it is resolved by treatment of the underlying medical condition.

fat: a mixture of triglycerides.

fat-controlled diet: a diet in which both the amount of fat *and* the type of fat are controlled.

fatfold test: a clinical test of body fatness in which the thickness of a fold of skin on the back of the arm (triceps), below the shoulder blade (subscapular), or in other places is measured with an instrument called a caliper. The older, less preferred, term for this is *skinfold test*.

fatty acid: a chain of carbon atoms with hydrogen attached.

fatty liver: an accumulation of fat in the liver. In PCM, fat accumulates in the liver because there is no protein available to form the lipoproteins that normally escort fat molecules in the blood.

fetal alcohol syndrome: the cluster of symptoms seen in an infant or child whose mother consumed excess alcohol during her pregnancy; includes mental and physical retardation with facial and other body deformities.

fiber: the portion of food that is found in the colon because we don't have the enzymes to digest it. See also the terms *crude fiber* and *dietary fiber*.

fistula (FIS-too-lah): an abnormal opening between two organs or from an organ to the skin.
fistula = pipe

flexibility: a component of fitness, the ability to bend without injury; it depends on the elasticity of muscles, tendons, and ligaments and on the condition of the joints.

fluorosis (floor-OH-sis): mottling of the tooth enamel from ingestion of too much fluoride during tooth development.

food preference list: a list of a person's likes and dislikes.

fortification: the addition of nutrients to a food, often in amounts much larger than might be found naturally in that food.

frame size: the size of a person's bones and musculature. A person with a large frame should weigh more than a person the same height with a small frame.

fructose: a monosaccharide; sometimes known as fruit sugar. Slightly sweeter than glucose and requires less energy to metabolize than glucose.
fruct = fruit

galactose: a monosaccharide; part of the disaccharide lactose.

galactosemia (ga-lac-toe-SEE-mee-uh): an inherited disorder characterized by a deficiency of one of several enzymes necessary to convert galactose to glucose in the body.

gallbladder: the organ that stores and concentrates bile. When it receives the signal that fat is present in the duodenum, the gallbladder contracts, and bile flows down the bile duct.

gangrene (GANG-green): death of tissue caused by lack of blood flow to the area.

gastric glands: exocrine glands in the stomach wall that secrete gastric juice into the stomach.
gastro = stomach

gastric juice: the secretion of the gastric glands. The principal enzymes are rennin (curdles milk protein, casein, and prepares it for pepsin action), pepsin (acts on proteins); and lipase (acts on emulsified fats).

gastritis: inflammation of the lining of the stomach.

GI tract: the gastrointestinal tract or alimentary canal; the principal organs are the stomach and intestines.
gastro = stomach
aliment = food

gliadin (GLIGH-ah-din): a fraction of the gluten protein.

gland: a cell or group of cells that secrete materials for special uses in the body. Glands may be **exocrine glands,** secreting their materials "out" (into the digestive tract or onto the surface of the skin) or **endocrine glands,** secreting their materials "in" (into the blood).
exo = outside
endo = inside
krine = to separate

glucose: a monosaccharide, the sugar common to all disaccharides and polysaccharides; sometimes known as blood sugar, sometimes as grape sugar; also called *dextrose*.

gluten (GLUE-ten): a vegetable protein found in wheat, oats, rye and barley.

glycerol (GLISS-er-ol): a small compound related to carbohydrates that can form the backbone of triglycerides and phospholipids.

glycosuria (GLIGH-cose-YOUR-ee-uh): sugar in the urine.
glyco = sweet

goiter (GOY-ter): an iodine-deficiency disease. Goiter caused by iodine deficiency is simple goiter.

goitrogen: a thyroid antagonist found in food causes *toxic goiter.*

gout (gowt): a metabolic disease in which crystals of uric acid precipitate in the joints.

granola: a cereal made from mixed oats and other grains that is often high in simple sugars and saturated fats.

granulated sugar: crystalline sucrose; 99.9% pure.

granuloma: (gran-you-LOH-mah): a granular tumor or growth.
granulum = little grain *oma* = tumor

green pills: pills containing dehydrated, crushed vegetable matter. One pill contains nutrients equal to those in one small forkful of fresh vegetables—minus losses incurred in processing.

GTF (glucose tolerance factor): a small organic compound containing chromium.

HDL: high-density lipoprotein. These lipoproteins seem to transport cholesterol back to the liver from peripheral cells. An alternative name is *alpha lipoprotein.*

heartburn: a burning pain felt behind the sternum that may spread into the neck and throat.

hemochromatosis (heem-oh-crome-a-TOCE-iss): iron overload characterized by deposits of iron-containing pigment in many tissues, with tissue damage. Hemochromatosis is a hereditary defect in iron metabolism.

hemodialysis (HE-mow-die-AL-ih-sis): removal of wastes from the blood by passing the blood outside the body through tubes made of semipermeable membranes submerged in a water solution.

hemoglobin: the oxygen-carrying protein of the red blood cells.
hemo = blood
globin = globular protein

hemorrhagic (hem-o-RAJ-ik) **disease:** the vitamin K deficiency disease in which blood fails to clot.

hemosiderosis (heem-oh-sid-er-OH-sis): iron overload characterized by excessive iron deposits in hemosiderin, the normal iron-storage protein.

hepatic coma: a state of unconsciousness that results from severe liver disease; also called *portal systemic encephalopathy.*

hepatitis (HEP-ah-TIE-tis): inflammation of the liver caused by a virus, alcohol, or drugs. Hepatitis can progress to cirrhosis.
hepat = liver
itis = inflammation

hiatal hernia: an outpouching of a portion of the stomach through the opening in the diaphragm through which the esophagus passes.

high-fructose corn syrup (HFCS): the predominant sweetener used in processed foods today. HFCS is mostly fructose; glucose makes up the balance.

high-quality protein: an easily digestible, complete protein whose amino acids fit the pattern needed by human beings.

histamine: a substance produced by cells of the immune system in reaction to an antigen. Histamine participates in causing the redness and swelling known as *inflammation.*

honey: sugar formed from nectar (mostly sucrose) gathered by bees. An enzyme splits the sucrose into glucose and fructose. Composition and flavor vary, but honey always contains a mixture of sucrose, fructose, and glucose.

hormone: a chemical messenger. Hormones are secreted by a variety of glands in the body in response to altered conditions. Each affects one or more target tissues or organs and elicits specific responses to restore normal conditions.

hunger: the physiological need to eat; a negative, unpleasant sensation.

hydrogenation: the process of adding hydrogen to unsaturated fat to make it more solid and resistant to chemical change.

hydrolyzed protein: an intact protein treated with acids or enzymes to yield a combination of free amino acids and short peptide chains. A *protein hydrolysate formula* contains hydrolyzed protein as a source of protein.

hydrostatic weighing: a clinical test of body fatness, also known as underwater weighing, in which the person is submerged and the displacement of water is measured. It is considered by many to be the most reliable method of determining body composition.

hyperactivity syndrome: in children: a cluster of symptoms including developmentally inappropriate inattention, impulsivity, and hyperactivity. Other important features are onset before age seven, duration of six months or more, and proven absence of mental illness or mental retardation. Other names associated with hyperactivity: *attention deficit disorder, hyperkinesis, minimal brain damage, minimal brain dysfunction, minor cerebral dysfunction.*

hyperammonemia (HIGH-per-am-moe-KNEE-mee-uh): elevated blood ammonia levels.

hyperlipidemia (HIGH-per-LIP-ih-DEE-mee-ah): elevated blood lipids.

hyperlipoproteinemia (HIGH-per-LIP-oh-PRO-teen-EE-mee-ah): elevated blood lipoproteins; often used interchangeably with hyperlipidemia.

hypertonic formula: a formula with an osmolality higher than that of blood serum.
hyper = greater, more

hypertrophy (high-PURR-tro-fee): an increase in size in response to use.

ideal weight: a misnomer; not the desirable but the average weight given in insurance tables for persons of a given sex and height—not necessarily ideal for a given individual.

ileocecal (ill-ee-oh-SEEK-ul) **valve:** sphincter muscle separating the small and large intestines.

ileum (ILL-ee-um): the last segment of the small intestine.

imitation food: a food nutritionally inferior to the food it imitates. By law, this term must appear on the label of a food if it contains less than 10 percent of the U.S. RDA of an essential nutrient found in the food it imitates.

inpatient: a person being treated or residing in a health care facility. Hospitals, nursing homes, rehabilitation centers, some eating disorder centers, and some drug and alcohol centers provide inpatient services.

intact protein formula: a liquid diet that contains a complete protein that has not been altered.

intermittent feeding by slow drip: delivery of a 4- to 6-hour volume of feeding solution over 20 to 30 minutes.

intestinal flora: the bacterial inhabitants of the GI tract.
flora = plant growth

intestinal juice: the secretion of the intestinal glands; contains enzymes for the digestion of carbohydrate and protein and a minor enzyme for fat digestion.

intravenous (IV) or parenteral: through a vein. *Parenteral nutrition* refers to the delivery of nutrients through a vein, bypassing the intestines.
intra = within
vena = vein
para = opposite
enteron = intestine

invert sugar: a mixture of glucose and fructose formed by the splitting of sucrose in a chemical process. Sold only in liquid form, sweeter than sucrose, invert sugar is used as an additive to help preserve food freshness and prevent shrinkage.

iron overload: toxicity from iron overdose. There are two types, hemochromatosis and hemosiderosis.

irritable bowel syndrome: a common GI disorder characterized by spasms of the colon. It is also called spastic colon, spastic constipation, spastic diarrhea, and mucous colitis.

isotonic formula: a formula with an osmolality similar to that of blood serum (300 mOsm). *iso* = the same
ton = tension.

IV catheter: the thin tube inserted into a vein through which nutrient solutions or medications can be given directly.

jaundice: bile pigments from the diseased liver spill into the blood and accumulate, causing the skin, whites of the eyes, and mucous membranes to become yellow.

jejunum (je-JOON-um): the first two-fifths of the small intestine beyond the duodenum.

junk food: a popular term used to denote foods that are "bad" for you, for example, foods high in salt, sugar, or fat.

kelp: a kind of seaweed used by the Japanese as a foodstuff. Kelp tablets are made from dehydrated kelp. The urine of people who use kelp has been found to contain raised concentrations of arsenic, a poison and possible carcinogen.

keratin (KERR-uh-tin): a water-insoluble protein; the normal protein of hair and nails. Keratin may be produced under abnormal conditions by cells that normally produce mucus. Keratin accumulation is known as **keratinization.** The progression of this condition to the extreme is **hyperkeratosis.**
hyper = too much

ketones (KEY-tones): a condensation product of fat metabolism produced when carbohydrate is not available.

ketonuria (KEE-tone-YOUR-ee-uh): ketones in the urine.

kwashiorkor (kwash-ee-OR-core, or kwash-ee-or-CORE): malnutrition caused by protein deficiency in the presence of adequate kcalories.

lactalbumin (lact-AL-byoo-min): the chief protein in human breast milk, as opposed to **casein** (CAY-seen), the chief protein in cow's milk.
lac = milk

lactic acid: a fragment produced from glucose during anaerobic metabolism. When oxygen becomes available, lactic acid can be completely broken down to carbon dioxide and water.

lactoferrin (lak-toe-FERR-in): a factor in breast milk that binds iron and keeps it from supporting the growth of the infant's intestinal bacteria, helps absorb iron, and helps kill bacteria.
fer = iron

lacto-ovo vegetarian: vegetarian who omits meat, fish, and poultry from their diets but use eggs, cheese, milk, and milk products.

lactose: a disaccharide composed of glucose and galactose; commonly known as milk sugar.
lact = milk

latent: the period in the course of a disease when the conditions are present but the symptoms have not begun to appear.
latens = lying hidden

LDL: low-density lipoprotein. This type of lipoprotein may be made by liver cells or derived from VLDL as cells remove triglycerides from them. An alternative name is **beta lipoprotein.**

lecithin: one of the phospholipids.

letdown reflex: the reflex that forces milk to the front of the breast when the infant begins to nurse.

limiting amino acid: the amino acid found in the shortest supply relative to the amounts needed for protein synthesis in the body.

lipase: a lipid-digesting enzyme secreted by the pancreas.

low birthweight (LBW): a birthweight of 5½ lb (2,500 g) or less, used as a predictor of poor health in the newborn and as a probable indicator of poor nutrition status of the mother during and/or before pregnancy. Normal birthweight is 6½ lb (3,000 g) or more.

low-fat diet: a diet in which the total amount of fat is limited.

lumen: the inner open space of a tube.

lymph (LIMF): The body's interstitial fluid, located between cells and outside the vascular system. Lymph consists of all the constituents of blood that can escape from the vascular system. It circulates in a loosely organized system of vessels and ducts known as the *lymphatic system.*

maltose: a disaccharide composed of two glucose units; sometimes known as malt sugar.

maple sugar: a sugar (mostly sucrose) purified from concentrated sap of the sugar maple tree. Maple sugar is expensive compared with other sweeteners.

marasmus: (ma-RAZZ-mus): malnutrition caused by simple starvation.

meat replacements: textured vegetable protein products formulated to look and taste like meat, fish, or poultry. Many of them are designed to match the known nutrient contents of animal-protein foods, but sometimes they fall short.

mechanical soft diet: a diet that excludes all foods difficult to chew or swallow; also called a **dental soft diet.**

medical record: a continuous written account of a client's medical care.

metabolism: the sum total of all the chemical reactions that go on in living cells.
meta = among
bole = change

microangiopathies (MY-crow-ANN-gee-OP-ah-thees): disorders of the capillaries, often seen in diabetes.

microcytic (my-cro-SIT-ic) **hypochromic** (high-po-KROME-ic) **anemia:** iron-deficiency anemia.
micro = small
cytic = cells
hypo = too little
chrom = color

microvilli (MY-cro-VILL-ee or MY-cro-VILL-eye): projections from the membranes of the cells of the villi. The singular form is *microvillus*.

milk allergy: the most common food allergy; caused by the protein in raw milk. Milk allergy is sometimes overcome by cooking the milk to denature the protein and sometimes "cured" by abstinence from and gradual reintroduction to milk.

milk anemia: iron-deficiency anemia caused by drinking so much milk that iron-rich foods are displaced from the diet.

modified or therapeutic diet: a regular diet that is adjusted to meet special nutrition needs. Such diets can be adjusted in consistency, total food energy, nutrients, amount of fluid, and number of meals or by the elimination of certain foods.

modular formulas: incomplete formulas that contain specific nutrients and are used as supplements.

molasses: a thick brown syrup, left over from sugar cane juice during sugar refining. It retains residual sugar and other by-products and a few minerals; blackstrap molasses contains significant amounts of calcium and iron—the iron from the machinery used to process it.

monounsaturated fatty acid: a fatty acid that has one point of unsaturation where hydrogens are missing, for example, oleic acid.

mucus (adjective mucous): a substance secreted by the epithelial cells of the mucosa.

mucus (MYOO-cuss): a mucopolysaccharide (relative of carbohydrate) secreted by cells of the stomach wall. The cellular lining of the stomach wall with its coat of mucus is known as the mucous membrane. (The noun is *mucus;* the adjective is *mucous.*)

muscular dystrophy (DIS-tro-fee): a hereditary disease in which the muscles gradually weaken; its most debilitating effects arise in the lungs.

muscular endurance: a component of fitness, the ability of a muscle to contract repeatedly within a given time without becoming exhausted.

muscular strength: a component of fitness, the ability of a muscle to work against resistance.

mutual supplementation: the strategy of combining two protein foods in a meal so that each food provides the essential amino acid(s) lacking in the other.

myoglobin: the oxygen-carrying protein of the muscle cells.
myo = muscle

natural food: an unprocessed food; a term often mistakenly used synonymously with "good for you."

night blindness: slow recovery of vision after flashes of bright light at night; an early symptom of vitamin A deficiency.

nitrogen balance: the amount of nitrogen consumed (N in) as compared with the amount of nitrogen excreted (N out) in a given period of time. The laboratory scientist can estimate the protein in a sample of food, body tissue, or excreta by measuring the nitrogen in it.

NPO: an order that means that nothing is to be given to the person orally (including food and medications). NPO stands for *nil per os,* which means "nothing by mouth." On the other hand, PO stands for *per os,* which means "by mouth" or "orally."

nutrient: a substance obtained from food and used in the body to promote growth, maintenance, or repair.

nutrient density: a characteristic of a food. A nutrient-dense food provides a high quantity (relative to need) of one or (preferably) several essential nutrients, with a small quantity (relative to need) of kcalories.

nutrition care plan: a strategy for translating nutrition assessment data into a plan for meeting the client's nutrient and nutrition education needs.

nutrition care process: an organized approach to problem solving that consists of five steps (assessing, analyzing, planning, implementing, and evaluating).

nutrition screening: the use of preliminary nutrition assessment techniques to identify people who are malnourished or who are at risk for malnutrition.

nutritional yeast: a food supplement containing B vitamins, iron, and protein that can be used to improve the quality of a vegetarian diet; also called brewer's yeast.

nutritious food: a food with high nutrient density.

obesity: excessive body fatness; often loosely defined as a condition of being overweight by 20 percent or more.

omega: the last letter of the Greek alphabet (ω), used by chemists to refer to the position of the last double bond in a fatty acid. The omega-6 fatty acids have their last double bond six carbons back along the chain; the omega-3 acids, three carbons back.

osmolality: the number of molecular and ionic particles (measured in osmoles) per kilogram of water in a solution.

osteomalacia (os-tee-o-mal-AY-shuh): the vitamin D deficiency disease in adults.
osteo = bone
mal = bad (soft)

ostomate (OSS-toh-mate): a person who has a surgically formed opening from the bowel to the outside of the body, bypassing the anus.

overt: out in the open, full-blown.
ouvrire = to open

overweight: body weight more than 10 percent above the average (insurance company table) weight.

oxidant: a compound (such as oxygen itself) that oxidizes other compounds.

oxidation: a type of chemical reaction. Oxidation reactions usually result in the release of energy. In chemical oxidation of nutrients, the energy released is largely chemical and mechanical; in oxidative combustion (burning), the energy released is mostly heat and light energy.

oxygen debt: a deficit of oxygen built up by the body during exercise when the cardiovascular system cannot deliver oxygen fast enough to the muscles to support aerobic metabolism; the debt must be repaid by rapid breathing after the activity slows down or stops.

palpitations: rapid fluttering or throbbing of the heart.

pancreatic (PAN-kree-AT-ic) **juice:** the exocrine secretion of the pancreas, containing enzymes for the digestion of carbohydrate, fat, and protein. Juice flows from the pancreas into the small intestine through the pancreatic duct. The pancreas also has an endocrine function, the secretion of insulin and other hormones.

pancreatitis (PAN-kree-uh-TIE-tis): inflammation of the pancreas.

pectin: carbohydrate fibers found in plant foods. Like cellulose, they are not attacked by human enzymes.

pellagra (pell-AY-gra): the niacin-deficiency disease.
pellis = skin
agra = seizure

pepsin: a protein-digesting enzyme (gastric protease) in the stomach. It circulates as a precursor, pepsinogen, and is converted to pepsin by the action of stomach acid.

peptic ulcer: an eroded lesion of the stomach (**gastric ulcer**) or duodenum (**duodenal ulcer**).

peripheral total parenteral nutrition (PTPN): the provision of nutrient solution that meets nutrient needs by peripheral vein.

peripheral vein: the smaller-diameter veins that bring blood to the extremities (arms and legs).

peristalsis (peri-STALL-sis): successive waves of involuntary muscular contraction passing along the walls of the intestine.
peri = around
stellein = wrap

peritoneal (PERR-ee-toe-NEE-al) **dialysis:** removal of wastes from the blood using the peritoneum as a semipermeable membrane.

pH: the concentration of hydrogen ions. The lower the pH, the stronger the acid. Thus pH 2 is a strong acid; pH 6 is a weak acid; pH 7 is neutral; a pH above 7 is alkaline.

phenylketonuria (FEN-ill-KEY-toe-NEW-ree-ah) **(PKU):** an inborn error of metabolism in which phenylalanine cannot be converted to tyrosine. Alternative metabolites of phenylalanine accumulate in the tissues, causing damage, and overflow into the urine.

phospholipid: a compound similar to a triglyceride but having choline (see Chapter 5) or another phosphorus-containing acid in place of one of the fatty acids.

pica (PIE-ka): a craving for nonfood substances; also known as *geophagia* (jee-oh-FAY-jee-uh) when referring to the clay-eating behavior.

pigment: a molecule capable of absorbing certain wavelengths of light. Pigments in the eye permit us to perceive different colors.

plaque: mounds of lipid material mixed with smooth muscle cells and calcium that are lodged in artery walls.

polypeptide: many amino acids bonded together. *Many* refers to ten or more. An intermediate string of between four and ten amino acids is an **oligopeptide.**
poly = many
oligo = few

portal hypertension: elevated blood pressure in the portal vein caused by obstructed blood flow through the liver.

postprandial or **reactive hypoglycemia:** low blood glucose within six hours after a meal; an overreaction to the carbohydrate in the meal; often treatable by diet.
post = after
prandium = meal

powdered bone, bone meal: two among many nutrient supplements intended to supply calcium and other bone minerals. Some bone meal has been found to contain high levels of lead.

precursor: a compound that can be converted into another compound. For example, carotene is a precursor of vitamin A.

preformed vitamin A: vitamin A in its active form.

pregnancy-induced hypertension (PIH), formerly known as **toxemia** (tox-EEM-ee-uh): a cluster of symptoms seen in pregnancy, including edema and often hypertension and kidney complications.
tox = poison
emia = in the blood

primary deficiency: a nutrient deficiency caused directly by lack of that nutrient in the diet.

processed food: any food subjected to a process, such as enrichment, refinement, fortification, alteration of texture, mixing, or cooking.

prognosis: the predicted course and outcome of a disease.
pro = ahead of time, before

protein: a compound composed of amino acids linked in a chain.

protein isolate: a type of intact protein; a protein with high biological value that has been separated from a source containing a variety of proteins. A *protein isolate formula* contains a protein isolate as the source of protein.

protein-kcalorie malnutrition: a deficiency of protein or kcalories or both, often

referred to as **PCM** and also as **PEM,** for **protein-energy malnutrition.**
mal = bad, poor

proteinuric: the loss of protein in the urine.

prothrombin time: the time it takes for the blood to clot. Both vitamin K deficiency and liver disease can prolong this time.

pulmonary edema: accumulation of fluid in the lungs.

pyloric (pie-LORE-ic) **sphincter:** sphincter muscle separating the stomach from the small intestine.
pylorus = gatekeeper

pyruvate (PIE-roo-vate): pyruvic acid, a compound derived from glucose and certain amino acids in metabolism. The term *pyruvate* means a salt of pyruvic acid. (Throughout this book the ending *ate* is used interchangeably with *-ic acid;* for our purposes they mean the same thing.)

radiation therapy: the use of radiation to arrest or destroy cancer cells.

ratchet effect: a popular term for the effect that repeated cycles of weight loss and gain without exercise have on body composition, in which the body fat content increases and kcaloric needs fall after each round, making the next round of weight loss harder. Also called the *yoyo effect.*

raw sugar: the first crop of crystals harvested during sugar processing. Raw sugar cannot be sold in the United States because it contains too much filth (dirt, insect fragments, and the like). Sugar sold domestically as raw sugar has actually gone through about half of the refining steps.

RDA: Recommended Dietary Allowances. The RDA are daily recommended intakes of nutrients intended to provide for individual variations among most normal, healthy people in the United States under usual environmental stresses.

RE (retinol equivalent): a measure of vitamin A activity; the amount of retinol that a vitamin A compound will yield after conversion in the body.

rectum: the muscular terminal part of the intestine from the sigmoid colon to the anus.

registered dietetic technician: a trained professional who has earned an associate degree or higher, has completed an ADA-approved Dietetic Technician program, has passed a national registration exam, and who assists in planning, implementing, and evaluating nutritional care.

registered dietitian (R.D.): a trained professional in dietetics with a bachelor's degree in nutrition or food science, a year's internship or the equivalent, and a passing score on the four-hour qualifying exam administered by the American or Canadian Dietetic Association.

renal failure: failure of the kidney's nephrons to maintain normal function.

requirement: the minimum amount of a nutrient that will just prevent the development of specific deficiency signs; distinguished from the RDA, which are recommended allowances that include a safety factor to provide for individual variability.

residue: the total amount of material in the colon; it includes undigested food, intestinal secretions, bacteria, and the turnover of intestinal cells.

residue: bulk in the colon that includes undigested food, intestinal secretions, bacteria, and cells shed from the intestinal lining.

respiratory acidosis: a condition of too much acid in the blood caused by failure of the lungs to ventilate properly. Excess acids are normally released from the lungs during exhalation; diseased lungs, however, are unable to perform this function adequately.

retina (RET-in-uh): the layer of light-sensitive cells lining the back of the inside of the eye; consists of rods and cones.

retinal (RET-in-al): the aldehyde form of vitamin A, active in the pigments of the eye.

retinol: one of the active forms of vitamin A, used as the standard for measuring vitamin A activity.

rheumatic (roo-MAT-ick) **heart disease:** a general term used to describe heart damage (often affecting the heart valves) that occurs due to rheumatic fever (caused by a bacterial infection).

rickets: the calcium deficiency (or vitamin D deficiency) disease in children.

RNI: Recommended Nutrient Intakes for Canadians: The RDA, The Canadian equivalent.

rooting reflex: the reflex that makes a newborn turn toward whichever cheek is touched and search for the nipple.

saliva: the secretion of the salivary glands; the principal enzyme is salivary amylase.

salt: a compound composed of charged particles (ions). Exceptions: a compound in which the positive ions are hydrogen ions (H+) is an acid; a compound in which the negative ions are hydroxyl ions (OH−) is a base.

satiety (sat-EYE-uh-tee): the feeling of fullness or satisfaction at the end of a meal that prompts a person to stop eating.

saturated fatty acid: a fatty acid carrying the maximum possible number of hydrogen atoms, for example, stearic acid. A *saturated fat* is composed of triglycerides in which all, or virtually all, of the fatty acids are saturated.

science of nutrition: the study of nutrients and of their ingestion, digestion, absorption, transport, metabolism, interaction, storage, and excretion. A broader definition includes the study of the environment and of human behavior as it relates to these processes.

scurvy: the vitamin C deficiency disease.

secondary deficiency: a deficiency caused by the body's inability to digest, absorb, or utilize a nutrient in the normal fashion, or by excess destruction or excretion of the nutrient.

segmentation: a periodic squeezing or partitioning of the intestine by its circular muscles.

selective menu: a menu from which clients select the foods they will receive while hospitalized. *House diets* are preselected by the dietary department.

semipermeable: more permeable to some substances (such as water) than to others (such as sodium and potassium). This condition is necessary for osmotic pressure to operate.
semi = half

set point: the point at which controls are set (for example, on a thermostat). In the case of body weight, the set point is that point above which the body tends to lose weight and below which it tends to gain weight.

shock: sudden, dramatic shift of fluid from the blood to the interstital space.

short bowel syndrome: a complex of symptoms that may include malabsorption, diarrhea, weight loss, hypocalcemia, hypomagnesemia, and anemia; it can occur whenever the absorptive surface of the small bowel is reduced.

simple carbohydrates: the monosaccharides (glucose, fructose, and galactose) and the disaccharides (sucrose, lactose, and maltose); also called the sugars.

spirulina: a kind of algae ("blue-green manna") said to contain large amounts of vitamin B_{12} and to suppress appetite. It does neither.

sports anemia: a temporary condition of low hemoglobin in the blood associated with the early stages of sports training or with other strenuous activity.

starch: a plant polysaccharide composed of glucose and digestible by humans.

stasis (STAY-sis): standing still. Normal actions of the intestines keep a steady stream of secretions flowing through them. Stasis in a blind loop allows bacteria to flourish.

steatorrhea (STEE-at-oh-REE-uh): fatty diarrhea characterized by stools that are foamy, greasy, and malodorous.

sterile: free of microorganisms, such as bacteria.

steroid (STARE-oid): a drug used to reduce tissue inflammation, to suppress the immune response, or to replace certain steroid hormones in people who cannot synthesize them.

sterol: a class of lipids. Cholesterol, vitamin D, and steroid hormones are examples.

sucrose: a disaccharide composed of glucose and fructose; commonly known as table sugar, beet sugar, or cane sugar.
sucro = sugar

superoxide dismutase (SOD): an antioxidant enzyme. Purified from animal tissues and sold in powder form, it is one of many fraudulent antiaging products on the market.

thrombosis: the blocking off of a blood vessel by a clot.

thrombus: a stationary clot.

total lymphocyte count: a count of the white blood cells; a measure of immune function that may or may not reflect nutrition status.

total parenteral nutrition (TPN): a method of meeting all nutrient needs by using large-diameter central veins.

trachea (TRAKE-ee-uh): windpipe.

transferrin: an iron-carrying protein in the blood. The concentration of this protein rises if the person's iron stores are depleted; it falls in protein malnutrition.

triglyceride (try-GLISS-er-ride): a compound composed of glycerol with three fatty acids attached to it.

tri = three
glyceride = a compound of glycerol

tripeptide: three amino acids bonded together.
tri = three

tube feedings: delivery of nutrients through a tube. *Enteral nutrition* refers to the delivery of nutrients into the intestines; oral diets and tube feedings are types of enteral nutrition.
enteron = intestine

turbinado (ter-bih-NOD-oh) **sugar:** raw (brown) sugar from which the filth has been washed; legal to sell in the United States.

ulcerative colitis: inflammation and ulceration of the colon.

underweight: body weight more than 10 percent below normal or average weight.

uremic (you-REE-mic) **syndrome:** a complex of symptoms seen late in renal failure, caused by the buildup of toxic waste products in the blood.

use-disuse principle: the principle that fitness develops in response to demand and diminishes in response to a lack of demand.

vegan: vegetarian who omits all animal products (including eggs, cheese, and milk) from the diet; also called strict vegetarian.

vegetarian diets: diets that omit meat or all animal flesh or all animal products.

villi (VILL-ee or VILL-eye): fingerlike projections from the folds of the small intestine. The singular form is *villus*.
villus = shaggy hair

VLDL: very-low-density lipoprotein. This type of lipoprotein is made by liver cells and to some extent by intestinal cells. An alternative name is **pre-beta** (pre-BAY-tuh) **lipoprotein.**

wasting syndrome: the pattern of failure to grow in children and reduced muscle mass, fat tissue, and blood protein levels in people of any age that frequently develop as a consequence of renal disease.

water-miscible (MISS-i-bull) **vitamins:** fat-soluble vitamins that readily mix with water and can be absorbed without fat.

wellness: the goal of the person who strives to realize his or her full mental, emotional, physical, interpersonal, social, and spiritual potential; this book also uses the term *optimal health*.

wheat germ: a part of the wheat grain, rich in nutrients.

white sugar: pure sucrose, produced by dissolving, concentrating, and recrystallizing raw sugar.

withdrawal reaction: a reaction to the withdrawal of a drug revealing in most cases that the user has become dependent.

INDEX

fasting, 435
food and, 26
modified diet for, 288t, 343t, 435–436
nocturnal, **432**
postprandial, 435
reactive, 435, 436
surgery and, 348t
symptoms of, **428**, 435, 436
Hypokalemia, 477
Hypothalamus, 137
Hypotonic solution, **136**
Hysterectomy, 139

Ideal body weight (IBW), 397, 406, 407–408, 429, 435
Idiopathic hypercalciuria, 509, **512**
Ileocecal valve, 66, **67**
Ileostomy, 348, 352–353, 461
Ileum, 66, **67**, 456–457, 459
Illness, see also Disease
children and, 294–295
effect of, on nutrition status, 282–284
the elderly and, 295–296
food as a source of, 301–303
nutrition and, 282–303
prevention of food-borne, 302t
protein-kcalorie malnutrition and, see
Protein-kcalorie malnutrition
Imitation food, 42, **45**, 48, 49
Immune systems
AIDS, see Acquired immune deficiency
disease (AIDS)
cancer and, 391
depressed, 267, 268, 282
food allergies and, 222
infections, see Infections
vitamin A and, 103t
vitamin E and, 107
zinc deficiency and, 149t
zinc toxicity and, 150t
Impotence, 96
Indigestion
fat malabsorption and, 453t
modified diet for, 288t, 342t, 343t, 350–351, 361, 362, 368
from poor eating habits, 71
Indoles, 392, 393
Induration, **267**
Infant Formula Act of 1980, 195
Infants
birthweight, 187, 198, 200
breastfed, see Breastfeeding
commercial baby foods, 201
diets of, 221
and excess protein, 56
first foods, 200–202
formula-fed, see Formula feeding
gestational age, **187**
GI tract of, 190

growth of, 198–199
iron intake, 221
meal plan for one-year-old, 202t
metabolism of, 199
nutrient needs compared with adult
nutrient needs, 199f
nutrition of, 198–203
with PKU, 445, 505, 506
premature, 107, **187**
and protein deficiency, 58, 59
vitamin C overdose, 124–125
vitamin E and, 107
vitamin K deficiency in, 110
Infections
AIDS and, 386
cirrhosis and, 494
diabetes and, 425, 428
diet for, 374t
drug use and, 224
gastritis caused by, 356
kidney stones and, 510
lung, 96
nephrotic syndrome and, 480
opportunistic, **386**
resistance to, 173
respiratory, 385–386
vitamin C and, 123, 124
vitamin deficiency and, 101–102, 103t
Inflammation, 222
Inflammatory bowel diseases
fat malabsorption and, 456–458
intestinal resection required, 459
modified diet for, 288t, 342t, 348, 374t, 422t, 451t, 457–458
TPN and, 324t
tube feedings and, 307t, 314
Initiative, 216
Inositol, 121
Inpatient, 285
Insulin, 54, **72**
actions of, 428t
administration of, **428**
for cancer patients, 383
chromium deficiency and, 154
diabetes and, 286, 423, 424, 426, 428–429, 430, 431, **432**, 433, 434, 455
dumping syndrome and, 436
human, **428**
hypoglycemia and, 435
in IV solution, 324
sugar and, 180
vitamin D and, 105
Insulin dependent diabetes mellitus
(IDDM), 286, see also Diabetes
Intercellular space, **54**
Intermittent claudication, **107**, 108t
Intermittent feeding by slow drip, **308**, 315
Internal systems, normal vs. malnourished, 208f
Interstitial fluid, **75**

Interstitial space, **54, 58**
Intestinal bypass surgery, **414**
Intestinal flora, **73, 109**
Intestinal juice, 72
Intestine, see also Digestive tract; GI tract
blind loop syndrome, 451t, 453t, 458
effects of alcohol on, 96
lactose intolerance, see Lactose intolerance
large intestine, 68f, 69f, 457
resection, 307t, 348t, 459
small intestine, 68f, 69f, 70, 72–75
Intracellular space, **54**
Intravascular space, **54**
Intravenous nutrition, 276
defined, **320**
ingredients of solution, 320, 321, 324–325
IV fat emulsions, 321–322, 324
for malnutrition, 493
nutrient content of IV solutions, 320–321, 322
for prolonged vomiting, 351
surgery and, 346, 347
Intrinsic factor, 120
Iodine, 135, 143, 150–151
Ions, 135–136, **138**
Iron, 143
absorption of, 123, 124, 144, 146, 147, 148, 190, 241, 367
alcoholism and, 146
anemia, see Anemia
breast milk and, **190**
calcium and, 299
deficiency, 144–146, **148**, 152, 154, **190**, 205–206, 207, 219, 241, 439, 457, 505, see also Anemia
and digestion, 69f
exercise and, 167–168
foods rich in, 146–147
heme, **146**
in infant formula, 195
intake needs, 113, 221
liver disease and, 146
losses, 144
measurement of, 12
need for, during lactation, 191
need for, during menstruation, 147–148, 218
need for, during pregnancy, 120, 185, 189
needs, 144, 146, 148
needs of infants, 199, 201
overload, 124, 146
preparations, 146
recommended intake, 45, 47, **148**
sources of, 5, 6t, 62, 146–147, **185**, 219, 221, 222
stores, 185, 198
supplements, 61, 120, 145, 146, 148, 168, 185, 189, 191, 197, 198, 299, 379, 439, 503
toxicity, 146

PHOTO CREDITS *(continued)*

Foundation; **202** Jacquelyn Nyenhuis; **203** Courtesy of H. Kaplan and V.P. Rabbach; **212** Michael Hayman, Stock Boston; **216** Corinne Cataldo; **219** (both) FourByFive collection; **226** Courtesy of the Eating Disorders Program at Sycamore Hospital, Miamisburg, OH; **237** (left) Courtesy of Gjon Mill; **239** Jacquelyn Nyenhuis; **244** Jacquelyn Nyenhuis; **246** ©Phil McCarten, PhotoEdit; **254** ©Mary Kate Denny, PhotoEdit; **258** (top) SIU, Photo Researchers, Inc.; (bottom) FourByFive/Robert Llewellyn; **263** Paul Crosby with cooperation from Group Health, Inc.; **272** (top) ©Stephen McBrady, InfoEdit; (bottom) Taurus Photos Inc.; **275** FourByFive/Robert Llewellyn; **282** ©Stephen McBrady, InfoEdit; **286** ©Michael Heron, Woodfin Camp & Associates; **291** ©Tony Freeman, PhotoEdit; **294** FourByFive collection; **317** Anthony Vanelli; **333** ©Valdimir Lange, The Image Bank; **336** Taurus Photos Inc.; **347** ©Hans Halberstadt, Photo Researchers Inc.; **366** ©Alan Oddie, PhotoEdit; **368** Courtesy of Humana Hospital, PhotoEdit; **375** Phil McCarten, PhotoEdit; **379** Reproduced with permission of *Nutrition Today* magazine, P.O. Box 1829, Annapolis MC, 21404, May/June 1981; **390** ©Phil McCarten, PhotoEdit; **409** Courtesy of Andreas Cahling; **415** ©Tony Freeman, PhotoEdit; **416** Ray Stanyard; **417** ©Richard Hutchings; **428** Paul Crosby; **429** Paul Crosby; **430** Anthony Vanelli; **431** Paul Crosby; **432** (both) ©Mary Kate Denny, PhotoEdit; **441** Anthony Vanelli; **444** ©Tony Freeman, PhotoEdit; **451** ©Mary Kate Denny, PhotoEdit; **464** Ray Stanyard; **472** Anthony Vanelli; **474** Anthony Vanelli; **475** ©Stephen McBrady, InfoEdit.

Nutrient	The RDA for an Adult Man (1968)	The RDA for an Adult Woman (1968)	The U.S. RDA
Nutrients that must appear on the label[a]			
protein (g), PER ≥ casein[b]	45	—	45
protein (g), PER < casein	65	55	65
vitamin A (RE)	1,000[c]	800[c]	1,000[c]
vitamin C (ascorbic acid) (mg)	60	55	60
thiamin (vitamin B_1) (mg)	1.4	1.0	1.5
riboflavin (vitamin B_2) (mg)	1.7	1.5	1.7
niacin (mg)	18	13	20
calcium (g)	0.8	0.8	1.0
iron (mg)	10	18	18
Nutrients that may appear on the label			
vitamin D (IU)	—	—	400
vitamin E (IU)	30	25	30
vitamin B_6 (mg)	2.0	2.0	2.0
folic acid (folacin) (mg)	0.4	0.4	0.4
vitamin B_{12} (μg)	6	6	6
phosphorus (g)	0.8	0.8	1.0
iodine (μg)	120	100	150
magnesium (mg)	350	300	400
zinc (mg)	—	—	15
copper (mg)	—	—	2
biotin (mg)	—	—	0.3
pantothenic acid (mg)	—	—	10

Source: Adapted from *Food Technology* 28(7): 5, 1974.
[a] whenever nutrition labeling is required.
[b] PER is an index of protein quality.
[c] 1,000 RE was originally expressed as 5,000 IU. 800 RE was orginally expressed as 4,000 IU.

As of 1980, the U.S. RDA numbers used on labels were still those taken from the 1968 RDA. There was no great need to update them because they still would be judged generous by any standard, and because the expense of converting labels to a different set of numbers would be too great to warrant the change.

The circled numbers are those chosen for the U.S. RDA from the adult male and female recommendations. In each case, the higher number is chosen.

In the case of thiamin, niacin, iodine, and magnesium the RDA for an adolescent boy is used because this is even higher than the adult RDA.

In the case of calcium and phosphorus, 1 g/day is used, more than the adult RDA. Pregnant and lactating women and rapidly growing teenagers have RDA even higher than this, but 1 g was considered generous enough for use as a standard for labels.

In the case of the last four nutrients—zinc, copper, biotin, and pantothenic acid, RDA had not been set as of 1968 but these nutrients were known to be essential. The agency set "guestimates" for these so that percent-of-U.S.-RDA labels could include them. As of 1980, all four of these nutrients were included in the RDA tables, but the U.S. RDA values were not changed to correspond; they were considered close enough already.

HOW TO DETERMINE YOUR FRAME SIZE BY ELBOW BREADTH

To make a simple approximation of your frame size:
Extend your arm and bend the forearm upwards at a 90-degree angle. Keep the fingers straight and turn the inside of your wrist away from your body. Place the thumb and index finger of your other hand on the two prominent bones on *either side* of your elbow. Measure the space between your fingers against a ruler or a tape measure.[a] Compare the measurements with the following standards.

These standards represent the elbow measurements for meduim-framed men and women of various heights. Measurements smaller than those listed indicate you have a small frame and larger measurements indicate a large frame.

Men		Women	
Height in 1-Inch Heels	*Elbow Breadth*	*Height in 1-Inch Heels*	*Elbow Breadth*
5 ft 2 inches to 5 ft 3 inches	2 ½ to 2 ⅞ inches	4 ft 10 inches to 4 ft 11 inches	2 ¼ to 2 ½ inches
5 ft 4 inches to 5 ft 7 inches	2 ⅝ to 2 ⅞ inches	5 ft 0 inches to 5 ft 3 inches	2 ¼ to 2 ½ inches
5 ft 8 inches to 5 ft 11 inches	2 ¾ to 3 inches	5 ft 4 inches to 5 ft 7 inches	2 ⅜ to 2 ⅝ inches
6 ft 0 inches to 6 ft 3 inches	2 ¾ to 3 ⅛ inches	5 ft 8 inches to 5 ft 11 inches	2 ⅜ to 2 ⅝ inches
6 ft 4 inches and over	2 ⅞ to 3 ¼ inches	6 ft 0 inches and over	2 ½ to 2 ¾ inches

[a] For the most accurate measurement, have your health care provider measure your elbow breadth with a caliper.
Source: Courtesy "Statistical Bulletin," Metropolitan Life Insurance Company.